Adult
Orthodontics

Adult Orthodontics

Second Edition

Edited by

Birte Melsen

1975-2013 Professor and Head of department of Orthodontics, Aarhus University, Denmark,
Visiting Professor, Program Affiliate Orthodontics (Part Time Faculty)

Cesare Luzi

Specialist in Orthodontics Aarhus University
Visiting Professor Università di Ferrara
Visiting Professor Università Cattolica del Sacro Cuore Roma
Diplomate European Board of Orthodontics
Diplomate Italian Board of Orthodontics
Private Practice, Via Gramsci 16, Rome, Italy

Companion Website: http://www.wiley.com/go/melsen-adult-orthodontics

WILEY Blackwell

This edition first published 2022
© 2022 John Wiley & Sons Ltd

Edition History
Blackwell Publishing Ltd. (1e, 2012)

Registered Offices
John Wiley & Sons, Inc., 111 River Street, Hoboken, NJ 07030, USA
John Wiley & Sons Ltd, The Atrium, Southern Gate, Chichester, West Sussex, PO19 8SQ, UK

Editorial Office
9600 Garsington Road, Oxford, OX4 2DQ, UK

For details of our global editorial offices, customer services and more information about Wiley products, visit us at www.wiley.com.

Wiley also publishes its books in a variety of electronic formats and by print-on-demand. Some content that appears in standard print versions of this book may not be available in other formats.

Library of Congress Cataloging-in-Publication Data
Names: Melsen, Birte, author. | Luzi, Cesare, 1975- author.
Title: Adult orthodontics / edited by Birte Melsen, Cesare Luzi.
Description: Second edition. | Hoboken : John Wiley & Sons, 2022. |
    Includes bibliographical references and index.
Identifiers: LCCN 2021053308 (print) | LCCN 2021053309 (ebook) | ISBN
    9781119775775 (hardback) | ISBN 9781119775782 (pdf) | ISBN 9781119775799
    (epub) | ISBN 9781119775805 (ebook)
Subjects: LCSH: Orthodontics.
Classification: LCC RK527 .A385 2022 (print) | LCC RK527 (ebook) | DDC
    617.6/43--dc23/eng/20211028
LC record available at https://lccn.loc.gov/2021053308
LC ebook record available at https://lccn.loc.gov/2021053309

Cover image: Courtesy of Delfino Allais, Valeria Costantini and Cesare Luzi
Cover design by Wiley

Set in 10/12 pt Minion by Integra Software Services, Pondicherry, India

Printed in Singapore
M114470_200622

Dedicate to all the people who helped us during the process

Contents

List of Contributors

Delfino Allais MSc
Certified Specialist in Orthodontics
Private Practice
Torino, Italy

Dorthe Arenholt Bindslev DDS, PHD
Certif.Specialist in Orthodontics
Chief Orthodontist (Silkeborg Community Dentistry)
Adj. Professor (Forensic Odontology)
Aarhus University Aarhus, Denmark

Vittorio Cacciafesta DDS, MSc, PhD
Private Practitioner
Milan, Italy and Stevenage, UK

Dr Pablo Echarri DDS
President of the Scientific Committee of Catalonian Dental
Association (COEC)
President of the Ibero-American Society of Lingual
Orthodontics (SIAOL)
Visiting Professor of Master in Orthodontics at the University
of Sevilla Barcelona, Spain

Fernando G. Exposto DDS, MS, PhD
Assistant Professor Section for Orofacial Pain and Jaw Function
Department of Dentistry and Oral Health Aarhus University
Aarhus, Denmark

Mauro Farella DDS, PhD
Professor of Orthodontics
Director of the Postgraduate Programme in Orthodontics
(DClinDent)
University of Otago, New Zealand

Giorgio Fiorelli MD, DDS
Specialist in Orthodontics, Orthodontic Department University
of Siena
School of Specialization/Postgraduate Master Course Siena,
Italy

Dr. Arturo Imbelloni, D.M.D.
CAGS Specialization in Prosthodontics, Boston University
CAGS Specialization in Periodontology, Boston University
Private Practice, Viale Mazzini 55, Rome, Italy

Jaume Janer DDS, MD
Certified Specialist in Orthodontics
Private Practice Barcelona, Spain

Dr Sonil Kalia B.D.S., L.D.S.R.C.S., MSc
Specialist in Orthodontics Aarhus University
Masters of Science – Orthodontics (University Aarhus–Denmark)
Visiting Lecturer in Orthodontics (Orthodontic Department
– University Aarhus–Denmark)
Private Practice Specialist Doctor in Orthodontics –
U.K. and Switzerland

Dr. Cesare Luzi DDS, MSc
Specialist in Orthodontics Aarhus University
Visiting Professor Università di Ferrara
Visiting Professor Università Cattolica del Sacro Cuore Roma
Diplomate European Board of Orthodontics
Diplomate Italian Board of Orthodontics
Private Practice, Via Gramsci 16, Rome, Italy

Emma Vila Mancho, DDS
Professor of the Master in Orthodontics and Dentofacial
Orthopaedics of Athenea Dental Institute - San Jorge
University, Spain

Marco A. Masioli PhD, MSc
Professor of Dentistry
Federal University of Espírito Santo (UFES)Vitoria, Brazil

Birte Melsen DDS Dr. Odont. Dr.h.c.
1975-2013 Professor and Head of department of
Orthodontics, Aarhus University, Denmark,
Visiting Professor, Program Affiliate Orthodontics (Part Time
Faculty)
College of Dentistry NYU New York Adjunct professor School
of Dentistry, M512 – The University of Western Australia

Rainer-Reginald Miethke Prof. emeritus
Visiting Professor Department of Orthodontics, Dentofacial,
Orthopedics and Pedodontics
Charité – Universitätsmedizin Berlin, Berlin, Germany
Part time practitioner ADENTICS – practice limited to
orthodontics

Francesco Milano DDS
Private Practice
Bologna, Italy

Laura Guerra Milano DDS
Certified Specialist in Orthodontics
Private Practice
Bologna, Italy

Sheldon Peck DDS, MScD
Adjunct Professor of Orthodontics School of Dentistry,
University of North Carolina
Chapel Hill, North Carolina, USA
Formerly Clinical Professor of Developmental Biology,
Harvard School of Dental Medicine
Boston, Massachusetts, USA
Deceased

Sabarinath Prasad DDS
Assistant Professor, Department of Orthodontics,
Hamdan Bin Mohammed College of Dental Medicine,
Dubai, United Arab Emirates

Gottfried Schmalza Prof. Dr. Dr. h. c. mult.
Department of Conservative Dentistry and Periodontology,
University Hospital Regensburg, Regensburg, Germany,
Department of Periodontology, University of Bern, Bern,
Switzerland

Peter Svensson DDS, PhD, Dr. Odont
Professor, Department of Clinical Oral Physiology
MINDLab, Center of Functionally Integrative Neuroscience,
Aarhus University Hospital,
School of Dentistry, Aarhus University, Aarhus, Denmark

Carlalberta Verna Dr. med. dent., PhD
Professor and Head Department of Paediatric Oral Heath and
Orthodontics
University Center for Dental Medicine UZB
University of Basel, Basel, Switzerland

About the Companion Website

This book is accompanied by a companion website for instructors:

http://www.wiley.com/go/melsen-adult-orthodontics

The website includes the following resources:

- PowerPoint slides
- Tables

Introduction

Working with the update of the book on adult orthodontics, I had to look back on the development within our discipline. In 1998 Carine Carels organised a symposium 'The future of orthodontics'.

The lectures given in that symposium were focused on research related to the influence of genetics and environmental factors two aspects are dominating over; TADS and Clear Aligners.

Another part of the symposium brought the attention to the increasing difficulties in using animal models when testing various treatment approaches.

The pro et contra related to randomised control trials was discussed and an attempt to quantify the need for treatment and to choose the optimal timing for treatment was illucidated.

Altogether, the sprit was high, but when looking at the developments occurring since the symposium in Leuven, they have deviated from the prediction with respect to several aspects. The development of orthodontics has, as most other disciplines, been fractioned and more parts have been outsourced. The companies have taken over. Orthodontists are no longer wire-benders the first, second and third order corrections are taken care of when buying the right preformed bracket. Given the current trends, many patients will receive orthodontic treatment by non-specialist dentists or without dentists at all. The number of adult and elderly patients is growing and one could envision orthodontists treating mostly patients with severe or complex malocclusions, with iatrogenic damages, or in need of re-retreatment.

There are several reasons for bending: to lower the force level, to control the first, second and third order corrections and to achieve the correct force system. While the force level can be lowered when choosing a different material and the prescription brackets can take care of the final position,

there is still a need for bending in order to obtain the correct force system. The latter is still valid.

Since the first version of Adult Orthodontics especially; TADS and Clear Aligners. But are they a blessing or a curse? However, the same development that has been taking over the medical world as orthodontics today "reification" in other words treating cases not patients. The number of publications with the keyword orthodontics are growing exponentially and the authors are paying to get published moving money from research to publishing. In the new version, we have chosen to present a survey of different TADs and aligners.

The advantages and disadvantages will be stressed. The definition of the treatment another topic that has been focussed on over the last decennia treatment should be individualised to achieve the goals.

The chapter on aligners is now including a history of the aligners and a description of the different types. We have focussed more on the possibility the mandibular repositioning and added a chapter on acceleration of tooth movement, another topic that has been focussed on over the last decennia. The number of Clear Aligner companies are growing every month and the different authors vary with respect to what problems they can solve.

Are we, maybe, focussing too much of the "hard" tissue and forgetting about the soft tissues, the muscle matrix and the tongue posture?

Just before submitting the book Sheldon Peck, who wrote the former introduction passed away. His interest reached from the history of orthodontics over clinical research. Let us recall a great colleague when we read the introduction to the first version.

I have been fortunate to have Dr Cesare Luzi as my co-editor. He has kept track on the delayed delivery from the co-authors who all have been overloaded with problems related to COVID-19. Some people manage to be present both for their family, their patients and their colleagues. He is one of those. Without him I would not have been able to complete this version in a period of a World dominated by lock-downs due to the pandemic COVID-19.

I thank all my co-authors for their contribution during these difficult times.

Introduction: More than a Century of Progress in Adult Orthodontic Treatment

Orthodontics for adults is not new. A hundred years ago and earlier, orthodontics was considered a division of prosthetics in the minds of most dentists. The problems related to the common loss of permanent teeth from uncontrolled caries were among the most frequent chief complaints of adult patients evaluated for 'orthodontia'. Unwitting extraction of posterior teeth during youth allowed adjacent teeth to tip into the spaces over time. Often, orthodontic uprighting of tipped teeth in adult patients was performed by the same doctor who afterwards prepared the teeth as anchor units for fixed or removable dental prostheses.

We are fortunate to have details of an adult orthodontic treatment performed by Edward H. Angle, MD, DDS (1855–1930), the man acknowledged worldwide as the first specialist in orthodontics. In addition to his skill at creating ingenious 'tooth-regulating' appliances, Angle was a bold and talented clinician. In 1901, a 38-year-old woman, Mrs A, came to him from Louisville, Kentucky, referred by her dentist. She was from a leading Kentucky family and she travelled 400 kilometres to Dr Angle's office in St. Louis, Missouri, because of his reputation as the 'world's best' clinical orthodontist.

Mrs A's four permanent first molars, all healthy, were 'sacrificed' at nine years of age by a dentist who said this course of action would prevent the development of malocclusion of the other teeth. She came to Dr Angle three decades later with severe tipping of the mandibular molars into the extraction sites (Figure 0.1a,b). In the maxillary dental arch, complete closure of the first molar sites had occurred with associated retroclination of the anterior teeth and loss of lip support. Furthermore, Angle reported that 'not only have the remaining teeth been rendered almost useless for mastication, but in recent years there has been chronic pericementitis, resulting from wrongly directed force from the molars in their tipped and abnormal positions' (Angle 1903, 1907).

A century ago, orthodontic treatment was not frequently undertaken for adult patients. Dentists perceived grave uncertainties of response and outcome associated with orthodontic tooth movement in adults, regardless of their absolute need for improved dental health. Even the great Dr Angle was doubtful in his prognosis for Mrs A, saying her age was 'the most advanced age recorded for such an extensive operation' (Angle 1903, 1907).

Nonetheless, Angle commenced a pre-prosthetic orthodontic treatment for his patient. He used his own design of nickel–silver fixed appliances to regain the lost spaces of the four first molars in preparation for fixed bridgework. First, Angle placed bands with buccal tubes (his 'D-bands') on the second molars. He then fabricated heavy labial arches ('E' arches) for insertion into the tubes to provide three-dimensional expansion of both dental arcades. In addition to regaining the lost molar spaces, he wanted to procline the anterior teeth, 'lengthen the bite' and give Mrs A's lips more support for better facial aesthetics. She was a very cooperative patient and all objectives were met within six months of treatment (Figure 0.2a,b). Angle was elated that her 'teeth were moved as easily and as rapidly as is usual in the case of a miss of eighteen, and with no unfavourable symptoms following the movement of any of the teeth' (Angle 1903, 1907). After active treatment, vulcanite removable plates were fitted for an additional six months of retention, until the teeth were set firmly enough in their new positions to receive space-filling bridgework from her dentist in Louisville.

Dr Angle was proud of Mrs A's treatment results and included her case in his published lectures and textbook (Angle 1903, 1907). In these written accounts, he described Mrs A as 38 years old. But in his private correspondence from 1899 to 1910 – recently available to us (Peck 2007) – he consistently referred to her as a woman aged 42 years.

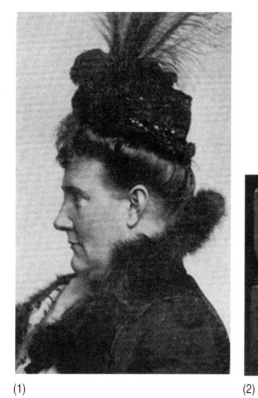

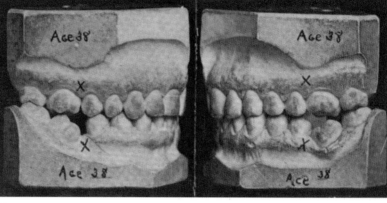

(1)

(2)

Fig. 0.1

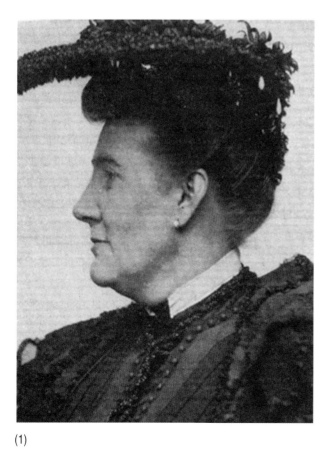

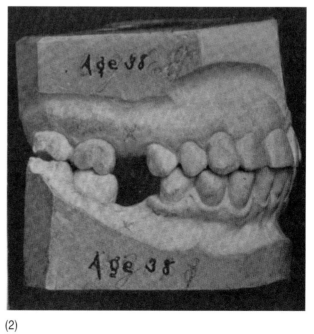

(1)

(2)

Fig. 0.2

Perhaps a sympathetic Angle made her appear four years younger in his professional publications as a concession to the vanity of this charming adult patient, whom his letters show he held in high esteem.

Today, adult orthodontics involves much more than regaining lost arch space. The enlightening chapters in this book demonstrate an unrestricted range of orthodontic

problems and solutions for the adult patient that more than match those associated with conventional adolescent treatments. Adult orthodontics demands additional skills, such as the ability to work with compromised dentitions and to accept less-than-ideal results as the best possible outcome in many cases.

We often have several choices in adult treatment plans. Sometimes financial cost becomes a significant factor from the adult patient's point of view. We must seriously attempt to weigh the costs of various treatment alternatives against the technical virtues of each. As socially sensitive clinicians, we must acknowledge differences within each society and between societies in the ability to absorb escalating costs of certain procedures. For example, consider the problem of a space resulting from the loss or absence of a tooth, which can be managed by either space-reopening or space-closing methods. Within a free-market healthcare system, the combined costs of pre-prosthetic orthodontics and a dental implant with crown are often greater than a full-treatment orthodontics fee. Thus, it may be economically prudent to manage the space in this instance with orthodontic closure rather than with a multidisciplinary prosthetic solution.

If we may speculate based on the historical record, Edward H. Angle would likely be very pleased with this elaborately designed book on adult orthodontics. It contains the elements he considered essential for solid scientific problem-solving. First, the diagnostic aspects and problems

are clearly defined. Then, various solutions and limitations are elucidated in the simplest terms possible, using case studies. Beautifully illustrated case reports are featured in a supplemental CD disk which is conveniently provided in a pocket on this book's inside cover. And finally, Angle greatly respected those who explained and thoughtfully encouraged new and promising materials, methods and techniques.

Birte Melsen is exceptionally well-suited to the task of orchestrating the production of a state-of-the-art text on adult orthodontics. She is both a biologic researcher and a talented, experienced clinician. She knows how to plan practical, biologically sound treatments and she has pioneered innovative therapeutic pathways. Dr Melsen, with the contributed expertise of her extremely capable team of hands-on authorities, has given us a book that will surely extend the boundaries of the specialist's abilities and vision in the management of complex adult orthodontic problems.

Sheldon Peck, DDS, MScD
Adjunct Professor of Orthodontics
School of Dentistry University of North Carolina Chapel
Hill, North Carolina, USA
(formerly Clinical Professor of Developmental Biology
Harvard School of Dental Medicine Boston,
Massachusetts, USA)

References

Angle EH (1903) Some basic principles in orthodontia. *Int Dent J* 24, 729–768.

Angle EH (1907) *Treatment of Malocclusion of the Teeth: Angle's System*, 7th edn, pp. 438–445. Philadelphia, PA: SS White Dental Manufacturing.

Peck S (ed.) (2007) *The World of Edward Hartley Angle, MD, DDS: His Letters, Accounts and Patents*, 4 volumes. Boston, MA: EH Angle Education and Research Foundation.

1

Potential Adult Orthodontic Patients – Who Are They?

Birte Melsen

Introduction

The number of adult patients receiving orthodontic treatment is increasing worldwide. According to the editor of the *Journal of Clinical Orthodontics*, the time when orthodontics was just for children is definitely over (Keim et al. 2005a, 2005b). The increase in the number of adult patients requesting orthodontic treatment is also reflected in European countries (Burgersdijk et al. 1991; Stenvik et al. 1996; Kerosuo et al. 2000). Vanarsdall and Musich (1994) listed five reasons for this change. Three concerned the improved capacity of the profession to treat problems in adult patients either only orthodontically or in combination with orthognathic surgery. Two points referred to the patient's desire to maintain their natural teeth.

Proffit (2000) explained that the increase in the number of adult patients seeking treatment was due to greater availability of information, and analysed the motivation necessary to seek orthodontic treatment as an adult. However, the patients referred to by Proffit are mostly well informed about the possibilities and limitations of orthodontic treatment, and while this assertion may be valid within certain socioeconomic groups in the USA, it is rarely the case in Europe. A possible explanation of this difference between the USA and Europe could be the marketing of orthodontics in the USA. In Europe, it is often ignorance and insecurity that characterise the adult patients seen in the orthodontist's office. Patients may come on their own initiative because they are dissatisfied with either the appearance of their teeth or their ability to chew, or due to a combination of both, or they may have been referred by their family dentist.

Who are the patients?

How can we characterise the adult population presenting to an orthodontic office? Adult patients can be classified according to several criteria. While they all share the fact that they are no longer growing, we must differentiate between young adults, who have recently stopped growing, and older adults, who have experienced deterioration of their dentition and changes in their occlusion over time (Figures 1.1 and 1.2).

Young adult patients are those who, from a professional point of view, should have been treated earlier, or those in whom optimal treatment can be carried out only after cessation of growth. Based on the importance of the impact of genetics on the final skeletal morphology (Savoye et al. 1998), it is frequently considered desirable to postpone treatment of severe skeletal deviations that can be recognised in other members of the family until adulthood, at which time surgical treatment can be carried out (Figure 1.3).

Some young adult patients with severe malocclusions should, however, have been treated earlier. Their malocclusion, which was not considered as an indication for treatment when younger, worsens with time and leads them to seek treatment as adults (Figures 1.2 and 1.4). Proffit (2006) diagrammatically illustrated where tooth movement alone can solve the problem, where tooth movements combined with growth modification are needed and where surgery is considered necessary. However, the lines indicating the limits should not be considered as sharp cut-off points, but rather as indicative of a 'grey zone' in which more than one treatment option can be considered (Figure 1.5). Cassidy et al. (1993) discussed making a decision about surgery based on the advantages and disadvantages of surgical and orthodontic approaches to the treatment of these patients. On the basis of analysis of post-treatment changes and a risk analysis, they concluded that conventional orthodontic treatment is a better choice in borderline cases.

Surgery should not be a substitute for orthodontic treatment, but when treatment is delayed beyond the time when growth modification is possible, surgery is often the only possible solution. A lack of treatment at the most convenient time thus adds to the number of surgical

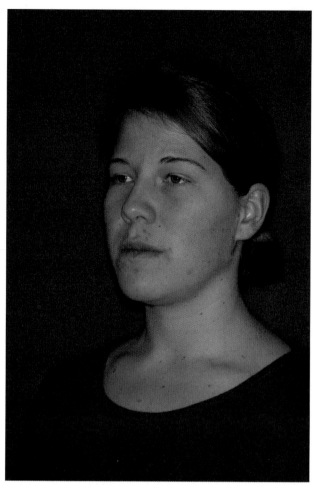

Fig. 1.3 Extraoral photograph of a young woman whose treatment was postponed until adulthood as a surgical solution was foreseen. The malocclusion had worsened over puberty, but since it was reflecting a family facial pattern, treatment was delayed until cessation of growth.

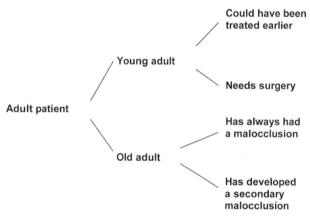

Fig. 1.1 Classification of adult patients.

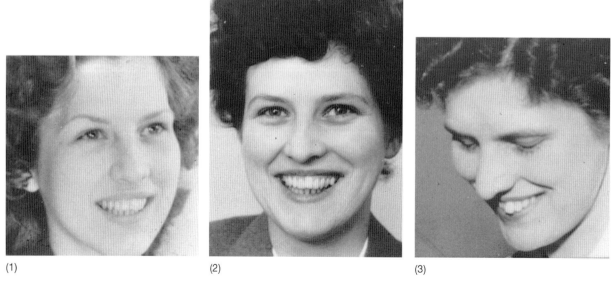

(1) (2) (3)

Fig. 1.2 (1)–(3) An adult patient demonstrating a gradual increase in overjet over time.

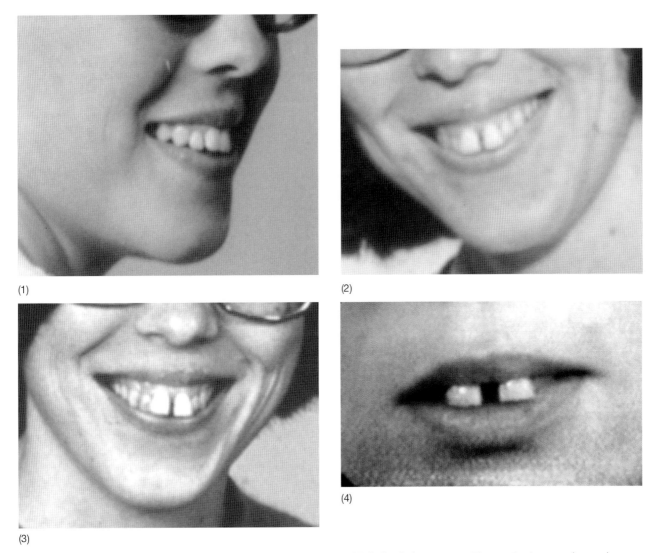

(1)

(2)

(3)

(4)

Fig. 1.4 (1)–(3) A slight increase in overjet which did not qualify for publicly funded treatment. The overjet increased over the years and a medial diastema developed, leading to a more severe malocclusion. (4) In addition to the increased overjet, there was extrusion of the upper incisors.

candidates. Another factor contributing to the increased demand for orthognathic surgery is the simplification of orthodontic techniques. The use of pre-adjusted brackets and the 'Straight-Wire Appliance' (SWA) has certain limitations and may contribute to the increased indication for orthognathic surgery. When the available mechanics are limited to 'straight wires' only, however, for patients in 'grey zone', the most suitable treatment option seems to be leaning more and more towards surgery (Burstone 1991).

Lack of availability or financial considerations may also be a reason for not having orthodontics at the optimal time. Third-party payments may have an impact on which children will be offered orthodontic treatment, and in several countries such as Denmark, the percentage of children who will be offered conventional orthodontic treatment is politically determined. Orthodontic treatment will not be performed if the severity of the malocclusion is below the criteria established by law (National Board of

Health 2003), and as a consequence the patient in Figure 1.4 might not be offered treatment today either.

Very few features of malocclusion reduce with time (Harris and Behrents 1988), with both Class II and Class III malocclusions becoming more severe (Figure 1.6). Therefore, if a skeletal deviation which could have been handled by growth modification is left to worsen until growth ceases, the only possible treatment may be a combination of orthodontics and surgery. A reason, although not acceptable, for the increase in the number of patients receiving orthognathic surgery is the fact that treatment comprising orthognathic surgery is frequently paid for by a third party, that is, insurance or public funds. This has led to a preference for a surgical solution in borderline patients who could be treated either with or without surgery. Third-party involvement in orthodontic services may thus result in the unfortunate development of an increase in the number of adult patients needing

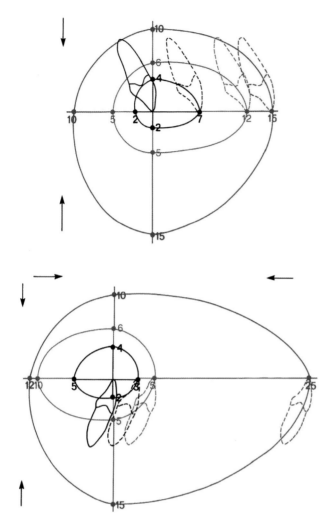

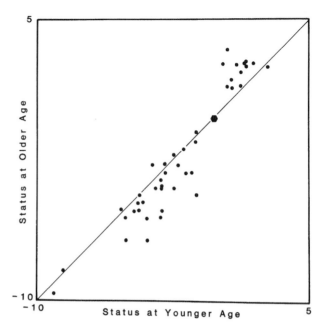

Fig. 1.6 Graphic illustration of the development of occlusion with age. Note that the Class II and Class III malocclusions have worsened. (Redrawn from Harris and Behrents 1988, with permission from Elsevier.)

Fig. 1.5 Diagrammatic illustration of the changes in incisor position in growing and non-growing individuals that are possible with orthodontic tooth movement, growth adaptation and orthognathic surgery. The teeth in the centre of the coordinate system illustrate the ideal position. The inner envelope of each diagram illustrates the possible correction that can be obtained by tooth movements alone. It should be noted that the envelope is elliptical in shape, as the limits of movement in the labial and lingual directions are not the same. Labial movement is easier in the maxilla, and lingual movement is easier in the mandible. The middle envelope indicates what can be achieved if orthodontic tooth movement is combined with growth modification. The outer envelope indicates the possibilities of treatment when surgery is performed. (From Proffit [2006], with permission from Elsevier.)

treatment when the indication for treatment depends on the severity of the malocclusion as based on static morphological criteria. Where the percentage of children who can be offered publicly funded treatment is determined politically, the orthodontist has only limited freedom in determining how the resources available should be used in the most efficient way (National Board of Health 2003). As a result, the orthodontist may opt not to treat the most

difficult cases but refer them to surgery, thus shifting the responsibility for these cases to another part of the health service. Excessive tightening of the criteria for reimbursing treatment costs may therefore increase rather than reduce the total costs for the 'third party' in the long run (Mavreas and Melsen 1995).

Older adult patients, over age 40, present with signs of ageing, deterioration or a dentition often characterised by extensive rehabilitation (Proffit 2000). The number of these patients is also increasing and the patients often present with a 'secondary malocclusion', that is, malocclusion that has developed or has worsened in adulthood. This may occur as a result of deterioration of the dentition and the periodontium due to poor dental care. The aetiology of these malocclusions will be dealt with in more detail in Chapter 3.

In addition to age, adult patients can also be classified based on reasons for the first consultation. Some patients may come on their own intuition; others are referred by family or friends or a general dentist. Family and friends may hear about the possible treatments offered by orthodontists or they may have noted an ongoing deterioration in the patient's occlusion, for example, increasing spacing or crowding. Aesthetics plays a major role as a motive for treatment among these patients (Figure 1.7). Functional problems related to speaking (Figure 1.8), chewing or temporomandibular disorder (TMD) symptoms are other motives for seeking orthodontic treatment. The family dentist may also refer a patient because he or she considers orthodontic treatment necessary in order to halt

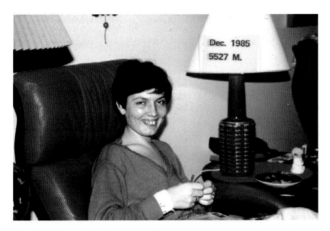

Fig. 1.7 This patient came with a photograph taken at home and declared, 'I was not aware that my teeth were sticking out that much'.

ongoing deterioration of a dentition or because the present tooth position and/or occlusion do not provide a satisfactory basis for planned prosthodontic rehabilitation (Figure 1.9).

An alternative classification of adult patients could therefore also be based on the chief complaint: aesthetics, function or difficulty in achieving suitable occlusal rehabilitation due to, for example, tooth malposition (Melsen and Agerbaek 1994).

Malocclusions detected by adult patients are generally confined to the anterior teeth and comprise spacing or crowding, often related to changes in the overjet and overbite. Factors of importance for development of secondary malocclusion within the masticatory apparatus are, among others, loss of one or more teeth in the buccal segments and periodontal disease. Both factors influence the internal balance (Figure 1.10).

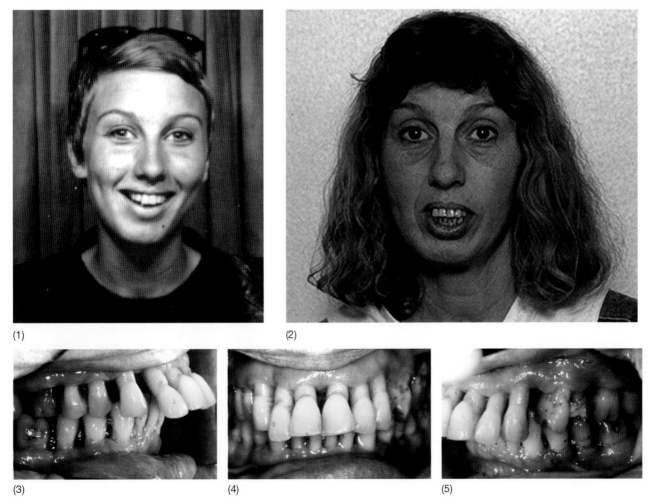

Fig. 1.8 (1) As a young person, this patient had been a singer. (2) With the increase in overjet, this was no longer possible, but it was not until she saw a periodontist that she became aware that something could be done about her occlusion. (3)–(5) The intraoral photographs demonstrated extreme periodontal involvement, elongated clinical crowns following periodontal surgery, flaring of the upper incisors and crowding of the lower incisors.

How do the patients express their needs?

Some adult patients indicate that they have desired treatment for some time, but for various reasons, it had not been possible – some would have grown up in areas where orthodontic services were not available; others would not have received treatment for financial reasons. With increasing availability of orthodontic services, the first type of adult patient may be less prevalent in the future. The increased sensitivity to deviation in appearance within many societies will eventually lead some patients to seek treatment (Lazaridou-Terzoudi et al. 2003). Appearance is becoming increasingly more important and the level of deviation from socially determined norms is reducing. This tendency is reflected in the increased desire for aesthetic treatment, including cosmetic surgery, orthodontics and aesthetic dentistry (Schweitzer 1989a, 1989b; Nathanson 1991; Matarasso 1997; Figueroa 2003).

Some patients who did not perceive a need for treatment earlier will, as a result of continuing deterioration of the dentition, find themselves no longer satisfied with the function or the appearance of their dentition. Some of these patients may have been treated earlier, but were not aware of the possibility for treatment or did not perceive a need for it until recently (Figure 1.11). The individual level of acceptance varies greatly. The mere thought of having to wear braces keeps some patients from consulting the orthodontist. Awareness of this problem within the profession has led to the development of various attempts to reduce or even totally avoid visibility of the necessary appliances. Placement of the appliances on the lingual side has been one way of preventing their being seen. Smaller-sized or transparent brackets have also made labial appliances more acceptable. The introduction of Invisalign® reflects the desire to develop and use orthodontic appliances that are not seen while in the mouth (Smith et al. 1986a, 1986b; Fontenelle 1991; Bishara and Fehr 1997; Sinha and

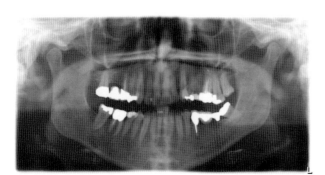

(1)

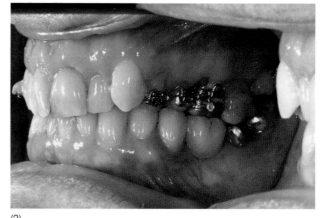

(2)

Fig. 1.9 (1) and (2) This patient had a bridge to replace the left first and second lower molars. The bridge was made after the upper molar had overerupted and the third molar had tipped mesially. The adverse direction of loading of the bridge led to fracture of the second premolar. The patient then required orthodontic treatment in addition to three implants. This could have been avoided had the bridge been fitted soon after the extraction.

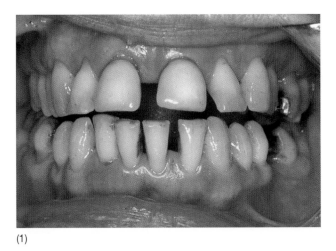
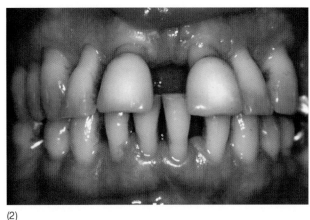

(1)   (2)

Fig. 1.10 (1) Patient who had 'always' had a diastema. However, it increased in size following the extraction of two lower molars. (2) Situation 2 years later.

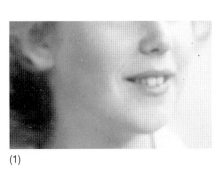
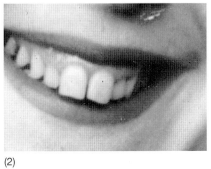
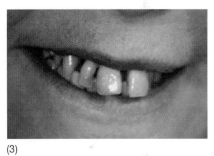

(1)   (2)   (3)

Fig. 1.11 (1)–(3) This patient brought in a series of personal photographs clearly demonstrating the development of a malocclusion. It was, however, not until the dentist explained that an incisor was at risk, but no replacement was possible due to the diastema that the patient requested treatment.

Nanda 1997; Norris et al. 2002; Vlaskalic and Boyd 2002; Wong 2002; Bollen et al. 2003; Joffe 2003; Wiechmann 2003; Wiechmann et al. 2003; Wheeler 2004; Eliades and Bourauel 2005; Nedwed and Miethke 2005; Turpin 2005). It is well known that most minor malocclusions become more pronounced with increasing age (Harris and Behrents 1988; Baumrind 1991).

The first visit

At the first consultation, on the one hand, adult patients may seem insecure due to lack of knowledge regarding the aetiology of their malocclusion and the available treatment alternatives. They are, on the other hand, conscious regarding their desire to improve the appearance or function of their teeth, but there may be some doubts and even a reluctance to undergo orthodontic treatment.

How can the orthodontist advise such patients?

Which malocclusions require orthodontic correction? Only scarce evidence indicates a relationship between the existence of a malocclusion and the prevalence of other dental problems such as caries, periodontal disease and gnathological problems (Gher 1998).

On this basis, how can the orthodontist give appropriate advice to the patient? Recently Johnston (2000) proposed that a need for treatment in this group of adult patients is not identical to the demand for treatment, and that the demand for improved aesthetics would usually be the main reason for undertaking treatment. This implies that the priority given by an individual patient to aesthetics determines his or her need for treatment. The present author does not share this opinion. The reasons for seeking an orthodontic consultation are often: fear of losing teeth; lack of the possibility of a fixed prosthodontic solution or functional problems. In any case, it is important to inform the patient of the likelihood of further deterioration of the malocclusion if left untreated.

Even a patient given adequate information may refrain from having treatment. If the patient is in doubt, it may be advisable to produce a set of study casts, preferably digital, and then observe the changes over one or more years. Based on the changes seen, the patient can then reconsider whether to initiate orthodontic treatment (Figure 1.12). Another

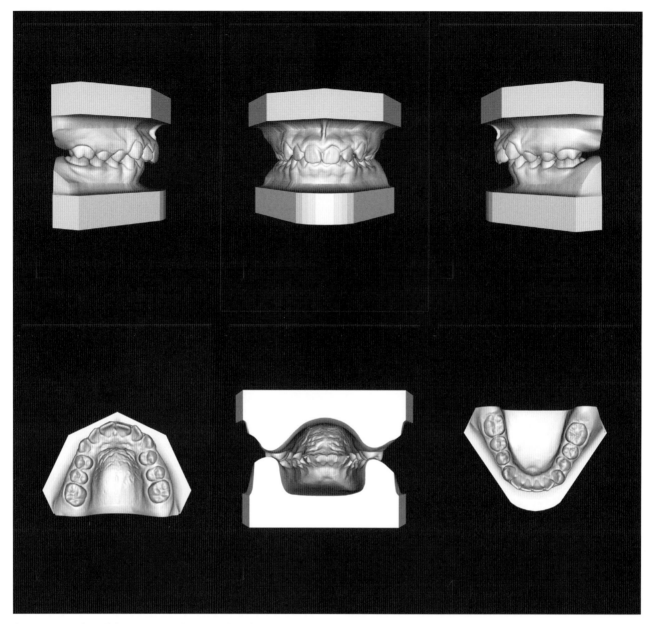

Fig. 1.12 Virtual models. Images can be printed or downloaded by the patient at home where she or he can discuss the problems with family and friends and also follow the eventual deterioration of the occlusion over time.

approach is to ask the patient to present with personal photographs from over his or her lifetime, which could illustrate the development of the malocclusion. Changes within the dentition occur slowly and it is often only when seeing together pictures taken after long intervals of time that patients realise what is happening.

Other patients will have noted changes in their dentition, and will describe either deterioration of a previously acceptable malocclusion or the development of a secondary malocclusion in relation to the loss of one or more teeth or periodontal disease. They may request intervention to prevent further development or treatment that can restore

the original occlusion. Should we fulfil this request or even establish an occlusion that is better than the original? Do these patients really need orthodontic treatment?

The event that triggers the patient to seek treatment may differ from patient to patient. The problems most frequently mentioned are related to flaring of the front teeth. A patient may have had an increased overjet as long as they can remember, but slow and gradual worsening, and the development of an anterior diastema, makes the situation unacceptable. A photograph taken at a social event may be the primary trigger (Figure 1.7). Comparison of this image with an earlier photograph would clearly demonstrate the aggravation of the situation and the patient may decide to seek treatment to stop this, or they may at least seek advice from an orthodontist.

Communicating with the patient

The first visit to the orthodontist may result in conflict (Kalia and Melsen 2001) between the orthodontist and the general dentist, between the patient and the orthodontist or even between the patient and the general dentist. The orthodontist may wonder why the patient was not referred earlier and remark on the rehabilitation that has been done so far, and even indicate that this may interfere with the solution considered best by the orthodontist. If the orthodontist approaches the general dentist for information on the patient's dental care and recent development, the

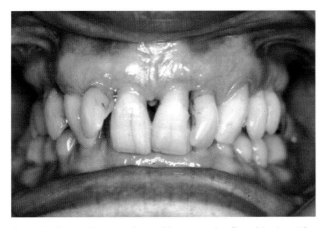

Fig. 1.13 The patient's main problem was the flared incisor. The patient was not aware of the deep bite and the crowding in the lower teeth.

general dentist may well consider it undesirable interference, especially when the patient consults an orthodontist without a referral from their general dentist. It may, however, also occur if the patient is referred to the orthodontist from the general dentist, but without sufficient information of the situation. The general dentist may not have worked up a comprehensive problem list, but used a single symptom as the basis of referral to the orthodontist. If the patient also perceives the cause of referral as a minor problem, the orthodontist's explanation of the situation may generate a problem. The patient in Figure 1.13 was referred for flaring of a single incisor without their being aware that this may be related to crowding in the lower jaw and a deepening of the bite. The patient may react negatively to the information about the complexity of the problem and confront their general dentist with the new information; this may create conflict between the patient and dentist. The patient may feel that he or she has been misinformed by the general dentist and therefore even choose to change their family dentist, or the patient may perceive the complexity of the problem as an overreaction from the orthodontist's side. This is particularly difficult in cases where previous prosthodontic work has to be redone following the treatment suggested by the orthodontist (Figure 1.14).

An orthodontic consultation may thus result in problems between the colleagues involved in the treatment. This can be further aggravated when a third colleague is consulted, for example, a periodontist, who may find that insufficient periodontal maintenance has contributed to the present situation. Neglect on the part of a colleague who has been taking care of a patient in the period when a secondary malocclusion has developed may result in negative feelings between the patient and the involved dentist.

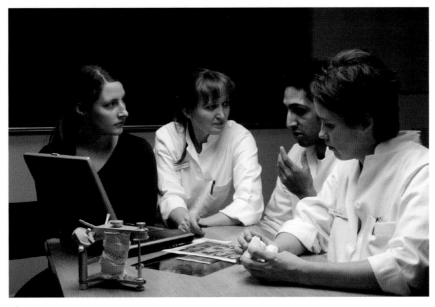

Fig. 1.14 A group of colleagues discussing possible treatment options with a patient.

The scenario that an apparently small problem can be a sign of a severe condition often occurs in other professions as well: 'The strange noise in my car proved to be the sign of a gearbox breaking down'. Pain in the arm can temporarily be alleviated with analgesics, but it may be a symptom of a severe heart condition. In the medical profession, it is not unusual to find patients with a simple problem where it turns out to be a symptom of a more complex disease. Why does it then seem so difficult for the dental profession to accept such a diagnosis?

In order to avoid conflicts related to adult patients, close teamwork between dental colleagues, maintaining a high level of communication, should be established. The information given to the patient by different colleagues should not be contradictory. The consequences of failing to give or giving insufficient information can lead to neglect on the patient's side; for instance, insufficient interest in replacing a tooth that was extracted.

A crucial requirement in relation to treatment planning where multiple disciplines are involved is agreeing on a common problem list and treatment plan in which there are no disagreements among the colleagues involved. Possible and unavoidable differences of opinion should be discussed, but never in front of the patient. The final problem list and the treatment plan agreed by all specialists should then be communicated to the patient and all dental colleagues involved.

The patient may desire a more detailed explanation of both the problem list and treatment plan (Boxes 1.1 and 1.2). This should be carried out by the team member who is in closest contact with the patient or by the one bringing the team together. The level of information must be the same among the team members and all data of importance for the treatment decision should be presented to the patient in a diplomatic way. When explaining the problem and possible treatment options to the patient, it is of the utmost importance also to explain the consequences of completing versus not completing the treatment.

Summary

Adult patients consulting the orthodontist present with a large variety of problems and a dentition often characterised by deterioration and extensive rehabilitation that may make treatment planning complicated. In most cases, the treatment will have to be done as a team approach because periodontal, functional and prosthodontic problems also have to be taken into consideration. The importance of good communication both between the involved team members and between the patient and the clinicians cannot be sufficiently stressed. Sharing information on the various treatment options with various specialities will improve the likelihood that patients receive the best possible outcome (Figure 1.14). It is, when explaining the treatment options to the patient, important to make it clear that all treatment results have to be maintained. The patient should not expect stability, but be aware that maintenance is important.

References

Baumrind S (1991) Prediction in the planning and conduct of orthodontic treatment. In Melsen B (ed.) *Current Controversies in Orthodontics*, pp. 25–44. Chicago, IL: Quintessence.

Bishara SE and Fehr DE (1997) Ceramic brackets: something old, something new, a review. *Semin Orthod* 3, 178–188.

Bollen AM, Huang G, King G, Hujoel P and Ma T (2003) Activation time and material stiffness of sequential removable orthodontic appliances. Part 1: ability to complete treatment. *Am J Orthod Dentofacial Orthop* 124, 496–501.

Burgersdijk R, Truin GJ, Frankenmolen F, Kalsbeek H, van't Hof M and Mulder J (1991) Malocclusion and orthodontic treatment need of 15–74-year-old Dutch adults. *Commun Dent Oral Epidemiol* 19, 64–67

Burstone CJ (1991) The biomechanical rationale of orthodontic therapy. In Melsen B (ed.) *Current Controversies in Orthodontics*, pp. 147–180. Chicago, IL: Quintessence.

Cassidy DW Jr, Herbosa EG, Rotskoff KS and Johnston LE Jr (1993) A comparison of surgery and orthodontics in 'borderline' adults with Class II, division 1 malocclusions. *Am J Orthod Dentofacial Orthop* 104, 455–470.

Eliades T and Bourauel C (2005) Intraoral aging of orthodontic materials: the picture we miss and its clinical relevance. *Am J Orthod Dentofacial Orthop* 127, 403–412.

Figueroa C (2003) Self-esteem and cosmetic surgery: is there a relationship between the two? *Plast Surg Nurs* 23, 21–24.

Fontenelle A (1991) Lingual orthodontics in adults. In Melsen B (ed.) *Current Controversies in Orthodontics*, pp. 219–268. Chicago, IL: Quintessence.

Gher ME (1998) Changing concepts. The effects of occlusion on periodontitis. *Dent Clin North Am* 42: 285–299.

Harris EF and Behrents RG (1988) The intrinsic stability of Class I molar relationship: a longitudinal study of untreated cases. *Am J Orthod Dentofacial Orthop* 94, 63–67.

Joffe L (2003) Invisalign: early experiences. *J Orthod* 30, 348–352.

Johnston LE (2000) Stop me before I write again… *Am J Orthod Dentofacial Orthop* 117, 540–542.

Kalia S and Melsen B (2001) Interdisciplinary approaches to adult orthodontic care. *J Orthod* 28, 191–196.

Keim RG, Gottlieb EL, Nelson AH, and Vogels DS III (2005a) 2005 JCO orthodontic practice study. Part 1: trends. *J Clin Orthod* 39, 641–650.

Keim RG, Gottlieb EL, Nelson AH, and Vogels DS III (2005b) 2005 JCO orthodontic practice study. Part 2. Practice success. *J Clin Orthod* 39, 687–695.

Kerosuo H, Kerosuo E, Niemi M, and Simola H (2000) The need for treatment and satisfaction with dental appearance among young Finnish adults with and without a history of orthodontic treatment. *J Clin Orthod* 61, 330–340.

Lazaridou-Terzoudi T, Kiyak HA, Moore R, Athanasiou AE, and Melsen B (2003) Long-term assessment of psychologic outcomes of orthognathic surgery. *J Oral Maxillofac Surg* 61, 545–552.

Matarasso A (1997) Facialplasty. *Dermatol Clin* 15, 649–658.

Mavreas D and Melsen B (1995) Financial consequences of reducing treatment availability in a publicly-funded orthodontic service. A decision analysis problem. *Br J Orthod* 22, 47–51.

Melsen B and Agerbaek N (1994) Orthodontics as an adjunct to rehabilitation. *Periodontol 2000* 4, 148–159.

Nathanson D (1991) Current developments in esthetic dentistry. *Curr Opin Dent* 1, 206–211.

National Board of Health, Denmark (2003) Bekendtgørelse nr. 1073 af 11. december om tandpleje.

Nedwed V and Miethke RR (2005) Motivation, acceptance and problems of Invisalign ((R)) patients. *J Orofac Orthop* 66, 162–173.

Norris RA, Brandt DJ, Crawford CH, and Fallah M (2002) Restorative and Invisalign: a new approach. *J Esthet Restor Dent* 14, 217–224.

Proffit WR (2000) Treatment for adults: special consideration in comprehensive treatment for adults. In Proffit WR (ed.) *Contemporary Orthodontics*, p. 648. St Louis, MO: Mosby.

Proffit WR (2006) Combined surgical and orthodontic treatment. In Proffit WR (ed.) *Contemporary Orthodontics*, p. 690, Fig. 17.4. St Louis, MO: Mosby.

Savoye I, Loos R, Carels C, Derom C and Vlietinck R (1998) A genetic study of anteroposterior and vertical facial proportions using modelfitting. *Angle Orthod* 68, 467–470.

Schweitzer I (1989a) The psychiatric assessment of the patient requesting facial surgery. *Aust N Z J Psychiatry* 23, 249–254.

Schweitzer I (1989b) The psychiatric assessment of the patient requesting facial surgery. *Aust N Z J Psychiatry* 23, 314.

Sinha PK and Nanda RS (1997) Esthetic orthodontic appliances and bonding concerns for adults. *Dent Clin North Am* 41, 89–109.

Smith JR, Gorman JC, Kurz C and Dunn RM (1986a) Keys to success in lingual therapy. *J Clin Orthod* 20, 604.

Smith JR, Gorman JC, Kurz C and Dunn RM (1986b) Keys to success in lingual therapy. Part 2. *J Clin Orthod* 20, 330–340.

Stenvik A, Espeland L, Berset GP, Eriksen HM and Zachrisson BU (1996) Need and desire for orthodontic (re-)treatment in 35-year-old Norwegians. *J Orofac Orthop* 57, 334–342.

Turpin DL (2005) Clinical trials needed to answer questions about Invisalign. *Am J Orthod Dentofacial Orthop* 127, 157–158.

Vanarsdall RL and Musich DR (1994) Adult orthodontics: diagnosis and treatment. In Graber L and Vanarsdall RL (eds) *Orthodontics Current Principles and Techniques*, 2nd edn, pp. 750–834. St Louis, MO: Mosby.

Vlaskalic V and Boyd RL (2002) Clinical evolution of the Invisalign appliance. *J Calif Dent Assoc* 30, 769–776.

Wheeler TT (2004) Invisalign material studies. *Am J Orthod Dentofacial Orthop* 125, 19A.

Wiechmann D (2003) A new bracket system for lingual orthodontic treatment. Part 2: first clinical experiences and further development. *J Orofac Orthop* 64, 372–388.

Wiechmann D, Rummel V, Thalheim A, Simon JS and Wiechmann L (2003) Customized brackets and archwires for lingual orthodontic treatment. *Am J Orthod Dentofacial Orthop* 124, 593–599.

Wong BH (2002) Invisalign A to Z. *Am J Orthod Dentofacial Orthop* 121, 540–541.

2

Diagnosis: Chief Complaint and Problem List

Birte Melsen, Marco A. Masioli

Introduction

The patient's chief complaint when first encountering the orthodontist is often far from the objective problem list envisioned by the clinician. In a recent comment, Bowman (2005) asked: Have you ever had a patient asking 'Can you just fix this tooth that is crooked?' (Figure 2.1)? Or they ask: 'Do you have to put braces on all my teeth?' Independent of the reason for the consultation, treatment options can only be discussed following the workup of a comprehensive problem list (Table 2.1).

Orthodontists generally perceive the problem list as the diagnosis. Whereas a diagnosis within other areas of medicine includes information regarding aetiology, pathogenesis and prognosis, this is not the case within orthodontics, as the signs and symptoms related to a specific malocclusion can have a large variety of causes. For example, increased overjet may be a sign of a skeletal discrepancy (maxillary prognathism or mandibular retrognathism) or a dentoalveolar condition. All of these can contribute to an increase in overjet. A problem list, by contrast, is the compilation of positive findings obtained from the interview,

the clinical examination and the analysis of the diagnostic records.

Workup of a problem list – the interview and chief complaint

Before compiling the problem list, the patient should be allowed to express, in his or her words, their problem and the stimulus or motivating factor that led to the consultation. Letting patients express themselves freely allows the orthodontist to get a better impression of the priority that the patient gives to their problem. Proffit and Ackerman (2000) recommended the use of a questionnaire for a parent accompanying a child to the orthodontist. In the case of an adult patient, a personal interview prompted by a few open-ended questions is preferable to a standard questionnaire. The way in which a patient explains their problem gives an indication of whether poor dental aesthetics or function ranks higher in their perception of the problem. The orthodontist should not try to influence the patient during this part of the interview.

Adult Orthodontics, Second Edition. Edited by Birte Melsen and Cesare Luzi.
© 2022 John Wiley & Sons Ltd. Published 2022 by John Wiley & Sons Ltd.
Companion Website: http://www.wiley.com/go/melsen-adult-orthodontics

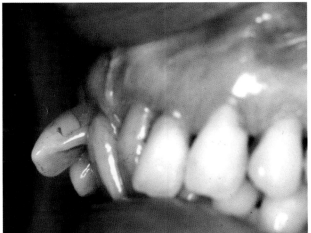

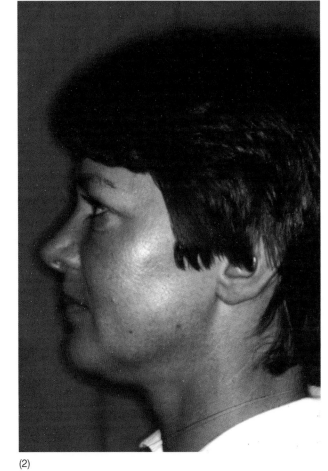

(1)   (2)

Fig. 2.1 (1) and (2) This patient was referred from the general dentist to the orthodontist for correction of flaring of the upper right lateral incisor. It is obvious that the flared incisor cannot be corrected without taking into consideration other problems such as the crowding and the deep bite.

Table 2.1 Chief complaint – 'My upper front tooth is sticking out and catching my lower lip. It is getting worse'.

Problem list	Solution
Extraoral examination	
Straight profile with a lip trap related to the upper right lateral incisor	Alignment of the lateral incisors following distalisation of 23 and 24
Functional analysis	
Traumatic occlusion on the incisors	Intrusion of upper incisors and proclination of lower incisors for reduction of the overbite. Coordination between structural position and intercuspation
The mandible forced back to a deep bite with impingement, muscle tenderness	
Intraoral analysis	
Missing teeth: 17 and 27	Have to be accepted
Total periodontitis: 16 and 15	Extraction: 16 and 15
Gingival dehiscence generally	Motivation and oral hygiene instruction
Motivation and oral hygiene instruction	Distalisation of 14, 13 and 12
Proclination and distal rotation: 21 and 22	Retroclination of 12, and proclination of 11, 21 and 22
Distal canine relationship, left side	Retraction of 14 and 13
Deep bite with impingement	Levelling and intrusion of upper and lower incisors

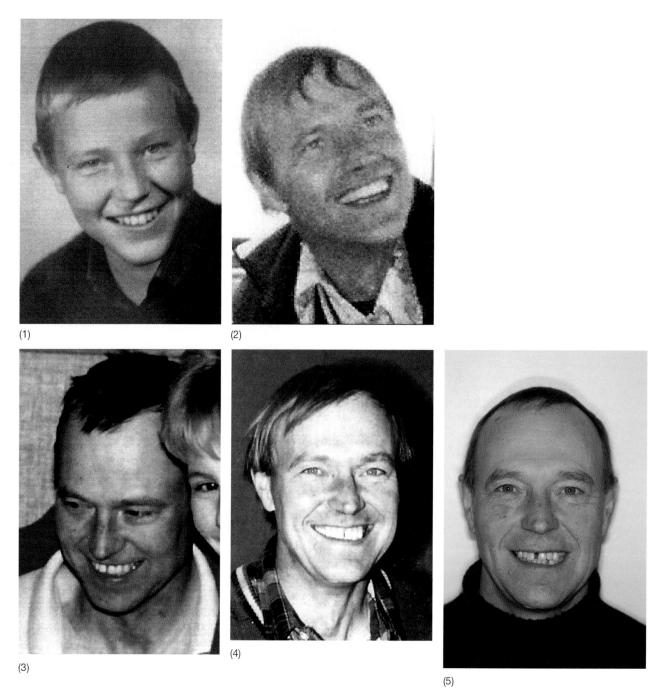

(1)

(2)

(3)

(4)

(5)

Fig. 2.2 (1)–(5) A patient with a major need for occlusal rehabilitation presented with this series of family photographs that clearly illustrated the gradual deterioration of his dentition. The patient had seen a family dentist regularly, but only at the last visit was he referred for an orthodontic consultation.

In the case where the malocclusion is described as developing over time, it is advisable to ask the patient to bring in an earlier photograph from which the smile can be evaluated. The gradually occurring changes demonstrated by means of the photographs can then be used while explaining the development of the malocclusion and when discussing the consequences of no intervention with the patient (Figure 2.2).

If the patient is referred by a general dentist or a colleague within another discipline, it would be important to know the attitude of the referring dentist to orthodontics. How has the dentist presented the problem to the patient? Why was the patient not referred before? Has the family dentist made any comments? Does the family have a 'new' dentist? If yes, why did the patient look for a new dentist?

Once patients have expressed their perceived problems, the orthodontist can start gathering the information required to propose a solution to the problem.

General health

Changes occurring in the occlusion may reflect general health. A thorough medical history is therefore needed both for the clarification of the aetiology and for prediction of the tissue reaction to the orthodontics. Patients may think that their general health problems are irrelevant to their dental problems, but information about previous diseases, for example, juvenile idiopathic arthritis or trauma to either soft or hard tissues, could contribute to clarification of the aetiology. Metabolic diseases and chronic medication may also have an influence. In this context, a medical health

questionnaire is useful, as the repeated questions may seem trivial when asked verbally (Figure 2.3).

Risk factors for periodontitis have been the subject of numerous studies and a multi-factorial aetiology is generally accepted (Papapanou 1999; Van Dyke and Sheilesh 2005). The role of systemic conditions and disorders in periodontal disease was discussed by Genco and Loe (1993) in a comprehensive review, focusing particularly on the impact of diabetes and smoking. The mechanism by which diabetes contributes to the periodontal breakdown was discussed by Lalla et al. (2000), and according to Taylor et al. (1998a, 1998b), who compared people with diabetes and healthy individuals, the odds ratio for progression of bone loss in the case of diabetes was 4.2.

Smoking is the other risk factor that routinely stands out when performing analysis of risk factors related to

---

MEDICAL HISTORY   **Date:**

Patient name: _____

Date of birth: _____

Name of physician: Office phone:

Address: Date of last exam:

1.   Do or did you have a general health problem? Yes ☐ No ☐

      If yes, please explain: _____

      _____

2.   Have you ever been hospitalized, had general anesthesia, or emergency room visits?

                             Yes ☐ No ☐

      If yes, please explain: _____

      _____

3.   Are you allergic to anykind of drugs, medical products (latex), or the environment (dust, mites, pollen, mold)?

                             Yes ☐ No ☐

      If yes, please explain: _____

      _____

4.   Do you take any medicine regularly? If yes please list dailymedications:

      _____

Fig. 2.3 The medical history form.

5.   Have you ever had or been treated by a physician for:

Problem	Yes	No	Don't know
Problems at birth			
Heart murmur			
Heart disease			
Rheumatic fever			
Anemia			
Sickle cell anemia			
Bleeding/hemophilia			
Blood transfusion			
Hepatitis			
AIDS or HIV+			
Tuberculosis			
Liver disease			
Kidney disease			
Diabetes			
Arthritis			
Cancer			
Cerebral palsy			
Seizures			
Asthma			
Osteoporosis			
Speech or hearing problems			
Eye problems/contact lenses			
Skin problems			
Tonsil/adenoid/sinus problems			
Sleep problems			
Emotional/behavior problems			
Radiation therapy			
Hormonal therapy			
Immune suppression			

Fig. 2.3 (Continued)

periodontal disease. A meta-analysis concluded that the odds ratio for developing periodontal disease is increased by smoking to 2.82 with a 95% confidence limit of 2.36–3.39 (Papapanou and Lindhe 2003). The causal effect of smoking is not known. It may be indirect, as smokers are generally more slender than their non-smoker counterparts, and, therefore, have lower bone density; smokers also in general have poorer oral hygiene than their non-smoker counterparts. On the other hand, it may also be a direct effect of the toxicity of tobacco smoke (Johnston 1994).

Other systemic risk factors include diseases or medications influencing the immune system, such as human immunodeficiency virus (HIV) infection and medications that lead to suppression of the immune system.

Clinical examination

The clinical examination includes extraoral examination, evaluation of the function of the masticatory system and intraoral examination and should be supplemented with findings from a review of photographs, dental casts and radiographs.

When listing the results of the examination, only positive findings should be listed and these should always appear in the same order (Box 2.1).

Box 2.1 Clinical examination

Extraoral
- En face
- Smile – lip line
- Profile
- Lips
- Midlines: nose; maxillary dental; mandibular dental; chin

Oral function
- Opening path
- Maximum opening
- Lateral movements
- Temporomandibular joints (TMJs)
- Muscles of mastication
- Tongue function
- Lip catch
- Mode of respiration
- Mode of swallowing

Intraoral
- Mucosa
- Dental status

Missing teeth
Morphological anomalies
Restorations
Attrition
Periodontal status
- Pathological pockets
- Recessions

Dental casts
- Positional anomalies; tipping; rotation
- Occlusion – sagittal, vertical, transverse

Space analysis
- Maxilla
- Mandible

Arch shape
- Maxilla
- Mandible

Cephalometric analysis

Extraoral examination

The face is first observed from the frontal view and apparent asymmetries noted. The relative widths of the eyes, the nose and the mouth are assessed and major deviations noted (Figure 2.4). The inter-inner-canthal distance in a harmonious face corresponds to the width of the nose, whereas the inter-iris width is equal to the width of the mouth (Figure 2.4). The vertical proportions can be measured both on the frontal and on the profile views. The division of the face into thirds has been accepted as a desirable norm for white Caucasians (Figure 2.5).

Exact measurements are of little value. 'Beauty is in the eye of the beholder' and the results of such analysis are partially subjective and can only act as a guide. Sagittally, a face can, based on white Caucasian norms, be characterised as convex, straight or concave (Figure 2.6). An impression of the mandibular inclination can be obtained by holding a straight instrument along the border of the mandible (Figure 2.7). Anthropometric measurements that have been published for different ethnic groups are characterised by large standard deviations and low reproducibility (Farkas and Kolar 1987; Farkas 1994), and many of our patients cannot be classified as belonging to one race only.

Most soft tissue analyses have focused on the two-dimensional profile and frontal images, but although both hard and soft tissues can now be analysed three-dimensionally, two-dimensional images still dominate our diagnostic routine (Arnett and Bergman 1993a, 1993b).

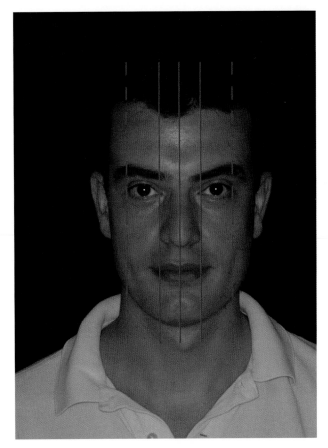

Fig. 2.4 Frontal view of a patient fulfilling the criteria of harmony. The inter-inner-canthal distance corresponds to the width of the nose. The symmetry of the face can be evaluated by drawing vertical lines through the medial and lateral aspects of the eyes.

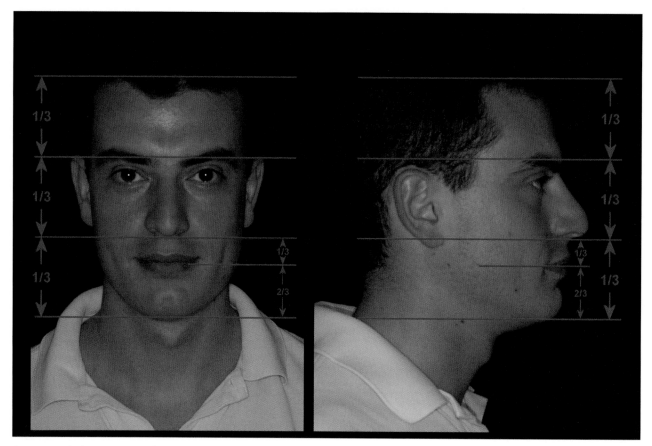

Fig. 2.5 Vertical proportion of the face seen en face and in profile view. The proportions indicated are the ideal values for white Caucasians.

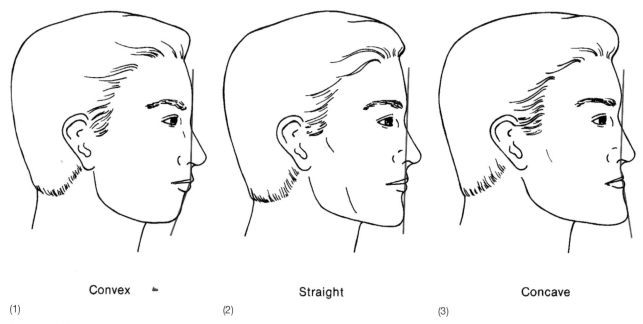

Convex   Straight   Concave

(1)   (2)   (3)

Fig. 2.6 Profiles representing different skeletal patterns. (1) The convex profile typically presents with a Class II malocclusion, whereas (3) the concave profile would be seen in a patient with a Class III malocclusion. In both cases, the deviation may be in either the position of the maxilla or in the position of the mandible. (2) The straight profile may likewise be due to bimaxillary retrusion or protrusion. (From Proffit and Ackerman (2000). Reproduced with permission from Elsevier.)

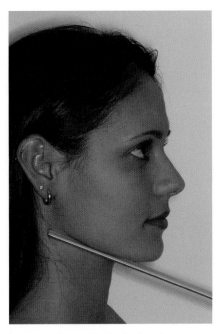

Fig. 2.7 Assessment of mandibular inclination.

Extraoral photographs

As the evaluation of the extraoral appearance has an increasing role in treatment planning, it is of paramount importance that photographs are taken in a way that they provide a valid record. The relative positions of patient, photographer and source of illumination should be taken into consideration. The ideal distance from the lens to the patient is 100 cm. With shorter distance, the image will be distorted (Figure 2.8). The facial photographs should include the neck and a part of the thorax. The background should be of a uniform colour, preferably light; however, some orthodontists prefer a blue or a black background, as it gives fewer problems with shadows. The patient should be upright with the lips in a relaxed position. In the case of insufficient lip closure, a photograph should also be taken with the lip strain necessary to obtain closure. The ears should be uncovered.

Vertically, the centre of the camera should be at the level of the Frankfort horizontal plane, in the midsagittal plane of the patient.

For the en face views, the patient should look at the superior part of the lens of the camera. A camera above or below this level will result in a distortion of the face (Figure 2.9). The light from the flash should be above the top of the

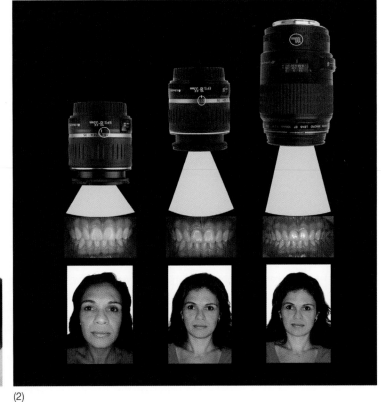

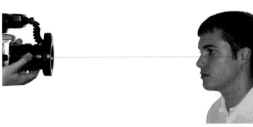

(1)   (2)

Fig. 2.8 (1) The lens focal distance for the extraoral images should be 1–1.5 m. (2) Frontal image taken with shorter lens focal distance leading to severe distortion.

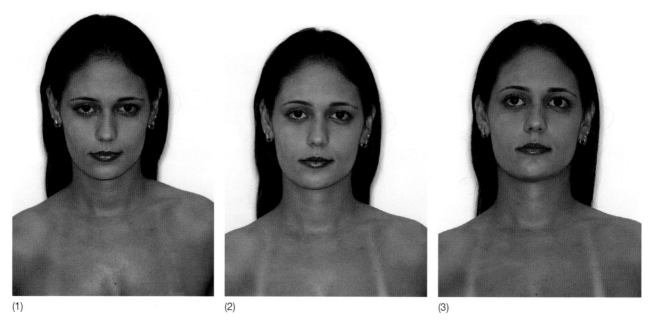

(1)   (2)   (3)

Fig. 2.9 Influence of the photographic technique on the extraoral image taken: (1) with the lens 10 cm above the height of the eyes of the patient, (2) at correct height and (3) 10 cm too low.

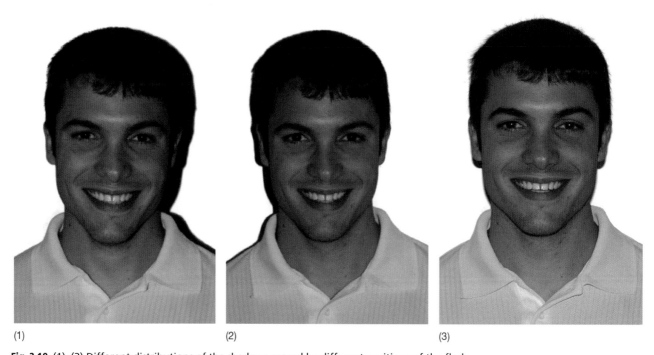

(1)   (2)   (3)

Fig. 2.10 (1)–(3) Different distributions of the shadows caused by different positions of the flash.

object (at 12 o'clock) in order to get the correct distribution of shadows (Figure 2.10).

On the profile images, the patient looks straight ahead, but turning the head just enough to see the eyelashes of the other side often gives a better impression of the profile (Figure 2.11). The illumination has to be oblique from the front with the flash turned towards the nares. This concentrates the shadows behind the head. Light from above produces shadows below the head (Figure 2.12), and

light from below will result in shadows above. Lateral illumination will lead to a shadow below the face and a pronounced nasolabial line (Figure 2.13). Thus, incorrect illumination results in unsatisfactory images.

Oblique 45° views are especially useful in the evaluation of midface deformities, and the projection of the nose relative to the rest of the face is also best evaluated on the oblique view (Figure 2.14). For all the images, a flash with low power connected to a photocell can be used to illuminate

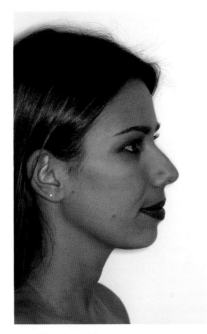

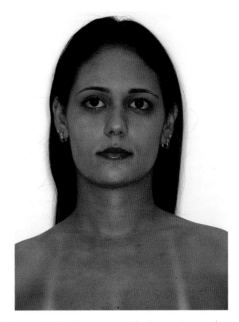

Fig. 2.13 Lateral illumination results in contours that are too sharp on one side.

Fig. 2.11 Natural head position.

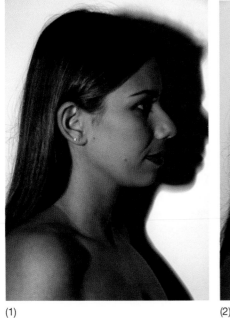

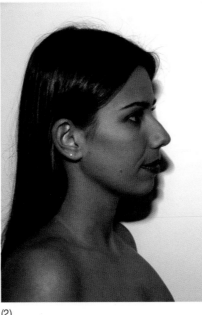

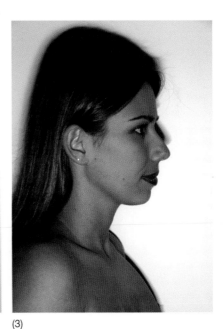

(1)   (2)   (3)

Fig. 2.12 Correct position of the lens, but wrong position of the flash: (1)–(3) Profile images.

the background wall, but the rules for the illumination of the object are still the same.

When evaluating extraoral images, both race and age have to be taken into consideration. Hellman (1921) described the difference in the slope of the face and showed that white Caucasians are frequently characterised by posterior divergence and Asians and black people have a higher prevalence of anterior divergence. These characteristics were not classified as problems, but as features of different ethnic groups. Age is also important, as both lip length and thickness are related to age (Figure 2.15) (Akgul and Toygar 2002).

When determining the treatment plan, the predicted changes can be simulated by various types of computer software. However, the accuracy and reliability of these systems are not yet sufficient for inclusion in routine diagnosis and treatment planning (Sameshima et al. 1997; Schultes et al. 1998; Kazandjian et al. 1999; Lu et al. 2003).

Function of the masticatory system

In order to avoid bias, function is evaluated before the occlusion is registered. A comprehensive examination of the temporomandibular joints (TMJs) and masticatory muscles is a crucial part of the clinical examination. The research diagnostic criteria (RDC) are widely used for the establishment of the problem list for patients with temporomandibular disorders (TMDs) (Le Resche et al. 1988; Dworkin et al. 2002) and are dealt with in Chapter 16.

Clinical examination of oral function should start with an assessment of the mandibular movement. The opening

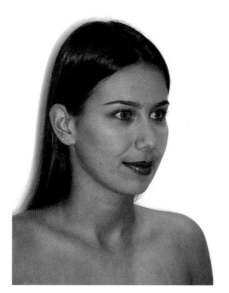

Fig. 2.14 Oblique 45° view in relaxed position.

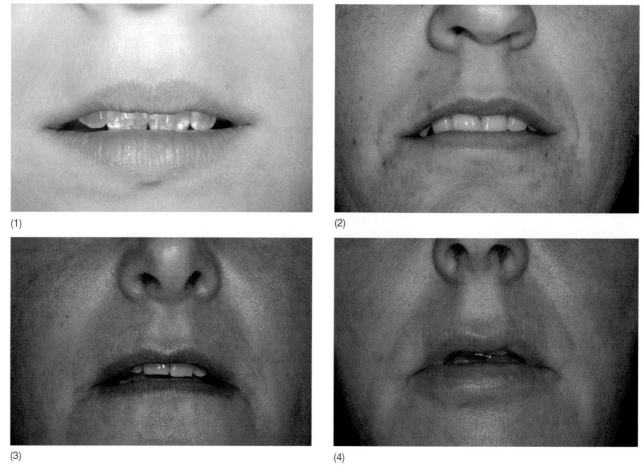

(1)

(2)

(3)

(4)

Fig. 2.15 Lip projection is a product both of lip thickness and dental protrusion. Due to age changes in the upper lip, less upper tooth substance is visible with increasing age: (1) 10 years of age, (2) 30 years, (3) 40 years and (4) 50 years.

movement should be observed and any asymmetry noted. Maximum opening and lateral movements and the difference between retruded position and maximum intercuspation should be measured. Freeway space is classified as increased, normal or reduced.

The TMJs should be examined with respect to clicking, with or without reduction in crepitation. Pain on palpation in the anterior, lateral or posterior aspects of the joint and on palpation of the masticatory muscles should be registered. An abnormal swallowing pattern or a localised abnormality in tongue pressure should be included in the problem list as should the patient's general respiratory habits and signs of parafunction such as bruxism.

Intraoral analysis – oral health

The evaluation of oral health includes an examination of the mucosa. Positive findings may lead to further examinations or referral to an oral pathologist. The dental status, which includes the number of teeth, fillings, restorations, active caries sites and teeth with dubious prognosis or inadequate restorations, is then registered. The intraoral examination is frequently combined with an evaluation of intraoral radiographs such as bitewings or panoramic radiographs and eventually supplemented with information obtained from the patient's general dentist.

The dental analysis includes an evaluation of: *tooth anomalies* such as deviation in number and shape; *eruption anomalies* such as ectopic teeth, transpositions, arrested eruption and ankylosis and *position anomalies*, including tipping, rotation and overeruption. Positional abnormalities and occlusal anomalies should be noted during the clinical examination or when analysing the study casts, since variation in projection of intraoral photographs has a significant impact on the evaluation of the findings (Figures 2.16 and 2.17).

The dental examination is followed by registration of the periodontal status, including the presence of plaque,

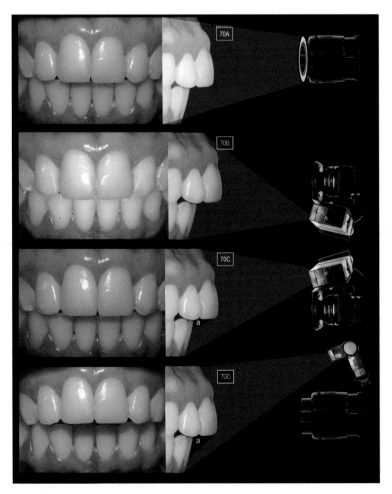

Fig. 2.16 An illustration of the influence of the camera position on the photograph produced.

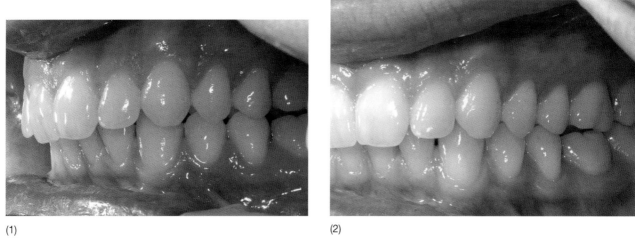

(1)   (2)

Fig. 2.17 (1) and (2) 'Photodontics': The change in the camera position changes the perception of the lateral occlusion.

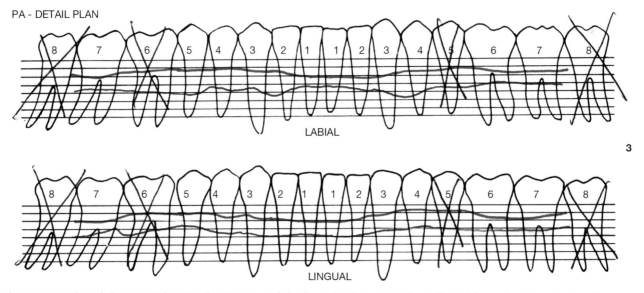

Fig. 2.18 Periodontal diagram indicating the gingiva and the bone level measures buccally and lingually in a patient with severe periodontal loss.

calculus, inflammation, pathological pockets and bony dehiscences, all of which should be noted on a periodontal chart. The level of marginal bone should be checked on the periapical X-ray and noted on the chart (Figure 2.18).

Any soft tissue problems such as a high labial frenum or any frena that might compromise the integrity of the marginal gingiva should be mentioned. The width of the keratinised gingiva should be noted if significantly reduced and also the biotype if the patient has extremely thin gingiva.

Evaluation of dental casts – arch form

Each cast is examined separately the arch form – the shape of the upper and the lower dental arches. For a detailed discussion of the arch form, see Chapter 5.

Occlusal analysis

The occlusion should be registered in all three planes of space both anteriorly and laterally, either on plaster casts or on virtual models (Figure 2.19) (Tomassetti et al. 2001; Santoro et al. 2003; Zilberman et al. 2003; Quimby et al.

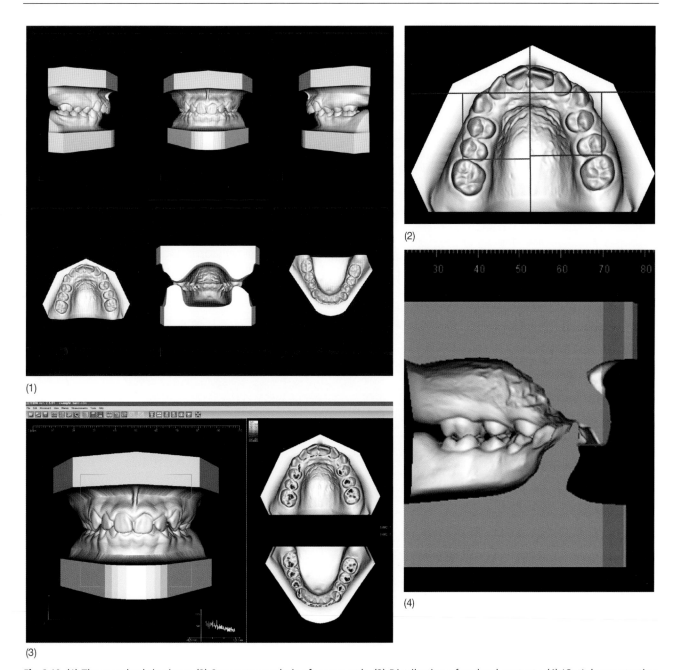

Fig. 2.19 (1) The standard six views. (2) Symmetry analysis of upper arch. (3) Distribution of occlusal contacts. (4) 'Cut' demonstrating the inclination of the incisors.

2004). Apart from practical advantages as storage and easy retrieval, virtual casts also have the advantage that they can be shared. This is of particular importance in relation to multidisciplinary treatments where colleagues simultaneously can access information regarding a common patient, including photographs, study casts and radiographs.

The sagittal occlusion is usually described in terms of the Angle classification, even though weaknesses of this classification system have been pointed out repeatedly (Tang and Wei 1993; Liu and Melsen 2001). To supplement the Angle classification, the molar relationship should also be studied from the lingual aspect. In this manner, it will be possible to distinguish between the distal occlusion caused by a mesial rotation of the molars and that due to a skeletal Class II relationship. Less discussion has taken place regarding the transverse and vertical deviations of occlusion. The Venn diagram developed by Ackerman and Profitt (1970) illustrates the possible combination of occlusal anomalies in the most didactic way. This diagram can therefore be recommended as an aide-memoire when evaluating occlusion (Figure 2.20).

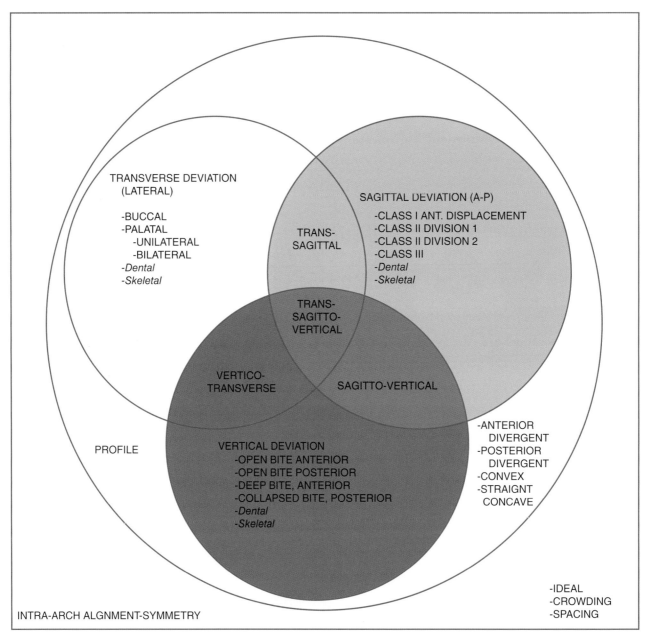

Fig. 2.20 The Venn diagram developed by Proffit and Ackerman. The diagram illustrates the combination of deviation in the three planes of space. (From Proffit [2000]. Reproduced with permission from Elsevier.)

Space analysis

The space requirements should be evaluated and included in the problem list, provided either spacing or crowding is present. Space analysis in the adult patient is not performed as described in most textbooks in relation to existing arch form, but is expressed in relation to the space in the arch as it is defined on the occlusogram, indicating the arch shape at the end of treatment (Figure 2.21). A useful measurement is the anterior ratio expressing the relationship between the sum of the mesiodistal measurements of the lower and the upper incisors.

Cephalometric analysis

In the adult patient, cephalometric analysis can be carried out on the head film as in young growing patients. However, its main use is in evaluating the need for extraction or space opening or in determining if the only treatment option will be orthognathic surgery.

All cephalometric analyses are characterised by moderate or low reproducibility flawed by the selection of the reference points (Baumrind and Frantz 1971). The head film in the adult patient will therefore be used only for a few measurements such as those related to assessment of relative

3-D TREATMENT OBJECTIVE

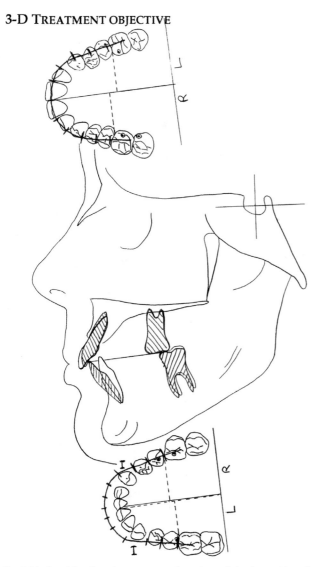

Fig. 2.21 Combined occlusogram and tracing of the lateral head film. The future arch form and position are indicated, and the mesiodistal width of the individual teeth is indicated on this arch form, in order to evaluate the need for space.

maxillary and mandibular prognathism (SNA, SNB, SN-Pg), and the inclination of the maxilla (NSL/NL) and of the mandible (NSL/ML). These may be supplemented by measurements of the incisor inclination, although the latter measurements are known to give rise to the largest errors, as all four incisors are usually superimposed. The limited value of conventional cephalometric analysis was demonstrated by Wylie et al. (1987), who compared five different analyses and concluded that different analyses resulted in different suggestions for surgery in the same patient. The inclination of the incisors is better assessed on virtual models 'cut' through each incisor (Figure 2.22).

The introduction of the cone-beam technique has changed the evaluation of the craniofacial skeleton. A comparison of the information retrievable from conventional head film, even of a good quality, with that obtained by

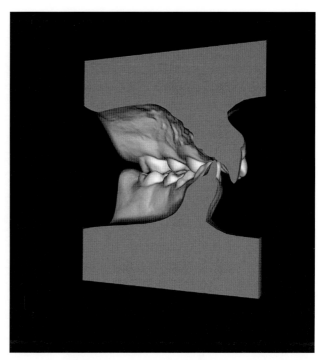

Fig. 2.22 Cut through upper incisors on a virtual model.

cone-beam imaging illustrated clearly that three-dimensional imaging results in a more valid diagnosis (Mah and Hatcher 2005; Redmond et al. 2005) (Figure 2.23).

The conventional cephalometric analysis can help to identify the origin of the malocclusion and, since the skeletal pattern of adult patients cannot be changed, to determine whether orthognathic surgery will be part of the treatment. However, the tracing of the head film combined with the occlusogram plays an important role in predicting the treatment goals and the determination of the necessary tooth movements.

Final problem list

The final problem list should only include positive findings. Proffit and Ackerman (2000) suggest listing the problems according to priority, but the problem list could also be presented in a standard sequence. This has the advantage that it is easy to detect where the problems are and, at the same time, where no deviations exist. Having completed the problem list, the orthodontist should indicate a tentative suggestion for a solution to each of the listed problems or whether the sign or symptom has to be accepted as no solution is possible (Table 2.1).

A problem list should not be mistaken as a description of the patient; it only should include true problems and perceived deviations from the norm. This list starts with a description of the patient's chief complaint: 'My teeth are migrating and I do not like that they are sticking out' or 'I do not like the space between my front teeth', or similar expressions expressed in the patient's own words. This

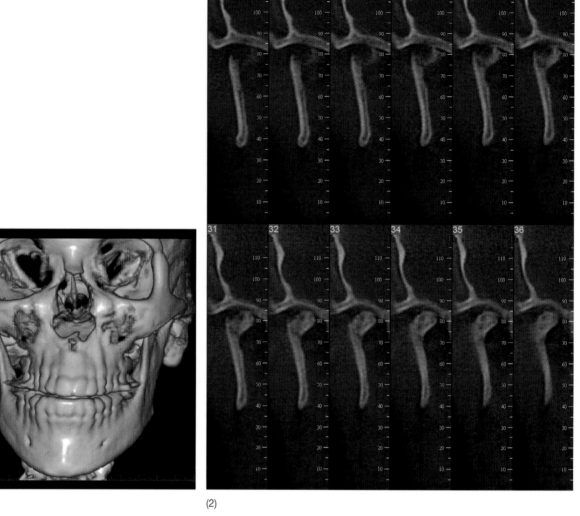

(1)   (2)

Fig. 2.23 (1) Cone-beam image of an adult patient with an open bite following an accident. The patient had pain in the right temporomandibular joint (TMJ). (2) The frontal tomogram of the TMJ revealed a fracture of the right joint and a medial displacement of the condyle. This was not observed in the conventional radiographs.

should be followed by the objective problem list based on the clinical examination and findings obtained from photographs and X-ray examinations. It is important that the problems are listed in the same sequence (Box 2.1), as an absence of a comment in relation to one or more of the points listed means that there is no anomaly.

A summary version of the treatment goal agreed on by clinician and patient is then produced in the form of a three-dimensional illustration produced by the combination of head film and occlusogram. This should also be presented to the dentist who will be responsible for the prosthodontic part of the treatment (Figure 2.21).

Indication for treatment

The indications for treatment should be added to the problem list and evaluated from a cost-benefit point of view. When discussing the treatment plan with the patient, it is also important to consider the long-term maintenance of the dentition after active treatment ends, and what should be done to prevent further deterioration of the dentition, as discussed in Chapter 19. Whether orthodontic treatment is carried out or not, age-related changes will continue to occur. The results of orthodontic treatment thus cannot be anticipated to be stable and must be maintained with the use of retainers. This includes both biological and mechanical maintenance. Biological maintenance comprises a strict protocol of periodontal health maintenance and optimisation of occlusal loadings through prosthodontic replacement of restorations not in harmony with the occlusion obtained by treatment. Mechanical maintenance will be dealt with in Chapter 19.

The presentation of the problem list – the tip of the iceberg

A major concern in treating adult patients is communicating the problem list to the patient. It is a difficult task to explain that what the patient perceives as a simple problem is the symptom of a highly complex situation. For example, on hearing that a simple complaint such as a diastema or the flaring of incisors is a symptom of a more severe malocclusion, patients may react in different ways. They may reject the complexity of the problem and opt for an immediate and easy solution. In the case of crowding, this may consist of extraction, or in the case of a deep bite, reduction in the height of incisors by grinding or posterior onlays that will leave the incisors to erupt even further. A compromise procedure may be chosen, as recommended by Zachrisson (2004a, 2004b), when treating elderly adult patients. In such cases, the limitations of the treatment goal should be made clear to the patient as should the influence of the treatment on the prognosis of the dentition.

The description of the patient's chief complaint, the reason for seeking an orthodontic consultant as well as a workup of a comprehensive problem list are the foundation stones on which treatment options are built and can be discussed. The following example illustrates the conflict between subjective and objective problems, between the chief complaint and the dentist's findings or, in other words, *treatment demand* and *treatment need*.

A 48-year-old woman experienced pain and developed an abscess above the upper left first molar when on vacation. She was given high dosages of antibiotics and was advised to see her dentist on returning home. She explained her acute problem and in addition mentioned that she had a bridge which repeatedly came loose: 'By the way, now that I am here, could you fix a bridge in the other side, since it has come loose several times?' Apart from these complaints, the patient was generally satisfied with her dentition. Asked about any other complaints, she explained that she frequently had headaches, which she ascribed to a stressful job situation.

Extraoral examination: The face appeared symmetrical in the frontal view with bimaxillary protrusion and incomplete lip seal (Figure 2.24). Functional analysis revealed traumatic occlusion in the first premolar region bilaterally and a sliding of the mandible to the left during closure. This resulted in a slightly asymmetrical occlusion and an asymmetrical condylar position, which was later confirmed by the large discrepancy between the posterior contours of

the right and left mandibular rami on the head film (Figure 2.24(10)). Palpation of the muscles revealed tenderness in the temporalis muscles on both sides.

Intraoral examination: Before carrying out any other analysis, it became obvious that the problems were more severe than anticipated by the patient. The upper right molar in which she had experienced pain had an abscess related to two roots with incomplete root fillings. The tooth could not be saved. In relation to the other chief complaint, the loose bridge, the radiographs demonstrated that beneath the crown on tooth 24 there was a very deep carious lesion involving part of the root and extending deep below the bone margin (Figure 2.24(4)).

An objective problem list was worked out on the basis of the clinical and functional examination, the radiographic analysis supplemented with a lateral head film and a set of articulator-mounted study casts. Apart from the chief complaints, the problem list included conditions that the patient did not want corrected, as well as problems for which no solution could be offered (see Table 2.2).

The comments of the patient when presented with the problem list were as follows:

- *Extraoral findings*: Incomplete lip seal. This was not of concern to the patient. She had had incompetent lips related to her bimaxillary protrusion for a long time and she liked her smile and accepted the situation as it was (Figure 2.24(1–3)).
- *Function*: Traumatic occlusion on the premolars on both sides, which had led to marked mobility of the teeth and bony dehiscence on the buccal aspect of 34 and 44, although without loss of attachment. Whenever the patient chewed, these teeth tipped slightly buccally. This had led to a very particular chewing pattern in order to avoid the traumatic occlusion. This may also in part explain her tension headache. However, she did not want to relate the headache to the dental situation and thought it would not be sensible to include this in the solution to her dental problems. The head film confirmed that the mandible was forced into an asymmetrical position on closure into maximal intercuspation. The patient's reaction was, however, that she had lived with this occlusion for many years and she would deal with the problem when it became acute. As of now she managed to avoid the traumatic occlusion by adapting her chewing pattern.
- *Dental status*: The dentition reflected extensive caries experience, but no active caries apart from the lesion in 24. Tooth 25 was missing and replaced by a bridge; 16 could not be saved. Apart from occlusal and Class II restorations, many teeth had cervical composite fillings in the defects generated by a too-aggressive mode of toothbrushing. The patient was not concerned about the irregular position of single teeth, but definitely wanted the missing teeth replaced.

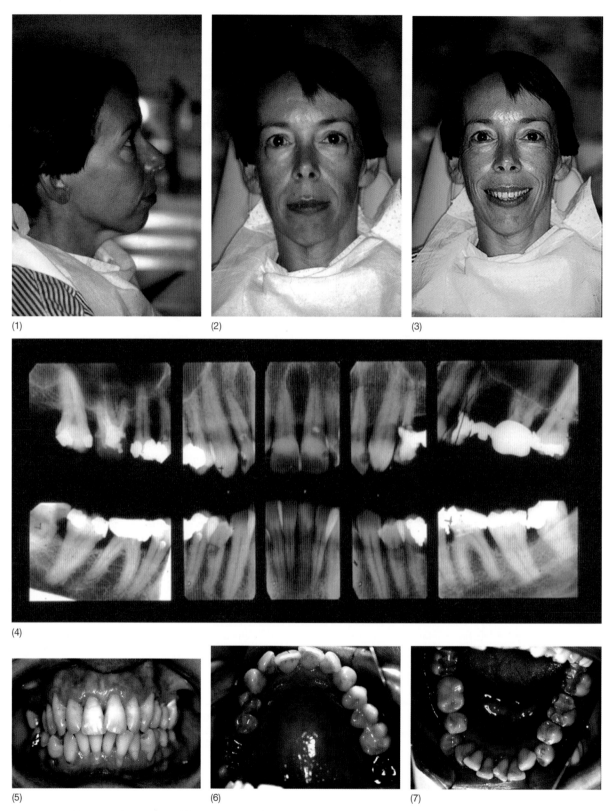

Fig. 2.24 Extraoral images of a 48-year-old patient seeing her dentist due to pain. (1)–(3) The patient has a bimaxillary protrusion and insufficient lip closure. (4) Periapical radiographs demonstrating two granulomas in relation to 16 and a deep carious lesion in 24. (5)–(9) Intraoral pictures revealing a neutral sagittal relationship with crowding in both arches and traumatic occlusion on the first lower premolars, which are in crossbite. (10) Lateral tracing demonstrating an asymmetry in the level of the posterior border of the mandible on the right and left sides as a possible sign of a forced bite. (11) Three-dimensional Visual Treatment Objective (3D VTO) made on a lateral tracing combined with an occlusogram. (12)–(14) Following the extraction of the 16 and 24, which could not be prevented, the second upper left molar was moved mesially in combination with distal rotation. Sectional mechanics were used simultaneously bilaterally to produce lingual root torque in the canines which had been in crossbite. In the lower jaw, 34 and 44 were extracted and levelling and space closure were performed with a continuous archwire. (15)–(21) Post-treatment views.

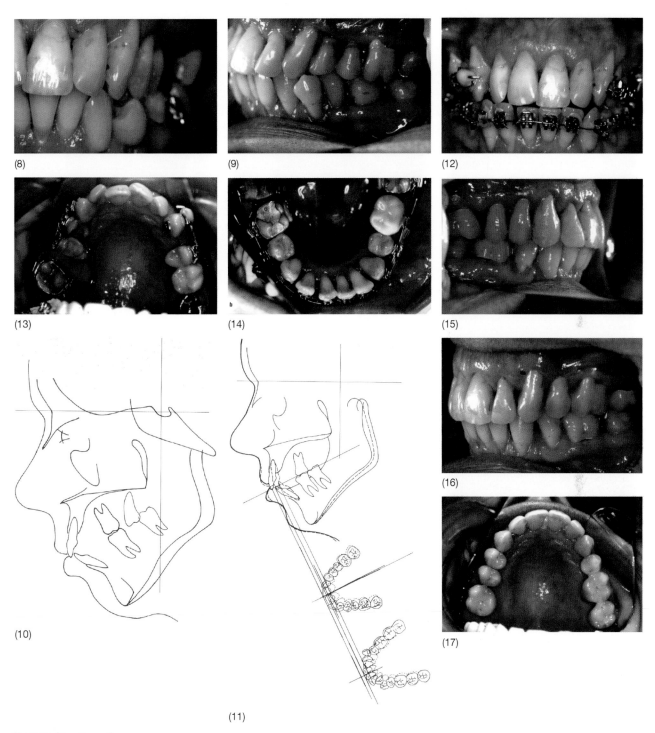

Fig. 2.24 (*Continued*)

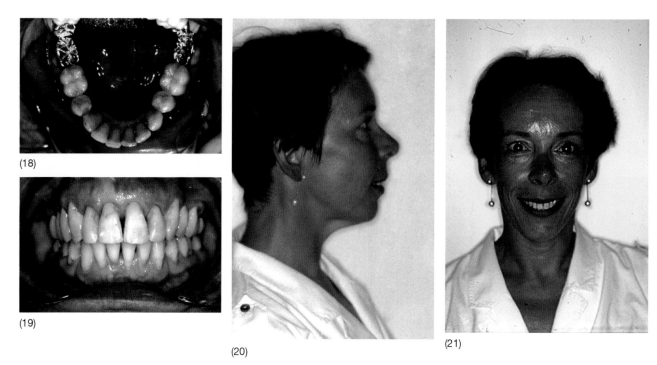

(18)

(19)

(20)

(21)

Fig. 2.24 (*Continued*)

Table 2.2 Chief complaint – 'I had toothache in my upper right molar and I have a loose bridge on the left side'.

Problem list	Solution
Extraoral examination	
Bimaxillary protrusion, insufficient lip closure	Reduction of protrusion through space closure following extraction of 16, 24, 34 and 44
Functional analysis	
Traumatic occlusion on lower first premolars	Extraction of 34 and 44
Laterally forced bite	Coordination between structural position and intercuspation
Muscle tenderness	
Intraoral analysis	
Missing tooth 25	Space closure
Teeth that cannot be saved: 16 and 24	
Gingival dehiscences	Have to be accepted
Bony recessions: 34 and 44	Extraction: 34 and 44
Bony fenestration apically: 13 and 23	Lingual root torque: 13 and 23
Irregular position and crowding of upper and lower anterior teeth	Levelling following extraction

- *Periodontal status*: In general, the periodontium was healthy, but was characterised by generalised gingival recession. The traumatic occlusion on the lower first premolar had led to loss of bone on the buccal aspect, resulting in increased mobility of these teeth. In the upper jaw, the traumatic occlusion had led to lingual tipping of the canines with bony fenestration in the apical region of 13 and 23. This was reflected in pain whenever she blew her nose because this entailed touching the apices of the canines. The patient's reaction was that she could simply avoid touching these

areas. The problem of bone dehiscence and associated gingival recession could not be treated, since buccal fillings were covering the exposed cementum. Therefore, they had to be accepted with possible replacement of the fillings.

- *Occlusion*: The patient had a neutral molar relationship, half-cusp distal canine relationship and bilateral crowding in the upper and lower jaws, especially in the incisal region of the lower jaw. When the problem list was presented, the possible solutions were explained to the patient, including potential extraction of the first premolars in the lower jaw which would be followed by levelling to resolve the traumatic occlusion. This would also take care of the lower arch crowding. However, the patient felt that all these problems had been there for so long that she saw no reason to treat the crowding and the thought of having to wear braces was unacceptable to her. Her only wish was to replace her missing teeth.

A 3D Visual Treatment Objective (VTO) was carried out to illustrate to the patient that the space left after extraction of 16, instead of being replaced with a bridge, could be closed by mesial movement of the second molar and slight distal movement of the premolar and canine (Figure 2.24(11)). This would allow for correction of the anterior crowding and lingual root torque of the canines. On the right side, the space left after extraction of the root of 24 could alleviate the problem of anterior crowding. If the two lower first premolars, which had severe loss of buccal bone, were extracted, the patient would end up with neutral molar relationship on both sides, no crowding and less protrusion. The treatment in the upper jaw would involve torquing the upper incisors as well. The prognosis, long- and short-term, the advantages and disadvantages of the prosthetic solution and the combined orthodontic–prosthetic solution were well explained, and the timescale of the treatment and the visibility of the appliance discussed. It was explained to the patient that the first part of the treatment could be done with segmental orthodontics and anterior brackets would be needed only for the last 3 months of treatment. The patient accepted this treatment plan.

The treatment was started with extraction of teeth 16 and 24, which could not be saved. The general practitioner separated 14 from the bridge extending from 24 to 26 and a bracket was bonded onto the pontic extending from 26. Following extensive cleansing and careful instructions, the first premolars in the lower jaw were extracted, after which the crowded lower incisors were left to unravel spontaneously for a few months (Figure 2.24(12–14)).

Space closure following extraction of 16 was performed from the lingual aspect, since the force system generated between a power arm on the second molar and the anterior segment would lead to combined distal rotation and mesial movement. Lingual root torque was added to the canine, which is part of the anterior segment. On the left side, space closure following extraction of 24 was done using type B anchorage (Burstone 1982). Also on this side, lingual root torque was applied to the canine. The orthodontic treatment was finished with a neutral canine relationship without spacing or crowding. The patient was referred back to the prosthodontist with a fully equilibrated splint that was used to maintain the jaw position, which at this time had been changing gradually following the extraction of the lower premolars that had been in traumatic occlusion. The patient was also now free of headaches. The occlusal surfaces that did not fit into the corrected occlusion were restored. The

patient thereby achieved full function after all the treatment, which had lasted less than 2 years, without any teeth at risk and without any periodontal problems. The gingival marginal recession was left untreated, as mucogingival surgery was not indicated due to the many composite fillings that had been done to cover the defects generated by poor tooth-brushing habits (Figure 2.24(17–21)).

The treatment planning had been *interdisciplinary*. The team included a dental hygienist, an orthodontist and a prosthodontist who also served as a gnathologist during the establishment of the mandibular position before the final occlusal adjustment.

In terms of cost-benefit analysis, the treatment compared positively with the one requested by the patient. She asked for restoration of the missing teeth which would have involved insertion of two bridges or three implants. Due to the quality of the bone, it is likely that bone augmentation would have been needed if this treatment had been chosen. Following the interdisciplinary treatment, including orthodontic treatment that lasted 18 months and subsequent occlusal rehabilitation that lasted 6 months, the patient had spent less money and had no teeth at risk. The treatment had aimed to solve the cause of the problem rather than simply alleviating the symptoms.

Concluding remarks

When seeing an adult patient, the chief complaint is most likely to represent the tip of an iceberg. The first task is therefore to explain to the patient the bigger picture and how the problem that led the patient to see the orthodontist fits into it, and to make it clear that limiting the treatment to 'the social six' may compromise long-term prognosis.

Another issue which has to be dealt with prior to initiating orthodontic treatment is the patient's expectations about the possible treatment. The key to successful orthodontic treatment of an adult patient lies in coordination of the patient's expectations with results that are realistically achievable, as well as ensuring the patient can fulfil the requirements of compliance with treatment, investment of the time needed and the economic resources needed for the treatment.

References

Ackerman JL and Proffit WR (1970) Treatment response as an aid in diagnosis and treatment planning. *Am J Orthod* 57, 490–496.

Akgul AA and Toygar TU (2002) Natural craniofacial changes in the third decade of life: a longitudinal study. *Am J Orthod Dentofacial Orthop* 122, 512–522.

Arnett GW and Bergman RT (1993a) Facial keys to orthodontic diagnosis and treatment planning. Part II. *Am J Orthod Dentofacial Orthop* 103, 395–411.

Arnett GW and Bergman RT (1993b) Facial keys to orthodontic diagnosis and treatment planning. Part I. *Am J Orthod Dentofacial Orthop* 103, 299–312.

Baumrind S and Frantz RC (1971) The reliability of head film measurements. 1. Landmark identification. *Am J Orthod* 60, 111–127.

Bowman SJ (2005) Comment: the social six: is that all there is? *Aust Orthod J* 21, 68–71.

Burstone CJ (1982) The segmented arch approach to space closure. *Am J Orthod* 82, 361–378.

Dworkin SF, Sherman J, Mancl L, Ohrbach R, LeResche L and Truelove E (2002) Reliability, validity, and clinical utility of the research diagnostic criteria for temporomandibular disorders axis II scales: depression, non-specific physical symptoms, and graded chronic pain. *J Orofac Pain* 16, 207–220.

Farkas LG (1994) *Anthropometry of the Head and Face in Medicine.* New York, NY: Raven Press.

Farkas LG and Kolar JC (1987) Anthropometrics and art in the aesthetics of women's faces. *Clin Plast Surg* 14, 599–616.

Genco RJ and Loe H (1993) The role of systemic conditions and disorders in periodontal disease. *Periodontol 2000* 2, 98–116.

Hellman M (1921) Variations in occlusion. *Dent Cosmos* 63, 608–619.

Johnston JD (1994) Smokers have less dense bones and fewer teeth. *J R Soc Health* 114, 265–269.

Kazandjian S, Sameshima GT, Champlin T and Sinclair PM (1999) Accuracy of video imaging for predicting the soft tissue profile after mandibular set-back surgery. *Am J Orthod Dentofacial Orthop* 115, 382–389.

Lalla E, Lamster IB, Drury S, Fu C and Schmidt AM (2000) Hyperglycemia, glycoxidation and receptor for advanced glycation endproducts: potential mechanisms underlying diabetic complications, including diabetes-associated periodontitis. *Periodontol 2000* 23, 50–62.

Le Resche L, Burgess J and Dworkin SF (1988) Reliability of visual analog and verbal descriptor scales for 'objective' measurement of temporomandibular disorder pain. *J Dent Res* 67, 33–36.

Liu D and Melsen B (2001) Reappraisal of Class II molar relationships diagnosed from the lingual side. *Clin Orthod Res* 4, 97–104.

Lu CH, Ko EW and Huang CS (2003) The accuracy of video imaging prediction in soft tissue outcome after bimaxillary orthognathic surgery. *J Oral Maxillofac Surg* 61, 333–342.

Mah JK and Hatcher D (2005) Craniofacial imaging in orthodontics. In Graber TM, Vanarsdall RL and Vig KLW (eds) *Orthodontics – Current Priciples and Techniques*, 4th edn, pp. 71–100. St Louis, MO: Mosby.

Papapanou PN (1999) Epidemiology of periodontal diseases: an update. *J Int Acad Periodontol* 1, 110–116.

Papapanou PN and Lindhe J (2003) Epidemiology of Periodontal Diseases. In Lindhe J, Karring T, Lang NP et al. (eds) *Clinical Periodontology and Implant Dentistry*, 4th edn, pp. 50–80. Munksgaard: Blackwell.

Proffit WR and Ackerman JL (2000) Orthodontic diagnosis: the development of problem list. In Proffit WR and Fields HW (eds) *Contemporary Orthodontics*, 3rd edn, pp. 147–195. St Louis, MO: Mosby.

Quimby ML, Vig KW, Rashid RG and Firestone AR (2004) The accuracy and reliability of measurements made on computer-based digital models. *Angle Orthod* 74, 298–303.

Redmond WR, Huang J, Buman A and Mah J (2005) The cutting edge. *J Clin Orthod* 39, 421–428.

Sameshima GT, Kawakami RK, Kaminishi RM and Sinclair PM (1997) Predicting soft tissue changes in maxillary impaction surgery: a comparison of two video imaging systems. *Angle Orthod* 67, 347–354.

Santoro M, Galkin S, Teredesai M, Nicolay OF and Cangialosi TJ (2003) Comparison of measurements made on digital and plaster models. *Am J Orthod Dentofacial Orthop* 124, 101–105.

Schultes G, Gaggl A and Karcher H (1998) Accuracy of cephalometric and video imaging program dentofacial planner plus in orthognathic surgical planning. *Comput Aided Surg* 3, 108–114.

Tang EL and Wei SH (1993) Recording and measuring malocclusion: a review of the literature. *Am J Orthod Dentofacial Orthop* 103, 344–351.

Taylor GW, Burt BA, Becker MP, Genco RJ and Shlossman M (1998a) Glycemic control and alveolar bone loss progression in type 2 diabetes. *Annals Periodontol* 3, 30–39.

Taylor GW, Burt BA, Becker MP, Genco RJ, Shlossman M, Knowler WC and Pettitt DJ (1998b) Non-insulin dependent diabetes mellitus and alveolar bone loss progression over 2 years. *J Periodontol* 69, 76–83.

Tomassetti JJ, Taloumis LJ, Denny JM and Fischer JR Jr (2001) A comparison of 3 computerized Bolton tooth-size analyses with a commonly used method. *Angle Orthod* 71, 351–357.

Van Dyke TE and Sheilesh D (2005) Risk factors for periodontitis. *J Int Acad Periodontol* 7, 3–7.

Wylie GA, Fish LC and Epker BN (1987) Cephalometrics: a comparison of five analyses currently used in the diagnosis of dentofacial deformities. *Int J Adult Orthod Orthog Surg* 2, 15–36.

Zachrisson BU (2004a) Actual damage to teeth and periodontal tissues with mesiodistal enamel reduction ('stripping'). *World J Orthod* 5, 178–183.

Zachrisson BU (2004b) First premolars substituting for maxillary canines–esthetic, periodontal and functional considerations. *World J Orthod* 5, 358–364.

Zilberman O, Huggare JA and Parikakis KA (2003) Evaluation of the validity of tooth size and arch width measurements using conventional and three-dimensional virtual orthodontic models. *Angle Orthod* 73, 301–306.

3

Aetiology

Birte Melsen

Introduction

Malocclusions registered among adult patients comprise two categories: the first, malocclusions that develop during the period of occlusal development and, if not corrected by interceptive treatments, may worsen with increasing age; the second, type, which is a result of the ongoing, age-related deterioration of the permanent dentition. Marks and Corn (1989) did not differentiate between malocclusions developing during different periods, but distinguished between malocclusions of dental and skeletal origins. Among the dental type, they listed intra-arch discrepancies, including malpositions of teeth. Both types of malocclusions can be considered as having both genetic and environmental origins, but in the case of the older adult patient, age-related tooth migrations occur as a result of deterioration, as well as different types of oral parafunction and dysfunction constitute important aetiological factors.

Biological background

Understanding of the aetiology of malocclusions requires a background knowledge of the biology related to the oral tissues and surrounding bone. In adult patients, this is even more important, as the reaction of the periodontal tissues to orthodontic tooth movement is age-related and influenced by both local and general pathological conditions.

The early development of the head and neck structures starts with the branchial arches, which are present from around weeks 5–6 of gestation. These prominences are composed of epithelium, which surrounds mesenchymal cells predominantly of neural crest origin. As the first branchial arch develops to form the mandibular and maxillary processes, the stomatodeum or primitive mouth cavity becomes prominent.

The development of the dentoalveolar region starts in the fourth week when neural crest cells migrate into the branchial arches, forming a band of ectomesenchyme under the epithelium of the primary oral cavity. Interaction between the ectomesenchyme and the epithelium initiates the subsequent formation of the dental lamina from which the tooth buds originate. The tooth bud passes through the cap stage to the bell stage in which the enamel organ, the dental lamina, the dental papilla and the dental follicle can be differentiated (Figure 3.1). The attachment apparatus with all its components will develop from this follicle. Once the crown has formed, root formation starts. Studies involving transplantation of a tooth germ to a different location clearly indicate that the development of the periodontium is completely dependent on the existence of

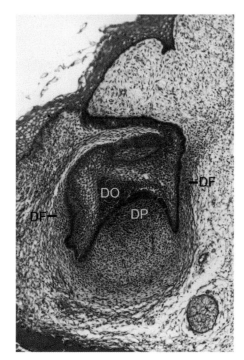

Fig. 3.1 Cap stage demonstrating the condensation of ectomesenchymal cells in relation to the dental epithelium, the dental organ (DO), from which the dental papilla (DP) that gives rise to the pulp and the dentine is formed. The dental follicle (DF) is seen surrounding the dental papilla and gives rise to the periodontal tissues. (Reproduced from Lindhe J, Karring T, Lang NP, eds. (2005) *Clinical Periodontology and Implant Dentistry*, 4th edn., with permission from Wiley-Blackwell.)

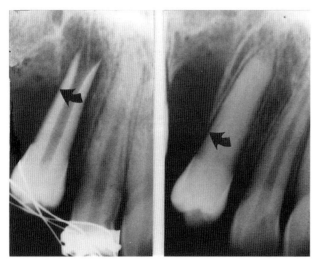

Fig. 3.2 An unerupted premolar transplanted to a canine region with severe loss of bone following an injury. It can be seen that bone formation has been induced during root formation. (Reproduced from Andreasen JO (1996) *Textbook and Color Atlas of Traumatic Injuries to the Teeth*, with permission from Wiley-Blackwell.)

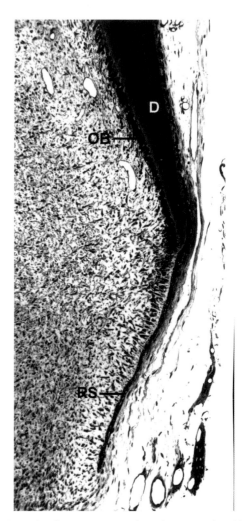

Fig. 3.3 Root development starts when the external and internal dental epithelia meet and proliferate as a double layer of cells, now named Hertwig's epithelial root sheath (RS). The inner epithelial cells differentiate into odontoblasts (OB) and start forming dentine (D). Formation of dentine continues in an apical direction and generates the framework for the root. (Courtesy of K. Josephsen, from Lindhe J, Karring T and Lang NP, eds. (2005) *Clinical Periodontology and Implant Dentistry*, 4th edn., with permission from Wiley-Blackwell.)

the dental follicle. When transplanted with its follicle, a tooth bud will give rise to periodontal tissues even in different locations (Kristerson and Andreasen 1984; Palmer and Lumsden 1987) (Figure 3.2).

The root formation and the formation of the periodontal tissues are closely interdependent and linked in time (Hammarstrom et al. 1996). At the point where the internal and the external dental epithelium cells meet and proliferate in an apical direction, Hertwig's epithelial root sheath is formed and projects in the future direction of the root (Figure 3.3). Local pathological processes affect root formation and its shape, length and direction of growth.

Table 3.1 Development anomalies of the teeth.

Initiation phase	Anodontia
	Oligodontia
	Supernumerary teeth
Bud stage	Microdontia
	Macrodontia
Cap stage	Dens invaginatus
	Gemination/Fusion
	Tubercle formation
	Apposition phase hypoplasia
	Hypocalcification
	Amelogenesis and dentinogenesis imperfecta
Root formation	Enamel pearls
	Root dilaceration

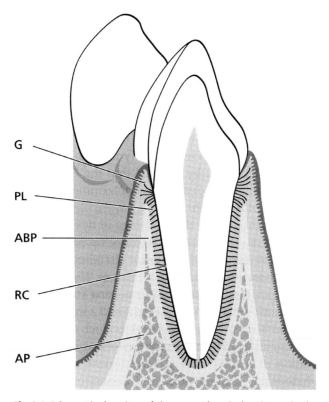

Fig. 3.4 Schematic drawing of the normal periodontium: gingiva (G), periodontal ligament (PL), root cementum (RC), alveolar bone (AB) and alveolar bone proper (ABP). (Reproduced from Lindhe J, Karring T and Lang NP, eds. (2005) *Clinical Periodontology and Implant Dentistry*, 4th edn., with permission from Wiley-Blackwell.)

Developmental anomalies can occur if disturbances occur during any of the stages of tooth development (Table 3.1). The periodontium, also defined as the attachment apparatus, surrounds the tooth and includes: the gingiva; the periodontal ligament; the cementum and the alveolar bone

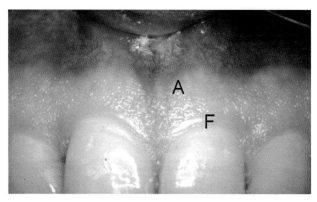

Fig. 3.5 Intraoral view demonstrating the healthy gingiva of a young individual. The gingiva immediately adjacent to the crown of the tooth is smooth and pale pink in colour. It is called the free gingiva (F), since it does not rest on alveolar bone. It is delineated from the attached gingiva by the free gingival groove, which also reflects the underlying cementoenamel junction. The attached gingiva (A) extends from this groove in an apical direction and merges with the free mucosa. The attached gingiva has a stippled appearance due to the small impressions on its surface.

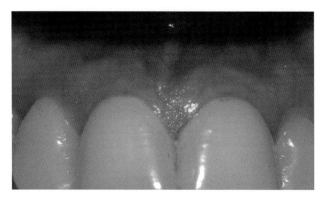

Fig. 3.6 Intraoral image of a 40-year-old woman. The free gingiva has disappeared.

(Figure 3.4). Both the development and the maintenance of the alveolar bone are closely associated with root development and the eruption of the teeth.

The gingiva is the part of the oral mucosa that covers the alveolar process and surrounds the teeth. The gingiva consists of epithelium covering underlying connective tissue called the lamina propria. The gingiva immediately adjacent to the teeth has been defined as free gingiva and this does not rest on bone (Figure 3.5). At the free gingival groove (F), which corresponds approximately to the marginal bone level, it continues apically as the attached gingiva (A). The free gingiva does not have the stippled appearance characterising the attached gingiva. It is pale and smooth and demarcates the cementoenamel junction in young individuals (Figure 3.5). In older adults, apical displacement of the gingival tissue leads to loss of the free gingiva (Figure

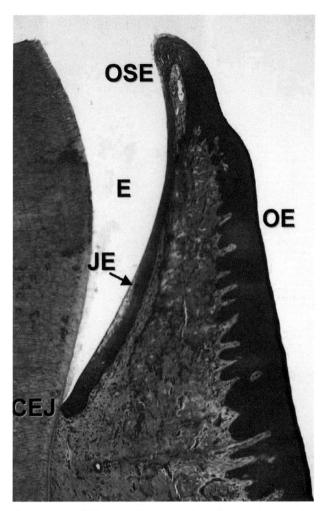

Fig. 3.7 Sagittal histological section through a tooth. It can be seen that the sulcular epithelium comprises only a few cell layers. E, enamel; JE, junctional epithelium; CEJ, cementoenamel junction; OE, oral epithelium and OSE, oral sulcular epithelium. (Reproduced from Lindhe J, Karring T and Lang NP, eds. (2005) *Clinical Periodontology and Implant Dentistry*, 4th edn., with permission from Wiley-Blackwell.)

3.6). The attached gingiva will consequently border the tooth and continue into the most marginal part of the pocket epithelium, the sulcular epithelium. This merges with the junctional epithelium that lines the pocket; it is not keratinised and is only a few cell layers thick (Figure 3.7). In young individuals, the junctional epithelium is attached to the enamel through a laminar structure resembling a basement membrane (Furseth et al. 1986a).

The attached gingiva extends from the gingival margin to the mucogingival junction from which it is sharply delineated by a scalloped line on the buccal aspect (Figure 3.8). Lingually, there is no sharp demarcation between gingiva and palatal mucosa. The attached gingiva has a typical stippled appearance in young individuals with a healthy gingiva.

The gingival epithelium covers the lamina propria, which consists of densely packed collagen fibres, vessels and nerves, and a small component of fibroblasts. According to their function, insertion and attachment, the fibres have been classified as: dentogingival fibres; dentoperiosteal and transseptal fibres (which extend from the cementum of one tooth to the cementum of the adjacent tooth); alveologingival fibres and the circular fibres circumscribing the tooth. The periodontal ligament is a continuation of the lamina propria and is dominated by collagen fibres that according to orientation and localisation are distinguished as alveolar crest fibres, horizontal fibres, oblique fibres and apical fibres (Figure 3.9). The total fibre system is subject to deterioration in many of the adult patients who present with loss of both periodontal attachment and teeth. The remaining components of the lamina propria comprise the matrix and the cells, predominantly fibroblasts, and also granulocytes, lymphoid cells and mast cells. The distribution of the cells depends on the health status of the gingiva. The function of the matrix is transportation of water, electrolytes, nutrients and metabolites between the cells.

The periodontal ligament connects the teeth with the alveolar bone and is a continuation of the lamina propria.

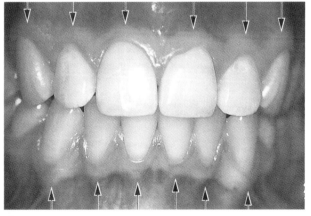

(1)

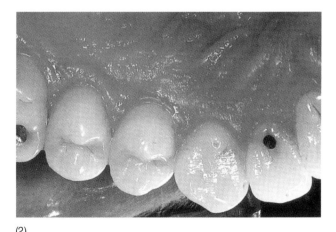

(2)

Fig. 3.8 (1) Buccal and (2) lingual intraoral views of the alveolar epithelium. On the buccal side, there is a sharp delineation between the keratinised and the non-keratinised gingiva. This is not the case on the lingual aspect. (Reproduced from Lindhe J, Karring T and Lang NP, eds. (2005) *Clinical Periodontology and Implant Dentistry*, 4th edn., with permission from Wiley-Blackwell.)

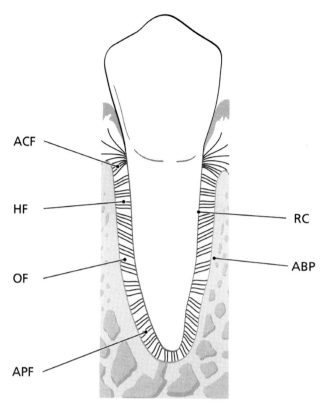

Fig. **3.9** Schematic drawing illustrating how the periodontal ligament is situated between the alveolar bone proper (ABP) and the root centrum (RC). The tooth is joined to the bone by bundles of collagen fibres which can be divided into the following main groups according to their arrangement: ACF, alveolar crest fibres; HF, horizontal fibres; OF, oblique fibres and APF, apical fibres. (Reproduced from Lindhe J, Karring T and Lang NP, eds. (2005) *Clinical Periodontology and Implant Dentistry*, 4th edn., with permission from Wiley-Blackwell.)

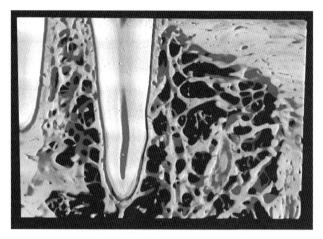

Fig. **3.10** Micro-computed tomography (CT) image illustrating that the width of the periodontal ligament is smallest in the middle of the root, probably corresponding to the centre of resistance of the tooth.

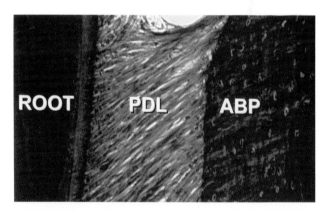

Fig. **3.11** Principal fibres extend from the bone in an apical direction to the cementum of the tooth. The fibres embedded into the cementum have a smaller diameter than the ones embedded into the alveolar wall. PDL, periodontal ligament; ABP, alveolar bone proper. (Reproduced from Lindhe J, Karring T and Lang NP, eds. (2005) *Clinical Periodontology and Implant Dentistry*, 4th edn., with permission from Wiley-Blackwell.)

The thickness of the periodontal ligament varies between 0.2 and 0.4 mm depending on its functional status. Also, within the individual tooth there is a variation, as the thickness of the periodontal ligament is minimum at the point around which the tooth tips when submitted to a force system acting on the crown (Figure 3.10) (Dalstra et al. 2006). The orientation of the collagen fibres in the periodontal ligament varies according to the location of the fibres. The majority are orientated so that they will be stretched when the tooth is loaded with occlusal forces, thereby generating the force system necessary for the maintenance of the alveolar bone (Figure 3.11). The fibres that extend from the cementum do not cross through the periodontal ligament but intertwine with those extending from the alveolar bone proper, making up the lamina dura (Figure 3.12).

The dentine and the cementum covering the root are formed simultaneously as the Hertwig's sheath is gradually fragmented and the ectomesenchymal cells from the dental follicle differentiate into cementoblasts. The first formed cementum is cellular and attached to the dentine via collagen fibres passing from the dentine. When the thickness of the cementum increases, some cementoblasts are incorporated into what will then become cellular cementum. The cementocytes are interconnected like the osteocytes in bone and also serve the same function as the osteocytes. Formation of the cellular cementum takes place during the functional period of the tooth; it undergoes a certain amount of turnover, for which reason it can also contribute to the repair of minor resorptive areas. A sign of the ongoing turnover is the presence of cutting cones (Williams 1984; Mobers 1991). From this cementum, fibres constituting the essential part of the attachment apparatus extend into the periodontal ligament. This extrinsic fibre system is generated by the fibroblasts of the periodontal ligament, while the internal fibre system, consisting of fibres oriented parallel to the long axis of the tooth, is formed by the cementoblasts.

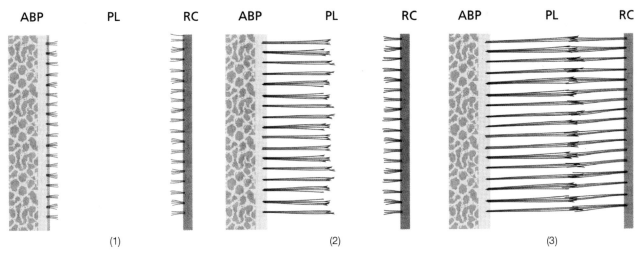

Fig. 3.12 (1)–(3) Drawing illustrating that periodontal fibres do not extend from the cementum to the alveolar wall and vice versa, but become intertwined in the middle of the periodontal ligament (PDL). ABP, alveolar bone proper; RC, root cementum. (Redrawn from Lindhe J, Karring T and Lang NP, eds. (2005) *Clinical Periodontology and Implant Dentistry*, 4th edn., with permission from Wiley-Blackwell.)

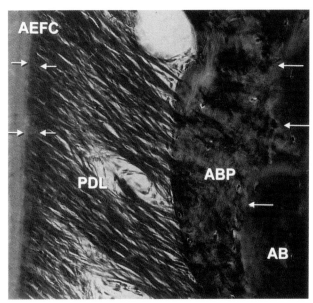

Fig. 3.13 Photomicrograph of a periodontal ligament (PDL) from an area where the root is covered with a cellular extrinsic fibre cementum (AEFC). Arrows indicate fibres inserted into the cementum covering the root and in the alveolar bone proper (ABP) of the other side. The structure of the alveolar bone proper woven bone can be distinguished from the more well-structured alveolar bone (AB) towards the right side of the image. (Reproduced from Lindhe J, Karring T and Lang NP, eds. (2005) *Clinical Periodontology and Implant Dentistry*, 4th edn., with permission from Wiley-Blackwell.)

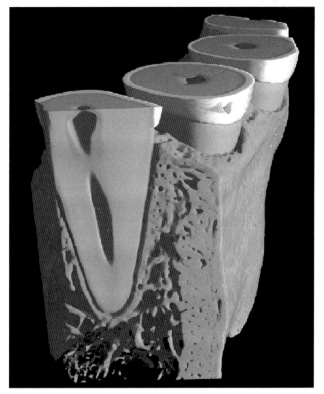

Fig. 3.14 Micro-computed tomography (CT) demonstrating the alveolar bone proper (ABP) as well as the surrounding trabecular bone (T).

Unlike bone, the turnover of cementum is more like a drift, resulting in gradual increase in thickness of the cellular cementum (Figure 3.13).

The alveolar bone is, based on its origin, separated into the alveolar bone proper adjacent to the teeth and the surrounding alveolar bone, which consists of trabecular bone and the cortical bone bordering the lingual and buccal aspects of the alveolar process and continuing as the cortical bone covering the basal parts of the jaws (Figures 3.10 and 3.14). The alveolar bone proper has also been termed lamina dura because of its radiographic appearance. However, three-dimensional images clearly show that the lamina dura

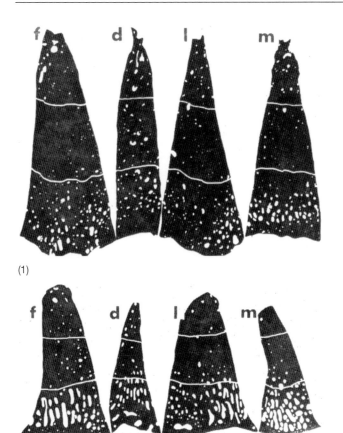

(1)

(2)

Fig. 3.15 (1) Image of an impression of a dry skull showing an alveolus with a normal bone level and (2) one characterised by marginal bone loss. The fenestrations in the alveolar wall are much more pronounced in the impression of the tooth socket with marginal bone loss, most likely due to the inflammation causing the bone loss.

is heavily perforated and that the term 'dura' is a mere projection phenomenon as seen in histological sections (Figures 3.15 and 3.16). The alveolar process including alveolar bone proper and the surrounding trabecular and or cortical bone is entirely dependent on the presence of teeth (Figure 3.17).

The quality and level of the bone reflect the function of the teeth, so that the bone surrounding non-functional teeth will exhibit a reduction in density and develop an inactive osteoporosis. In addition, eruption may occur when no opposing teeth are present (Picton 1964). The marginal bone level is displaced in an apical direction with age (Figure 3.15). The buccal part of the alveolar bone may be very thin and will with increasing age exhibit both fenestrations and dehiscences. Whereas fenestrations may be related to skeletal morphology, dehiscences are frequently pathological in origin.

The periodontium, as the word indicates, surrounds the teeth and constitutes the tissue delivering support to the tooth. In the case of sufficient support, the teeth exhibit only limited mobility and the thickness of the periodontal ligament is maintained within narrow limits (Lindhe et al. 1997). The level of connective tissue attachment into the cementum of the root determines to a large extent the mobility of the tooth. The marginal bone level is highly, although not uniformly, correlated to the level of attachment.

Aetiology of malocclusions in adults

The aetiology of malocclusions presented by adult patients consists of the same genetic and environmental factors as in young patients, but, in addition, the ongoing age-related

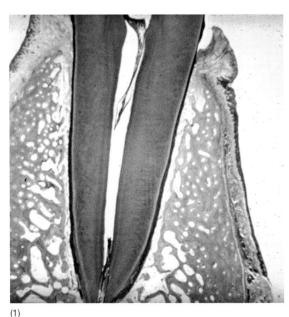

(1)

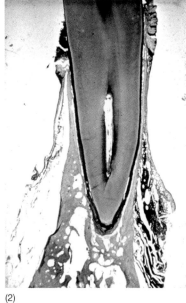

(2)

Fig. 3.16 (1) Buccolingual sections of an incisor from a patient with a brachycephalic skull and (2) from an individual with a dolichocephalic skull. (Courtesy of Birgit Ellegård.)

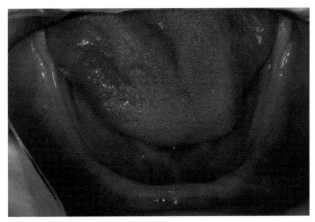

(1)

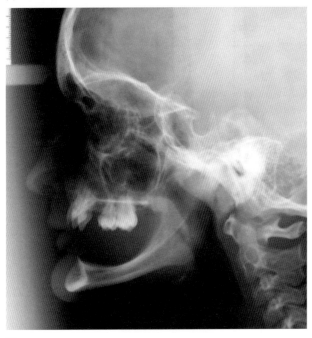

(2)

Fig. 3.17 (1) The dependency of the alveolar process on the presence of teeth is clearly demonstrated in this patient with anodontia. (2) Head film of a patient with total agenesis and, as a consequence, absence of the alveolar processes. (Courtesy of H. Gjoerup.)

degeneration, both general and local, contributes to the development of so-called secondary malocclusions.

Analyses of cephalometric variables on radiographs of skulls from various periods have demonstrated that over the past millennia changes have occurred predominantly in the dentoalveolar area and are related to alterations in lifestyle (Carlson 1976; Carlson and Van Gerven 1977). This was also confirmed by Varrela (1992), who studied the development of the craniofacial structures over the past four centuries, and by Vyslozil et al. (1996), who compared cephalograms of Austrian soldiers killed in the late eighteenth century with those obtained from soldiers a 100 years later. The

differences between the two groups in the latter study were also predominantly dentoalveolar.

Although growth modification in growing individuals is recognised as a legitimate treatment principle, it is generally accepted that the changes achievable in the basal structures are minor and frequently limited to the removal of detrimental environmental influences and dysfunction, thus enhancing the adaptation of the dentoalveolar structures to the existing skeletal basis. In adults, moderate skeletal changes have been generated by the Herbst appliance (Ruf and Pancherz 1999, 2004; Paulsen and Karle 2000; Kitai et al. 2002). It remains to be shown whether the condylar growth demonstrated is later replaced by dentoalveolar modelling.

Whereas the contribution of hereditary and environmental factors to the malocclusions seen in young patients is not yet fully known and remains under intense discussion, it is evident that the secondary malocclusion observed in the older patients is a product of general and local age-related changes.

Age-related changes in the skeleton

The skeleton is in a dynamic state (Frost 1990a, 1990b, 1992), undergoing continuous changes. These changes include both a reduction of the absolute volume of bone as a result of remodelling and change in the outer shape of the bones as a result of modelling. Throughout life, the human skeleton is renewed by a sequence of bone resorption followed by formation (remodelling). Since the rate of resorption is higher than the rate of apposition (formation), the relative extension of resorption surfaces is always lower than that of apposition (formation surfaces) even in a state of balance (Brockstedt et al. 1993; Eriksen et al. 1994). The temporal sequence of resorption and subsequent apposition has been defined as a remodelling cycle (Figure 3.18). As a response to a biochemical or mechanical stimulus, recruitment and activation of osteoclasts will turn a given site into a resorptive area. In cortical bone, a resorption tunnel (also termed a cutting cone) is created and Howship's lacunae are formed by the osteoclasts. On the trabecular bone surfaces, the remodelling sites are called packets (Kragstrup et al. 1982, 1983a, 1983b; Kragstrup and Melsen 1983). The remodelling follows the same pattern at both sites. After the first phase of resorption, the osteoclasts have been described to be substituted by mononuclear resorptive cells that continue the resorption until the predetermined depth has been reached (Eriksen 1993; Eriksen et al. 1994). At this stage there is a reversal and the site is occupied by pre-osteoblasts that differentiate into active osteoblasts, which start the synthesis of osteoid. The osteoid will later mineralise and form an entity of bone called the bone structural unit, the BSU (osteon), also known as the basic multicellular unit (BMU, Figure 3.19; Frost 1983, 1992).

Due to ongoing remodelling, a certain volume of bone is resorbed but not re-formed. This volume of bone is called the

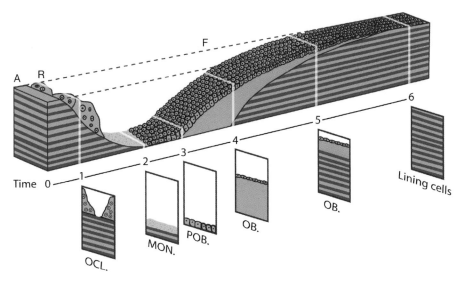

Fig. 3.18 Remodelling cycle starting with an activation (A) followed by a resorption (R), ending with formation (F). OCL: osteoclasts; MON: monocytes; POB: pre-osteoclasts and OB: osteoblast. (Courtesy of E Fink Eriksen.)

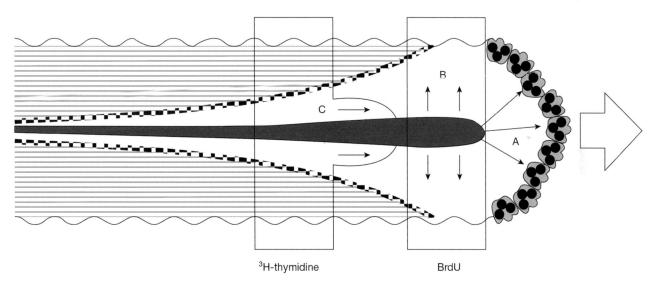

Fig. 3.19 A schematic diagram of a cutting/filling cone illustrating the pattern of distribution of osteoclastic (zone A) and osteogenic (zone B) cells. The proliferating cells were labelled in the DNA synthesis phase twice: (H^3)-thymidine 7 days and bromodeoxyuridine 1 hour before tissue sampling. The cells originallyy labelled with H^3-thymidine have formed osteoblasts and maintained the perivascular proliferative pool of osteogenic cells (zone C). H^3–thymidine-labelled precursors of osteoclasts are seen in the zone marked A. The bromodioxyuracil-labelled osteoblast precursors marked 1 hour before sampling are localised in the zone marked B. The experiment is consistent with a marrow origin for preosteoclasts and demonstrates that osteoblasts are derived from a proliferating population of perivascular connective tissue cells. The bone structural unit of cortical bone (BSU) is the Haversian system with its cutting cone where the resorption occurs. (Courtesy of EW Roberts.)

remodelling space, and is dependent on the frequency of activation of new foci of resorption, the depth of the individual resorption sites and the length of both the resorptive and the formative periods. An increased activation frequency will result in a larger remodelling space, that is, reversible bone loss. This may occur due to changes in hormonal balance because of disease or some medications and may influence the resistance to spontaneous tooth migration.

A small amount of irreversible bone loss may occur as the result of a negative balance in relation to the amount of bone resorbed and later re-formed at each BSU, and if the activation frequency (turnover) is high, bone loss will be accelerated. Permanent loss of trabecular bone may also occur if a resorption lacuna perforates a trabeculum, whereby no surface for subsequent formation is available. Besides a reduction in bone volume, perforations also lead to a distortion of the trabecular architecture, reducing the bone strength dramatically with an increased risk of fractures (Vesterby 1993a, 1993b). The risk of trabecular perforations depends on the activation frequency, depth of the resorption lacunae and the thickness of the trabeculae (Melsen 1978; Mosekilde 1990).

The physiology of remodelling has been discussed by Parfitt (1996). He differentiates between the need for remodelling of cortical and trabecular bones. The cortical bone has previously been assigned mainly load-bearing properties, whereas the trabecular bone has been described as more actively involved in the mineral homeostasis and in the generation of a favourable microenvironment for the haematopoietic system. Nevertheless, since the description of Wolff's law, it has been recognised that both cortical and cancellous bones are organised to facilitate load transfer (Meyer 1867). This also applies to alveolar bone (Verna et al. 1999).

The turnover of the cortical bone has been reported to be lower than that of trabecular bone (Melsen 1978; Kragstrup et al. 1982; Eriksen 1993). This perception has been used within orthodontics when moving roots into cortical bone with the purpose of obtaining 'cortical anchorage' (Ricketts 1976; Urias and Mustafa 2005). The difference in remodelling can, however, to some degree, be explained by the method by which the bone turnover is estimated. Trabecular bone remodelling is usually estimated based on the surface-defined activation frequency and not corrected for the surface to volume ratio. Since this ratio is five times higher for trabecular bone than for cortical bone, the trabecular bone could have high turnover in spite of a low intensity of absolute bone replacement (Foldes et al. 1991). At least three different reasons for the ongoing remodelling have been described:

- To allow the bone to serve as a mineral store (mainly calcium) for the maintenance of a normal calcium homeostasis.
- To allow repair of microfractures and ensure viability of the osteocytes.
- To allow changes in bone architecture in response to changes in mechanical demands.

The highest bone turnover rate is found in the axial cancellous bone and estimated to be 15–35% per year. From a mechanical point of view, this does by far exceed the remodelling necessary for the maintenance of an acceptable mean age of the BSUs. The relative importance of mechanical and metabolic needs for remodelling does clearly vary within the different regions of the skeleton. The high turnover of the axial skeleton has thus been ascribed to its role in calcium homeostasis. However, this was not confirmed by Parfitt (1996), who claimed that there is no evidence that trabecular bone in the appendicular skeleton participates to a significant extent in the metabolic functions of the skeleton – neither in homeostasis nor in haematopoiesis.

Normal calcium homeostasis does not completely depend on the net calcium loss from bone, but also on renal reabsorption, which is under the control of the parathyroid hormone (PTH), and intestinal calcium absorption, which depends on the presence of vitamin D. An equilibrium is obtained when a balance exists between the influx and outflux of calcium at the quiescent bone surfaces. The calcium level is determined by the effect of the PTH on the bone-lining cells. This mechanism depends on the rapid blood flow close to the bone surface. In addition, retention of water in the superficial layer of bone is important for the diffusion of minerals. Only a high rate of remodelling can ensure this. With increasing age, the secondary mineralisation slows down, and due to crystal enlargement, water is displaced, which reduces the capacity of rapid mineral exchange. The hypermineralised surfaces therefore have to be remodelled in order to allow the bone to maintain its role in the calcium homeostasis. The stimulus for this remodelling is however unknown. It has, by contrast, been demonstrated that a drop in the plasma-free calcium level leads to an increase in the secretion of PTH and not only an increased activation frequency but also higher activity among existing osteoclasts.

The second function of remodelling ensures that new bone constantly replaces old bone that would otherwise compromise the functional capacity of the skeleton. The repetitive cyclical loading, which occurs in bone during normal function, for example, chewing, would in the long run result in fatigue damage if the constant renewal of bone did not provide a means by which bone that has undergone microdamage is replaced. The role of the microdamage in relation to orthodontic tooth movement will be discussed later. The targeted remodelling is still not fully elucidated, but it has been suggested that the osteocytes play an important role in the detection of microcracks (Marotti 2000). The osteocytes have been described to transmit changes in strain in the surrounding bone to the nearest bone surface (Parfitt 1996). The type of signal is, however, not fully understood.

The most well-known age-related change occurring in the skeleton is the general bone loss. The rate and magnitude of bone loss vary, but it occurs all over the skeleton. The loss is about 1% a year between 25 and 75 years of age (Parfitt et al. 1983) (Figure 3.20). All bone loss takes place on one of the internal surfaces of bone and the rate depends on both the negative balance at each BSU and on the activation frequency. Cortical thinning seems to be a result of deeper penetration of the cortical BMUs, which may vary between different sites, and although attempts have been made to explain these differences based on differences in local strain, this does not account for all the variation. The general pattern is that there is a negative balance on the endocortical surface and a positive balance on the periosteal surface so that the diameter of the long bones increases with age.

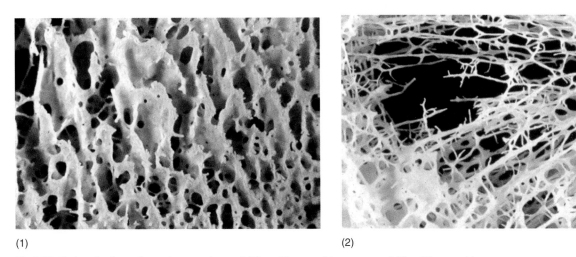

(1)   (2)

Fig. 3.20 Trabecular bone from the vertebrae of (1) an 18-year-old woman and (2) a 60-year-old woman.

When Jeffcoat et al. (1996) discussed the relationship between oral and systemic bone loss, they stressed that several of the same risk factors were present. Kribbs et al. (1983a, 1983b) reported a strong correlation between total bone mass and dental bone mass in women. The same group also found that mandibular bone mass was more closely related to that of the whole skeleton than to age. Habets et al. (1988) studied biopsies from 74 patients with severe mandibular ridge resorption and verified that these patients had osteopenia. But Klemetti and Vainio (1993) failed to establish a correlation between alveolar bone loss and general bone mass. Krall et al. (1994, 1997), who analysed the mineral density at the spine and the radius, found that alveolar bone was significantly correlated to the number of teeth present, but not to the bone of the appendicular skeleton. This was corroborated by Verna et al. (1999), who found that the bone mass in the maxilla and in the mandible was only vaguely correlated to the bone mass of the iliac crest. On the other hand, functional occlusion did have a significant impact on the quality of the alveolar bone.

It can thus be concluded that although the general bone mass has a certain influence, other factors such as mechanical demands play an important role in the maintenance of the quantity and density of the alveolar bone. The development of the alveolar process is completely dependent on the eruption of teeth (Furseth et al. 1986b; Lindhe et al. 1997), but the bone quality is related to the functional demands and also to the morphology of the craniofacial skeleton and the occlusal relationship (Figure 3.16). The influence of the craniofacial morphology on the alveolar bone is not only seen in adults with a functioning dentition but also reflected in the loss of the alveolar process in edentulous patients (Tallgren and Solow 1991). The influence of function on the bone structure of the alveolar process was clearly demonstrated by Picton (1964), who extracted teeth in one quadrant in monkeys and compared the bone density around teeth in occlusion and those without occlusion. In

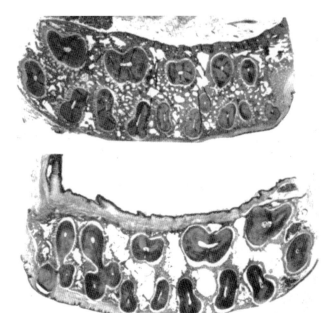

Fig. 3.21 Two horizontal sections of the maxilla. The occluding teeth were extracted and as a consequence the density of the surrounding bone decreased dramatically. (Reproduced from Picton DCA (1969) The effect of external forces on the periodontium. In: Melcher AH and Bowen WH, eds. *Biology of the Periodontium*. London: Academic Press. Reproduced with permission from Elsevier.)

relation to the latter, the bone surrounding teeth without occlusal contacts clearly suffered from inactivity osteoporosis (Figure 3.21).

Whereas the bone mass seems to be under control of local functional demands, the bone turnover in the different sites of the skeleton including the jaws was shown to be significantly correlated (Verna 2002). Therefore, systemic diseases influencing bone metabolism can be expected to influence the alveolar bone as well. The effect of systemic diseases may manifest as a reduction in the resistance to spontaneous tooth migration due to reduced density of the alveolar bone and due to an increased risk of developing periodontal diseases.

The most common disease associated with a rapidly progressing bone loss of the alveolar bone due to an aggressive form of periodontal disease is diabetes mellitus. According to Jeffcoat et al. (1996), a full understanding of the mechanism does not exist, but it seems to be a common finding that individuals with diabetes have an increased risk of periodontal disease and severe alveolar bone loss (Zachariasen 1991; Iacopino 1995; Lalla et al. 1998; Papapanou 1999). The disease seems to be triggered by the presence of hyperglycaemia, which leads to non-enzymatic glycation and oxidation of proteins and lipids, which then result in formation of advanced glycation end products. These may alter the phenotype of the macrophages, which may be responsible for inducing inflammatory tissue destruction including alveolar bone loss.

In relation to systemic diseases, it may not always be the disease itself but the long-term medications that lead to alveolar bone loss. Von Wowern et al. (1992) studied the mineral content in the forearm and in the mandible in patients with acute nephrotic syndrome treated with steroids and found that the degree of osteopenia was correlated in the two sites.

Increased bone turnover related to, for example, hyperthyroidism or secondary hyperparathyroidism will reduce the resistance to spontaneous tooth migration and may as such be a contributing factor to a change in occlusion. The same applies to patients with chronic medication that suppresses the immune system. This may be the case in patients who are prepared for or have had transplants, for example, of the cornea and/or the kidneys. It can be anticipated that the proportion of older patients with metabolic disease or on chronic medications that influence the bone metabolism is increasing (Kalia et al. 2004). Finally, non-pathological events such as pregnancy also influence bone turnover, and it has been documented that progesterone influences the biosynthesis of prostaglandins, leading to inflammation and secondary bone loss. Contraceptives may for the same reason increase the risk. Sweet and Butler (1977) reported a significant higher incidence of osteitis in relation to removal of third molars among women on oral contraception than in a control group. The biggest risk is, however, the increased activation frequency in relation to menopause that will increase the rate of bone loss in a reversible manner as the remodelling space is increased. This may reduce the resistance to spontaneous tooth migration.

Among the medication-induced changes in bone turnover, the influence of bisphosphonates is increasingly focused on (Delmas 2000, 2002). Their role is in the treatment of osteoporosis, as they are known to inhibit protein tyrosine phosphatases, which are necessary elements for osteoclast formation. In addition, the bisphosphonates seem to induce osteoclast apoptosis (Rogers 2004). Research on bisphosphonates initially concentrated on reduced osteoclastic activity and the increased rate of apoptosis of the osteoclasts. It was only recently that the effect on osteoblast activity has been analysed. A histomorphometric study of femurs and tibias from rats treated with bisphosphonates for 17 days clearly demonstrated that the bisphosphonates affect osteoblast activity significantly, not only reducing resorption but also bone formation (Iwata et al. 2006). This may explain the steady increase in case reports of patients presenting with osteonecrosis following treatment with various versions of these drugs (Migliorati et al. 2005; Farrugia et al. 2006; Mortensen et al. 2007). It can be hypothesised that the increased mean age of single trabecula may lead to an increased fracture risk, and as the oral mucosa is thin and frequently submitted to trauma from the oral environment, it may facilitate infection leading to osteonecrosis. The trauma may also be in relation to a dental intervention, an extraction or the insertion of an implant. The increasing number of case reports stresses the severity of the problem and the difficulty in treating these patients. At present, there is no advice apart from treating very conservatively and refraining from any treatment that may lead to exposure of bone.

Age-related changes in the craniofacial skeleton

The occlusion changes with age, but age-related changes in the craniofacial skeleton have also been described. Reich and Dannhauer (1996) analysed more than 10,000 head films and found that with age there was an increase in the prognathism of both jaws along with an anterior rotation of the mandible leading to a decrease in the lower facial height. Based on an anthropometric analysis of Caucasian skulls, Bartlett et al. (1992) concluded that the reduction of facial height and the increased depth of the face were strongly associated with tooth loss. Forward and downward displacement of the hard tissue pogonion, and retroclination of the lower incisors, leading to the development of mandibular dentoalveolar retrognathism was also reported by Driscoll-Gilliland et al. (2001). These authors demonstrated that the age-related changes in the craniofacial skeleton were smaller in cases with Angle's Class I relationship than in cases of either Class II or Class III dental relationships. This corroborated the findings of Harris and Behrents (1988).

Dysfunction can result in excessive wear and abrasion of the dentition contributes to the reduction in anterior face height and a deepening of the bite (Figure 3.22).

Although some of the malocclusions in adult patients reflect changes in the facial skeleton, the majority are a product of tooth migration caused predominantly by local changes in the dentition. General changes in the skeleton can, however, contribute indirectly, as they may have an influence on the quality and quantity of the alveolar bone.

Age-related changes in the local environment

Local age-related changes are a predominant feature in the explanation of the changes in dentition leading to development or aggravation of a malocclusion in adulthood. The decrease in periodontal support is frequently the underlying reason. The apical displacement of the marginal bone level has been described as an age-related change, but there is pronounced variation and the phenomenon is clearly related to the presence and severity of periodontal disease (Beck 1996).

Whereas the 1960s and 1970s were dominated by the view that periodontal disease should be considered a major

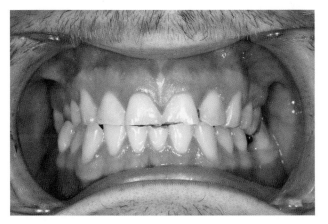

Fig. 3.22 A patient who following extraction of carious posterior teeth developed severe bruxism, leading to a deepening of the bite and reduction in the size of the incisors.

global public health problem (Scherp 1964), recent epidemiological research indicates that periodontal disease seems to be more site-specific than age-related. A small percentage of all individuals within a certain age group seem to account for the majority of sites with major attachment loss (Baelum et al. 1986).

A modest but generalised reduction in the marginal bone level is, however, also seen in patients who do not have periodontal disease. In the early mixed dentition, the cementoenamel junction of the permanent teeth is situated below the marginal bone and is thus not visible. In the young adult, the bone level changes so that there is a physiological gap between the junction and the bone level (Waerhaug and Steen 1952), and with increasing age this gap increases in a variable way (Figure 3.23).

Intra-age variation is mainly determined by four factors

Although there is a relationship between inflammation and attachment loss, the impact of plaque and calculus on the attachment level has still not been clearly elucidated. It has long been known that only a vague, if any, relationship exists between plaque, gingival inflammation and attachment loss in young individuals. In adults, the strength of this relationship increases with age and Shei et al. (1959) demonstrated that marginal bone loss is closely related to gingival inflammation in the adult patient above a certain age. These authors showed that the relation between the gingival and the periodontal status was not correlated in a young adult group, whereas oral hygiene and marginal bone levels were

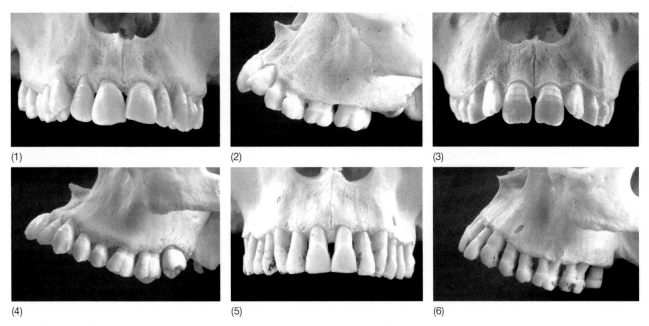

Fig. 3.23 Skull collection demonstrating the increase in the distance between the enamel and the cementum and the marginal bone level. (1) and (2) Mixed dentition. (3) and (4) Young adult. (5) and (6) Older adult with general periodontal disease.

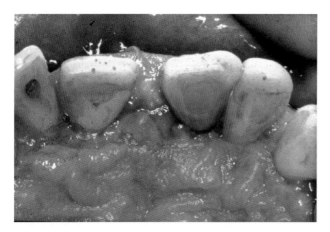

Fig. 3.24 Patient with a marked inflammation lingual to the upper incisors in spite of satisfactory oral hygiene due to impingement of the gingiva related to a deep bite.

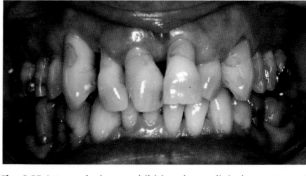

Fig. 3.25 Intraoral views exhibiting long clinical crowns and many gingival fillings. The long clinical crowns were the result of use of an incorrect brushing technique and the fillings were done to fill the defects generated by brushing with a hard toothbrush.

highly correlated above age 25, a correlation that became stronger with increasing age. This was confirmed by Holm-Pedersen et al. (1975), who compared the effect of lack of oral hygiene in a group of young adults (20–25 years old) and a group of mature adults (40–50 years old) and found that both plaque accumulation and inflammation in the gingival crevicular fluid were highly age-dependent. For a more detailed description, see Chapter 11.

With apical displacement of the marginal bone level, the quality of the bone seems to change as the alveolar wall undergoes changes leading to an increasing number of fenestrations. This consequently influences the location of the centre of resistance and thereby the stress/strain distribution in the case of loading, whether from the forces of occlusion or those applied by means of an orthodontic appliance (Birn 1966) (Figure 3.15).

The second factor of importance with regard to the local status of the periodontium is related to the occlusion. Traumatic occlusion may lead to a reduction in the marginal bone and a widening of the periodontal ligament. This will, however, lead to attachment loss only if there is concomitant inflammation (Glickman 1965, 1967; Meitner 1975; Karring et al. 1982). In such cases, the addition of occlusal trauma will cause the attachment loss to progress more rapidly (Macapanpan and Weinmann 1954; Glickman and Smulow 1965).

Trauma to the gingival margin in the form of gingival impingement also sets the stage for more rapid progression of existing periodontal disease. Direct impingement of the gingival margin is not compatible with an inflammation-free periodontium and will lead to the continued destruction of the marginal periodontium in the region (Figure 3.24).

Bruxism and other parafunctions that result in alterations in tooth morphology and crown length may contribute to the development of a secondary malocclusion. The parafunction may be caused by or lead to functional and periodontal problems (Figure 3.22). Lastly, iatrogenic factors may also influence the local environment; for example, trauma generated at the marginal gingiva from an incorrect or aggressive tooth-brushing technique. Patients with severe periodontal problems caused by poor oral hygiene in some areas may exhibit recession of the gingival margin caused by incorrect brushing or the application of too much pressure while brushing (Figure 3.25).

Consequences of deterioration of the dentition

With a reduced periodontium, the centre of resistance of the tooth or group of teeth is displaced apically, due to which the functional forces acting on the crowns of the teeth may generate moments leading to migration of the teeth. The migration of the anterior teeth lead to spacing, increased overjet and a deepening of the bite. Due to the conical form of their roots, even horizontal forces acting on these teeth lead to a combination of sagittal and vertical movements. This may continue to occur as a vicious circle. The deepening of the bite may on its own lead to impingement and gingival trauma. The latter may make the need for treatment evident to the patient. Another consequence of a deepening bite is an increase in crowding of the lower incisors, which secondarily will make maintenance difficult or impossible (Figure 3.26).

Apart from the tooth migration caused by the change in the position of the centre of resistance, another reason for development of secondary malocclusions is the unavoidable extraction of one or more permanent teeth due to caries or its sequelae. The loss of continuity of the dental arch may also lead to migration of the adjacent teeth if no replacement is inserted, and the possible consequence is a collapse of the bite, that is, bite deepening leading to the abovementioned vicious circle. Loss of the posterior teeth will often lead to extrusion of the opposing teeth and tipping and rotation of the adjacent teeth. The patient in Figure 3.27 had the lower

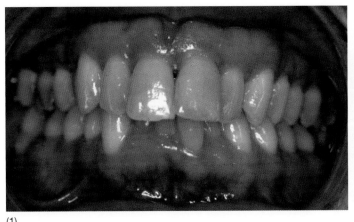

(1)

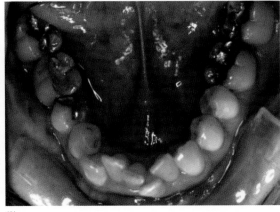

(2)

Fig. 3.26 This patient has had deepening of the bite and increasing crowding in the lower arch. It was now difficult to maintain satisfactory oral hygiene in this region.

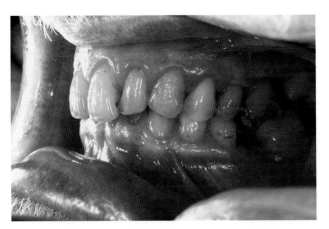

Fig. 3.27 Following the loss of 36, the anterior teeth have tipped distally into the extraction space resulting in a deep bite; 37 has tipped mesially and 26 has supraerupted into the extraction space.

first molar extracted. Subsequently, the upper molar started to erupt and the teeth neighbouring the extraction space tipped into it.

As a secondary effect, extraction, which is not followed by replacement, may lead to a change in function. Loss of the posterior teeth may result in increased activity of the tongue, which potentially can result in the development of anterior spacing. The appearance of spaces between the exposed roots following gingival retraction may likewise lead to a vicious circle in which tongue pressure leads to an increase in the spacing. It is, nevertheless, still common to encounter major, invasive oral rehabilitation treatments that could have been simplified if orthodontics had been involved as part of the treatment (Figure 3.28).

In sum, the orthodontic problems presented by adults are rarely unique, but only one of many symptoms reflecting a more complex problem related to general metabolic changes related to age and/or disease in combination with a degenerating chewing organ. In relation to the treatment

plan, it is therefore of the utmost importance that the aetiology is discussed and factors contributing to the development of the patient's problem are discussed, as well as the necessity for maintenance of the treatment result.

Case reports

To the author's knowledge, there is no published evidence based on comprehensive prospective studies to corroborate the abovementioned development of secondary malocclusions, and hence this rationale is based on retrospective observations. When asked to describe the development of their problem, most patients can demonstrate the influence of the deterioration of the dentition on their face and smile by means of personal photographs taken over the years. Two typical examples are described in the following text.

Aggravation of an existing malocclusion

The patient shown in Figure 1.4 (see Chapter 1) was concerned about a large median diastema. When asked to explain its development, she presented three photographs. The first photograph was taken at the age of 18 when she was finishing high school and clearly demonstrates that she had an increased overjet, which she did not perceive as a malocclusion requiring treatment. The second picture taken 6 years later at the time of her first pregnancy shows the development of a median diastema. This diastema is clearly increased in the third picture taken during the second pregnancy. At the time when the patient requested orthodontic treatment, the diastema had further worsened and the lower crowding was clearly contributing to the increased overjet. Contributing factors to the aggravation of the patient's malocclusion were in this case both the increased bone turnover related to the pregnancy and the initial overjet, which was too large to allow for normal lip closure (see Figure 1.4 in Chapter 1).

The patient in Figure 3.29 showed us her wedding picture, in which she presented, in her perception, an absolutely

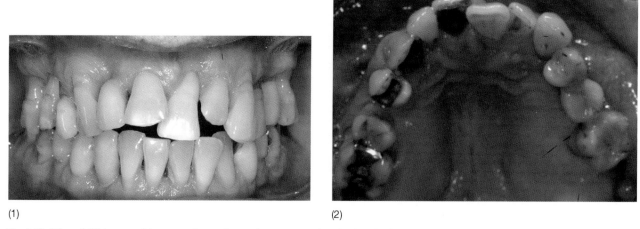

(1) (2)

Fig. 3.28 (1) and (2) Intraoral images of a patient who presented with the chief complaint that the anterior teeth were migrating forward. This had started when the lateral incisor was lost and a bonded bridge was inserted. This treatment would generate a major problem if an orthodontic correction of the progressive malocclusion was attempted.

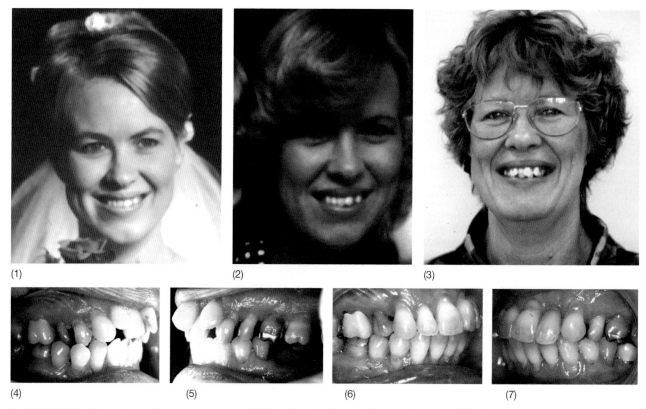

(1) (2) (3)

(4) (5) (6) (7)

Fig. 3.29 (1) Wedding picture of a young woman exhibiting irregularities of the anterior teeth. (2) The irregularity worsened over the years. (3)–(5) Situation following extraction of two lower molars. An anterior open bite had developed. (6) and (7) Following orthodontic treatment and the insertion of an implant to replace 36.

acceptable occlusion. It was characterised by a mild crowding and a small functional open bite. The later photographs demonstrated increased crowding and also the development of an increased overjet and a functional open bite. When she was seen at the orthodontic department, she had lost a few posterior teeth, which may also have contributed to the increase in tongue pressure (Figure 3.29).

Development of secondary malocclusion

The patient in Figure 3.30 was deeply concerned when the orthodontist first saw him. He had observed the deterioration of his dentition, but it was not until he changed dentists that he realised that there might be a solution to his dental problem. His previous dentist had never diagnosed his periodontal problems. When he finally changed dentists and

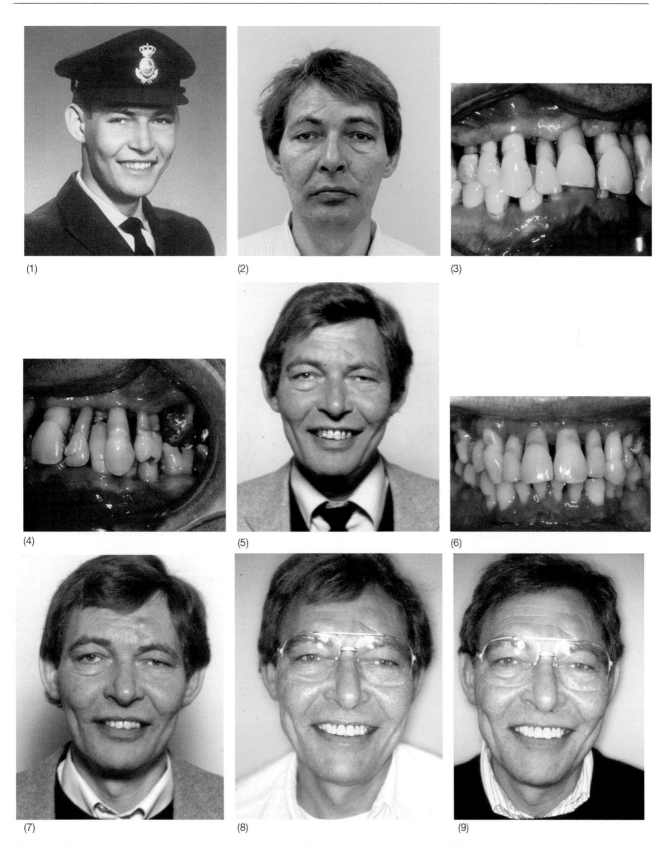

Fig. 3.30 (1) A smiling young man in his air-force uniform. (2) Twenty years later, it was difficult to provoke a smile. (3) and (4) This was understandable, as untreated, progressive periodontal disease had led to the extrusion and migration of all his teeth. (5) and (6) The smile returned when the malocclusion was corrected. (7) and (8) Five years after treatment. (9) Ten years after treatment.

had periodontal surgery, the severity of his marginal bone loss became evident. The patient was at this time no longer able to chew and afraid of occluding his teeth, as they were very mobile. This lead to not only a tension headache but also most likely a reduction in the bone density in the absence of normal occlusal loading (Figure 3.30).

Conclusion

The older adult patient seeking orthodontic treatment most frequently presents with an occlusion that is related to the deterioration, which is now exceeding the acceptable. The malocclusions detected by the patient are concentrated in the front teeth and comprise spacing or crowding often related to changes in the overjet and overbite. Factors of importance for the development or aggravation of the malocclusion are reduction in general and local resistance to spontaneous tooth migration.

References

Baelum V, Fejerskov O and Karring T (1986) Oral hygiene, gingivitis and periodontal breakdown in adult Tanzanians. *J Periodont Res* 21, 221–232.

Bartlett SP, Grossman R and Whitaker LA (1992) Age-related changes of the craniofacial skeleton: an anthropometric and histologic analysis. *Plast Reconstr Surg* 90, 592–600.

Beck JD (1996) Periodontal implications: older adults. *Ann Periodontol* 1, 322–357.

Birn H (1966) The vascular supply of the periodontal membrane. An investigation of the number and size of perforations in the alveolar wall. *J Periodont Res* 1, 51–68.

Brockstedt H, Kassem M, Eriksen EF, Mosekilde L and Melsen F (1993) Age- and sex-related changes in iliac cortical bone mass and remodeling. *Bone* 14, 681–691.

Carlson DS (1976) Temporal variation in prehistoric Nubian crania. *Am J Phys Anthropol* 45, 467–484.

Carlson DS and Van Gerven DP (1977) Masticatory function and post-Pleistocene evolution in Nubia. *Am J Phys Anthropol* 46, 495–506.

Dalstra M, Cattaneo PM and Beckmann F (2006) Synchrotron radiation-based micro-tomography of alveolar support tissues. *Orthod Craniofac Res* 9, 199–205.

Delmas PD (2000) How does antiresorptive therapy decrease the risk of fracture in women with osteoporosis? *Bone* 27, 1–3.

Delmas PD (2002) Treatment of postmenopausal osteoporosis. *Lancet* 359, 2018–2026.

Driscoll-Gilliland J, Buschang PH and Behrents RG (2001) An evaluation of growth and stability in untreated and treated subjects. *Am J Orthod Dentofacial Orthop* 120, 588–597.

Eriksen EF (1993) Assessment of erosion depth by lamellar counting. *Bone* 14, 443–447.

Eriksen EF, Axelrod DW and Melsen F (1994) *Bone Histomorphometry*. New York, NY: Raven Press, Ltd.

Farrugia MC, Summerlin DJ, Krowiak E, Huntley T, Freeman S, Borrowdale R and Tomich C (2006) Osteonecrosis of the mandible or maxilla associated with the use of new generation bisphosphonates. *Laryngoscope* 116, 115–120.

Foldes J, Parfitt AM, Shih MS, Rao DS and Kleerekoper M (1991) Structural and geometric changes in iliac bone: relationship to normal aging and osteoporosis. *J Bone Miner Res* 6, 759–766.

Frost HM (1983) Bone histomorphometry: choice of marking agent and labeling schedule. In Recker RR (ed.) *Bone Histomorphometry: Techniques and Interpretation*, pp. 37–52. Boca Raton, FL: CRC Press.

Frost HM (1990a) Skeletal structural adaptations to mechanical usage (SATMU): 1. Redefining Wolff's law: the bone modeling problem. *Anat Rec* 226, 403–413.

Frost HM (1990b) Skeletal structural adaptations to mechanical usage (SATMU): 2. Redefining Wolff's law: the remodeling problem. *Anat Rec* 226, 414–422.

Frost HM (1992) Perspectives: bone's mechanical usage windows. *Bone Miner* 19, 257–271.

Furseth R, Selvig KA and Mjör IA (1986a) The periodontium. In Mjör IA and Fejerskov O (eds) *Human Oral Embryology and Histology*, 1st edn, pp. 131–175. Copenhagen: Munksgaard.

Furseth R, Selvig KA and Mjör IA (1986b) The periodontium. In Mjör IA and Fejerskov O (eds) *Human Oral Embryology and Histology*, 1st edn, pp. 131–175. Copenhagen: Munksgaard.

Glickman I (1965) Clinical significance of trauma from occlusion. *J Am Dent Assoc* 70, 607–618.

Glickman I (1967) Occlusion and the periodontium. *J Dent Res* 46, 53–59.

Glickman I and Smulow JB (1965) Effect of excenssive occlusal forces upon the pathway of gingival inflammation in humans. *J Periodontol* 36, 141–147.

Habets LL, Bras J and van Merkesteyn JP (1988) Mandibular atrophy and metabolic bone loss. Histomorphometry of iliac crest biopsies in 74 patients. *Int J Oral Maxillofac Surg* 17, 325–329.

Hammarstrom L, Alatli I and Fong CD (1996) Origins of cementum. *Oral Dis* 2, 63–69.

Harris EF and Behrents RG (1988) The intrinsic stability of Class I molar relationship: a longitudinal study of untreated cases. *Am J Orthod Dentofacial Orthop* 94, 63–67.

Holm-Pedersen P, Agerbaek N and Theilade E (1975) Experimental gingivitis in young and elderly individuals. *J Clin Periodontol* 2, 14–24.

Iacopino AM (1995) Diabetic periodontitis: possible lipid-induced defect in tissue repair through alteration of macrophage phenotype and function. *Oral Dis* 1, 214–229.

Iwata K, Li J, Follet H, Phipps RJ and Burr DB (2006) Bisphosphonates suppress periosteal osteoblast activity independently of resorption in rat femur and tibia. *Bone* 39, 1053–1058.

Jeffcoat MK, Reddy MS and DeCarlo AA (1996) Oral bone loss and systemic ostepenia. In Marcus R, Zfeldman D and Kelsey J (eds) *Osteoporosis*, pp. 969–990. San Diego: Academic Press, Inc.

Kalia S, Melsen B and Verna C (2004) Tissue reaction to orthodontic tooth movement in acute and chronic corticosteroid treatment. *Orthod Craniofac Res* 7, 26–34.

Karring T, Nyman S, Thilander B and Magnusson I (1982) Bone regeneration in orthodontically produced alveolar bone dehiscences. *J Periodontal Res* 17, 309–315.

Kitai N, Kreiborg S, Bakke M, Paulsen HU, Moller E, Darvann TA, Pedersen H and Takada K (2002) Three-dimensional magnetic resonance image of the mandible and masticatory muscles in a case of juvenile chronic arthritis treated with the Herbst appliance. *Angle Orthod* 72, 81–87.

Klemetti E and Vainio P (1993) Effect of bone mineral density in skeleton and mandible on extraction of teeth and clinical alveolar height. *J Prosthet Dent* 70, 21–25.

Kragstrup J, Gundersen HJ, Melsen F and Mosekilde L (1982) Estimation of the three-dimensional wall thickness of completed remodeling sites in iliac trabecular bone. *Metab Bone Dis Relat Res* 4, 113–119.

Kragstrup J and Melsen F (1983) Three-dimensional morphology of trabecular bone osteons reconstructed from serial sections. *Metab Bone Dis Relat Res* 5, 127–130.

Kragstrup J, Melsen F and Mosekilde L (1983a) Thickness of bone formed at remodeling sites in normal human iliac trabecular bone: variations with age and sex. *Metab Bone Dis Relat Res* 5, 17–21.

Kragstrup J, Melsen F and Mosekilde L (1983b) Thickness of lamellae in normal human iliac trabecular bone. *Metab Bone Dis Relat Res* 4, 291–295.

Krall EA, Wson-Hughes B, Hannan MT, Wilson PW and Kiel DP (1997) Postmenopausal estrogen replacement and tooth retention. *Am J Med* 102, 536–542.

Krall EA, Wson-Hughes B, Papas A and Garcia RI (1994) Tooth loss and skeletal bone density in healthy postmenopausal women. *Osteoporosis Int* 4, 104–109.

Kribbs PJ, Smith DE and Chesnut CH III (1983a) Oral findings in osteoporosis. Part I: measurement of mandibular bone density. *J Prosthet Dent* 50, 576–579.

Kribbs PJ, Smith DE and Chesnut CH III (1983b) Oral findings in osteoporosis. Part II: relationship between residual ridge and alveolar bone resorption and generalized skeletal osteopenia. *J Prosthet Dent* 50, 719–724.

Kristerson L and Andreasen JO (1984) Autotransplantation and replantation of tooth germs in monkeys. Effect of damage to the dental follicle and position of transplant in the alveolus. *Int J Oral Surg* 13, 324–333.

Lalla E, Lamster IB, Feit M, Huang L and Schmidt AM (1998) A murine model of accelerated periodontal disease in diabetes. *J Periodontal Res* 33, 387–399.

Lindhe J, Karring T and Araújo M (1997) Anatomy of the periodontium. In Lindhe J, Karring T and Lang NP (eds) *Clinical Periodontology and Implant Dentistry*, 4th edn, pp. 3–49. Munksgaard: Blackwell.

Macapanpan LC and Weinmann JP (1954) The influence of injury to the periodontal membrane on the spread of gingival inflammation. *J Dent Res* 33, 263–272.

Marks MH and Corn H (1989) *Atlas of Adult Orthodontics. Functional and Esthetic Enhancement*. Philadelphia, PA: ea and Febiger.

Marotti G (2000) The osteocyte as a wiring transmission system. *J Musculoskel Neuron Interact* 1, 133–136.

Meitner S (1975) Co-destructive factors of marginal periodontitis and repetitive mechanical injury. *J Dent Res* 54 Spec no C, C78–C85.

Melsen F (1978) *Histomorphometric Analysis of Iliac Bone in Normal and Pathological Conditions*. Denmark: Aarhus University.

Meyer GH (1867) Architectur der spongiosa. *Arch Anat Physiol Wissensch* 34, 615–628.

Migliorati CA, Casiglia J, Epstein J, Jacobsen PL, Siegel MA and Woo SB (2005) Managing the care of patients with bisphosphonate-associated osteonecrosis: an American Academy of Oral Medicine position paper. *J Am Dent Assoc* 136, 1658–1668.

Mobers S (1991) *Annual Variation in Root Resorption of Deer Teeth*. Aarhus: University of Aarhus.

Mortensen M, Lawson W and Montazem A (2007) Osteonecrosis of the jaw associated with bisphosphonate use: presentation of seven cases and literature review. *Laryngoscope* 117, 30–34.

Mosekilde L (1990) Consequences of the remodelling process for vertebral trabecular bone structure: a scanning electron microscopy study (uncoupling of unloaded structures). *Bone Miner* 10, 13–35.

Palmer RM and Lumsden AG (1987) Development of periodontal ligament and alveolar bone in homografted recombinations of enamel organs and papillary, pulpal and follicular mesenchyme in the mouse. *Arch Oral Biol* 32, 281–289.

Papapanou PN (1999) Epidemiology of periodontal diseases: an update. *J Int Acad Periodontol* 1, 110–116.

Parfitt AM (1996) Skeletal heterogeneity and the purposes of bone remodeling: implications for the understanding of osteoporosis. In Marcus R, Zfeldman D and Kelsey J (eds) *Osteoporosis*, pp. 315–329. San Diego: Academic Press, Inc.

Parfitt AM, Mathews CH, Villanueva AR, Kleerekoper M, Frame B and Rao DS (1983) Relationships between surface, volume, and thickness of iliac trabecular bone in aging and in osteoporosis. Implications for the microanatomic and cellular mechanisms of bone loss. *J Clin Invest* 72, 1396–1409.

Paulsen HU and Karle A (2000) Computer tomographic and radiographic changes in the temporomandibular joints of two young adults with occlusal asymmetry, treated with the Herbst appliance. *Eur J Orthod* 22, 649–656.

Picton DC (1964) The effect of repeated thrusts on normal axial tooth morbility. *Arch Oral Biol* 16, 55–64.

Reich U and Dannhauer KH (1996) Craniofacial morphology of orthodontically untreated patients living in Saxony, Germany. *J Orofac Orthop* 57, 246–258.

Ricketts RM (1976) Bioprogressive therapy as an answer to orthodontic needs. Part II. *Am J Orthod* 70, 359–397.

Rogers MJ (2004) From molds and macrophages to mevalonate: a decade of progress in understanding the molecular mode of action of bisphosphonates. *Calcif Tissue Int* 75, 451–461.

Ruf S and Pancherz H (1999) Dentoskeletal effects and facial profile changes in young adults treated with the Herbst appliance. *Angle Orthod* 69, 239–246.

Ruf S and Pancherz H (2004) Orthognathic surgery and dentofacial orthopedics in adult Class II Division 1 treatment: mandibular sagittal split osteotomy versus Herbst appliance. *Am J Orthod Dentofacial Orthop* 126, 140–152.

Scherp HW (1964) Current concepts in periodontal diseases research: epidemiological contributions. *J Am Dent Assoc* 68, 667–675.

Shei O, Waerhaug J, Lovdal A and Arnulf A (1959) A alveolar bone loss as related to oral hygeine and age. *J Periodontol* 26, 7–16.

Sweet JB and Butler DP (1977) Increased incidence of postoperative localized osteitis in mandibular third molar surgery associated with patients using oral contraceptives. *Am J Obstet Gynecol* 127, 518–519.

Tallgren A and Solow B (1991) Age differences in adult dentoalveolar heights. *Eur J Orthod* 13, 149–156.

Urias D and Mustafa FI (2005) Anchorage control in bioprogressive vs straight-wire treatment. *Angle Orthod* 75, 987–992.

Varrela J (1992) Dimensional variation of craniofacial structures in relation to changing masticatory-functional demands. *Eur J Orthod* 14, 31–36.

Verna C (2002) *Root Resorption Curing Orthodontic Tooth Movement under Different Metabolic Conditions in Rats*. Aarhus: University of Aarhus.

Verna C, Melsen B and Melsen F (1999) Differences in static cortical bone remodeling parameters in human mandible and iliac crest. *Bone* 25, 577–583.

Vesterby A (1993a) Marrow space star volume can reveal change of trabecular connectivity. *Bone* 14, 193–197.

Vesterby A (1993b) Star volume in bone research. A histomorphometric analysis of trabecular bone structure using vertical sections. *Anat Rec* 235, 325–334.

von Wowern N, Klausen B and Olgaard K (1992) Steroid-induced mandibular bone loss in relation to marginal periodontal changes. *J Clin Periodontol* 19, 182–186.

Vyslozil O, Jonke E and Kritscher H (1996) Akzeleration und Zahnengstand. Eine kieferorthopädisch-anthropometrische Vergleichsuntersuchung – Anhang: Die Bedeutung von Augustin Weisbach für die Anthropologie Österreichs. *Österreiche Dentisten-Zeitung* 97/A, 169–217.

Waerhaug J and Steen E (1952) The presence or absence of bacteria in gingival pockets and the reaction in healthy pockets to certain pure cultures; a bacteriological and histological investigation. *Odontologisk Tidskrift* 60, 1–24.

Williams S (1984) A histomorphometric study of orthodontically induced root resorption. *Eur J Orthod* 6, 35–47.

Zachariasen RD (1991) Diabetes mellitus and periodontal disease. Compendium 12;324, 326–328.

4

Interdisciplinary versus Multidisciplinary Treatments

Birte Melsen

Interdisciplinary or multidisciplinary treatments

When treating an adult patient, orthodontics will, in the majority of cases, be only part of the patient's need for dental treatment. A few decades ago, it was more the rule than the exception that at the end of life people had none or very few remaining natural teeth, with or without removable dentures, depending on the society they lived in. However, during the past 10 years, it has become increasingly more unacceptable to wear a removable denture in the so-called First World (Wostmann et al. 2005). As a consequence of the reduction in caries and the treatment of periodontal disease, an increasing number of elderly people still have several natural teeth (DeBiase and Austin 2003; Pyle and Stoller 2003). This has resulted in an increase in the potential population seeking solutions for a secondary malocclusion. As noted in previous chapters, a secondary malocclusion may develop as a consequence of age-related changes in general resistance, or in the local environment, due to wear, loss of one or more teeth or periodontal disease. With the changes in the constraints, spontaneous tooth migration may take place and lead to the development of secondary malocclusions. These cannot be treated as isolated phenomena and orthodontics will be but one component in the re-establishment of an aesthetically and functionally satisfactory dentition. This can only be achieved by collaborative working of several disciplines.

Recent developments within periodontal and conservative dentistry have led to a redefinition of the treatment goal. Within periodontology, the treatment goal is no longer limited to arrest of the destructive process but to re-establish lost periodontium through the principle of guided regeneration and/or application of growth factors (Venezia et al. 2004). The use of guided tissue regeneration (GTR), which also serves as a barrier ensuring new bone formation adjacent to implants (Pretorius et al. 2005), and the application of biochemical compounds with osteogenic potential have impacted on the possible treatment strategies for degenerating dentitions (Terranova and Wikesjo 1987; Hammarstrom 1997; Gestrelius et al. 2000; King 2001). Within prosthodontics, lost teeth that were usually replaced by dentures or bridges are nowadays more frequently being replaced by intraosseous implants. In the presence of a malocclusion, orthodontics is a necessary component of the total treatment, which involves collaboration between different specialities. The approach to the treatment may be multidisciplinary or interdisciplinary.

Many of the references retrieved from PubMed by using the keyword 'multidisciplinary' do not differ from those retrieved by using the keyword 'interdisciplinary'. In October 2011, 132 references fulfilled the search for 'adult orthodontics and interdisciplinary', whereas 184 references were displayed when the search was done on 'adult orthodontics and multidisciplinary'. There was, however, no significant difference in the content. Of the papers with the keyword interdisciplinary, 89 were case reports, as were 124 of the references with the keyword multidisciplinary. No randomised clinical trials were published and the (Spear et al. 1997; Willems et al. 1999) 28 review papers found with the keyword multidisciplinary focused on special considerations in dental rehabilitation (Vanarsdall 1989; Diedrich 1996; Shroff et al. 1996; Margolis 1997). Several papers appeared under both searches (Meistrell 1988; Celenza and Mantzikos 1996; Roberts 1997; Narcisi and DiPerna 1999; Willems et al. 1999).

No attention seems to have been specifically paid to differentiating between the words interdisciplinary and multidisciplinary. There is, however, a significant difference in the meaning of the words. The word multidisciplinary indicates solely that more than one discipline is involved – the act to be performed is composed of several different branches of learning. The word interdisciplinary, on the other hand, indicates an interaction between the involved disciplines, an interaction which is required both in the planning phase and during treatment. Interdisciplinarity requires a team which is highly interactive. Whereas the ability of the involved colleagues to treat is limited to one area, interdisciplinarity requires a high level of information, not only within one's own speciality but also about the state of the art of all the involved disciplines. Important issues here are clear agreement about the distribution of responsibilities and shared knowledge of the patient's expectations.

In the case of failed or no interaction, each of the involved colleagues will see the problem from their own angle only and may not have a full understanding of the different disciplines involved. The result of multidisciplinary treatment can therefore never be better than the sum of the contribution of each of the colleagues. A lack of insight in the total treatment may lead to an inappropriate sequence of treatment events or even prevent delivery of the optimal treatment. For example, the chosen site for an implant may be inconvenient from the orthodontic point of view, as the occlusion following the orthodontic treatment was not foreseen (Figure 4.1). Likewise, teeth that are required to be extracted as part of the orthodontic treatment might be submitted to endodontic or prosthetic treatment (Figure 4.2).

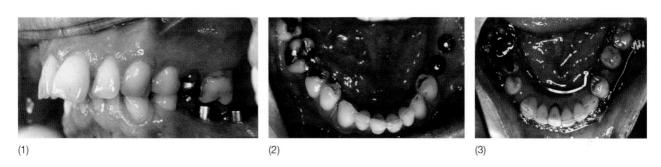

(1) (2) (3)

Fig. 4.1 (1) and (2) This patient had two implants placed before referral for orthodontics. (3) Following the correction of the arch form, it can be seen that the placement of the implants interfered with the optimal orthodontic treatment, as the implants were either too far distal for space closure or too far mesial for a reasonable replacement option distal to the canines.

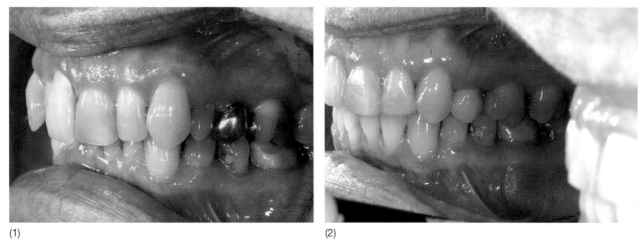

(1) (2)

Fig. 4.2 (1) This patient had an incisor and a premolar crown made shortly before a referral for orthodontic treatment. (2) The crowned premolar was extracted to allow correction of the increased overjet, and the crowned incisor was extruded and the crown then needed to be replaced.

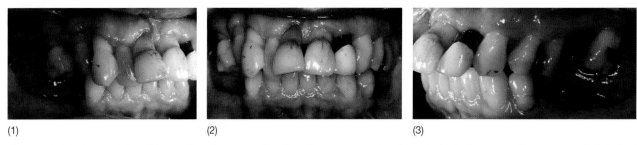

(1)   (2)   (3)

Fig. 4.3 (1)–(3) The dentition did not allow for conventional anchorage, so a wire through the infrazygomatic crest provided skeletal anchorage against which the anterior teeth were retracted. (See also Chapter 8.)

During an interdisciplinary interaction, it will not only become clear how each discipline can contribute to the solution of a problem, but also expand the capacity of each discipline and thereby often make the impossible possible. Figure 4.3 illustrates this situation. A partially edentulous patient was referred to the orthodontic department, as her incisors were drifting more and more forward. She had undergone periodontal treatment and had at the time of referral a healthy periodontium and no pathological pockets. The remaining teeth had, however, much reduced periodontal support and when the periodontist suggested retraction and intrusion of the upper anterior teeth, the first question from the orthodontist was: 'Against what? Which teeth can be used as anchorage?' There were none.

The extremely weak molars tipped forward within a week when loaded with a force of 50 cN. The periodontist, on the other hand, was not discouraged. She pointed to the zygomatic arch and asked: 'Can we find anchorage in that region? Why not try?' A surgical wire was inserted into a small hole made through the zygomatic arch. The wires were loaded immediately and served as anchorage for the retraction and intrusion of the incisors. Fourteen more patients were treated in the same way. There were, however, several inherent drawbacks in the method: only a very limited range of force direction could be obtained (Melsen et al. 1998), and the insertion procedure was a surgical intervention which required particular skills. Therefore, this method was replaced with the use of a mini-implant that could be easily inserted (Costa et al. 1998). The mini-implants could be used in other areas of the mouth too and soon a number of intraosseous anchorage systems saw the light (Melsen 2004, 2005; Melsen and Verna 2005). If the periodontist had not asked the orthodontist to perform the impossible, skeletal anchorage would not have been developed at that time.

Another example of how the interaction between the periodontist and the orthodontist can be of benefit for the patient is that the tissue reaction generated by the orthodontist in relation to tooth movement can be utilised by the periodontist in the generation of new attachment. This topic will be discussed in detail in Chapter 11 (Melsen and Agerbaek 1994).

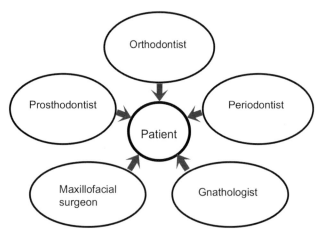

Fig. 4.4 The disciplines frequently involved in the treatment of adult patients.

Establishment of an interdisciplinary team

The establishment of an interdisciplinary approach requires not only close communication between colleagues but also mutual respect and confidence. Usually the team includes a periodontist, a prosthodontist and an orthodontist, which may be assisted by a gnathologist and a maxillofacial surgeon. In relation to the diagnosis, a radiologist may be needed and if parafunctions or muscular tensions cannot be managed satisfactorily, a physiotherapist may be needed (Figure 4.4). In addition, the collaboration of medical specialities may be needed.

The collaboration starts when the problems are listed. The patient's chief complaint will often be of an aesthetic nature. This fact, however, does not exclude the need in any adult patient for drawing up a comprehensive problem list.

The problem list is developed by dentists from the different disciplines involved and includes, in addition to the orthodontic findings, necessary features from the patient's general physical and psychological health profile, findings related to function, the periodontium and the dental status. The materials used for the interdisciplinary discussion comprise the results of the clinical examination, analysis of photographs and X-rays and if relevant the

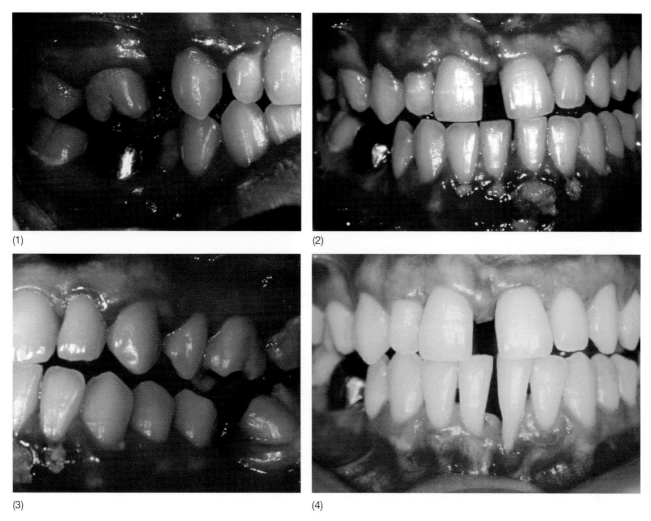

(1)

(2)

(3)

(4)

Fig. 4.5 (1)–(3) Patient with a median diastema (see also Chapter 13). The oral status and dental hygiene led the dentist to reject even any thought of orthodontics. (4) Following professional cleansing and instructions, the patient, however, learnt to maintain meticulous hygiene and eventually had the desired orthodontic, periodontal and prosthodontic treatment. Patient treated by F. Milano.

results of other special investigations such as the bite force, jaw tracking and electromyography (EMG). It is during the workup of the treatment goal that mutual inspiration between team members may allow the limits for the possible to be shifted.

Dentists are frequently prejudiced when judging a new patient. This attitude may influence the suggested treatment plan. The first look, however, may give an erroneous impression of the patient as illustrated in the following example (Figure 4.5): A young patient presented with a wish of having a median diastema closed. Looking at the patient, the first thought may be: 'How did the patient get the idea of an orthodontic treatment?' Massive calculus deposits were present in the lower jaw and a clinician's initial impression might be that the patient had no wish or ability to maintain the oral hygiene levels necessary for major dental treatment. Photographs were obtained, and following cleansing and scaling, the patient was given thorough instructions in the

tooth-brushing technique he was required to follow for maintaining satisfactory oral hygiene.

It was explained to the patient that the tooth-brushing programme, which varies from individual to individual, was his own responsibility and that probably nobody ever explained to him how it should be done. The reaction to the instruction was excellent.

Based on an examination of the study casts, it was explained to the patient that closure of the diastema would not be a simple affair, which could be done in isolation, but that space would need to be created for a premolar in the region of 14. The crowding in the lower jaw needed to be resolved with space closure in the area where a lower molar had been extracted. A precondition for initiating the treatment, however, would be maintenance of good oral hygiene. For a detailed description of this treatment, see Chapter 11.

Following the workup of the problem list and devising the tentative treatment plan, all the different aspects of the

Table 4.1 Chief complaint: diastema between the upper anterior teeth (Figure 4.5).

Problem	Solution
Extraoral	
Function:	
Simple tongue pressure	Close the diastema and replace the missing teeth
Intraoral	
Massive amount of calculus in the lower incisor region	Professional cleansing
Periodontal recession: 31, 32 and 41 buccally	Free graft in the lower incisor region
Reduced keratinised gingiva: 31, 33, 41 and 44	
Missing teeth: 18, 15, 14, 25, 28, 36 and 38	Upper jaw: Closure of the medial diastema and opening of space for a bridge to replace 14
Major restoration: 46	
Occlusion; lateral open bite	
Overbite: 0 mm	LJ: correction of crowding in right side, closure of space for 35
Crossbite: 26/37	
Space: upper jaw crowding (right), diastema Front: lower jaw crowding (right), spacing (left)	Correction of arch form to correct crossbite
	Correction of positional and occlusal deviation, carry out a visual treatment objective (VTO)

Prognosis: depends on the periodontal health.

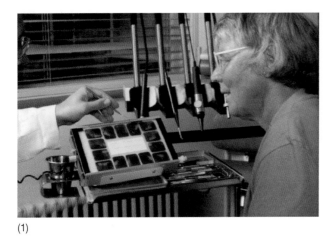
(1)

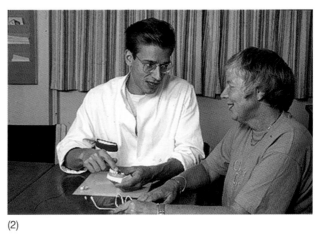
(2)

Fig. 4.6 One person, a doctor or a dental hygienist, can, with the help of (1) radiographs and (2) a model, explain to the patient the treatment alternatives, the time frame and the costs related to the different alternatives, as well as the consequences of no treatment.

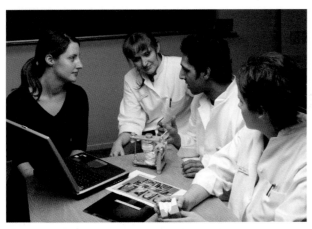

Fig. 4.7 Group of colleagues talking to a patient. This might be overwhelming and having one person communicate the treatment alternatives to the patient is often preferred.

problem list have to be explained carefully to the patient. As in the above-mentioned case, the patient should be aware of the interrelationships between the problems and how different signs or symptoms may reflect the same underlying problem. It should further be mentioned which of the listed problems may be left untreated or just had to be accepted as they could not be treated. Table 4.1 shows an example of a problem list and the suggested solutions.

One team member is chosen to explain the problem list to the patient and ensure that the patient feels comfortable with the treatment choice (Figures 4.6 and 4.7). When alternative treatment plans are presented, the patient should be informed of the advantages and the disadvantages of each individual treatment plan. Maintenance or extraction of teeth with a dubious prognosis, simple or more complex orthodontic treatment, and more or less extensive prosthodontics may be among the alternatives. A lack of the necessary information or contradictory information will have a negative impact on the patient's attitude to the treatment. The roles and the responsibility of the team members in this collaboration should at this point be clearly defined.

The digital records may be given to the patient so that they have an opportunity to discuss their problem with family and friends before making the sometimes rather difficult decision from among the different solutions offered to them. The amount of information provided can never be too much. A patient must be kept fully informed before, during and after treatment.

Treatment sequence

Once the patient has accepted a treatment plan, the choice should be communicated to the participating team and a tentative time schedule worked out and added to the patient's file. Where all the team members are not geographically located in the same dental office, a short but comprehensive summary of the problem list and the treatment goal decided on should be made available to all the team members. Transfer of data and information over the Internet now often replace face-to-face meetings, but remember that being acquainted with one's colleagues, sharing of information and mutual respect are the preconditions for the success of the professional interaction.

Depending on the degree of deterioration of the dentition and the age of the patient, the orthodontic treatment is preceded by different types of dental care. It is crucial for the orthodontic treatment that the biological environment is healthy, which is why periodontal treatment varying from careful monitoring of hygiene to more complicated periodontal surgery attempting to generate new attachment is always necessary. The orthodontic treatment will frequently be followed by restorative work ranging from adjustment of a single occlusal surface to major occlusal rehabilitation.

Essential and optional treatment procedures

Essential treatment

The procedures involved when treating adult patients with a deteriorating dentition can be divided into two categories: essential and optional procedures (Box 4.1). The pre-decided sequence of procedures must be followed, since the next step can only be followed if the previous one was successful.

Since a healthy periodontium is essential, the first part of every treatment should be professional cleansing and scaling, oral hygiene instruction and motivation. The last is most important during treatment and for the maintenance of the result following orthodontic treatment (Figure 4.8).

No periodontal surgery should be carried out if the oral hygiene is not absolutely perfect. Periodontal surgery may result in iatrogenic damage if it is not followed by maintenance of good oral hygiene. There should not be any attempt to influence the mandibular position with a splint before the essential procedures are carried out. The final treatment depends on the effect of the oral prophylaxis. A healthy periodontium is important and active pathological

---

Box 4.1   Overview of essential and optional procedures

Essential procedures:
- Oral prophylaxis
- Restorative treatment
- Endodontics
- Extractions
- Provisional restorations

Optional procedures:
- Periodontal surgery
- Gnathological splint
- Implants
- Orthodontic therapy: major/minor
- Implants
- Prosthetic rehabilitation
- Implants
- Orthognathic surgery

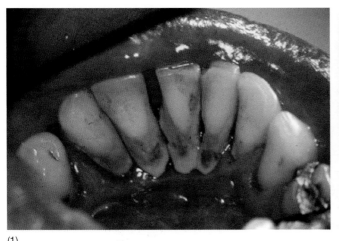 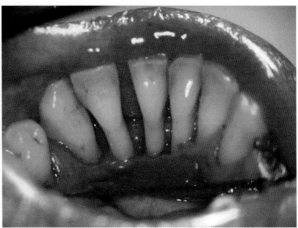

(1)   (2)

Fig. 4.8 A patient desiring orthodontic treatment as he had observed an increase in the spacing in his lower teeth. (1) The pre-treatment situation. (2) Situation following treatment with a dental hygienist.

processes such as caries and endodontic problems should be all treated before orthodontics is commenced. However, it is important not to perform any permanent occlusal restorations at this stage, as the occlusal relationship will most likely change because of the orthodontic treatment.

Extraction of teeth should only be done if the oral hygiene is such that we can anticipate that space closure can be achieved without any iatrogenic damage and that the teeth to be extracted cannot serve as temporary anchorage (see Chapter 8). Major orthodontic work should be planned only if the necessary pre-conditions are present: a healthy periodontium, healthy general metabolism and the willingness to undergo the necessary post-orthodontic prosthodontic restorations and maintenance. Before the orthodontic treatment, only provisional restorations, for example, to serve as anchorage, should be done.

Optional procedures

These procedures should only be performed following successful finishing of the essential procedures, that is, the establishment of a healthy oral environment. The requirement of absence of pathological pockets may be perceived as controversial seen in the light of the tendency towards conservative treatment and the demonstration of maintenance of deep pockets over many years (Badersten et al. 1985). This more conservative approach to periodontal treatment is well recognised, but does not apply to teeth that should be moved orthodontically. The tissue reaction generated by the orthodontic force systems is basically comparable to that of inflammation in a sterile environment, and it is crucial that it does not develop into a bacterial-induced inflammation, which would lead to loss of attachment and alveolar bone. Inflammation even on a subclinical level is not acceptable, and the periodontium cannot be 100% healthy in the presence of necrotic cementum. The periodontal surgery needed to reduce the pocket depth in the case of horizontal bone loss may include apical repositioning of the marginal gingiva. This may be unacceptable to the patient, as the surgical procedure results in elongation of the clinical crowns. However, further mucogingival surgery may reduce this problem (see Chapter 13). Vertical bone loss leading to pockets can successfully be treated by the application of the principles of GTR or with the addition of growth factors such as Emdogain[*] (Wang et al. 2005).

It is important to note that even in cases where the periodontium looks healthy, inflammation may exist and manifest as bleeding on probing. The inability for deep scaling to lead to a perfectly clean root was demonstrated by Waerhaug (1952). He performed meticulous scaling of teeth which were later to be extracted. In the case of teeth with no pockets greater than 3 mm, he was successful, but in teeth where the pockets were 3–5 mm deep, the success rate was down to 60%. In the case of pockets deeper than 5 mm, the roots could not be cleaned efficiently through a blind curettage alone. In the presence of pockets between 3 and 5 mm deep, not even half of the roots were completely

clean (Table 4.2). This is illustrated in Figure 4.9, where the lateral incisor has been scaled carefully by a very well-known and capable periodontist. Nevertheless, the bleeding on probing persisted and only when a modified Widman flap surgery was performed was it demonstrated that necrotic cementum and calculus were still present on the root surface. Figure 4.10 demonstrates the effect of combined periodontal and endodontic treatment leading to repair, making possible the subsequent orthodontic treatment. It is

Table 4.2 Rate of success or (Waerhaug 1952) failure as the result of subgingival plaque control in relation to pocket depth.[*]

	Pocket depth 3 mm		Pocket depth 3–5 mm		Pocket depth >5 mm		Total	
	No.	%	No.	%	No.	%	No.	%
Success	52	83	36	39	6	11	94	44
Failure	11	17	56	61	51	89	118	56
Total	63	100	92	100	57	100	212	100

[*]Evaluated on 212 surfaces of 53 teeth.

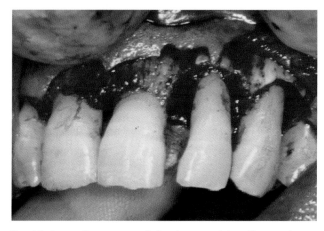

Fig. 4.9 Open flap surgery following careful scaling and root planing. Note that necrotic cementum is still present following closed scaling. (Courtesy of B Ellegård.)

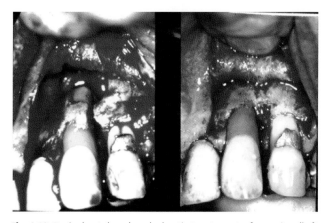

Fig. 4.10 Periodontal and endodontic treatment of a canine (left panel); 6 months later, the tooth is ready for orthodontic treatment (right panel). (Courtesy of B Ellegård.)

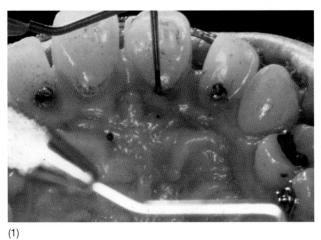
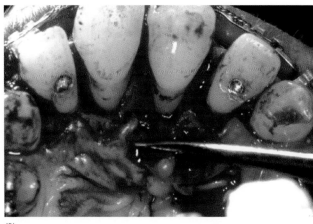

(1) (2)

Fig. 4.11 (1) Patient in whom it was decided to initiate orthodontic treatment in spite of pockets more than 3–4-mm deep, encouraged by the healthy appearance of the gingiva. (2) During treatment, swelling and bleeding on probing nevertheless developed lingual to the upper incisors. An open flap surgery revealed calculus and necrotic cementum on the lingual aspect of the incisors that had not been removed during the blind root planing carried out before the orthodontic treatment commenced.

thus important that pockets are treated before orthodontic treatment is initiated, especially if the orthodontic treatment involves intrusive movements.

The importance of reduction of pockets is illustrated by the example of the patient in Figure 4.11, who seemed to have perfect oral hygiene despite shallow pockets. However, bleeding on probing was seen following activation of the orthodontic appliance for intrusion and retraction of the spaced upper incisors. A modified Widman flap surgery in this case also showed that calculus had been left behind.

Only when this was removed could the orthodontic treatment be continued.

In relation to periodontal treatment, several opinions are presented in the literature on whether the grafting should be done before or after orthodontics. Free grafting, which is now less popular, will often lead to a patch with a different colour, since the palatal mucosa is paler than the mucosa in the area where it is grafted (Figure 4.12). Whenever possible, it is therefore an advantage to use a connective tissue graft, or, if a free graft is absolutely necessary, to do it before orthodontics, since the remodelling during orthodontics may reduce the colour difference (see Chapter 13).

In most patients, several treatment options are possible. The solution to the patient's problem may include either major or minor orthodontic therapy. Major orthodontic therapy leads to less need for restorative/prosthodontic treatment, whereas minor orthodontics results in the need for more extensive prosthodontic rehabilitation. It is important to consider the patient's expectations when determining the treatment strategy. Based on the explanation of the advantages and disadvantages of the different alternatives, the patient has to make the final decision. In patients where implants can serve as anchorage, these can be inserted at the beginning of treatment, but the position of the implants should be carefully planned bearing in mind

the planned tooth movements. In some cases, space has to be created and the alveolar process developed to allow insertion of a dental implant. In patients in whom orthognathic surgery is anticipated, the necessary

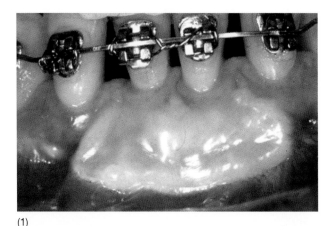

(1)

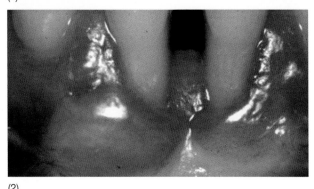

(2)

Fig. 4.12 (1) Results of a free gingival graft after orthodontic treatment; the colour difference is unfortunate. (2) Results of a free gingival graft done before orthodontic treatment; the colour difference is less obvious.

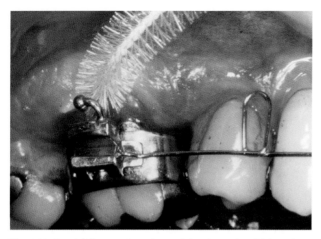

Fig. 4.13 Special instructions in oral hygiene should be given once the appliance is in place.

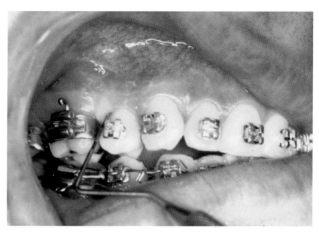

Fig. 4.14 Bands and brackets should not interfere with optimal cleaning of the gingival margin. Example of a band preventing proper cleansing.

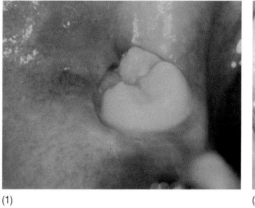

(1)

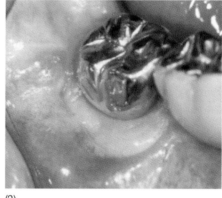

(2)

Fig. 4.15 (1) and (2) Patient in whom a retained third molar was brought forward orthodontically into the arch; the tooth was surrounded by non-attached gingiva. Several grafts had to be placed before the tooth could be considered suitable as a bridge abutment.

orthodontic treatment should be planned in collaboration with the maxillofacial surgeon.

Interaction during treatment

During the orthodontic treatment phase, it is important that patients are able to maintain perfect oral hygiene. This may require repeated instructions, since the placement of fixed appliances would make the usual brushing routine insufficient and a new routine has to be taught. It is also important that bands and/or brackets are placed in such a manner that the patient can maintain good oral hygiene (Figures 4.13 and 4.14).

Post-orthodontic treatment

Following the orthodontic treatment phase, further periodontal surgery may be needed before prosthodontic rehabilitation can be done. This is exemplified by the case in

Figure 4.15, treated by a collaborative effort between Dr Milano and Dr Guerra (see Chapter 13). The patient had lost several teeth in the lower jaw, but a third molar was retained. This third molar was moved forward but into a site without attached gingiva. The tooth was thus not acceptable as an abutment for a bridge, and advanced periodontal surgery was performed before a bridge could finally be made.

Patient satisfaction

The patient's satisfaction is related to the level of information provided. It depends on how well the discrepancy between treatment need and treatment demand has been resolved before initiating treatment. The orthodontist needs to know the patient's expectations regarding treatment time, discomfort and cost, and it is important to define the treatment goal according to the patient's expectations.

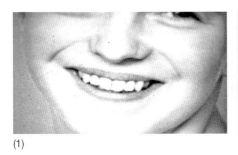
(1)
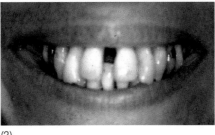
(2)
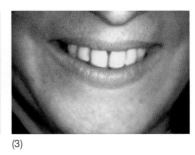
(3)

Fig. 4.16 (1) Patient with pleasing smile at the age of 25. (2) At the age of 46, the picture had changed. (3) The pleasant smile re-established following orthodontic treatment.

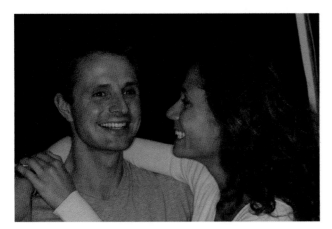

Fig. 4.17 Smile at the world and the world smiles at you.

Patient satisfaction will be highest if the patient's expectations are slightly lower than the delivered result. This is illustrated in Figure 4.16, where the deterioration of the patient's dental status from the age of 26 to the age of 52 can be appreciated. The patient came to the orthodontist after successful periodontal treatment. In spite of healthy periodontal status, the patient was not satisfied with either the function or the aesthetics of her dentition. Although much could be done to improve the situation, it was important to make it clear to the patient that orthodontic treatment would not be able to reproduce the smile she had had at a younger age. The treatment result, however, did improve her smile considerably and the black triangle between the incisors following treatment did not concern the patient, since it was not visible when she was smiling.

The patient's acceptance of her or his smile is an important factor for quality of life. People who like their smile are known to smile more frequently. Victor Borge, a famous Danish comedian, once said: 'A smile is the shortest distance between two people' (Figure 4.17).

Examples of interdisciplinary cases

For examples of interdisciplinary case studies, please refer to the companion website at www.wiley.com/go/melsen.

References

Badersten A, Nilveus R and Egelberg J (1985) Effect of nonsurgical periodontal therapy. VII. Bleeding, suppuration and probing depth in sites with probing attachment loss. *J Clin Periodontol* 12(6), 432–440.

Celenza F Jr and Mantzikos TG (1996) Periodontal and restorative considerations of molar uprighting. *Compend Contin Educ Dent* 17(3), 294–296, 298.

Costa A, Raffainl M and Melsen B (1998) Miniscrews as orthodontic anchorage: a preliminary report. *Int J Adult Orthod Orthog Surg* 13(3), 201–209.

DeBiase CB and Austin SL (2003) Oral health and older adults. *J Dent Hyg* 77(2), 125–145.

Diedrich P (1996) Preprosthetic orthodontics. *J Orofac Orthop* 57(2), 102–116.

Gestrelius S, Lyngstadaas SP and Hammarstrom L (2000) Emdogain–periodontal regeneration based on biomimicry. *Clin Oral Investig* 4(2), 120–125.

Hammarstrom L (1997) Enamel matrix, cementum development and regeneration. *J Clin Periodontol* 24(9 Pt 2), 658–668.

King GN (2001) New regenerative technologies: rationale and potential for periodontal regeneration: 2. Growth factors. *Dent Update* 28(2), 60–65.

Margolis MJ (1997) Esthetic considerations in orthodontic treatment of adults. *Dent Clin North Am* 41(1), 29–48.

Meistrell ME Jr (1988) Treatment objectives and planning in compromised adult cases. *Dent Clin North Am* 32(3), 551–569.

Melsen B (2004) Is the intraoral-extradental anchorage changing the spectrum of orthodontics? In McNamara JA Jr (ed.) *Implants, Microimplants, Onplants and Transplants: New Answers to Old Questions in Orthodontics*, 1st edn, pp. 41–68. Ann Arbor: University of Michigan.

Melsen B (2005) Mini-implants: where are we? *J Clin Orthod* 39(9), 539–547.

Melsen B and Agerbaek N (1994) Orthodontics as an adjunct to rehabilitation. *Periodontology 2000* 4, 148–159.

Melsen B, Petersen JK and Costa A (1998) Zygoma ligatures: an alternative form of maxillary anchorage. *J Clin Orthod* 32(3), 154–158.

Melsen B and Verna C (2005) Miniscrew implants: the Aarhus anchorage system. *Semin Orthod* 11, 24–31.

Narcisi EM and DiPerna JA (1999) Multidisciplinary full-mouth restoration with porcelain veneers and laboratory-fabricated resin inlays. *Pract Periodontics Aesthet Dent* 11(6), 721–728.

Pretorius JA, Melsen B, Nel JC and Germishuys PJ (2005) A histomorphometric evaluation of factors influencing the healing of bony defects surrounding implants. *Int J Oral Maxillofac Surg* 20(3), 387–398.

Pyle MA and Stoller EP (2003) Oral health disparities among the elderly: interdisciplinary challenges for the future. *J Dent Educ* 67(12), 1327–1336.

Roberts WE (1997) Adjunctive orthodontic therapy in adults over 50 years of age. Clinical management of compensated, partially edentulous malocclusion. *J Indiana Dent Assoc* 76(2), 33–38, 40.

Shroff B, Siegel SM, Feldman S and Siegel SC (1996) Combined orthodontic and prosthetic therapy. Special considerations. *Dent Clin North Am* 40(4), 911–943.

Spear FM, Mathews DM and Kokich VG (1997) Interdisciplinary management of single-tooth implants. *Semin Orthod* 3(1), 45–72.

Terranova VP and Wikesjo UM (1987) Extracellular matrices and polypeptide growth factors as mediators of functions of cells of the periodontium. A review. *J Periodontol* 58(6), 371–380.

Vanarsdall RL (1989) Orthodontics. Provisional restorations and appliances. *Dent Clin North Am* 33(3), 479–496.

Venezia E, Goldstein M, Boyan BD and Schwartz Z (2004) The use of enamel matrix derivative in the treatment of periodontal defects: a literature review and meta-analysis. *Crit Rev Oral Biol Med* 15(6), 382–402.

Waerhaug J (1952) The gingival pocket; anatomy, pathology, deepening and elimination. *Odontologisk Tidskrift* 60, 1–186.

Wang HL, Greenwell H, Fiorellini J, Giannobile W, Offenbacher S, Salkin L, Townsend C, Sheridan P Genco RJ and Research, Science and Therapy Committee (2005) Periodontal regeneration. *J Periodontol* 76(9): 1601–1622.

Willems G, Carels CE, Naert IE and van SD (1999) Interdisciplinary treatment planning for orthodontic-prosthetic implant anchorage in a partially edentulous patient. *Clin Oral Implants Res* 10(4), 331–337.

Wostmann B, Budtz-Jorgensen E, Jepson N, Mushimoto E, Palmqvist S, Sofou A and Owall B (2005) Indications for removable partial dentures: a literature review. *Int J Prosthodont* 18(2), 139–145.

5

Treatment Planning: The 3D VTO

Birte Melsen, Giorgio Fiorelli

Determining the treatment goal using the occlusogram

Once a patient decides to have treatment, detailed treatment planning has to be carried out. However, before the necessary appliance can be chosen, the treatment goal has to be established. This can be done by the workup of a three-dimensional visual treatment objective (3D VTO), which consists of an occlusogram combined with the tracing of a head film or by simulating the desired tooth movements on virtual models. In adult patients, in whom no growth-related changes are expected to influence the treatment result, the tooth movements necessary to achieve the treatment goal can therefore be more clearly defined.

The combination of an occlusogram and a cephalogram was used by Bjork and Skieller (1972) to illustrate the skeletal and dental changes occurring during growth. Their occlusograms were produced from drawings of photographs or photocopies of the study casts.

The conventional occlusogram described by Burstone and Marcotte (2000) was based on an image of the study casts or an occlusal view of virtual models, and the intermaxillary relationship was maintained with an alginate or silicone bite while trimming the study casts.

Purpose of occlusograms

- Assessment of the occlusal relationship.
- Estimation of space conditions.
- Estimation of arch length and width.
- Estimation of tooth movements in all three planes of space when combined with a profile tracing.
- Estimation of anchorage requirements.
- Assessment of tooth-size discrepancies.
- Estimation of necessary force systems.

In adult patients, the occlusogram is usually done using the habitual occlusal relation between the jaws. If mandibular repositioning or surgery is planned, this relationship should be modified accordingly. Once the jaw relation has been decided, the occlusogram can in combination with a cephalogram be used to illustrate tooth displacements in three dimensions. Over the past years, intraoral scans have become more popular (Aragón et al. 2016; Ellakany et al. 2020; Kwon et al. 2021) and will without doubt completely replace plaster models. Different companies offer virtual model analysis software that can clearly replace stone casts. Xiao et al. (2020) who described the integration of photos, cone beam computerized tomography (CBCT) images and virtual models presented the last development.

However, as many colleagues still use plaster models, we have chosen to maintain the description of the production of an occlusogram manually.

Adult Orthodontics, Second Edition. Edited by Birte Melsen and Cesare Luzi.
© 2022 John Wiley & Sons Ltd. Published 2022 by John Wiley & Sons Ltd.
Companion Website: http://www.wiley.com/go/melsen-adult-orthodontics

Production of an occlusogram: manual procedure and general concepts

In order to create the occlusogram manually, the study casts are placed into occlusion with a thin piece of silk (Hanel Articulating Silk®) inserted between the upper and lower casts to localise the occlusal intermaxillary contacts (Figure 5.1).

The following structures should be outlined:

Gingival contours of the teeth.
Incisal ridges and buccal cusp ridges.
Central grooves and cusp tips.
Palatal rugae and the mid-palatal raphe.
Reference points used when superimposing the upper and the lower occlusogram (Figure 5.2).
Once the images are drawn or printed on transparent paper, the upper and lower arches can be superimposed on the occlusal contacts (Figure 5.3).

Determination of the midline

The first step when producing virtual treatment objectives (VTOs) is to determine the position of the post-treatment dental midline either on the upper or on the lower dental cast. The dental arch in which the least number of corrections are required is usually selected to determine the midline. The

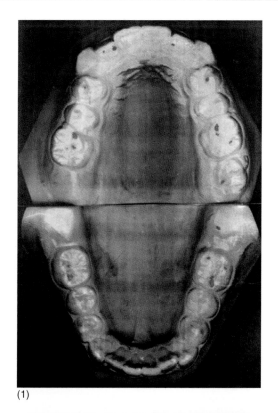

(1)

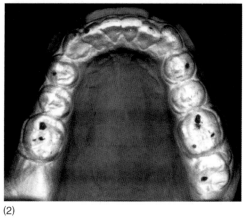

(2)

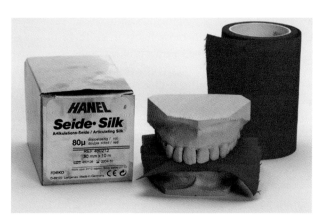

Fig. 5.1 Study casts in occlusion with red silk for localising the occlusal contacts.

Fig. 5.2 Occlusograms copied on transparent paper with occlusal contacts indicated (1) upper and (2) lower arches. (3) Transparents of the two arches superimposed.

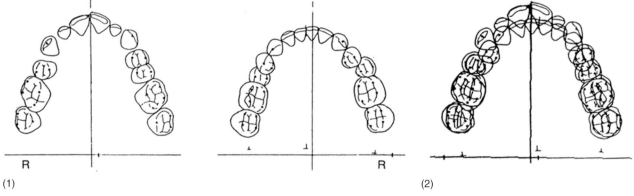

(1)   (2)

Fig. 5.3 (1) Hand-drawn occlusograms: (a) maxilla and (b) mandible. (2) Occlusograms superimposed on the occlusal contact points. The superimposed occlusograms demonstrated a midline discrepancy localized to the lower arch.

anterior dental midline should if possible coincide with the facial midline that is determined from a frontal view of the patient (Figure 5). Burstone and Marcotte (2000) showed that defining the dental midlines solely based on skeletal measurements can be considered invalid, as no symmetry exists between the bilateral landmarks (Figure 5.4). The most frequently used midline is therefore defined as the perpendicular to the midpoint of the interpupillary line (Figure 5.5).

The facial midline will be indicated as a point on the occlusogram. Once the dental midline has been determined on one arch, it will be transferred to the other arch by superimposing the occlusograms on the occlusal contact points (Figure 5.3).

However, when determining the anterior dental midline, the mesiodistal inclination of the incisors should be taken into consideration. Burstone therefore introduced the apical base midline, the position of which will influence the forces necessary to reach the ideal incisor position (Figure 5.6).

When heading for a symmetrical arch, the midline, drawn on the image of the occlusal view of the dental arches, represents an important reference when determining the treatment goal. In most patients, without facial asymmetry, the raphe mediana represents the posterior midline, which divides the dental arch into two mirror-like semi-arches. In this case, the symmetry line can be simply constructed by folding the occlusogram as showed in Figure 5.7. This midline will also be the geometrical midline.

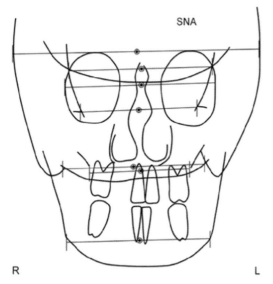

Fig. 5.4 Frontal radiograph on which bilateral landmarks and the midpoints are indicated. Note the large variation in the midpoint at different levels of the face. This variation frequently makes it impossible to construct a facial midline based on the radiograph. (From Burstone and Marcotte 2000. Reproduced with permission from Quintessence Publishing Co Inc., Chicago.)

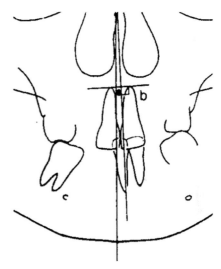

Fig. 5.6 Apical midline illustrating the influence of tipped incisors.

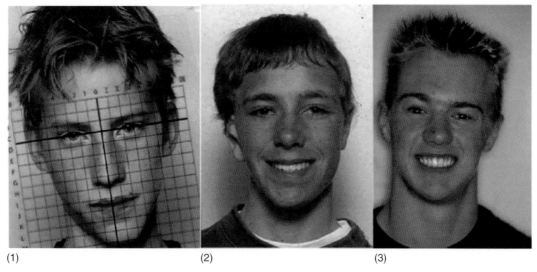

Fig. 5.5 (1) Patient with an obvious asymmetry. The facial midline can in this case be defined as the perpendicular to the midpoint of the interpupillary line. (2) This was also done in this patient with hemifacial microsomia. (3) In this patient with plagiocephaly, the occlusal plane was aligned to the true horizontal and the dental midlines were adjusted to the nose. Note that the asymmetry is more apparent.

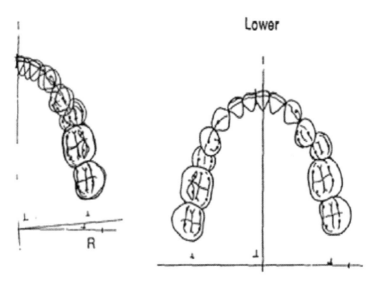

Fig. 5.7 The geometrical midline can be ascertained by folding the occlusogram, so that the molars of the two sides are superimposed. This can only be done if no local tooth movements have occurred. The geometrical midline can also be determined in relation to the virtual models with special software which can select two symmetrically located points in the lateral regions.

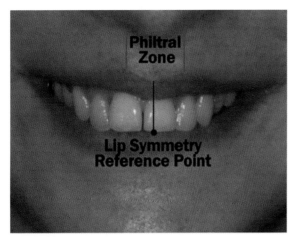

Fig. 5.8 The lip symmetry reference point showing a deviation of the upper dental midline to the right of the prolabial midline. This point can be indicated on the occlusal view and used as a reference to decide the dental midline line. This smile shows an asymmetric display of the two upper canines, with the right positioned more anteriorly than the left one, thus demonstrating the need for an asymmetrical sagittal movement of these teeth.

The geometric midline is defined by folding the occlusogram, so that the molars on one side cover the contralateral molars, provided they are not rotated or tipped. If this is the case, a simulation of the upright, non-rotated position should be assumed. When on the other hand, one side is wider than the other, as seen in Figure 5.7, the geometrical midline will deviate from the raphe.

The advantage of using the geometrical midline is that it allows for application of symmetrical mechanics. It is, however, necessary to ascertain that the dental midline is identical with or very close to facial midline. When the interpupillary line is used as a reference and the occlusal plane is planned to be parallel to this line, the face will seem less asymmetrical than when the occlusal plane is parallel to the true horizontal (Figure 5.5). The predicted anterior reference point and the dental midline should correspond to the midpoint of the interpupillary line and may be modified with regard to major asymmetries in other parts of the face, especially asymmetries of the nose. As a supplement to the facial midline, the lip symmetry (Figure 5.8) can be used a reference.

Some patients with a relative symmetrical face exhibit asymmetries including dental midline discrepancy, different sagittal relationship and different arch width of the two sides (Figure 5.9). When setting the treatment goal, the most important issue is that the canines are placed symmetrical even if the posterior part of the arch is asymmetrical. It is the clinician's task to determine if a correction is possible by displacement of teeth or if surgery is required.

Combining the occlusogram with the head film

The transfer is done using the following way: the functional occlusal plane must be indicated on the tracing. The functional occlusal plane may be defined perpendicular to the long axis of the premolars as recommended by Burstone and Marcotte (2000). This would, however, require a tomogram or a 45 degree image. An alternative would be a line extending from the distal occlusal contact point of the lower molars to a point indicating the desired overbite. A perpendicular is then constructed to this plane from the most prominent point of the lower and the upper incisors.

Next, two lines parallel to the occlusal plane are drawn one above and one below the cephalometric tracing, and the upper and lower occlusograms are placed with the symmetry axis superimposed to these lines. The sagittal position of the occlusograms is determined by the position of the anterior teeth, which should correspond in the cephalometric tracing and on the occlusograms (Figure 5.10).

Upper   Lower

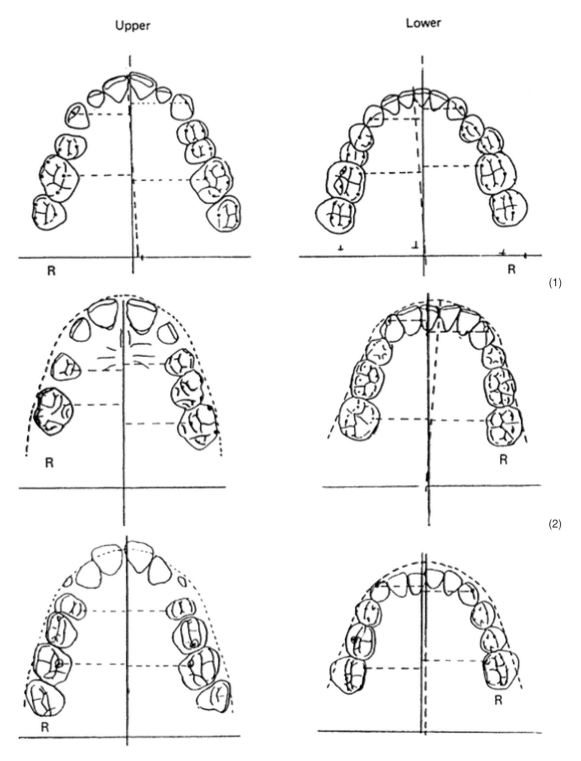

(1)

(2)

Fig. 5.9 Examples of occlusograms: (1) On the occlusogram of the upper arch, the midline corresponding to the median raphe, the anatomical midline is indicated. This patient had a Class II division 1 malocclusion with a deviation of the lower midline. The maxillary arch is slightly rotated to the right and the mandibular arch to the left. Both arches demonstrate dental sagittal and transverse asymmetries. As a consequence of the agenesis of the second upper right premolar, the molar has drifted, tipped and rotated forward. Continuous line: facial midline; dotted line: geometrical midline. The dental and the anatomical midlines correspond almost in the upper jaw but when transferred to the lower arch, a dental midline discrepancy can be detected. The geometrical midline is indicated with a dotted line on the lower occlusogram. (2) A patient with a crossbite on the right side and a lower midline shift to the right. The lower arch is rotated to the right. Continuous line: facial midline; dotted line: geometrical midline. (3) Occlusogram of a patient with a Class II division 1 malocclusion and a symmetrical upper arch. The lower arch is rotated to the right. The asymmetrical molar position has resulted in a negative leeway on the right side. Dotted lines: planned arch form.

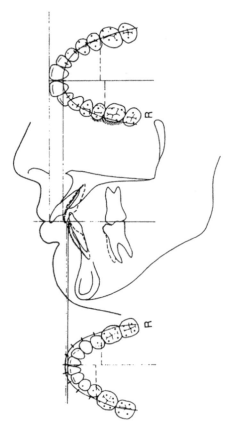

Fig. 5.10 Combination of the head film and the occlusogram. Two upper premolars are previewed, in the lower arch two premolars are already missing. The midlines are parallel to the occlusal plane.

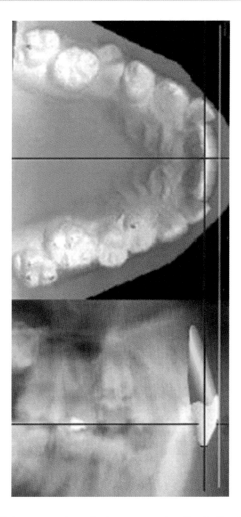

Fig. 5.11 In cases where incisors are retroclined, the incision point is not the most prominent point of the tooth seen on the lateral head film. When combining the lateral cephalogram and occlusal views of the dental arch, it has to be decided whether to use the most prominent point or incision when constructing the perpendicular to the occlusal plane. However, it is important to be consistent when choosing the point where the perpendicular line should intersect the midline of the dental arch and the incisors on the cephalogram. In this example the incision is used as reference and indicated as the blue line passing through the incisal edge, although the most prominent point is more anteriorly and closer to the gingival contour.

Alternatively, the perpendicular line can be drawn through the incisal edge, which is not necessarily the most prominent point of the tooth contour (Figure 5.11). The lower occlusogram is placed in the same way below the tracing. The midlines of the occlusograms will then be parallel to the occlusal plane.

Planning the anterior dental movements

The planning of the tooth movements is an iterative process that starts with the positioning of the upper incisor on the tracing. Although the position of the lower central incisor in relation to the mandibular plane (basal bone) has generally been used as the foundation for treatment planning, this traditional definition is not based on any scientific evidence. The standard deviation within an untreated population in Scandinavia is 7°, indicating that the inclination of the lower incisors may vary between 80° and 118° in 95% of the population (Bjork and Skieller 1972). The variation was even larger when several ethnic groups were pooled. A case–control study has demonstrated that the lower incisors could be proclaimed without any adverse effects on the periodontium (Allais and Melsen 2003; Melsen and Allais 2005). Since the upper incisors have a larger impact on the facial

appearance, it is important that defining the treatment goal starts with the desired position of these teeth. Both the inclination and the vertical position are of importance. As a guideline, the incisal edge in adult persons should be 2–3 mm below the relaxed upper lip (Al Wazzan 2004). In younger individuals, however, greater exposure of the incisors is recommended, as the length of the upper lip increases with age (Burstone and Marcotte 2000).

Once the upper incisors have been correctly positioned, the required movements of the lower incisors can be determined (Figure 5.12). If the amounts of tooth movements required to achieve this goal are considered unrealistic, the displacement of the upper incisors must be adjusted until an acceptable position of the lower incisors is established. The predicted and desired positions of the upper and lower incisors are then transferred to the occlusogram.

In adult patients, it is frequently desirable to correct an excessive overjet by the labial movement of the lower incisors, as retraction of the upper incisors will often influence the orofacial projection negatively, making the patient look older due to the increase in the nasolabial angle and the loss of support to the upper lip.

Due to the risk of ending with insufficient exposure of the upper incisor crowns, several orthodontists have believed that intrusion of upper incisors should be avoided. This is, however, not always possible, as there are often beneficial effects of intruding over erupted periodontally damaged upper incisors. It is also important to consider the possibility of intrusion and/or proclination of lower incisors when correcting a deep bite (Melsen and Allais 2005).

Defining the shape and dimension of the dental arches

Next, the dental arches must be defined. In the absence of transverse problems, no changes are indicated when the planned arches are drawn using the contact points on the occlusogram, in order to maintain the existing arch width (Figure 5.13). This step is similar in both the manual and computerised procedures.

If no transverse problems are present, no changes are indicated when the arches are drawn through the contact points on the occlusograms, thus maintaining the position of the posterior arches (Figure 5.13). Burstone and Marcotte (2000) suggested the drawing of three different arches: one indicating the shape of the needed arch wire, one through the buccal cusps and one through the contact points (Figure 5.14).

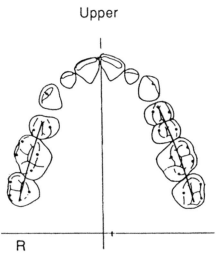

Fig. 5.13 A line is drawn through the contact points of both buccal segments on the image of the study cast. In the illustration, a premolar is missing on one side and the arch width is slightly different on the two sides. If no changes are planned to the arch width, the arch shape will be as indicated here through the contact points.

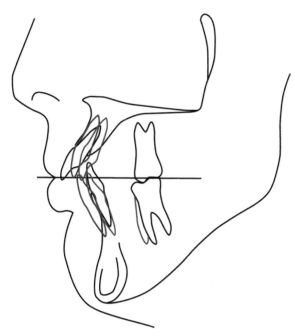

Fig. 5.12 Once the placement of the upper incisors has been determined, the movements of the lower incisors can be simulated in order to obtain a desirable incisor relationship. If the desired position of the upper incisors (red) requires too much forward movement of the lower incisors, a new compromise position (blue) should be determined for the upper incisors.

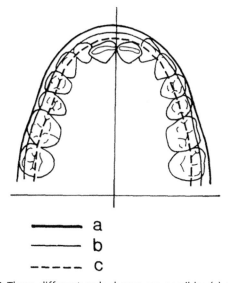

Fig. 5.14 Three different arch shapes are possible: (a) the arch form of the preformed arch wire; (b) an arch form passing through the buccal cusps and (c) an arch form passing through the contact points, which is the arch form used for the space evaluation.

The next step is to mark the mesiodistal dimension of each tooth on the final or desired arch shape, starting with the central incisors. Upon reaching the molars, a space estimation, negative or positive, can be assessed (Figure 5.15). This part can be done by software available from several companies.

If a space deficiency is present, two solutions are possible: reduction of tooth substance and creation of space, which can be obtained in different ways:

1) The incisor position can be modified to increase in arch length by a labial movement of the incisors: 1 mm of labial movement may provide up to 2 mm of space.
2) Increase in arch width, by transverse arch expansion either skeletal or dental.
3) Distal movement of posterior teeth. At this stage, it has to be evaluated whether the space that can be gained by space creation is sufficient to resolve dental crowding.
4) Reduction in tooth substance by interproximal reduction or extractions is necessary (Ballard and Sheridan 1996).

If the patient presents with spacing resulting from agenesis or loss of deteriorated dental elements, space closure and replacement are the possibilities and alternative solutions that should be discussed with other members of the treatment team before presented to the patient.

The computerised occlusogram

The treatment goals and the 3D VTO are essential parts of any individualised treatment plan, as these allow for the definition of the necessary force systems to obtain the desired tooth movements.

To facilitate the treatment planning which may be relatively time-consuming, Fiorelli and Melsen in 1999 proposed the development of a software.

The first version of a computerised occlusogram (1998) was based on the occlusal views of the dental casts and of the lateral cephalogram captured with a flatbed scanner. This method followed the same steps as the manual procedure described in the earlier text. Later (2006), the software imported directly model images together with tooth sizes and positions (She et al. 2021).

The steps followed by the current software after the acquisitions of the models and the lateral cephalogram images, both of which can be virtual, are:

● Midline decision (Figure 5.16).
● Alignment of the occlusal view of the models in relation to the lateral cephalometric (Figure 5.17) or sagittal cut of the virtual models (Figure 5.18).
● Definition of the desired position of the anterior teeth (Figure 5.19).
● Outline of the transverse dimension and the shape of the arches where interproximal contact points will be aligned (Figure 5.20).

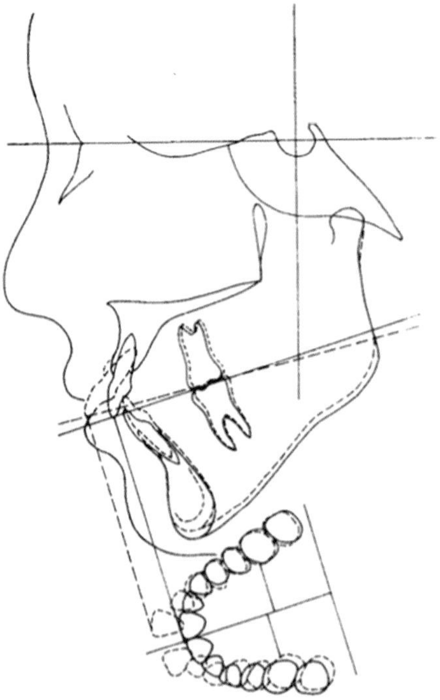

Fig. 5.15 Combined occlusogram and tracing of the head film of a patient in whom the treatment involved extraction of two premolars and retraction and intrusion of the upper incisors. In the lower arch, two premolars had already been extracted.

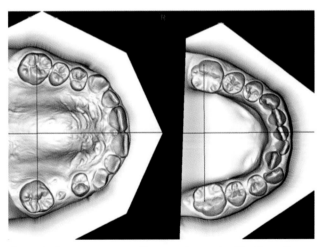

Fig. 5.16 The two symmetry lines are determined by the software by indicating two points, in one of the two arches that should be considered symmetrical. In this case, these are corresponding to the centres of the upper first molar crowns. In this way, the molars and the upper arch are to be considered symmetrical in relation to the constructed symmetry lines, while in the lower arch, an asymmetrical contraction or expansion is needed to restore symmetry.

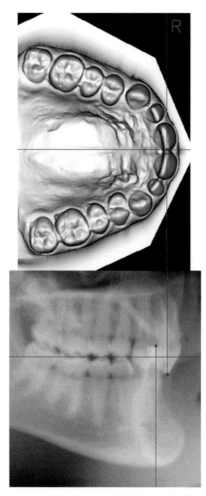

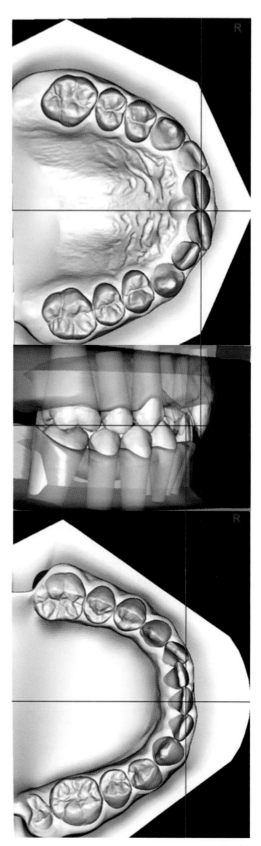

Fig. 5.17 Corresponding reference points are indicated on both the occlusal view of the models and on the lateral cephalometric image, to let the software align these views with the occlusal plane and the symmetry lines placed in parallel.

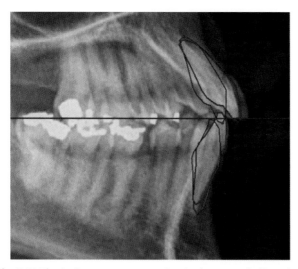

Fig. 5.19 The incisor contours, previously drawn and aligned to the occlusal views, are dragged on the screen from their initial (blue) to the desired (red) position to define the treatment goal in this area.

Fig. 5.18 In case that the lateral cephalogram is not available, a virtual model can be used for proper alignment of the models and the decision of the movement of the anterior teeth.

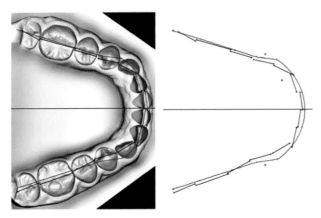
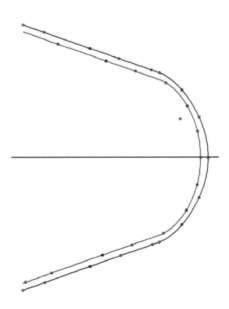

Fig. 5.20 T3DO occlusogram software showing the necessary dental movements represented by segment displacement. The initial position of the teeth is identified by the position of their mesiodistal contact points. These points are connected by the blue lines. It should be imagined how each blue segment (tooth) should be moved in order to reach its final alignment in the red arch. The software allows hiding or showing the model image in the background.

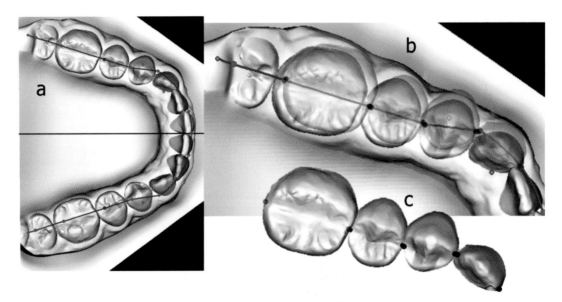

Fig. 5.21 The same alignment shown in Figure 5.23 can be represented graphically, by superimposing the images of the teeth along the occlusogram arch. (a) Mesiodistal dimensions of the teeth are represented along the arch created with the previous steps. The blue point represents the point of contact mesial to the first molar, the red one the point of contact mesial to the canine. (b) Detail of the predicted movements in quadrant 3. The contour of the teeth is superimposed aligning their mesiodistal extremities with the point of contacts that are already marked along the arch. In this way, the needed movements, representing the treatment goals, can be appreciated. A moderate expansion and a minimal mesial movement are expected for all teeth, besides the mesial rotation of 3.3. (c) Estimated final alignment (in two dimensions) from 3.6 to 3.3.

Once these inputs are given, the teeth dimensions that are imported from the digital models are indicated along predetermined arch form. In this way, it is possible to estimate the needed movements on the occlusal view in two dimensions (Figures 5.21 and 5.22) and the final relation between the two arches.

The first outcome can be modified by changing the input made by changing the dental dimension or removing/adding dental units.

Once the treatment plan has been decided, a summary sheet can also be created to represent the essentials of the treatment goal (Figure 5.23).

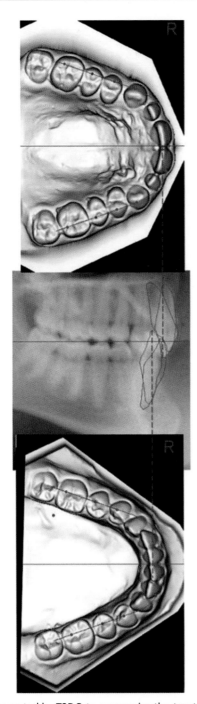

STANDARD MEASUREMENTS

OverJet & OverBite
- OvJ: 2,2
- OvB: 4,1

Upper Incisors
- Buccal displacement: 1,9
- Intrusion: 1,7
- Buccal Inclination: 17,8°
- Start: 88,7°
- Predicted: 106,5°

Lower incisors
- Buccal displacement:3
- Intrusion: 2,5
- Buccal Inclination: 12,4°
- Start: 93,9°
- Predicted: 106,3°

Maxilla
- No Movement

Mandible
- No Movement

Transversal Dimensions
- Upper Interpremolar distance(4-4): 37,3mm
- Lower Interpremolar distance(4-4): 30,8mm
- Upper Intermolar distance(6-6): 47,3mm
- Lower Intermolar distance(6-6): 41,0mm

Sagittal Symmetry
- Upper canine sagittal symmetry
- Canine sagittal asymmetry: 43 distal to 33 of 0,6mm
- Molar sagittal asymmetry: 16 distal to 26 of - 1,0mm
- Molar sagittal asymmetry: 46 distal to 36 of 2,2mm

Fig. 5.22 Sheet generated by T3DO to summarise the treatment plan.

The steps described in the earlier text lead basically to the same results provided by the manual procedure, even if the speed of execution, precision, and adjustability of the outcomes are superior. In many cases, the orthodontist may decide to limit the analysis to this 2D evaluation.

However, the use of digital models can widen the possibilities of establishing the treatment goal to a real 3D simulation. In this way, some of the limitations inherent of the 2D analysis, where it is not possible to evaluate some aspects of the treatment, are outdone.

When these elements are considered essential to the establishment of the treatment goal, the occlusogram procedure should be completed giving the software more inputs in order to create a reference arch in three dimensions within the dental models.

To achieve these results, the orthodontist must indicate the final arch position in the sagittal and frontal views and the desired curve of Spee (Figure 5.24). It is important to underline that this information should be given considering the actual position of the teeth in the facial structure (Figure 5.25).

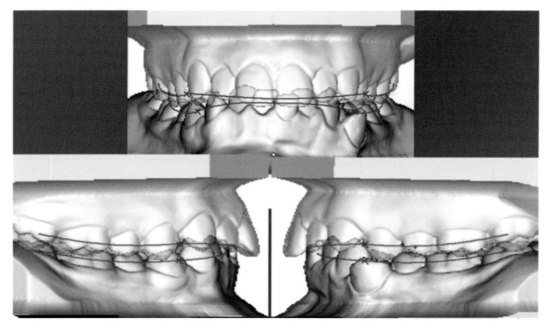

Fig. 5.23 T3D occlusogram. In order to produce a full three-dimensional visualisation of the occlusogram arches, the user must provide input parameters for the curve of Spee and shape of the arch as seen in the frontal view.

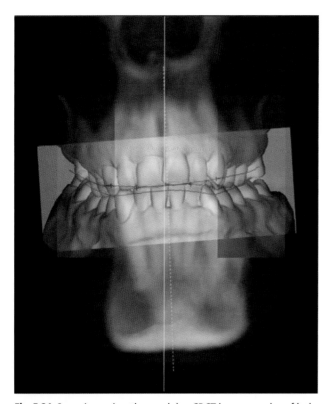

Fig. 5.24 Superimposing the model, a CBCT image can be of help to plan the vertical position of posterior teeth on the two sides to obtain an occlusal plane properly orientated in the frontal plane. In this case, an intrusion of the posterior teeth on the right side would be needed to correct the posterior cant of the occlusal plane.

Once the 3D occlusogram arch is embedded into the digital models it is possible to have a full 3D visualisation of all needed dental movements with the option of generating a semiautomatic virtual setup of the final dental position; if the virtual models have a segmentation of the teeth as individual objects, it will be also possible to see the planned movements in three dimensions for all teeth (Figure 5.26).

In conclusion, the advantages of the computerised procedure are a reduction in execution time, improved accuracy and, especially, the possibility of simulating different treatment options by changing only a single input parameter. In fact, once a treatment simulation has been completed, the clinician may explore other possibilities by simply changing the final desired position of the upper incisors on the lateral cephalogram, the arch size or shape, the symmetry line or the extraction/non-extraction strategy. With a single change in just one of these parameters, the software will recalculate the whole treatment.

Responding to patients' needs

The success of orthodontic treatment in adult patients depends largely on how the team works together. Referring to the car industry, Iacocca stated that success depends on having a good product, that the product can be delivered and that you love your customer (Iacocca and Novak 1986). So a car has to be reliable, has a good design and reasonable cost, and fulfils the customer's need. A sports car would not fulfil the needs of a family of four children. Loving your

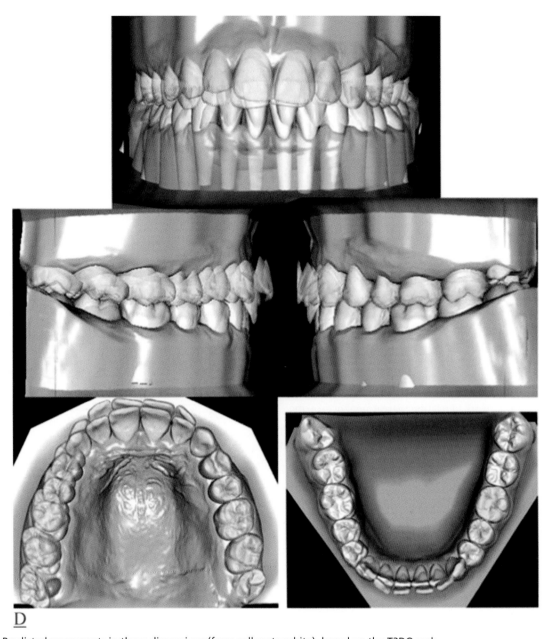

D

Fig. 5.25 Predicted movements in three dimensions (from yellow to white), based on the T3DO arch.

customer means recognising their needs. Transferring Iacocca's notion to the situation of an orthodontist treating the adult patients, we need to identify our patients' needs, know their expectations and explain the alternatives in such a manner that a realistic treatment goal will be able to fulfil the expectations of the patient. The possible goal is dependent on the framework mentioned and the ability of the orthodontist.

In adult treatment planning, the interaction between the prosthodontist, the periodontist and the orthodontist is of utmost importance. When evaluating how space problems

are resolved, the prognosis of each tooth has to be considered. It has to be determined which teeth should be maintained and which teeth should be extracted. A poor prognosis may be due to reduced periodontal support, or the need for or the presence of large restorations. The iterative treatment planning may result in several alternative plans, for which the advantages and the disadvantages of each have to be carefully evaluated before a final decision is taken.

Several alternative treatment plans can be explored and compared more easily with the computerised procedure. The relative contribution anticipated by the individual specialists can therefore be optimised. All the specialists should reach a consensus before meeting the patient, as the success of the adult orthodontic treatment is fully dependent on their collaborative efforts. Alternative solutions should be discussed. During these discussions, the patient's expectations can be addressed as best as possible, as the satisfaction depends on whether realistic expectations are fulfilled.

Orthodontic treatment: art or science?

The scientific nature of orthodontics was evaluated by Melsen (2020). She concluded that orthodontics has very little to do with science, which is normally characterised by the definition of a hypothesis that has to be either supported or rejected. The purpose of her paper was to re-analyse the controversies related to the same words used differently within bone biology and orthodontics. The definition of the treatment goal is based on perception of beauty; the trend to focus on efficacy and marketing more than on treatment of the individual patients and finally on the isolation of the effect of the orthodontic appliance from growth and function and the lack of understanding the word 'stability'.

Orthodontic treatment is usually carried out in phases often related more to the appliance than to the stage of treatment. This may work in relation to treatment of growing individuals, whereas a stage in adult patients is defined by specifying tooth movements. Some phases have to be kept separate, as the interaction may result in an unfavourable force system.

Planning of orthodontic treatment of adult patients is rarely done by the orthodontist alone, but involves interaction with other professions and foremost the periodontologist.

Adult treatment frequently requires the use of individually designed appliances and full 3D control of individual tooth movements. Besides, special considerations are required concerning anchorage. Techniques used successfully in children, such as the straight-wire approach, may prove problematic in the treatment of adult patients with mutilated dentitions. Whereas the result of orthodontic treatment in children is an expression of a combination of growth and the treatment itself, the treatment results in adult patients are more directly an expression of the effects of the force systems generated by the appliances and the forces of normal and abnormal functions.

References

Al Wazzan KA (2004) The visible portion of anterior teeth at rest. *J Contemp Dent Pract* 5, 53–62.

Allais D and Melsen B (2003) Does labial movement of lower incisors influence the level of the gingival margin? A case-control study of adult orthodontic patients. *Eur J Orthod* 25, 343–352.

Aragón MLC, Pontes LF, Bichara LM, Flores-Mir C and Normando D (2016) Validity and reliability of intraoral scanners compared to conventional gypsum models measurements: a systematic review. *Eur J Orthod* Aug;38(4), 429–434.

Ballard R and Sheridan JJ (1996) Air-rotor stripping with the Essix anterior anchor. *J Clin Orthod* 30, 371–373.

Bjork A and Skieller V (1972) Facial development and tooth eruption. An implant study at the age of puberty. *Am J Orthod* 62, 339–383.

Burstone CJ and Marcotte MR (2000) The treatment midline. In Burstone CJ and Marcotte MR (eds) *Problem Solving in Orthodontics. Goal Oriented Treatment Strategies*, pp. 145–178. Chicago, IL: Quintessence.

Ellakany P, Al-Harbi F, Tantawi ME and Mohsen C (2020) Evaluation of the accuracy of digital and 3D-printed casts compared with conventional stone casts. *J Prosthet Dent* Dec 8;S0022-3913(20)30623-5.

Fiorelli G and Melsen B (1999) The "3D Occlusogram" software. *Am J Orthod Dentofacial Orthop* 116(3), 363–368.

Iacocca L and Novak W (1986) *Iacocca: An Autobiography*, reissue edn. USA and Canada: Bantam Books.

Kwon M, Cho Y, Kim D-W, Kim M, Kim Y-J and Chang M (2021) Full-arch accuracy of five intraoral scanners: *In vivo* analysis of trueness and precision. *Korean J Ortho* Mar 25;51(2), 95–104.

Marcotte MR (1976) The use of the occlusogram in planning orthodontic treatment. *Am J Orthod* 69(6), 655–667.

McLaughlin RP and Bennett JC (1999) The dental VTO: an analysis of orthodontic tooth movement. *J Clin Orthod* Jul;33(7), 394–403.

Melsen B (2020) Where do we come from? Where are we going? *World Fed Orthod* Oct;9(3S), S74–S78.

Melsen B and Allais D (2005) Factors of importance for the development of dehiscences during labial movement of mandibular incisors: a retrospective study of adult orthodontic patients. *Am J Orthod Dentofacial Orthop* 127, 552–561.

She F, Abuneviciute A and Fiorelli G (2021) Visualizing treatment objectives and treatment planning using 2D and 3D occlusograms. In Retrouvey J-M and Abdallah M-N (eds) *3d Diagnosis and Treatment Planning in Orthodontics*, pp. 195–238. SpringerVerlag.

Xiao Z, Liu Z and Gu Y (2020) Integration of digital maxillary dental casts with 3D facial images in orthodontic patients: a three-dimensional validation study. *Angle Orthod* 90(3), 397–404.

6

Tissue Reaction

Carlalberta Verna, Birte Melsen

Orthopaedic effects

The treatment principles applicable to adult patients are basically limited to tooth movements and orthognathic surgery. However, some orthopaedic effects have been demonstrated clinically even in adult patients when using Herbst appliances and/or forward posturing.

The Herbst appliance

Condylar changes and modelling of the glenoid fossa following Herbst treatment have been demonstrated in both young and adult non-human primates (Woodside et al. 1987; Voudouris et al. 2003a, 2003b). Although the hyperactivity of the lateral pterygoid muscle does not correlate to growth modifications, the reciprocal stretch of the ligament connecting the condyle to the fossa may play a role in new bone formation.

Minor skeletal discrepancies in young adults can be corrected with Herbst appliance treatment. Paulsen and Karle (2000) treated two 20-year-old patients with Class II malocclusions using the Herbst appliance and found new

bone formation at the condyles. Distocranial bone apposition was visible both on the orthopantomograms and by means of computer tomography (CT). This is consistent with Ruf and Pancherz' (1999) findings, which demonstrated that efficiency of the Herbst appliance in the correction of Class II malocclusions was maximum after the pubertal growth spurt. Evidence of modelling of the temporomandibular joints (TMJs), the condyles as well as the articular fossae in young adults was confirmed by magnetic resonance and three-dimensional X-rays (Fig. 6.1). According to Ruf and Pancherz (1999), Herbst treatment could be a possible alternative to orthognathic surgery in borderline adult skeletal Class II cases.

Forward posturing

The capacity for the TMJ to model even in adult individuals is confirmed by the successful clinical results of forward posturing therapy suggested by Korn (personal communication, 2006; see Case 1 below). He demonstrated that mandibular forward posturing could be considered an alternative to surgery in patients declining surgery. Coordinating the arches so that they fit together when the mandible is postured forward resulted in a dual bite at first but, at the 5-year follow-up, the patient's mandible could no longer be forced back into the retruded contact position. However, the precise tissue reactions at the condyles and the articular fossae still remain to be elucidated.

Case 1: Adult patient before and after forward posturing of the mandible (courtesy of Dr M Korn)

A 47-year-old woman with a Class II division 1 malocclusion, mutilated dentition with loss of all second molars, and chronic temporomandibular disorder presented with unsatisfactory veneers that had been constructed to correct the

Adult Orthodontics, Second Edition. Edited by Birte Melsen and Cesare Luzi.
© 2022 John Wiley & Sons Ltd. Published 2022 by John Wiley & Sons Ltd.
Companion Website: http://www.wiley.com/go/melsen-adult-orthodontics

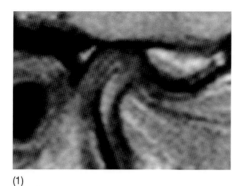

(1)

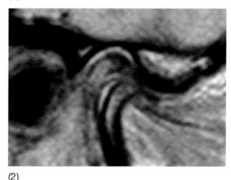

(2)

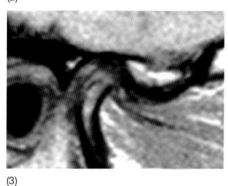

(3)

Fig. 6.1 (1-3) Magnetic resonance image of the temporomandibular joint tissue after Herbst appliance treatment in an adult patient. Note the tissue modelling at the condylar and fossa levels. (Courtesy of Professor S Ruf.).

attritions and mask the existing crowding without orthodontics. The patient did not want to have orthognathic surgery and was given a bite plane for 11 months while she participated in a forward posture training programme. Intra-arch orthodontic tooth movement was carried out as if she was to have orthognathic surgery, but instead of orthognathic surgery, the patient trained her mandible to posture forward in a dual bite Class I relationship. At the end of treatment, she was unable to move the mandible posteriorly into its original position. Eight years following treatment, the Class I relationship was maintained and the patient had no dual bite.

Palatal expansion

The dental arches can be expanded by opening the midpalatal suture or by modelling of the alveolar processes. With the establishment of the occlusion of the permanent teeth, the midpalatal suture shows tight bony interdigitation and expansion here becomes difficult (Melsen 1975; Persson and Thilander 1977; Knaup et al. 2004) (Fig. 6.2).

Rapid palatal expansion is performed with a cemented appliance and the skeletal contribution to the treatment result depends on the degree of opening of the suture. A histological study carried out on biopsies of the midpalatal suture following rapid palatal expansion (Hyrax) demonstrated that in children in the mixed dentition the suture opened. The increase in number of osteoblasts and osteoid formation indicated stimulation of growth, which then allowed establishment of the correct transverse relationship. Once tight interdigitation is established, rapid palatal expansion is achieved by fracture within or adjacent to the suture (Melsen 1972). As a consequence of the difficulty in widening of the suture, surgical-assisted rapid maxillary expansion (SARME) was introduced. By facilitating the separation of the two maxillary halves, the load on the posterior teeth and thereby the risk of creating buccal dehiscences is reduced. Tissue reaction at the suture following SARME or following the fracture resulting from the activation of the rapid expansion screw is comparable with that in distraction osteogenesis.

Depending on the magnitude of expansion, haemorrhage in the suture will occur. According to Chang, the vascular invasion by the blood clot is crucial for the new bone formation, due to the major osteogenic role of the paravascular cells (Chang et al. 1997). A recent study confirmed the role of the blood clot in healing, by showing that thrombin-related peptide accelerated the regeneration of bone following distraction osteogenesis (Amir et al. 2007). However, the stressed periosteum also plays a role in the healing process as tensile strain initiates the differentiation of the periosteal cells into osteogenic cells (Kanno et al. 2005). Although the risk of buccal dehiscence is reduced by using the SARME, the potential risk of periodontal damage between the upper central incisors should be taken into consideration (Cureton and Cuenin 1999).

Orthodontic effects in adult patients

Tissue reaction to orthodontic loading

The tissue reaction to the application of an orthodontic force is the result of the interaction between the mechanical perturbation generated by the orthodontic appliance and the modelling and remodelling of the alveolar bone. The clinician can control the force system delivered by the appliance. The tissues that are affected by the mechanical loading comprise: the root surface, the periodontal ligament (PDL) and the alveolar bone. Each tissue has its own cellular and extracellular elements and mechanical properties, and behaviour is controlled by both local and systemic factors (Verna et al. 1999).

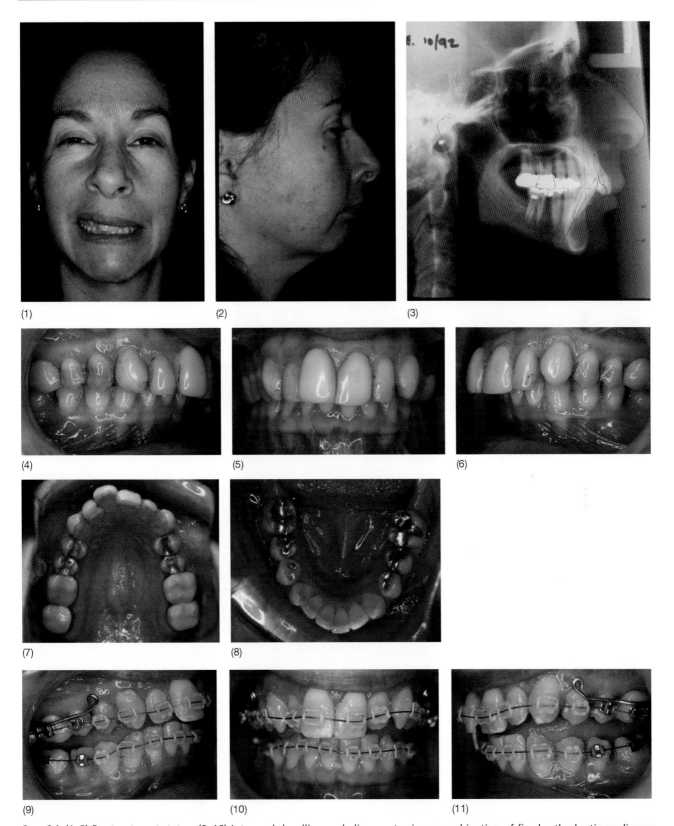

Case 6.1 (1–8) Pre-treatment status. (9–16) Intra-arch levelling and alignment using a combination of fixed orthodontic appliances and a bite plane. (17–23) End of treatment status. A dual bite has been established. (24–28) Five years following treatment. The mandible can no longer be forced back into a Class II relationship.

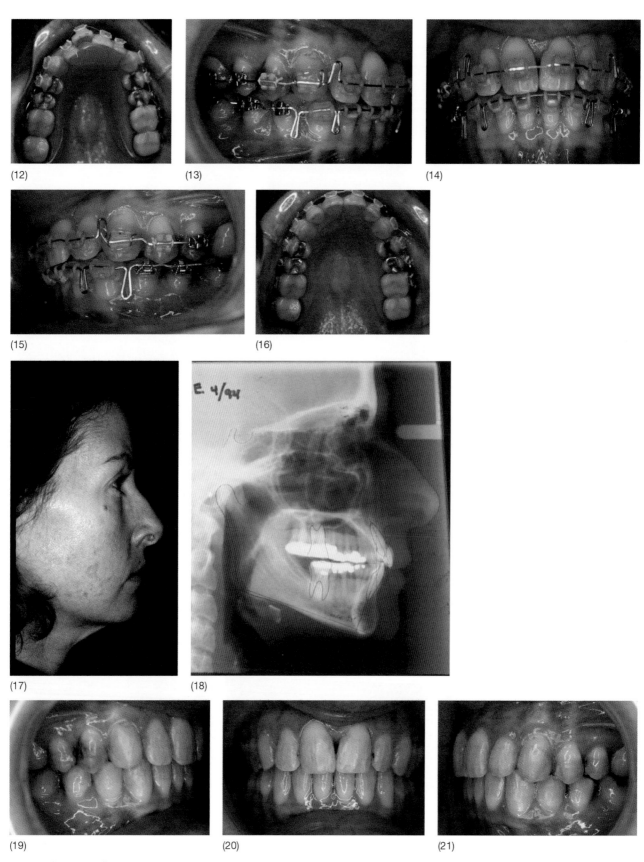

(12)

(13)

(14)

(15)

(16)

(17)

(18)

(19)

(20)

(21)

Case 6.1 (*Continued*)

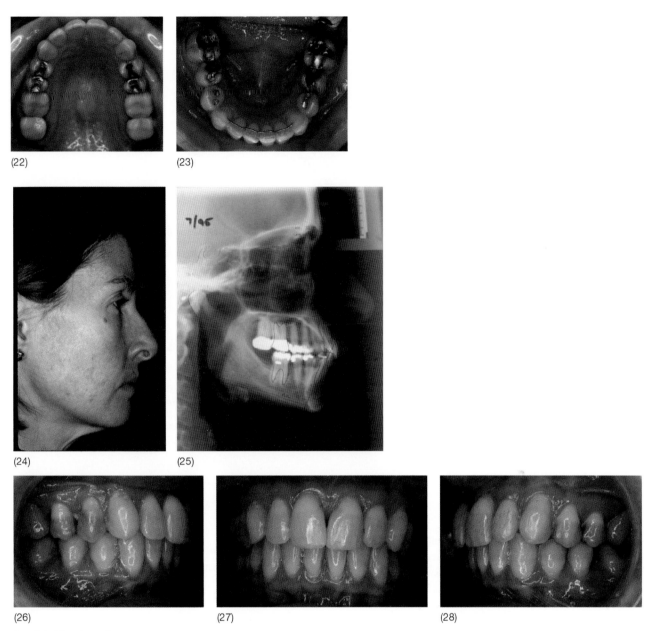

(22)   (23)

(24)   (25)

(26)   (27)   (28)

Case 6.1 (*Continued*)

Orthodontic tooth movement is a particular model of mechanical loading, due to the fact that the applied force to the teeth is transmitted to the alveolar bone via the PDL, whose mechanical properties are complicated by its nonisotropic structure. The reaction of the alveolar wall leading to tooth displacement has typically been ascribed as secondary to the reaction of the PDL. However, tooth movement depends on the turnover of the alveolar bone surrounding the PDL and this interaction is still a matter of debate in the field of orthodontic research. We still do not know all steps in the cascade of events that transform a mechanical perturbation into a biological reaction. Based on cellular research, the traditional discussion about pressure and tension has become irrelevant, as cells can hardly discriminate between pressure and tension, and instead react to difference in strain (Ehrlich and Lanyon 2002; Benjamin and Hillen 2003).

When treating adult patients, special attention should be paid to physiological age-related changes (Barnett and Rowe 1986; Jager 1996; Krall et al. 1997; Johnson et al. 2002; Jonasson 2005; Misawa-Kageyama et al. 2007) as well as changes related to metabolic diseases and chronic medication, both being more frequent in adult patients (Johnson et al. 2002; Verna et al. 2003, 2006; Kalia et al. 2004). In addition to the variation related to age, the response to identical stimuli varies considerably between individuals. Experiments carried out on dogs have clearly confirmed this clinical observation (Pilon et al. 1996; von Bohl et al. 2004a).

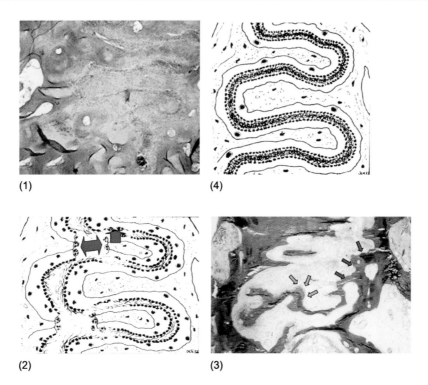

(1)   (4)

(2)   (3)

Fig. 6.2 1) Histological image of the midpalatal suture obtained at vautopsy from a 14 year old girl. Note the severe interdigitation illustrated in the drawing in 2). 3) A drawing illustrating the results of an expansion of a heavily interdigitated suture. The expansion would most likely lead to fractures of the bony extensions into the suture. A repair of these fractures are reflected in the presence of osteoclasts as indicated with the red arrows. 4) Histological image of a biopsy retrieved 6 weeks after expansion. Note the repair of fractures generated during the expansion. *Trans Eur Orthod Soc* 499–507 with kind permission the European Society.

The classical pressure–tension model

Within the classical view of the tissue reaction to orthodontic force systems, a clear distinction has been made between pressure and tension zones (Reitan and Rygh 1994). On the application of a force, within minutes, the tooth will be displaced inside the PDL with compression of the tissues in the direction of the tooth movement. On the tension side, widening of the PDL occurs and, within hours, the diameter of the blood vessels increases.

Based on electron microscopic studies, an outflow of blood constituents occurs in areas where the pressure leads to obstruction of blood vessels. Fibroblasts exhibited swelling of endoplasmic reticulum followed by rupture of the cytoplasmic membrane and loss of cytoplasm (Rygh and Brudvik 1995). Collagen fibrils in the PDL, nevertheless, retain their banded appearance but the glassy appearance of these areas gave this process the name hyalinization, which is in fact a sterile necrosis caused by the ischaemia. The hyalinized zone is removed by macrophages without a ruffled border. The tooth will not move until the bone covered by hyalinized PDL is resorbed by osteoclasts recruited from the bone marrow spaces of the spongiosa (or from the subcortical marrow if no spongiosa is present; Figure 6.3) (Baron 1975a). Once the undermining or

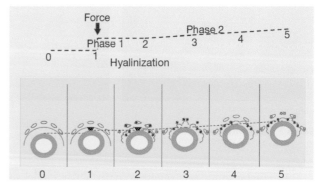

Fig. 6.3 Tooth movement through bone. When hyalinization occurs (1), the tooth does not move until the hyalinized tissue is removed via indirect resorption (2). In areas where no hyalinization occurs, bone is resorbed by osteoclasts recruited from the periodontal ligament, via direct resorption. (With permission from Verna C (2000) Biology of dental movement. In Melsen B and Fiorelli G (eds) *Biomechanics in Orthodontics, A Multimedia Textbook*, pp. 38–67. Arezzo, Italy: Libra Ortodonzia).

indirect resorption has reached the alveolar wall, the tooth will become loose, and resorption in the direction of the tooth movement can continue in the case of a light force as frontal or direct resorption, with osteoclasts acting directly on the alveolar wall. If, however, the force level is still high

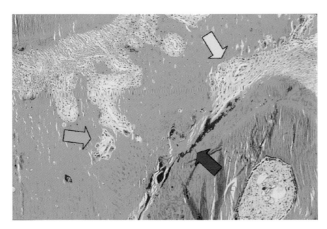

Fig. 6.4 Histological transverse section of the first root of a rat upper molar after 21 days of orthodontic force application. When the periodontal ligament is overcompressed, hyalinization occurs (red arrow) and the bone adjacent to the hyalinized tissue is resorbed by osteoclasts recruited from the marrow spaces (green arrow). The width of the periodontal ligament is not as wide as in the areas where bone resorption is carried out by the periodontal ligament cells (yellow arrow). (With permission from Verna C (2000) Biology of dental movement. In Melsen B and Fiorelli G (eds) *Biomechanics in Orthodontics, A Multimedia Textbook*, pp. 38–67. Arezzo, Italy: Libra Ortodonzia).

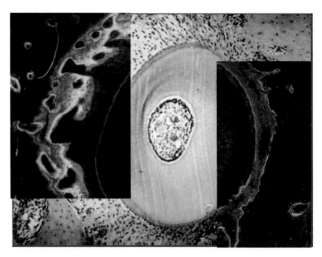

Fig. 6.5 Bone formation markers (tetracycline in yellow and calcein in green) observed in alveolar bone of a rat after the application of an orthodontic load. Note the lack of bone markers on the scalloped bone surface, typical of bone resorption in the direction of the force (right side). On the other side, a wide strip of bone markers, typical of new bone formation is seen. (With permission from Verna C (2000) Biology of dental movement. In Melsen B and Fiorelli G (eds) Biomechanics in Orthodontics, A Multimedia Textbook, pp. 38–67. Arezzo, Italy: Libra Ortodonzia).

enough to cause local ischaemia, renewed hyalinization and indirect resorption from the marrow spaces may occur (Fig. 6.4). Following the movement of the tooth, bone apposition is seen on the tension side (Fig. 6.5).

The so-called pressure-tension theory has been considered the state of the art and numerous studies have adopted this approach (Fig. 6.6). However, the notion of changes in the pressure within the PDL has also been questioned. Based on the physical properties of the PDL, that is, since it acts as a continuous hydrostatic system, Bien (1966) claimed that it is physically impossible to generate areas of specific pressure or tension within the PDL. Consequently, the initial distribution of the forces within the PDL is not constant and changes cannot be maintained. This view has been supported by Isaacson et al. (1993). Nanda and Heller (1979) have also questioned the determinant role of the PDL, showing that a biophysical modification of the PDL before tooth movement did not change the tissue reaction of the alveolar wall. They concluded that the distortion of the bone might be the primary stimulus for the cascade of events leading to the modelling of the alveolus.

No clear consensus has been reached concerning the relative contribution of the displacement of the tooth within the PDL and of bone bending to the initial tooth movement. Some authors ascribe a substantial role in initial tooth movement to bone bending (Roberts et al. 1992). The role played by bone bending may be proportional to the initially applied force (Grimm 1972). This notion was in contradiction to Storey (1973), who studied rodents and concluded that bone bending is substantially irrelevant, being even smaller

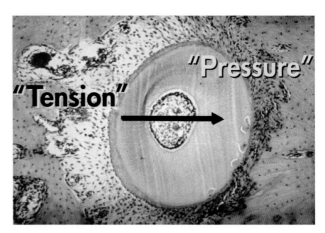

Fig. 6.6 Initial tooth movement following the application of the force in the direction indicated by the arrow. In the direction of the force, the periodontal ligament (PDL) becomes initially narrow and according to the distribution of the stresses, direct or indirect resorption occurs. This area has always been termed as the pressure area. On the opposite side, widening of the PDL is observed and cellular activity is characterized by bone apposition. This area has traditionally been termed as the tension side. (With permission from Verna C (2000) Biology of dental movement. In Melsen B and Fiorelli G (eds) *Biomechanics in Orthodontics, A Multimedia Textbook*, pp. 38–67. Arezzo, Italy: Libra Ortodonzia).

than the threshold of 0.1 mm detectable by the instruments. The methodological problem related to the differentiation between displacement within the PDL and bone bending makes it difficult to draw substantive conclusions. In spite of the different approaches and problems noted, the framework of pressure and tension areas is still a dominant theory.

A different approach to the analysis of the tissue reactions would be to start from the mechanical load, and follow the cascade occurring in the two main compartments (the PDL and the alveolar bone) separately until the same final result has been reached, i.e. modelling/ remodelling of the supporting tissues. The PDL has traditionally been considered the tissue from which resorption and formation of bone were orchestrated. This is surprising since it is well known that the principal detectors of mechanical strains in bone are the osteocytes.

Periodontal Ligament

Intermittent occlusal forces resulting in tension of the periodontal fibres are necessary for the maintenance of the alveolar bone. When these occlusal forces are absent, the density of the alveolar bone is dramatically reduced (see Chapter 3, Fig. 3.21) (Picton 1964).

Loadings with a different direction or duration than those occurring during normal function result in a permanent displacement of the tooth within the viscoelastic PDL. The change in the stress/strain distribution leads to a change in the fluid distribution and, due to the oblique alveolar surface, a horizontal force will result in a shearing, leading to extrusion. This effect has been referred to as the cone effect and depends on the inclination of the alveolar wall. It is usually resisted by the supracrestal fibres, but when the PDL is compromised, extrusion may occur. In adult patients with marginal bone loss, this effect will be more pronounced, and the applied force should have a small intrusive component to avoid extrusion (Fig. 6.7).

When an orthodontic load is applied the periodontal fibres, the PDL cells, and the extracellular matrix (ECM) are submitted to a deformation and a reduction in mechanical strength, particularly on the compression side (Fukui 1993). These changes are also present on adjacent teeth (Ki 1990) but are rapidly restored with retention (Fukui et al. 2003).

In vitro studies have shown that cell deformation is related to metabolic activity (Chicurel et al. 1998). The cytoskeleton represents a possible transducer of mechanical loading by means of the interaction with the ECM via the binding glycoprotein integrins (Talic et al. 2004). It has been demonstrated that cells use tensegrity architecture for their organization, that is, cells are hard-wired to respond immediately to mechanical stresses transmitted through cell surface receptors (Fig. 6.8). The cytoskeleton is physically coupled to the extracellular matrix thus tuning cellular response at a gene regulation level (Ingber 1997). From this perspective, the integrity of the cell membrane in the mechanotransduction pathway is taken into consideration, since it has been demonstrated that trauma facilitates mechano sensitivity (Wan et al. 1999), and PDL cells have been found to experience membrane disruption and resealing on

application of orthodontic force (Orellana-Lezcano et al. 2005).

Displacement of the fluid within the PDL generates shear stresses and to experience membrane disruption and resealing contributes to membrane deformation (Bien 1966). The dynamic of fluids in the PDL is mainly sustained by the vascular system that provides the PDL with essential cells and oxygen necessary for its remodelling (Rygh et al. 1986). Fifty percent of the PDL volume is occupied by blood vessels, with the highest percentage adjacent to the bony side. In the area of pressure, partial or complete occlusion of vessels leading to hyalinization is observed after 24 hours, whereas on the tension side, blood vessels are dilated. After 7 days of treatment, in the area of pressure, vascularization is re-established by invasion of vascular structures into the hyalinized areas whereas on the tension side, increased blood supply is still present (Khouw and Goldhaber 1970). The changes in density and distribution of blood vessels during tooth movement have been shown to be related to changes in the neural response (Vandevska-Radunovic et al. 1997).

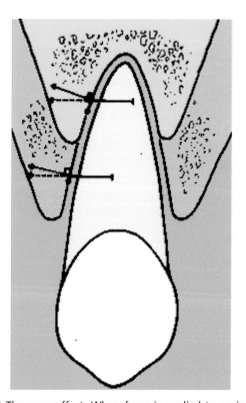

Fig. 6.7 The cone effect. When force is applied to an inclined plane there is resolution of the force into horizontal and vertical components. The vertical force is usually resisted by the supracrestal fibres, but when the periodontal ligament is compromised, extrusion is possible. (With permission from Verna C (2000) Biology of dental movement. In Melsen B and Fiorelli G (eds) *Biomechanics in Orthodontics, A Multimedia Textbook*, pp. 38–67. Arezzo, Italy: Libra Ortodonzia).

The cell pool assigned to anabolic activities includes PDL fibroblasts, osteoblasts and cementoblasts. The osteoprogenitor cells reside in the environment of the blood vessels in the area of the PDL close to the alveolar wall. Pavlin and Gluhak-Heinrich (2001) concluded that the induction of differentiation and increase in cell function are the primary responses to osteogenic loading, and suggested that the mechanical signal may be targeting osteoblast precursors without the initial proliferative response. The final result is an increased production of collagen, increased ECM synthesis, up-regulation of anti-apoptotic factors and increased matrix metalloproteinase 8 (MMP-8) production, as detected in crevicular fluid (Danciu et al. 2004; Ingman et al. 2005). Catabolic activity occurs in osteoclasts originating from the hemopoietic system by the differentiation of the monocyte series. The first resorbing cells on the alveolar wall are osteoclasts, the origin of which has been attributed to post-mitotic fusion of pre-osteoclasts

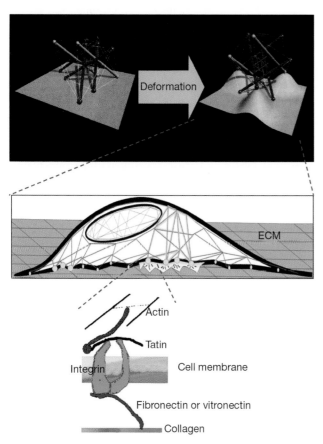

Fig. 6.8 Schematization of the architectural organization of cells following tensegrity. Secondary to mechanical perturbation, the extracellular matrix (ECM) is deformed along with the cell surface (top panel). Cells adhere to the ECM via integrin (middle panel), proteins that connect the ECM with the internal cytoskeleton (bottom panel). The cytoskeleton that supports the cell architecture is thus modified and transmits the signal at the nuclear level. (Modified from Ingber DE (1998) The architecture of life. Sci Am 278, 48–57, with permission from Scientific American).

from the cell pool present in the PDL (Tsay et al. 1999). According to Rody et al. (2001), the clasts originated from the bone marrow, where a significant increase in proliferation is already evident on the first day of loading (Fig. 6.9).

Biochemically, the mechanical perturbation causes an up-regulation of prostaglandins, release of nitric oxide (NO), and regulation of the expression of endothelial nitric oxide synthase (ecNOS). Both NO and prostaglandins are assumed to work as second messengers in the transduction pathway (Burger and Klein-Nulen 1999). The release of substance P by the sensory nerve endings in the PDL enhances prostaglandins release, leucocyte migration and secretion of lymphokines and the subsequent significant rise in levels of intracellular second messengers (cAMP, cGMP) (Davidovitch et al. 1988; Yamashiro et al. 2000). Together with prostaglandins, leukotrienes are mediators of orthodontic tooth movement, stimulating bone resorption and promoting the production of collagenase by fibroblasts that invade the hyalinized zones. This phenomenon together with a stimulation of movement of calcium in the cell has been suggested to be the mechanism by which leukotrienes enhance the remodelling of the PDL (Mohammed et al. 1989). Cytokines, soluble low-weight molecules secreted by most nucleated cells, modulate bone remodelling, coordinating metabolic responses from neighbouring cells. Among the cytokines, those that can influence connective tissue remodelling include interleukins (ILs), tumour necrosis factor (TNF) and its ligand family, interferons (IFNs), polypeptide growth factors (PGF) and colony stimulating factors (CSF).

Bone

When teeth are submitted to a force the surrounding alveolar bone undergoes deformation which is inversely proportional to the distance from the tooth apex (Asundi and Kishen 2000). Due to the stiff nature of intact *in vivo* bone,

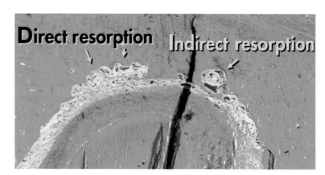

Fig. 6.9 Paraocclusal section of a rat root after 21 days of orthodontic force application. Both direct and indirect resorption can be present on the pressure side, depending on the local stress–strain distribution of the forces. (With permission from Verna C (2000) Biology of dental movement. In Melsen B and Fiorelli G (eds) *Biomechanics in Orthodontics, A Multimedia Textbook*, pp. 38–67. Arezzo, Italy: Libra Ortodonzia).

mechanical loads are translated to strains in the order of 0.2% (Burr et al. 1996).

Two types of activity in bone occur throughout life, modelling and remodelling. Adding to the confusion, orthodontists have applied only the word remodelling to cover both phenomena. Modelling is the dominant biological activity during growth, where it leads to changes in bone size and shape. Modelling is largely controlled by genetic programming and also by functional loads, and less so by systemic metabolic stimuli. In adult life, modelling causes the physiological drift of the alveolar socket and induces structural adaptation of bone to different mechanical demands (Frost 1990a). During tooth displacement the PDL width and bone thickness is maintained through coordinated resorption and apposition, thus resulting in

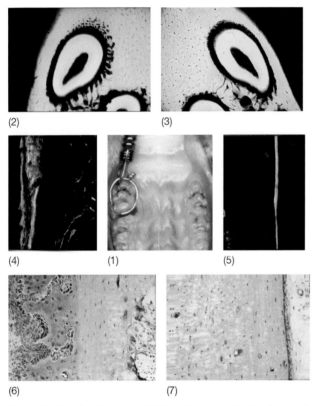

(2)   (3)

(4)   (1)   (5)

(6)   (7)

Fig. 6.10 Alveolar bone modelling during orthodontic tooth movement. After the application of 25 g of force a mesial tipping is produced in a rat first molar (1). After 14 days of treatment, the microradiographic analysis shows new bone formation ahead of the tooth on the treated side (2) compared with the untreated side (3). On the buccal side, new periosteal bone formation is observed, as shown by the wide strips of bone markers (4). Green = calcein, yellow = tetracycline. (5) Note the thin lines of bone markers on the untreated buccal side in contrast to the treated side. (6) Treated side at a higher magnification with toluidine-blue staining reveals intense new bone formation by active osteoblasts. (7) The untreated side does not show any new bone formation. (With permission from Verna C (2000) Biology of dental movement. In Melsen B and Fiorelli G (eds) *Biomechanics in Orthodontics, A Multimedia textbook*, pp. 38–67. Arezzo, Italy: Libra Ortodonzia).

drift of the whole alveolus (Baron 1975b) (Fig. 6.10). From animal studies, however, it seems that the process is more complex (Vignery and Baron 1980; Tran Van et al. 1982; Baron et al. 1984; King et al. 1992; Keeling et al. 1993; Melsen 1999). Bone formation has also been demonstrated in the direction of the force and bone resorption on the so-called tension side (Mohri et al. 1991; King et al. 1992; Zaffe and Verna 1995) . The presence of markers of both resorption and formation activities throughout the whole alveolar bone is well in agreement with the interaction between osteoblasts and osteoclasts seen in relation to the remodelling process (Fig. 6.11).

Remodelling occurs in discrete locations, involving a sequence of resorption and subsequent formation, spatially and temporally coupled, by the basic multicellular unit (BMU) (Frost 1964). Remodelling enables bone to adapt to mechanical stresses, minimizing fatigue damages, and is influenced by the action of hormones and cytokines (Mori and Burr 1993; Frost 1998). Synchronized initiation of numerous BMUs characterizes both pressure and tension sides.

The bone remodelling sequence is composed of four phases: activation, resorption, reversal and formation (Fig. 6.12). In the activation phase, lining cells change from a pancake-like to a cuboidal shape, the pre-osteoblasts, and secrete receptor activator of nuclear factor κ-B (RANK) ligand (RANKL), which remains bound to the cell surface. RANK receptors are present on cell membrane of preosteoclasts recruited from the bone marrow, which on activation by RANKL, fuse and differentiate into mature multinucleated osteoclasts and resorb bone. The resorption of bone also occurs as the result of inhibitory activities towards osteoblasts, as in the case of the release of sclerostin that inhibits bone formation and enhance osteoblast apoptosis (Winkler et al. 2003). At the same time, osteoprotegerin (OPG, a free-floating decoy receptor belonging to the TNF family) can bind the RANKL, thus preventing the activation of the RANK. The RANK-RANKL mechanism

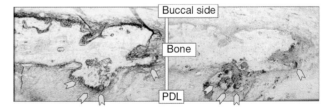

Fig. 6.11 Alveolar bone on the buccal side of a rat tooth after 14 days of orthodontic treatment. On the side facing the periodontal ligament (arrows) staining is positive for both alkaline phosphatase, i.e. bone formation (dark blue, left panel), and acid phosphatase, i.e. bone resorption (red, right panel). (With permission from Verna C (2000) Biology of dental movement. In Melsen B and Fiorelli G (eds) *Biomechanics in Orthodontics, A Multimedia Textbook*, pp. 38–67. Arezzo, Italy: Libra Ortodonzia).

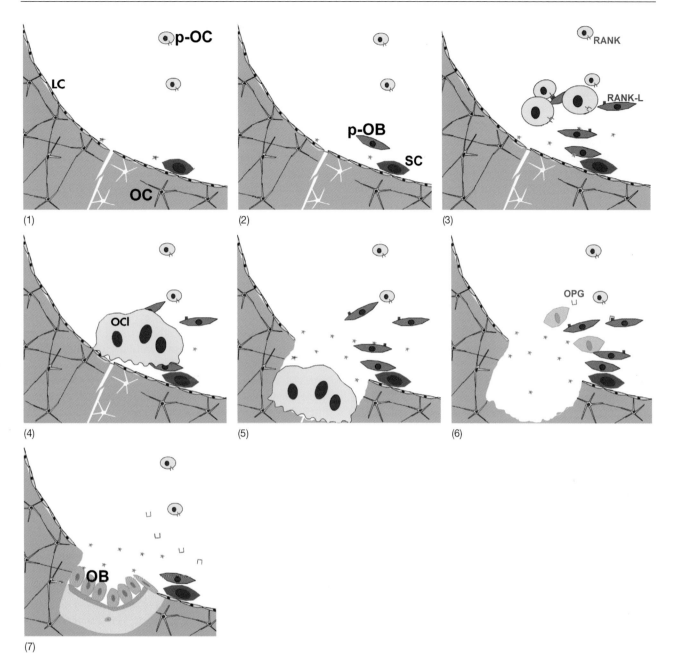

Fig. 6.12 (1) On a quiescent bone surface, osteocytes (OC) secrete sclerostin (*), which inhibits Wnt (protein that activate cell membrane receptors) signalling in cells near the surface. Pre-osteoclasts (p-OC) circulate in the bone marrow. A sudden stress results in a micro-crack. The osteocyte underneath the crack undergoes apoptosis. Osteocytes detect strains and secrete factors, including growth factors, prostaglandins and nitric oxide. LC = lining cells. (2) The stromal cells (SC) are now released from sclerostin inhibition and exposed to interleukin-1. They generate pre-osteoblasts. Stromal cells also secrete mononuclear phagocyte colony-stimulating factor (M-CSF), which helps generate the pre-osteoclasts. * = releasing factors. (3) The pre-osteoblasts proliferate and also secrete more factors, such as Wnt, interleukins and bone morphogenetic proteins. The pre-osteoblasts start to express receptor activator for nuclear factor κ-B ligand (RANK-L) on their surface. Pre-osteoclasts have RANK receptors on their surface. The activated pre-osteoclasts fuse to form an osteoclast. (4,5) The lining cells change shape and expose the collagen. The osteoclasts bind to the bone matrix with integrins and secrete acid cathepsin K to resorb the bone. Bone resorption at this spot takes about 2 weeks. Bone-derived growth factors, insulin-like growth factor (IGF) and transforming growth factor (TGF)-β are released. (6) Preosteoblast proliferate and mature into osteoblasts, which stops producing RANK-L and secrete OPG (osteoprotegerin) instead. The OPG binds to RANK, which blocks activation of the pre-osteoclasts. (7) The osteoblasts lining the resorption cavity secrete osteoid and then mineralize it to fill in the cavity in 3–4 months. The matrix also contains other proteins and growth factors, such as IGF and TGF-β. Some osteoblasts become osteocytes, some become lining cells, and the rest undergo apoptosis. Meanwhile, new osteocytes are establishing intercellular connections with older ones and after they are embedded in the new bone they secrete sclerostin and inhibit the surface cells. The microdamage is thus repaired. The new matrix will accumulate mineral and increase in density for about 3 years. (Reproduced with permission of Prof S Ott from Osteoporosis and Bone Physiology http://courses.washington.edu/bonephys).

has been shown to be present in the PDL and is enhanced by mechanical loading (Ogasawara et al. 2004). Local delivery of RANKL has been shown to accelerate tooth movement. The up-regulation of RANKL induced by orthodontic force has been shown to be dependent on the presence of PGE_2, which is released by osteoblasts and oste-ocytes (Kanzaki et al. 2006). Following orthodontic load, Kanzaki et al. (2004) found that the lack of OPG induced a significantly higher level of bone resorption in the compression area, while the delivery of OPG reduced tooth movement rate.

Bone resorption lasts for about 2 weeks after which the osteoclasts undergo programmed cell death or apoptosis. In the reversal phase mononuclear phagocyte cells come in contact with bone, completing the resorption and deepening the lacunae (Eriksen et al. 1994). Pre-osteoblasts migrate into the resorbed cavity and differentiate into osteoblasts. The border between the resorbed old bone and the new formed bone is called the cement line or reversal line. Fibroblasts also migrate towards the cement line and secrete thin collagen fibrils around which osteoblasts start synthesizing osteoid. The fibrils are then embedded into bone matrix and the subsequent mineralization firmly anchors them into the new bone (Saffar et al. 1997).

Bone formation needs the differentiation of preosteoblasts into osteoblasts. The former are probably attracted by the bone-derived growth factor transforming growth factor (TGF)-β. This derived from marrow stromal cells, which can differentiate into either adipocytes or osteoblasts. The active, secreting osteoblasts then synthesize layers of osteoid and slowly refill the cavity. Through a positive feedback mechanism, they also secrete growth factors, oste- opontin, osteocalcin, and other proteins such as IGF-1 IL-6, bone morphogenetic proteins (BMPs) and fibroblast growth factor (FBF), which aims to stimulate osteoblast activity. When the osteoid thickness reaches about 6 μm, the mineralization process starts and after about 4 months, the resorption cavity is refilled with new bone with closely packed mineral crystals and subsequent increase in bone density.

Both modelling drift and remodelling are involved in the displacement of the alveolus. The cascade of events that transforms the applied force to the cellular reaction necessary for the displacement of the alveolus has been the subject of a multiple studies.

Bending of hydrated bone caused displacement of the extracellular fluids through inter-crystalline matrix spaces, and streaming generated potentials (SGPs) can be measured (Weinbaum et al. 1994). The electrical charges generated by SGPs may affect osteocytic somatic processes that, via a secondary message or low resistance gap junctions, transmit the signal to the osteoblasts and lining cells by the network (Cowin et al. 1991) (Fig. 6.13). At the same time, other streaming potentials generated by the interstitial fluid amplify the message (Burger and Klein-Nulen 1999).

As when loading a fluid-filled sponge, the interstitial fluid flows through the lacunar-canalicular network. Since osteocytes cell membranes and processes are located within the lacunar-canalicular network, they are directly subjected to the interstitial fluid's shear stress in loading conditions (Klein-Nulend et al. 2005). As stretch-activated ion channels have been found on bone cells, a direct mechanical deformation of the cell membrane cannot be excluded and any disruption in the tension of the extracellularly exposed integrin would transmit a signal to the osteocyte nucleus (Duncan and Turner 1995). It has recently been reported that bone cells possess primary cilia that project from the cell surface. They deflect during fluid flow and are required for osteogenic and bone resorptive responses to dynamic fluid flow (Malone et al. 2007). Nicolella et al. (2005) maintained that the osteocyte can modify the size of its lacunae and the diameter of its canaliculi, thereby modifying the bone fluid dramatically. For the same rate of bone fluid flow within canaliculi, a narrower canal diameter would increase shear stress, while widening the canal would decrease shear stress. This may explain why the ageing skeleton is less responsive to strain. Using a digital image correlation strain measurement technique, it has been found that macroscopic strains of about 0.2% amplified over 15 times at the osteocyte lacuna level. Strain patterns were highly heterogeneous and in some locations generated microdamage around osteocyte lacuna.

Microdamage increases with fatigue load at physiological levels and will result in bone remodelling and osteocyte apoptosis (Noble 2003). There is an increasing focus on the role of micro-cracks and microdamage in the initiation of bone resorption during orthodontic tooth movement. Verna et al. (2004) showed a significant increase in crack density in the direction of force after 1 days of treatment. Micro-cracks could therefore represent the first damage induced by orthodontic force (Verna et al. 2004). The generation of micro-cracks with the application of an orthodontic force is even more likely considering that the surface over which the forces are distributed (what has been called the lamina dura in the literature) is characterized by a series of rather small bony spicules (Fig. 6.14).

A new theory and its terminology

Based on orthopaedic research, it is common knowledge that loading leads to increased density of bone and that unloading, as in the case of space travel, leads to decreased bone density. It therefore seems controversial that the ortho-dontists associate compression with resorption.

The change in shape observed subsequent to loading in long bones is a result of apposition on the compressed side and resorption on the side on which tension prevails. A link between change in shape and biological activity in the alveolar bone was indicated by Epker and Frost (1965), who suggested that the control of the location of resorption and formation is related to the change in surface curvature of the alveolar walls. During tooth movement, the so-called 'pressure' side become flattened (less concave) and the opposite side tends to be more concave, as it is pulled by the periodontal fibres under tension (Fig. 6.15). Finite element analysis (FEA) has been used to study the load transfer of an orthodontic load from the tooth to the alveolar wall. The pressure and tension zones are observed only when the PDL is modelled as a solid with a linear relationship between load and deformation. However, it is unrealistic to assume that the PDL acts as a solid, due to its viscoelastic nature. When the material properties are realistically considered with regard to physical properties and morphology, it becomes clear that the stimulus to the alveolus cannot be explained in terms of pressure and tension. When applying

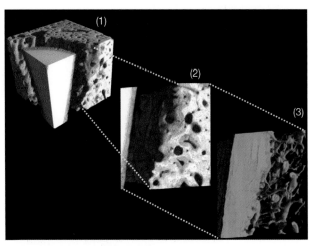

Fig. 6.14 (1) Three-dimensional reconstruction following high-resolution micro-CT scan of the molar root and the surrounding alveolar bone. (2) Detail of the tooth–bone interface with a false-colouring of the soft tissues. The dark grey layer represents less mineralized, newly formed bone. (3) Close-up of the soft tissues, showing the fine network of fibres and vessels penetrating the alveolar bone.

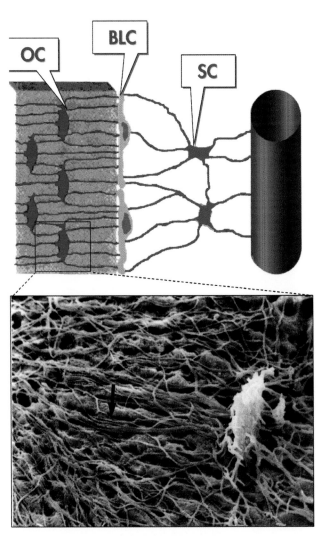

Fig. 6.13 Schematization of the wire transmission mechanism. The cells of the osteogenic lineage (stromal cells (SC), osteoblasts or bone lining cells (BLC), osteocytes (OC)) are connected through a functional syncytium that allows osteocytes to act as sensors of mechanical stresses. The cellular interaction is thus not only based on volume transmission (paracrine and endocrine stimulation), but also on wire transmission, as in neuronal communication. (With permission of Marotti G (1996) Int J Anat Embriol 101(4), and Firenze University Press (2000) J Musculoskelet Neuron Interact 1(2), 133–136).

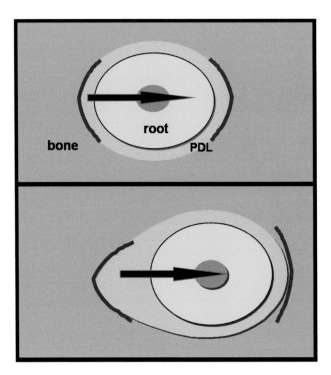

Fig. 6.15 Schematic illustration of the deformation of the alveolar bone in the horizontal plane after the application of an orthodontic force towards the right hand side. At the side towards which the tooth is moving, bone surface tends to be less concave, since the periodontal ligament fibres are not pulling. On the side from which the tooth is moving, bone surface tends to be more concave, since the PDL fibres are stretched. On the less concave bone surface, resorption prevails; on the concave surface, bone formation usually occurs. The changes in shape of the bone surface are called local strain operators and control the biological behaviour in mechanically induced modelling. (With permission from Verna C (2000) Biology of dental movement. In Melsen B and Fiorelli G (eds) *Biomechanics in Orthodontics, A Multimedia textbook*, pp. 38–67. Arezzo, Italy: Libra Ortodonzia).

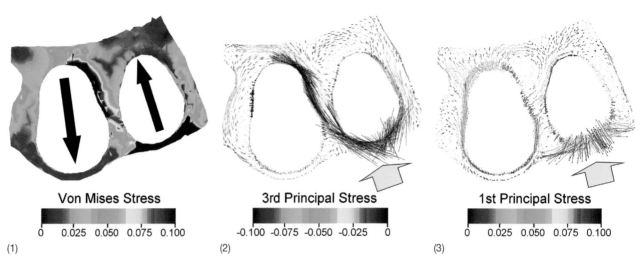

Fig. 6.16 Finite element study of a canine and a premolar in a coronal section of the alveolar bone, when a tipping movement is simulated in the direction of the arrow, with material properties assumed to be non-linear. Stress concentration described by Von Mises' stresses shows the lowest values in the direction of the force, while the contrary is observed on the opposite side (1). Compressive stresses are the lowest in the direction of the force (2), and tensile stresses (3) show the opposite trend. Notice that compressive and tensile stresses are simultaneously present in the same area (yellow arrow). (Cattaneo P et al. (2005) The finite element method: a tool to study orthodontic tooth movement. J Dent Res 84(5), 428–433. Copyright © 2005, Reprinted by permission of SAGE Publications).

low forces and considering the non-linear properties of the PDL, tension is by far more predominant than pressure (Cattaneo et al. 2005). On the 'pressure' side, the fibres of the PDL become curled up and practically no stresses are transferred onto the alveolar wall. The frontal, direct resorption can therefore be perceived as resorption caused by remodelling, as the strain will be below the minimum effective strain (MES) defined by Frost (1990b). This perception has been corroborated by the observation that even minimal forces are sufficient to initiate the cascade leading to tooth movement (Weinstein et al. 1963; Ren et al. 2004). As depicted in Figure 6.16, no tension and very little compressive strain are present in the bone in the direction of the force. In the alveolar wall, the tensile stresses generated by the pulling of the PDL fibres are transformed into compressive hoop stresses analogous to the principle of the roman arch. This means that both tensile and compressive stresses co-exist in the 'tension' side. In this perspective, the PDL acts as a bone distractor device with potential implication in bone regeneration, particularly needed in the often deteriorated dentition of adult patients (Fig. 6.17).

Direct frontal resorption rarely occurs at the beginning of a tooth movement and, as the lamina dura is not a smooth surface, areas of hyalinization may be found throughout the entire tooth movement even with light forces (von Bohl et al. 2004a). Empty osteocyte lacunae are observed in the alveolar walls beneath the hyalinization, although osteocytes of the adjacent alveolar bone seemed to be intact. Studies using specific apoptosis markers have shown signs of degeneration and apoptosis and a lack of lining cells

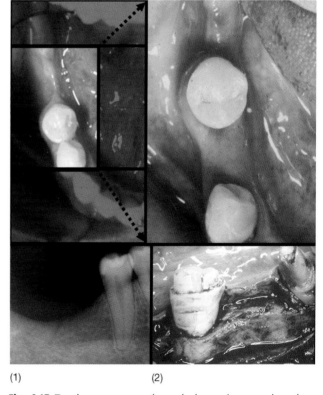

Fig. 6.17 Tooth movement through bone in an edentulous alveolar crest, where no bone is present (1, top and bottom). Alveolar drift allows for the movement of the whole alveolus (2, top panel), and the osteogenic potential of the periodontal ligament (PDL) is fully expressed in the formation of the new bone (2, bottom panel). (Courtesy of A. Fontenelle).

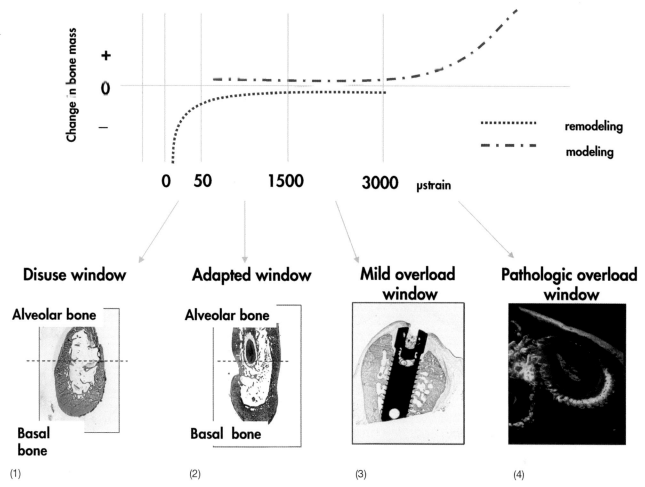

Fig. 6.18 Describing the mechanical usage of bone, Frost defines four 'windows' according to the increasing size of bone strain, where remodelling, modelling and the rapid acceleratory phenomenon (RAP) occur to different extents. (1) The acute disuse window, where remodelling increases up to five times and no remodelling or RAP activities are present. The minimum effective strain for remodelling (MESr) is in this case 50–100 µstrain. It can be the case in resorption of edentulous crests. (2) The adapted window (between 50–100 and 1000–1500 µstrain), where BMUs equalize resorption and formation, no remodelling or RAP. This tends to conserve bone and its strength. This occurs during normal mechanical usage. (3) Mild overuse window (between 1000–1500 and 3000 µstrain), where lamellar drifts usually occurs, with normal formation of BMUs, no RAP and little microdamage. The minimum effective strain is (MESm), in this case, 1500 µstrain. It is usually the case of adaptation of bones to growth and in strain caused by some dental implants (modelling). (4) Pathological overload window (>3000 µstrain), where microdamage occurs and BMUs increase in the repair process. At the same time, BMUs increase because of a RAP phenomenon and woven bone drift occurs. The MESp (minimum effective strain pathological) is in this case 3000 µstrain. Excessive orthodontic forces can easily cause such a reaction, with the result of a weakening of bone structure. At about 25 000 µstrain, the bone's ultimate capacity to bear strain is reached and fracture occurs. Some non-mechanical factors (genes, hormones, vitamin, minerals, drugs and other agents) seem to be able to modify the above listed MES thresholds (Frost 1998), thus explaining the onset of some diseases. (With permission from Verna C (2000) Biology of dental movement. In Melsen B and Fiorelli G (eds) *Biomechanics in Orthodontics, A Multimedia Textbook*, pp. 38–67. Arezzo, Italy: Libra Ortodonzia).

(Hamaya et al. 2002). Based on these findings, it would be more reasonable to perceive indirect resorption as a repair process. The word pressure is probably still appropriate to use in cases of high concentration of forces over small surfaces, where blood pressure is overcome, blood vessels and PDL constituents are compressed, and root surface is separated from alveolar bone only by areas of hyalinization.

In accordance with more recent research, the words pressure and tension should be avoided, and instead the tissue reaction related to the stress/strain distribution described in the mechanostat theory of Frost (2003) (Fig. 6.18) should be used. According to this theory the woven bone commonly observed ahead of the tooth and on the periosteal surface can be considered a rapid acceleratory phenomenon (RAP), i.e. a healing process (Melsen 1999; Verna 1999) (Fig. 6.19).

Tooth movement can be performed 'with bone' or 'through bone'. When the tooth is moved in a mesiodistal direction, this generally does not represent a problem. However, particular attention should be paid when the

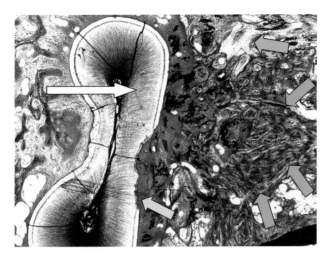

Fig. 6.19 Horizontal section of a monkey mandibular molar after the application of an orthodontic load (white arrow). Note the formation of woven bone in the direction of the force, as a sign of rapid acceleratory phenomenon tissue repair (green arrows). Woven bone is less dense than old bone (blue arrow). Root resorption (yellow arrow) also occurs on the so-called compression side.

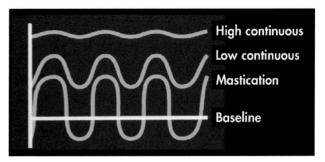

Fig. 6.20 The rhythmic activity of mastication interferes with the type of force delivered by the appliance. The lighter the force is the larger is the influence of the chewing activities, as shown by this diagram. In other words, the so- called continuous light forces are in reality intermittent due to the interference of mastication. On the other hand, the use of high forces ensures a better constancy of delivery, as the forces of mastication do not interfere with them. However, continuous forces are more detrimental for the periodontal ligament than intermittent forces. (With permission from Verna C (2000) Biology of dental movement. In Melsen B and Fiorelli G (eds) *Biomechanics in Orthodontics, A Multimedia Textbook*, pp. 38–67. Arezzo, Italy: Libra Ortodonzia).

movement has to generate modelling of the alveolar process to move teeth outside their given envelope, since success of this treatment depends on the movement 'with bone'. In case of movement against cortical bone, hyalinization should be minimized in order to obtain direct resorption (Baron 1975b). In case of a thin cortex and hyalinization, indirect resorption will occur from the periosteal surface, resulting in the generation of bone fenestration. The classification of tooth movement as 'with bone' or 'through bone' can be revised in a loading history perspective:

- 'With bone': the mechanical load is within the very narrow 'mild overload window' (1500-3000 microstrain). Lamellar bone formation drift and only little microdamage.
- 'Through' bone: the mechanical load exceeds the 3000 microstrain, being in the 'pathological overload window'. Hyalinization of the PDL, ischaemia-induced necrosis of the lining cells and microdamage of the bone in the direction of the force will be repaired by increased BMU activation frequency and destruction of alveolar wall.

The modelling of the alveolar process generated when a tooth is moved 'with bone' enables the clinician to perform tooth movement otherwise considered impossible (Fig. 6.17).

Orthodontist-related factors

The local stress/strain distribution is determined by the line of action of the force, which can be monitored by variation in the moment-to-force ratio delivered at the bracket. The variables controlled by the orthodontist include the magnitude, the distribution, the timing of the application, whether continuously or intermittent, and the duration of the treatment.

Force delivery regimens have been classified as continuous, interrupted continuous or intermittent (Reitan and Rygh 1994). At the tissue level, variation in the stress/strain distribution is a product of the interaction of the applied force system with the variation caused by functions such as chewing and swallowing (Fig. 6.20). The individual stimulus has to be above the threshold for the initial reaction and the duration of the stimulus long enough to initiate the cascade of biological reactions. Due to the viscoelastic nature of the PDL, the magnitude and the duration of the stimulus are mutually dependent. As little as 4gr of force seems to be a sufficient stimulus if interaction from the surrounding environment is removed (Weinstein et al. 1963) and trying to identify an optimal force level for efficient orthodontic tooth movement is probably not possible as too many confounding factors are involved (Melsen et al. 2007). Nikolai estimated that the value of capillary blood pressure (between 20 and 47gr/cm^2) is the limit beyond which necrosis occurs, following the total ischemia of the PDL (Nikolai 1975). The magnitude of the applied load has to be chosen with respect to the individual variation in the supporting structures.

Fixed appliances deliver continuous forces but, provided the force level is kept low, a fluctuation in the stress/strain distribution in the periodontium is still occurring as a result of function, and the biological reaction is thus simulating the one generated by an intermittent force. Only in the case of a stainless steel wire and a short interbracket distance will the PDL perceive the orthodontic force system as continuous (Andersen et al. 1991). The terms continuous and intermittent should therefore be reconsidered. Lanyon and Rubin demonstrated that a continuous load did not trigger a biological reaction, while intermittent loads are sufficient to maintain bone architecture (Lanyon and Rubin 1984). It is likely that the increase in rate of tooth movement observed with lower forces is a reflection of the intermittent force system perceived by the periodontium.

Patient-related factors

Age

The tooth-supporting tissues are influenced by age (Fig. 6.21). At the PDL level, the turnover of collagen and proliferative activities of fibroblast-like cells decrease with age (Kyomen and Tanne 1997). In addition, the ratio of ground substance to collagen as well as the cell population (fibroblasts, osteoblasts and cementoblasts) increases with age (Manson and Lucas 1962). As a consequence, it has been observed that the initial tissue reaction to the orthodontic force system is delayed.

Also the relative extent of bone surface covered by 'active' osteoblasts seems to be smaller and the number of osteoclasts seems to be fewer in adult than in young patients (Melsen and Mosekilde 1980; Jager 1996). In older individuals, the marrow spaces are smaller, with fewer cells, and the alveolar walls are mainly composed by dense lamellar bone with few openings into the marrow spaces (Jager 1996). The delayed or absent compensatory bone formation at the periosteal margin observed with age can lead to loss of alveolar crestal height and increased risk of bone dehiscences. Cortical porosity in the mandible has been found to increase with age (Manson and Lucas 1962). The age-related marginal bone loss may be worsened in case of pathological changes in bone metabolism nd/or in progressive periodontal disease.

The tissue reactions required for orthodontic tooth movement are not age-dependent but make a difference to the treatment options relevant to young and adult patients. Forces used in adults should be lower than in children, especially at the beginning of tooth movement, as the pool of cells available to initiate the cascade of biological events is smaller. In a study on crestal bone height before and during treatment in adolescents and adults, Harris and Baker (1990) found a greater loss of bone in the adults, but the major differences were found at the start of treatment. This underlines the importance of a careful evaluation of the periodontal status before the treatment, and that the orthodontic treatment itself, if carefully performed, is not a risk *per se* (Harris and Baker 1990). In rats the rate of tooth movement is higher and the lag time shorter in young than in adult rats (Bridges et al. 1988), corresponding to the delayed bone formation in adults reported by Reitan (1951) and by a lower responsiveness of cytokine levels in the crevicular fluid of adult rats after orthodontic load (Ren et al. 2002). Another explanation for the longer lag time in adult rats may be the narrower PDL in adult rats, which makes it more vulnerable to hyalinization (Kabasawa et al. 1996). According to the findings of Ren et al. (2003) tooth movement, once it has started, can be equally efficient in young persons and adults.

Metabolic changes

The reaction of the alveolar bone to the orthodontic force system interacts with the ongoing bone remodelling, which is influenced by systemic factors. Since the prevalence of patients with metabolic disease taking long-term medications increases with age, the influence of bone metabolism on orthodontic tooth movement is particularly important when dealing with adult patients (Table 6.1).

Experimentally, the rate of tooth movement has been enhanced secondary to an increase in bone turnover generated by deprivation of oestrogen as in relation to menopause or after ovariectomy (Yamashiro et al. 1994; Arslan et al. 2007). Administration of oestrogen will on the other hand neutralize the effect of deprivation and decrease the rate of tooth movement. Pregnancy (Hellsing and Hammarstrom 1991) and lactation increase the rate of bone turnover and of tooth movement, as does a low calcium diet, possibly due to secondary hyperparathyroidism (Goldie and King 1984). High bone turnover can also be induced by the administration of thyroid hormone and, as anticipated, enhance tooth movement (Verna et al. 2000). Local

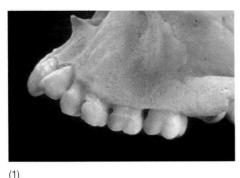
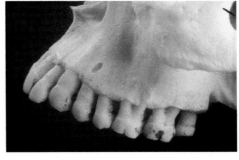

(1) (2)

Fig. 6.21 Maxillary bone from a young (1) and an adult (2) skull. Note the horizontal bone loss that has occurred with age in the adult bone when compared with the younger skull. (With permission from Melsen B and Fiorelli G (eds) (2000) *Biomechanics in Orthodontics, A Multimedia Textbook*, pp. 38–67. Arezzo, Italy: Libra Ortodonzia).

Table 6.1 Effects of systemic factors and drugs on induced tooth movement (modified from Gameiro et al. 2007).

	Effects on bone metabolism	Effects on tooth movement
Oestrogen	↓bone resorption	↓tooth movement
Androgen	↓bone resorption	unproven
Relaxin	↑bone resorption	↑tooth movement
Thyroid hormones	↑rate of bone remodelling	↑tooth movement
	↑bone resorption	↓root resorption
Parathyroid hormone	↑bone resorption	↑tooth movement
Vitamin D	↑rate of bone remodelling	↑tooth movement
	↑bone resorption	
Non-steroidal anti-inflammatory drugs		
Aspirin	↓bone resorption	↓tooth movement
Diclofenac	↓bone resorption	↓tooth movement
Ibuprofen	↓bone resorption	↓tooth movement
Indometacin	↓bone resorption	↓tooth movement
Celecoxib	↓bone resorption (in vitro)	No influence
Corticosteroids	↑bone resorption (chronic use)	↑tooth movement
Bisphosphonates	↓bone resorption	↓tooth movement
Paracetamol (acetaminophen)	Unproven	No influence

enhancement of resorption by injection of prostaglandins has been suggested by Yamasaki et al. (1984), a technique that has not been adopted in routine practice due to the pain associated with the procedure and to the fact that the coupling between resorption and formation has not been clarified.

Many adult patients take steroids for various reasons but the effect on tooth movement will be dependent on the duration of the administration as corticosteroid treatment initially has an inhibitory effect on bone turnover but subsequently leads to secondary hyperparathyroidism (Kalia et al. 2004).

Vitamin D administration has been found to increase tooth movement rate (Takano-Yamamoto et al. 1992).

Frequently used non-steroidal anti-inflammatory drugs have been shown to delay tooth movements due to their interference with the synthesis of prostaglandins. The analgesic that has been found not to interfere clinically with tooth movement is paracetamol (acetaminophen) (Mohammed et al. 1989; Kehoe et al. 1996; Arias and Marquez-Orozco 2007).

An increasing number of older patients are treated for osteoporosis with bisphosphonates. Originally bisphosphonates were used in the treatment of metabolic bone diseases and neoplasms localized to bone. Due to their increased use in the treatment of osteoporosis, adult potential orthodontic patients may be under bisphosphonate treatment. The action of the bisphosphonates is to reduce proliferation and inhibit osteoclast function and to induce osteoblasts to produce osteoclast-inhibiting factors. The effect of bisphosphonates has extensively been described as a reduction in resorption activity, but there is a general suppression of the turnover, since the alteration also includes the formative part of the remodelling cycle (Follet et al. 2007). With prolonged use, the average age of single units increases and, as a result, there is increased brittleness and accumulation of micro-damage.

As the number of patients treated with various types of bisphosphonate can be expected to increase, it is considered crucial that orthodontists take a thorough medication history in patients. The effect of bisphosphonates depends on the dosage and the duration of treatment. In low-risk patients, i.e. when the medication is given orally and for short duration, it can be expected that tooth movement will be considerably slowed down and compromise treatment. When there is a realistic risk of an adverse effect, major orthodontics should be avoided. A call for a proactive approach to bisphosphonate treatment was made by Zahrowski (2007), who recommended medication screening, patient counselling, informed consent, and, perhaps, changes in the offered treatment plans.

One adverse effect of bisphosphonates has been the development of osteonecrosis of the jaw bone, of which 60% developed secondary to dental interventions. A recent review reported that the majority of cases with jaw necrosis were of patients with cancer with bone metastasis, who received intravenous administration of bisphosphonates, although patients who had received the drug orally for osteoporosis were also reported to have osteonecrosis of the jaws (Woo et al. 2006). Before the focus on the iatrogenic damage caused by these drugs, bisphosphonates were injected to effect a significant reduction in the number of osteoclasts to reduce root resorption and enhance stability subperiosteally (Adachi et al. 1994; Igarashi et al. 1994, 1996; Liu et al. 2004).

Orthodontically induced apical root resorption

External root resorption is a known phenomenon associated with orthodontic treatment (Killiany 2002; Segal et al. 2004). Several potential risk factors relating both to the individual patient and to the treatment have been suggested as causative of root resorption, but direct causal factors have not been identified yet (Vlaskalic et al. 1998).

Among the patient-related factors, a possible role of genetics, immune system, and medical history has been suggested (Baumrind et al. 1996; Harris et al. 1997).

However, most studies have focused on treatment-related factors. In a recent meta-analysis, Segal et al. (2004) found that mean apical root resorption was strongly correlated with total apical displacement (r = 0.822) and treatment duration (r = 0.852), thus indicating that the total distance the apex has to be moved and the treatment duration should be considered risk factors.

The type of appliance used for a treatment also influences the risk of root resorption. Fixed appliances are more detrimental than removable appliances (Linge and Linge 1991). Also the force level applied has an influence, as forces exceeding the optimal capillary blood pressure cause periodontal ischaemia, which can lead to root resorption (Harry and Sims 1982). Root resorption has generally been measured unidimensionally or at the most bidimensionally but when root resorption was expressed volumetrically it became even more evident that high forces generate 3.31-fold greater total resorption than light forces (Chan and Darendeliler 2004) (Fig. 6.22). However, Maltha et al. (2004) found that force regimen and duration of treatment have a larger influence on root resorption than force magnitude both on two- and three-dimensional examination. Continuous forces were found to be more detrimental than intermittent force and it was found that superelastic wires resulted in more resorption than stainless steel (Acar et al. 1999) Not only the extent of root resorption but also the depths of the cavities were influenced by the type of wire used, as the volume of the resorption craters were 140 times greater when superelastic wires were used rather than stainless steel (Weiland 2003).

Interruption of treatment for 2–3 months in patients with root resorption decreases the amount of root resorption (Levander et al. 1994). Among the types of tooth movement, intrusion has been implicated as having the largest risk, but when performed with light forces the resorption is negligible, without influencing the prognosis, even in adult patients with periodontally damaged teeth (Melsen et al. 1989). Parker et al. found that intrusion with lingual root torque is a risk factor for root resorption, while distal bodily retraction, extrusion and lingual crown tipping had no discernible effect (Parker and Harris 1998). Jiggling movements have been linked to root resorption and the finding that more root resorption occurs with use of intermaxillary elastics, especially on teeth that are directly loaded, may confirm this hypothesis (Mirabella and Artun 1995).

A question thus arises about a higher susceptibility of adult patients to root resorption as the cementum is wider, the PDL is thinner, and the vascular and proliferative activities are reduced (Kyomen and Tanne 1997). Harris et al. (1990) did not find any difference between young and adult treated patients but many adults had larger amount of root resorption before treatment. In conclusion, once a careful examination of the patient is performed, the risk of root resorption in the adult patient does not represent a limiting factor for orthodontic treatment.

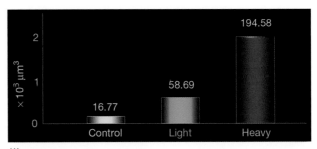

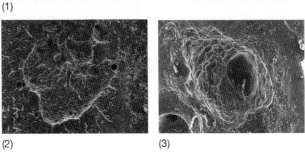

Fig. 6.22 (1) Mean volume of resorption of roots of premolars after the application of light and heavy forces. Orthodontic force induced root resorption compared with no treatment. Moreover, the heavy forces induce significantly more resorption than light forces. (2) and (3) show the three-dimensional reconstruction of resorption lacuna in case of light and heavy force application, respectively. (Courtesy of A Darendeliler).

References

Acar A, Canyurek U, Kocaaga M and Erverdi N (1999) Continuous vs. discontinuous force application and root resorption. *Angle Orthod* 69, 159–163.

Adachi H, Igarashi K, Mitani H and Shinoda H (1994) Effects of topical administration of a bisphosphonate (risedronate) on orthodontic tooth movements in rats. *J Dent Res* 73, 1478–1486.

Amir LR, Li G, Schoenmaker T, Everts V and Bronckers AL (2007) Effect of thrombin peptide 508 (TP508) on bone healing during distraction osteogenesis in rabbit tibia. *Cell Tissue Res* 330, 35–44.

Andersen KL, Mortensen HT, Pedersen EH and Melsen B (1991) Determination of stress levels and profiles in the periodontal ligament by means of an improved three-dimensional finite element model for various types of orthodontic and natural force systems. *J Biomed Eng* 13, 293–303.

Arias OR and Marquez-Orozco MC (2007) Aspirin, Acetaminophen and ibuprofen: their effects on orthodontic tooth movement. *Am J Orthod Dentofacial Orthop* 130, 364–370.

Arslan SG, Arslan H, Ketani A and Hamamci O (2007) Effects of estrogen deficiency on tooth movement after force application: an experimental study in ovariectomized rats. *Acta Odontol Scand* 65, 319–323.

Asundi A and Kishen A (2000) A strain gauge and photoelastic analysis of in vivo strain and in vitro stress distribution in human dental supporting structures. *Arch Oral Biol* 45, 543–550.

Barnett NA and Rowe DJ (1986) A comparison of alveolar bone in young and aged mice. *J. Periodontol* 57, 447–452.

Baron R (1975a) Histophysiologie des reaction tissulaires au cours du deplacement orthodontique. In Chateau M (ed.) *Orthopedie Dentofaciale. Bases Fondamentales*, pp. 328–364. Paris: J Prélat.

Baron R (1975b) Remodeling of alveolar bone in spontaneous and induced tooth displacement. *Revue D Orthopedie Dento Faciale* 9, 309–325.

Baron R, Tross R and Vignery A (1984) Evidence of sequential remodeling in rat trabecular bone: morphology, dynamic histomorphometry, and changes during skeletal maturation. *Anat Rec* 208, 137–145.

Baumrind S, Korn EL and Boyd RL (1996) Apical root resorption in orthodontically treated adults. *Am J Orthod Dentofacial Orthop* 110, 311–320.

Benjamin M and Hillen B (2003) Mechanical influences on cells, tissues and organs 'Mechanical Morphogenesis'. *Eur J Morphol* 41, 3–7.

Bien SM (1966) Hydrodynamic damping of tooth movement. *J Dent Res* 45, 907–914.

Bridges T, King G and Mohammed A (1988) The effect of age on tooth movement and mineral density in the alveolar tissues of the rat. *Am J Orthod Dentofacial Orthop* 93, 245–250.

Burger EH and Klein-Nulen J (1999) Responses of bone cells to biomechanical forces in vitro. *Adv Dent Res* 13, 93–98.

Burr DB, Milgrom C, Fyhrie D, Forwood M, Nyska M, Finestone A, Hoshaw S, Saiag E and Simkin A (1996) In vivo measurement of human tibial strains during vigorous activity. *Bone* 18, 405–410.

Cattaneo PM, Dalstra M and Melsen B (2005) The finite element method: a tool to study orthodontic tooth movement. *J Dent Res* 84, 428–433.

Chan EK and Darendeliler MA (2004) Exploring the third dimension in root resorption. *Orthod Craniofac Res* 7, 64–70.

Chang HN, Garetto LP, Potter RH, Katona TR, Lee CH and Roberts WE (1997) Angiogenesis and osteogenesis in an orthopedically expanded suture. *Am J Orthod Dentofacial Orthop* 111, 382–390.

Chicurel ME, Singer RH, Meyer CJ and Ingber DE (1998) Integrin binding and mechanical tension induce movement of mRNA and ribosomes to focal adhesions. *Nature* 392, 730–733.

Cowin SC, Moss-Salentijn L and Moss ML (1991) Candidates for the mechanosensory system in bone. *J. Biomed Eng* 113, 191–197.

Cureton SL and Cuenin M (1999) Surgically assisted rapid palatal expansion: orthodontic preparation for clinical success. *Am J Orthod Dentofacial Orthop* 116, 46–59.

Danciu TE, Gagari E, Adam RM, Damoulis PD and Freeman MR (2004) Mechanical strain delivers anti-apoptotic and proliferative signals to gingival fibroblasts. *J. Dent Res* 83, 596–601.

Davidovitch Z, Nicolay OF, Ngan PW and Shanfeld JL (1988) Neurotransmitters, cytokines, and the control of alveolar bone remodeling in orthodontics. *Dent Clin North Am* 32, 411–435.

Duncan RL and Turner CH (1995) Mechanotransduction and the functional response of bone to mechanical strain. *Calcif Tissue Int* 57, 344–358.

Ehrlich PJ and Lanyon LE (2002) Mechanical strain and bone cell function: a review. *Osteoporos Int* 13, 688–700.

Epker BN and Frost HM (1965) Correlation of bone resorption and formation with the physical behavior of loaded bone. *J. Dent Res* 44, 33–41.

Eriksen EF, Axelrod DW and Melsen F (1994) *Bone Histomorphometry*. New York, NY: Raven Press.

Follet H, Li J, Phipps RJ, Hui S, Condon K and Burr DB (2007) Risedronate and alendronate suppress osteocyte apoptosis following cyclic fatigue loading. *Bone* 40, 1172–1177.

Frost HM (1964) Dynamics of bone remodeling. In Frost HM (ed.) *Bone Biodynamics*, pp. 315–333. Boston, MA: Little, Brown.

Frost HM (1990a) Skeletal structural adaptations to mechanical usage (SATMU): 1. Redefining Wolff's law: the bone modeling problem. *Anat Rec* 226, 403–413.

Frost HM (1990b) Skeletal structural adaptations to mechanical usage (SATMU): 2. Redefining Wolff's law: the remodeling problem. *Anat Rec* 226, 414–422.

Frost HM (1998) A brief review for orthopedic surgeons: fatigue damage (microdamage) in bone (its determinants and clinical implications). *J Orthop Sci* 3, 272–281.

Frost HM (2003) Bone's mechanostat: a 2003 update. *Anat Rec A Discov Mol Cell Evol Biol* 275, 1081–1101.

Fukui T (1993) Analysis of stress-strain curves in the rat molar periodontal ligament after application of orthodontic force. *Am J Orthod Dentofacial Orthop* 104, 27–35.

Fukui T, Yamane A, Komatsu K and Chiba M (2003) Restoration of mechanical strength and morphological features of the periodontal ligament following orthodontic retention in the rat mandibular first molar. *Eur J Orthod* 25, 167–174.

Gameiro GH, Pereira-Neto JS, Magnani MB and Nouer DF (2007) The influence of drugs and systemic factors on orthodontic tooth movement. *J Clin Orthod* 41, 73–78.

Goldie RS and King GJ (1984) Root resorption and tooth movement in orthodontically treated, calcium-deficient, and lactating rats. *Am J Orthod* 85, 424–430.

Grimm FM (1972) Bone bending, a feature of orthodontic tooth movement. *Am J Orthod* 62, 384–393.

Hamaya M, Mizoguchi I, Sakakura Y, Yajima T and Abiko Y (2002) Cell death of osteocytes occurs in rat alveolar bone during experimental tooth movement. *Calcif Tissue Int* 70, 117–126.

Harris EF and Baker WC (1990) Loss of root length and crestal bone height before and during treatment in adolescent and adult orthodontic patients. *Am J Orthod Dentofacial Orthop* 98, 463–469.

Harris EF, Kineret SE and Tolley EA (1997) A heritable component for external apical root resorption in patients treated orthodontically. *Am J Orthod Dentofacial Orthop* 111, 301–309.

Harry MR and Sims MR (1982) Root resorption in bicuspid intrusion. A scanning electron microscope study. *Angle Orthod* 52, 235–258.

Heller IJ and Nanda R (1979) Effect of metabolic alteration of periodontal fibers on orthodontic tooth movement. An experimental study. *Am J Orthod* 75, 239–258.

Hellsing E and Hammarström L (1991) The effects of pregnancy and fluoride on orthodontic tooth movements in rats. *Eur J Orthod* 13, 223–230.

Igarashi K, Adachi H, Mitani H and Shinoda H (1996) Inhibitory effect of the topical administration of a bisphosphonate (risedronate) on root resorption incident to orthodontic tooth movement in rats. *J Dent Res* 75, 1644–1649.

Igarashi K, Mitani H, Adachi H and Shinoda H (1994) Anchorage and retentive effects of a bisphosphonate (AHBuBP) on tooth movements in rats. *Am J Orthod Dentofacial Orthop* 106, 279–289.

Ingber DE (1997) Tensegrity: the architectural basis of cellular mechanotransduction. *Annu Rev Physiol* 59, 575–599.

Ingman T, Apajalahti S, Mantyla P, Savolainen P and Sorsa T (2005) Matrix metalloproteinase-1 and -8 in gingival crevicular fluid during orthodontic tooth movement: a pilot study during 1 month of follow-up after fixed appliance activation. *Eur J Orthod* 27, 202–207.

Isaacson RJ, Lindauer SJ and Davidovitch M (1993) On tooth movement. *Angle Orthod* 63, 305–309.

Jager A (1996) Histomorphometric study of age-related changes in re-modelling activity of human desmodontal bone. *J Anat* 189(Pt 2), 257–264.

Johnson RB, Gilbert JA, Cooper RC, Parsell DE, Stewart BA, Dai X, Nick TG, Streckfus CF, Butler RA and Boring JG (2002) Effect of estrogen deficiency on skeletal and alveolar bone density in sheep. *J Periodontol* 73, 383–391.

Jonasson G (2005) Mandibular alveolar bone mass, structure and thickness in relation to skeletal bone density in dentate women. *Swed Dent J Suppl* 177, 1–63.

Kabasawa M, Ejiri S, Hanada K and Ozawa H (1996) Effect of age on physiologic and mechanically stressed rat alveolar bone: a cytologic and histochemical study. *Int J Adult Orthodon Orthognath Surg* 11, 313–327.

Kalia S, Melsen B and Verna C (2004) Tissue reaction to orthodontic tooth movement in acute and chronic corticosteroid treatment. *Orthod Craniofac Res* 7, 26–34.

Kanno T, Takahashi T, Ariyoshi W, Tsujisawa T, Haga M and Nishihara T (2005) Tensile mechanical strain up-regulates Runx2 and osteogenic factor expression in human periosteal cells: implications for distraction osteogenesis. *J. Oral Maxillofac Surg* 63, 499–504.

Kanzaki H, Chiba M, Arai K, Takahashi I, Haruyama N, Nishimura M and Mitani H (2006) Local RANKL gene transfer to the periodontal tissue accelerates orthodontic tooth movement. *Gene Ther* 13, 678–685.

Kanzaki H, Chiba M, Takahashi I, Haruyama N, Nishimura M and Mitani H (2004) Local OPG gene transfer to periodontal tissue inhibits orthodontic tooth movement. *J Dent Res* 83, 920–925.

Keeling SD, King GJ, McCoy EA and Valdez M (1993) Serum and alveolar bone phosphatase changes reflect bone turnover during orthodontic tooth movement. *Am J Orthod Dentofacial Orthop* 103, 320–326.

Kehoe MJ, Cohen SM, Zarrinnia K and Cowan A (1996) The effect of acetaminophen, ibuprofen, and misoprostol on prostaglandin E2 synthesis and the degree and rate of orthodontic tooth movement. *Angle Orthod* 66, 339–349.

Khouw FE and Goldhaber P (1970) Changes in vasculature of the periodontium associated with tooth movement in the rhesus monkey and dog. *Arch Oral Biol* 15, 1125–1132.

Ki HR (1990) The effects of orthodontic forces on the mechanical properties of the periodontal ligament in the rat maxillary molars. *Am J Orthod Dentofacial Orthop* 98, 533–543.

Killiany DM (2002) Root resorption caused by orthodontic treatment: review of literature from 1998 to 2001 for evidence. *Prog Orthod* 3, 2–5.

King GJ, Keeling SD and Wronski TJ (1992) Histomorphological and chemical study of alveolar bone turnover in response to orthodontic tipping. In Carlson DS and Goldstein SA (eds) *Bone Biodinamics in Orthodontic and Orthopedic Treatment*, pp. 281–297. Ann Arbor, MI: Center for Human Growth and Development.

Klein-Nulend J, Bacabac RG and Mullender MG (2005) Mechanobiology of bone tissue. *Pathol Biol (Paris)* 53, 576–580.

Knaup B, Yildizhan F and Wehrbein H (2004) Age-related changes in the midpalatal suture. A histomorphometric study. *J Orofac Orthop* 65, 467–474.

Krall EA, Wson-hughes B, Mt H, PW W and DP K (1997) Postmenopausal estrogen replacement and tooth retention. *Am J Med* 102, 536–542.

Kyomen S and Tanne K (1997) Influences of aging changes in proliferative rate of PDL cells during experimental tooth movement in rats. *Angle Orthod* 67, 67–72.

Lanyon LE and Rubin CT (1984) Static vs dynamic loads as an influence on bone remodelling. *J Biomech* 17, 897–905.

Levander E, Malmgren O and Eliasson S (1994) Evaluation of root resorption in relation to two orthodontic treatment regimes. A clinical experimental study. *Eur J Orthod* 16, 223–228.

Linge L and Linge BO (1991) Patient characteristics and treatment variables associated with apical root resorption during orthodontic treatment. *Am J Orthod Dentofacial Orthop* 99, 35–43.

Liu L, Igarashi K, Haruyama N, Saeki S, Shinoda H and Mitani H (2004) Effects of local administration of clodronate on orthodontic tooth movement and root resorption in rats. *Eur J Orthod* 26, 469–473.

Malone AM, Anderson CT, Tummala P, Kwon RY, Johnston TR, Stearns T and Jacobs CR (2007) Primary cilia mediate mechanosensing in bone cells by a calcium-independent mechanism. *Proc Natl Acad Sci U S A* 104, 13325–13330.

Maltha JC, van Leeuwen EJ, Dijkman GE and Kuijpers-Jagtman AM (2004) Incidence and severity of root resorption in orthodontically moved premolars in dogs. *Orthod Craniofac Res* 7, 115–121.

Manson JD and Lucas RB (1962) A microradiographic study of age changes in the human mandible. *Arch Oral Biol* 7, 761–769.

Melsen B (1972) A histological study of the influence of sutural morphology and skeletal maturation on rapid palatal expansion in children. *Trans Eur Orthod Soc* 499–507.

Melsen B (1975) Palatal growth studied on human autopsy material. A histologic microradiographic study. *Am J Orthod* 68, 42–54.

Melsen B (1999) Biological reaction of alveolar bone to orthodontic tooth movement. *Angle Orthod* 69, 151–158.

Melsen B, Agerbaek N and Markenstam G (1989) Intrusion of incisors in adult patients with marginal bone loss. *Am J Orthod Dentofacial Orthop* 96, 232–241.

Melsen B, Cattaneo PM, Dalstra M and Kraft DC (2007) The importance of force levels in relation to tooth movement. *Semin Orthod* 13, 220–233.

Melsen F and Mosekilde L (1980) Trabecular bone mineralization lag time determined by tetracycline double-labeling in normal and certain pathological conditions. *Acta Pathol Microbiol Scand A Pathol* 88, 83–88.

Mirabella AD and Artun J (1995) Risk factors for apical root resorption of maxillary anterior teeth in adult orthodontic patients. *Am J Orthod Dentofacial Orthop* 108, 48–55.

Misawa-Kageyama Y, Kageyama T, Moriyama K, Kurihara S, Yagasaki H, Deguchi T, Ozawa H and Sahara N (2007) Histomorphometric study on the effects of age on orthodontic tooth movement and alveolar bone turnover in rats. *Eur J Oral Sci* 115, 124–130.

Mohammed AH, Tatakis DN and Dziak R (1989) Leukotrienes in orthodontic tooth movement. *Am J Orthod Dentofacial Orthop* 95, 231–237.

Mohri T, Hanada K and Osawa H (1991) Coupling of resorption and formation on bone remodeling sequence in orthodontic tooth movement: a histochemical study. *J Bone Miner Metab* 9, 57–69.

Mori S and Burr DB (1993) Increased intracortical remodeling following fatigue damage. *Bone* 14, 103–109.

Nicolella DP, Bonewald LF, Moravits DE and Lankford J (2005) Measurement of microstructural strain in cortical bone. *Eur J Morphol* 42, 23–29.

Nikolai RJ (1975) On optimum orthodontic force theory as applied to canine retraction. *Am J Orthod* 68, 290–302.

Noble B (2003) Bone microdamage and cell apoptosis. *Eur Cell Mater* 6, 46–56.

Ogasawara T, Yoshimine Y, Kiyoshima T, Kobayashi I, Matsuo K, Akamine A and Sakai H (2004) In situ expression of RANKL, RANK, osteoprotegerin and cytokines in osteoclasts of rat periodontal tissue. *J Periodontal Res* 39, 42–49.

Orellana-Lezcano MF, Major PW, McNeil PL and Borke JL (2005) Temporary loss of plasma membrane integrity in orthodontic tooth movement. *Orthod Craniofac Res* 8, 106–113.

Ott S, Osteoporosis and Bone physiology http://courses.washington.edu/bonephys/ophome.html © 1998-2010 by Susan Ott, MD Updated Sept 14, 2010.

Parker RJ and Harris EF (1998) Directions of orthodontic tooth movements associated with external apical root resorption of the maxillary central incisor. *Am J Orthod Dentofacial Orthop* 114, 677–683.

Paulsen HU and Karle A (2000) Computer tomographic and radiographic changes in the temporomandibular joints of two young adults with occlusal asymmetry, treated with the Herbst appliance. *Eur J Orthod* 22, 649–656.

Pavlin D and Gluhak-Heinrich J (2001) Effect of mechanical loading on periodontal cells. *Crit Rev Oral Biol Med* 12, 414–424.

Persson M and Thilander B (1977) Palatal suture closure in man from 15 to 35 years of age. *Am J Orthod* 72, 42–52.

Picton DC (1964) The effect of repeated thrusts on normal axial tooth mobility. *Arch Oral Biol* 16, 55–64.

Pilon JJ, Kuijpers-Jagtman AM and Maltha JC (1996) Magnitude of orthodontic forces and rate of bodily tooth movement. An experimental study. *Am J Orthod Dentofacial Orthop* 110, 16–23.

Reitan K (1951) The tissue reaction as related to the functional factor. *Dent Rec (London)* 71, 173–183.

Reitan K and Rygh P (1994) Biomechanical principles and reactions. In Graber TM and Vanarsdall RL (eds) *Orthodontics: Current Orthodontic Concept and Techniques*, 2nd edn., pp. 96–192. St Louis: Mosby.

Ren Y, Maltha JC, 't Hof MA and Kuijpers-Jagtman AM (2003) Age effect on orthodontic tooth movement in rats. *J Dent Res* 82, 38–42.

Ren Y, Maltha JC, Van 't Hof MA and AM K-J (2004) Optimum force magnitude for orthodontic tooth movement: a math- ematic model. *Am J Orthod Dentofacial Orthop* 125, 71–77.

Ren Y, Maltha JC, Van't Hof MA, Von Den Hoff JW, Kuijpers-Jagtman AM and Zhang D (2002) Cytokine levels in crevicular fluid are less responsive to orthodontic force in adults than in juveniles. *J Clin Periodontol* 29, 757–762.

Roberts WE, Garetto LP and Katona TR (1992) Principles of orthodontic biomechanics: metabolic and mechanical control mechanisms. In Carlson DS and Goldstein SA (eds) *Bone Biodynamics in Orthodontic and Orthopedic Treatment*, pp. 1[27], 189–255. University of Michigan, Ann Arbor: Center for Human Growth and Development. Craniofacial Growth Series.

Rody WJ Jr, King GJ and Gu G (2001) Osteoclast recruitment to sites of compression in orthodontic tooth movement. *Am J Orthod Dentofacial Orthop* 120, 477–489.

Ruf S and Pancherz H (1999) Dentoskeletal effects and facial profile changes in young adults treated with the Herbst appliance. *Angle Orthod* 69, 239–246.

Rygh P, Bowling K, Hovlandsdal L and Williams S (1986) Activation of the vascular system: a main mediator of periodontal fiber remodeling in orthodontic tooth movement. *Am J Orthod* 89, 453–468.

Rygh P and Brudvik P (1995) The histological responses of the periodontal ligament to horizontal orthodontic loads. In Berkovitz BKB and Newman HB (eds) *The Periodontal Ligament in Health and Disease*, 2nd edn., pp. 243–258. St Louis, MI: Mosby-Yearbook.

Saffar JL, Lasfargues JJ and Cherrau M (1997) Alveolar bone and the alveolar process: the socket that is never stable. *Periodontol 2000* 13, 76–90.

Segal GR, Schiffman PH and Tuncay OC (2004) Meta analysis of the treatment-related factors of external apical root resorption. *Orthod Craniofac Res* 7, 71–78.

Storey E (1973) The nature of tooth movement. *Am J Orthod* 63, 292–314.

Takano-Yamamoto T, Kawakami M and Yamashiro T (1992) Effect of age on the rate of tooth movement in combination with local use of 1,25(OH)2D3 and mechanical force in the rat. *J Dent Res* 71, 1487–1492.

Talic N, Evans CA, Daniel JC, George A and Zaki AM (2004) Immunohistochemical localization of alphavbeta3 integrin receptor during experimental tooth movement. *Am J Orthod Dentofacial Orthop* 125, 178–184.

Tran Van PT, Vignery A and Baron R (1982) Cellular kinetics of the bone remodeling sequence in the rat. *Anat Rec* 202, 445–451.

Tsay TP, Chen MH and Oyen OJ (1999) Osteoclast activation and recruitment after application of orthodontic force. *Am J Orthod Dentofacial Orthop* 115, 323–330.

Vandevska-Radunovic V, Kvinnsland S and Kvinnsland IH (1997) Effect of experimental tooth movement on nerve fibres immunoreactive to calcitonin gene-related peptide, protein gene product 9.5, and blood vessel density and distribution in rats. *Eur J Orthod* 19, 517–529.

Verna C (1999) *The Influence of Different Bone Turnover Rates on the Tissue Reactions to Orthodontic Load*. Denmark: Aarhus University, Department of Orthodontics.

Verna C, Dalstra M, Lee TC, Cattaneo PM and Melsen B (2004) Microcracks in the alveolar bone following orthodontic tooth movement: a morphological and morphometric study. *Eur J Orthod* 26, 459–467.

Verna C, Dalstra M and Melsen B (2000) The rate and the type of orthodontic tooth movement is influenced by bone turnover in a rat model. *Eur J Orthod* 22, 343–352.

Verna C, Dalstra M and Melsen B (2003) Bone turnover rate in rats does not influence root resorption induced by orthodontic treatment. *Eur J Orthod* 25, 359–363.

Verna C, Hartig LE, Kalia S and Melsen B (2006) Influence of steroid drugs on orthodontically induced root resorption. *Orthod Craniofac Res* 9, 57–62.

Verna C, Zaffe D and Siciliani G (1999) Histomorphometric study of bone reactions during orthodontic tooth movements in rats. *Bone* 24, 371–379.

Vignery A and Baron R (1980) Dynamic histomorphometry of alveolar bone remodeling in the adult rat. *Anat Rec* 196, 191–200.

Vlaskalic V, Boyd RL and Baumrind S (1998) Etiology and sequelae of root resorption. *Semin Orthod* 4, 124–131.

von Bohl M, Maltha J, Von DHH and Kuijpers-Jagtman AM (2004b) Changes in the periodontal ligament after experimental tooth movement using high and low continuous forces in beagle dogs. *Angle Orthod* 74, 16–25.

von Bohl M, Maltha JC, Von Den Hoff JW and Kuijpers-Jagtman AM (2004a) Focal hyalinization during experimental tooth movement in beagle dogs. *Am J Orthod Dentofacial Orthop* 125, 615–623.

Voudouris JC, Woodside DG, Altuna G, Angelopoulos G, Bourque PJ, Lacouture CY and Kuftinec MM (2003a) Condyle-fossa modifications and muscle interactions during Herbst treatment, Part 2. Results and conclusions. *Am J Orthod Dentofacial Orthop* 124, 13–29.

Voudouris JC, Woodside DG, Altuna G, Kuftinec MM, Angelopoulos G and Bourque PJ (2003b) Condyle-fossa modifications and muscle interactions during herbst treatment, part 1. New technological methods. *Am J Orthod Dentofacial Orthop* 123, 604–613.

Wan X, Juranka P and Morris CE (1999) Activation of mechanosensitive currents in traumatized membrane. *Am J Physiol* 276, C318–C327.

Weiland F (2003) Constant versus dissipating forces in orthodontics: the effect on initial tooth movement and root resorption. *Eur J Orthod* 25, 335–342.

Weinbaum S, Cowin SC and Zeng Y (1994) A model for the excitation of osteocytes by mechanical loading-induced bone fluid shear stresses. *J Biomech* 27, 339–360.

Weinstein S, Haack DC, Morris LY, Snyder BB and Attaway HE (1963) On an equilibrium theory of tooth position. *Am J Orthod* 33, 1–26.

Winkler DG, Sutherland MK, Geoghegan JC, Yu C, Hayes T, Skonier JE, Shpektor D, Jonas M, Kovacevich BR, Staehling-Hampton K, Appleby M, Brunkow ME and Latham JA (2003) Osteocyte control of bone formation via sclerostin, a novel BMP antagonist. *EMBO J* 22, 6267–6276.

Woo SB, Hellstein JW and Kalmar JR (2006) Narrative [corrected] review: bisphosphonates and osteonecrosis of the jaws. *Ann Intern Med* 144, 753–761.

Woodside DG, Metaxas A and Altuna G (1987) The influence of functional appliance therapy on glenoid fossa remodeling. *Am J Orthod Dentofacial Orthop* 92, 181–198.

Yamasaki K, Shibata Y, Imai S, Tani Y, Shibasaki Y and Fukuhara T (1984) Clinical application of prostaglandin E1 (PGE1) upon orthodontic tooth movement. *Am J Orthod* 85, 508–518.

Yamashiro T, Fujiyama K, Fujiyoshi Y, Inaguma N and Takano-Yamamoto T (2000) Inferior alveolar nerve transection inhibits increase in osteoclast appearance during experimental tooth movement. *Bone* 26, 663–669.

Yamashiro T, Sakuda M and Takano-Yamamoto T (1994) Experimental tooth movement in ovariectomozed rats. *J Dent Res* 73(JADR Abst), 148.

Zaffe D and Verna C (1995) Acid and alkaline phosphatase activities in rat's alveolar bone experimentally loaded by orthodontical forces. *Ital J Miner Electrol Metab* 9(Suppl 1[2]), 11.

Zahrowski JJ (2007) Bisphosphonate treatment: an orthodontic concern calling for a proactive approach. *Am J Orthod Dentofacial Orthop* 131, 311–320.

7

Appliance Design

Birte Melsen, Delfino Allais, Giorgio Fiorelli

Introduction

When selecting an appliance for orthodontic treatment of adult patients, it is important to recognise the limitations caused by general or local loss of periodontium due to missing teeth and prosthetic replacements which have to be maintained. The absence of growth conversely allows for a more precise prediction of the treatment result, as a change of jaw's relation can only be done by surgery or mandibular repositioning. While the surgical intervention can change the position of both jaws and teeth, tooth movement can be done either before or after surgery. In relation to repositioning, tooth movements necessary to allow for the adaptation of the two arches have to be done before the repositioning, while movements to adapt the two arches have to be done after it is clear that the neuro-muscular adaptation to repositioning is possible.

Treatment goal definition

The treatment goal definition should always be based on a well-determined mandibular position and a definition of the desired dental movements, as described in Chapter 5.

Mandibular position

Although the habitual occlusion has to be maintained during treatment of the majority of adult patients, some patients need a correction of the intermaxillary relation. This can be achieved either with surgical intervention in one or both jaws or in some cases by changing the position of the condyles in the glenoid fossa (mandibular repositioning).

Many patients can adapt to a wide range of positions without developing any articular or muscular discomfort. Fiorelli et al. (2018) found that it was possible to correct, or reduce, a Class II relationship or an asymmetry in 60% of a sample of adult patients by repositioning the mandible.

According to these authors, it was possible to identify the patients that could be repositioned through a 3-month clinical adaptation test. This was done when the initial adaptation of the arches necessary for surgery was performed. Examples of this approach are shown in Chapter 6 and this chapter (in the patient shown in Figure 7.1).

The currently available evidence suggests that occlusion plays a limited role concerning the onset and development of temporomandibular dysfunctions (TMDs) (Luther 2007; Türp and Schindler 2012, Chapter 16). For this reason, a change of the mandibular position, and the following orthodontic treatment, should nowadays rarely be done to treat TMDs.

Dental movements

Once the skeletal relationship is established, the dental displacement necessary to achieve the treatment goal can be

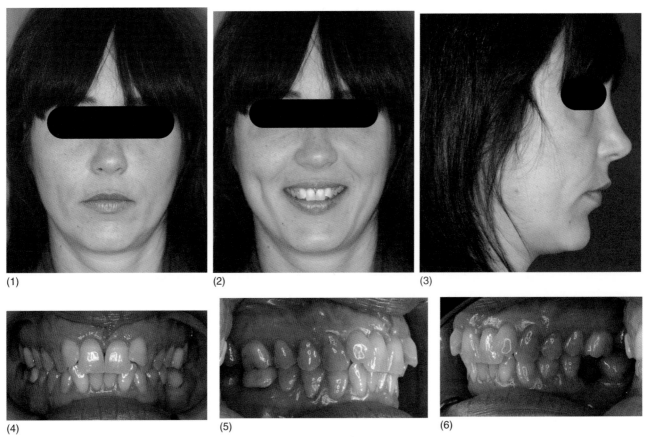

(1) (2) (3)

(4) (5) (6)

Fig. 7.1 (1)–(3) Face, smile and profile of a 42-year-old female patient, whose chief complaint was the malalignment of upper anterior teeth. The profile shows a retruded chin; however, the soft tissues determine a good harmony of the profile. (4)–(8) Intraoral images show dental Class II relations, upper and lower crowding, 'V'-shaped dental arches with transversal contraction of canines and premolars, palatally inclined upper central incisors and mesial inclination of tooth 3.7 due to the loss of 3.6. Tooth 4.6 was later extracted by her dentist who considered this element not recoverable. Note that due to the palatally inclined central incisors, a minimal overjet is present and, therefore, the mandibular anterior repositioning is not possible at the beginning of the treatment. (9) Lateral head film, confirming the Class II skeletal relations. (10) The CBCT images of the joints show both condyles with an intact cortical bone. The condylar position is on both sides quite posterior. This finding indicates the possibility of an anterior repositioning despite the steep eminence slope. (11) Mandibular protrusion of 3 mm done on digital models using a virtual articulator (Ortolab DDP software). This jaw movement is blocked by interferences on the anterior teeth (blue areas); however, this relation between the jaws was used for the treatment planning. (12) Occlusogram performed using T3DO software (IOSS GmbH). The virtual models with a mandibular protrusion were used to produce this treatment plan. The images show the needed movements of expansion especially in the first premolar area and also the desired anterior inclination of upper central incisors. (13) and (14) The treatment started with an upper transversal expansion and a proclination of the central incisors to facilitate the following anterior mandibular repositioning. In these images, we see a lateral view comparison, (13) before and (14) after repositioning. The amount of mandibular repositioning can be appreciated, with the canine relation that is in (14) a full Class I. At this time, the case was evaluated for stability with lack of dual bite, and the temporo-mandibular joint sign and symptoms for 3 months, without modifying posterior contacts. The Triad Gel onlay was never broken or detached demonstrating a full adaptation to the new occlusion. The patient was consistently biting with the modified jaw relations and no symptoms or sign of the TMD appeared. At this point, the treatment continued with the aim of stabilising the new jaw relation and correcting the residual malalignments. (15) Eighteen months after starting of the treatment, a CBCT was repeated to check the condylar position. The lateral view of the skull shows improved skeletal relations, the normal inclination of the anterior teeth with correct overjet and overbite. (16) The joint images show how in full occlusion the condyles are now resting along the slope of the eminence. (17)–(19) The case at the end of active treatment lasted 22 months. Face, smile and profile. The profile shows a significant forward positioning of the chin with an improvement in its aesthetics. (20)–(24) Intraoral picture showing a normal overjet and overbite with canine in Class I relation. Second lower molars are now uprighted and implants should be inserted mesial to them. The patient started to wear Essix retainers at night and was visited in the retention period once a year. The use of retainers was reduced progressively in the following years. (25)–(27) Follow-up six years after the end of treatment. Patient at the age of 51. Face, smile and profile, showing the maintenance of the profile. (28)–(32) Intra-oral pictures, showing good stability of the occlusion. The patient is wearing occasionally her Essix retainers, while she did not have lower implants as recommended.

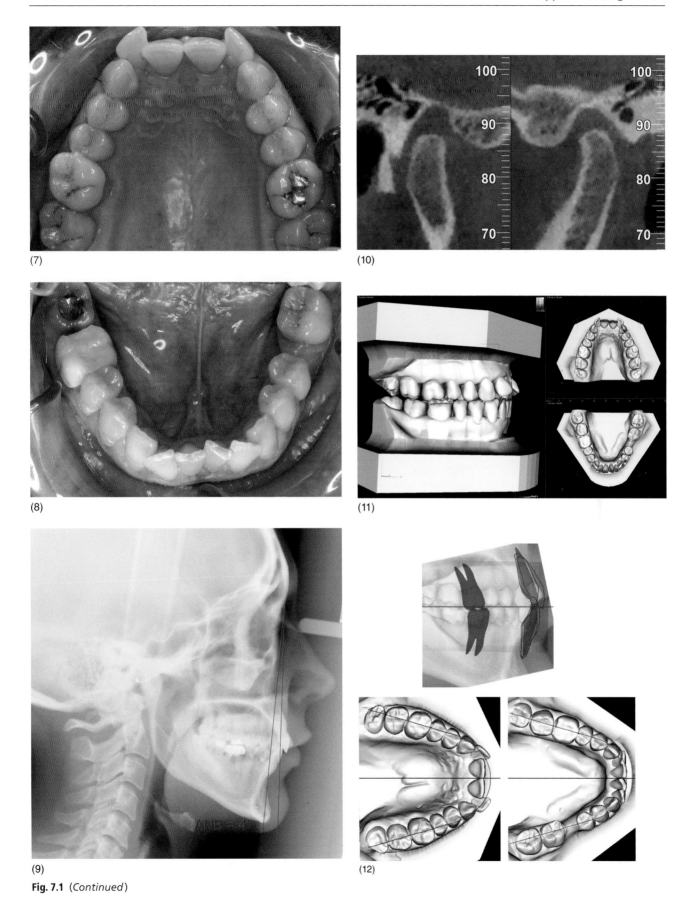

(7)

(10)

(8)

(11)

(9)

(12)

Fig. 7.1 (*Continued*)

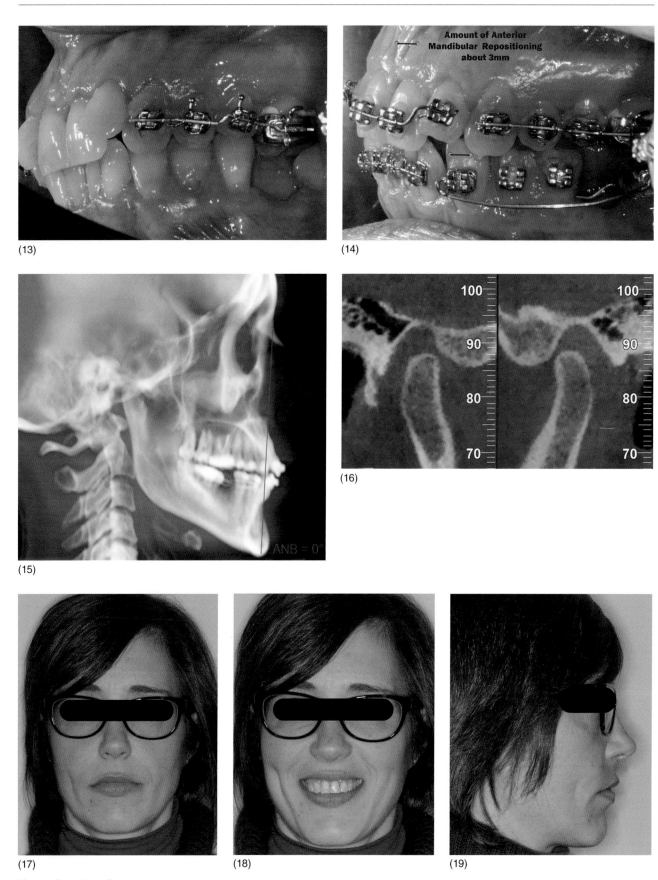

(13)

(14)

Amount of Anterior
Mandibular Repositioning
about 3mm

(15)

ANB = 0°

(16)

100 100
90 90
80 80
70 70

(17)

(18)

(19)

Fig. 7.1 (*Continued*)

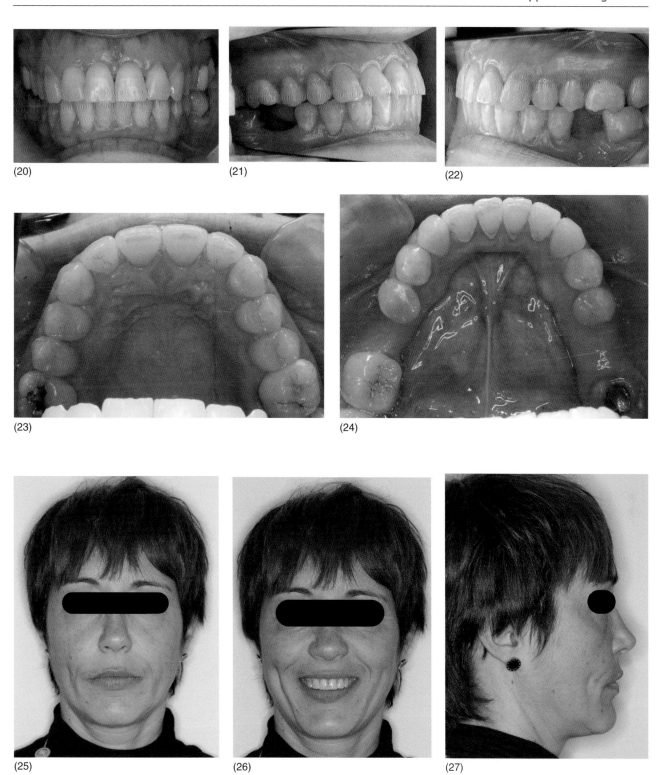

(20)

(21)

(22)

(23)

(24)

(25)

(26)

(27)

Fig. 7.1 (*Continued*)

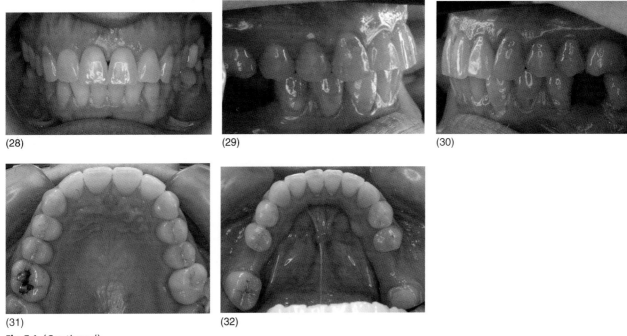

(28)　(29)　(30)

(31)　(32)

Fig. 7.1 (*Continued*)

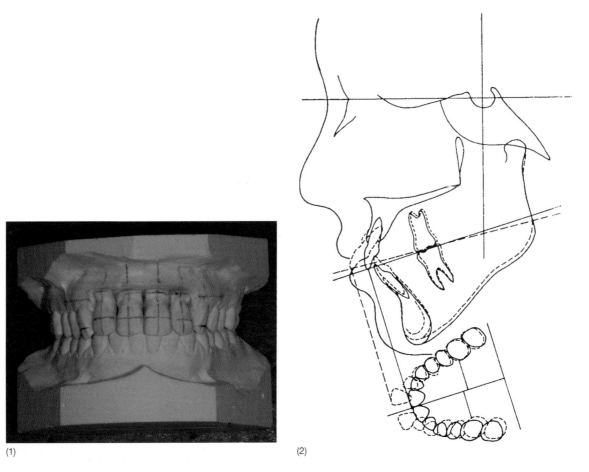

(1)　(2)

Figure 7.2 (1) A setup made from study casts. Note the grid drawn before the teeth are moved. This allows the dentist to appreciate the exact movement performed on the setup. In this case, the upper incisors have been intruded and retracted. (2) Treatment goal illustrated on a combination of an occlusogram and a tracing of the head film. The flaring and spacing of the upper incisors will be corrected by extraction of one upper premolar followed by retraction of the four incisors.

defined. The force system needed to generate the planned movements then has to be calculated. The direction and location of the line of action of the applied force determine how and in which direction the individual tooth or groups of teeth will move. Apart from the forces resulting from the orthodontic appliance, the treatment result will also be influenced by the soft tissue matrix, that is, the balance between the internal and the external muscle matrices, and the occlusal forces.

The planned tooth movements in three planes of space can be done on a diagnostic setup of study casts (Figure 7.2(1)), or a combination of a tracing of a head film and occlusogram (Figure 7.2(2)) or a setup on virtual models generated by a scan performed intraorally, of impressions or study casts (Mah and Sachdeva 2001; Sachdeva 2001; Santoro et al. 2001, 2003; Vlaskalic and Boyd 2002; Freshwater 2003; Joffe 2003, 2004; Zilberman et al. 2003; Dalstra and Melsen 2009). The setup is frequently done by orthodontic companies with only minimal interaction with the orthodontist and without detailed information about how the final occlusion can be achieved. The treatment plan and appliance design are not separable, since the prescription or even the appliance is provided with the setup. The orthodontist aims for a good occlusion without knowing how the individual teeth will achieve their final position. An analogy would be: 'I wish to spend my vacation in the snow, but I do not know whether the travel agency has sent me to, Mount Cook or Mont Blanc'. The setup, whether real or virtual, should include information about the movement of each tooth or group of teeth in all three planes of space. If the combination of a head film and an occlusogram or a virtual model is used, the tooth movements can be visualised in all three planes. For a more detailed description, see Chapter 5. In relation to the movement of teeth on virtual models, a set of coordinates should indicate the displacement.

Definition of the necessary force system

A force acting on a tooth can be represented as a vector defined in relation to a given coordinate system by its magnitude, its point and line of application, as well as its direction and orientation (Figure 7.3).

Tooth movements can be translations, rotations or various combinations of translation and rotation. According to the line of action of the force vector, Hocevar (1981, 1987) defined four types of horizontal tooth movement in the sagittal plane (Figure 7.4). A force passing through the bracket results in uncontrolled tipping. When the force passes halfway between the centre of resistance (CR) of the tooth and the bracket, the resulting movement is so-called controlled tipping with the centre of rotation close to the tooth apex. A force passing through the CR generates translation, and further apical displacement of the line of action of the force leads to root movement with the centre of rotation in the crown area. Similar classifications of tooth movement can be made in other planes of space (Christiansen and Burstone 1969; Kusy and Tulloch 1986).

Application of the correct line of action is a pre-condition for well-controlled tooth movement. In cases in which the major part of the planned tooth movement will occur in one plane of space, it may be sufficient to define the line of action in that particular plane of space (Figure 7.5).

The localisation of the line of action in relation to the CR of the tooth or the group of teeth will determine the relative contribution of translation and rotation to the total movement, and thus determine the centre of rotation for the total movement (Figure 7.6). The perpendicular distance from the CR to the line of action expresses the moment-to-force ratio at the CR, thus the relative amount of rotation and translation of the movement. A change in the moment-to-force ratio can be obtained by displacement of the point of force application or by adding a moment to the bracket (Figure 7.7).

According to the law of physics, the stress distribution in a solid object is uniquely related to the position and incidence of the line of action of an applied force and to the specific characteristics of the material. Since the dental movement can be considered a biological adaptation to the applied stress and it is related to the stress distribution, it is therefore reasonable to say that there is a unique relation between the line of action of the applied force and the dental movement. However, the same line of action can be generated by a multiplicity of appliances. To facilitate the estimation of the force system needed for a specific movement, a special Dental Movement Analysis (DMA) software was developed in the late nineties and updated later on. Based on relations between the localisation of the centre of rotation and the applied force system (Burstone and Pryputniewicz 1980; Burstone 1991), DMA can simulate

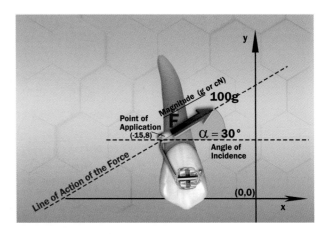

Fig. 7.3 The force can be described as a vector in a coordinate system. Four parameters are necessary to define a force: the magnitude is indicated by the length of a vector in a coordinate system with an arbitrary scale. The point of force application and the angle of incidence define the line of action of the force. The orientation of the arrowhead indicates its direction, thereby completing the force definition.

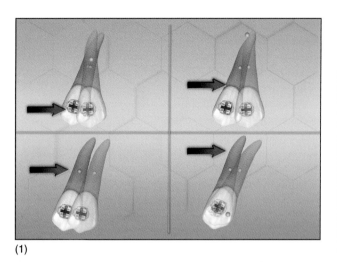

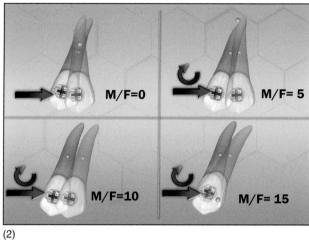

(1)   (2)

Fig. 7.4 (1) The four types of sagittal movements of a canine as defined by Hocevar (1981), with the corresponding line of action of the force. (2) Same classification, but with the force system defined with respect to the bracket. It should be kept in mind that the values of the M/F ratio described here are not to be considered an absolute reference for any kind of movement, since the distance between the bracket and the centre of resistance can change dramatically if a force with a different magnitude is applied.

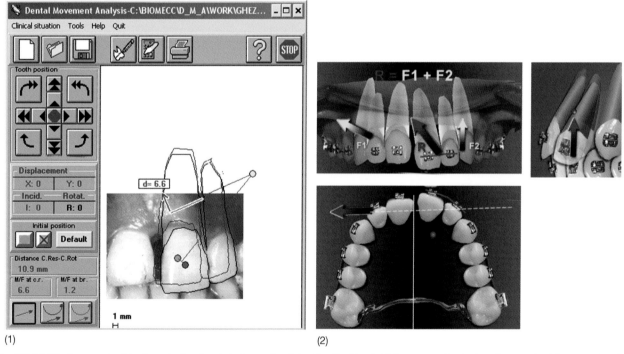

(1)   (2)

Fig. 7.5 (1) Displacement of incisors in the frontal plane, simulated by the Dental Movement Analysis software. In this example, the software simulates the movement of teeth 21 and 22 as a single unit in two dimensions. The yellow circle is the desired centre of rotation. The red arrows represent the single force that should be applied in order to obtain the displayed movement. (2) Three-dimensional analysis of a force system. Two different vectors (F1 and F2) are applied and the resultant force (R) is shown in the frontal, occlusal and sagittal planes, as is the estimated position of the centre of resistance of the active unit. This type of analysis allows a detailed prediction of dental movement.

any dental movement in two dimensions and visualise the line of action needed with respect to either the bracket or the CR (Fiorelli and Melsen 1999) (Figure 7.5(1)). 3D evaluations can be also done by repeating the movement analysis in different planes (Figure 7.5(2)).

The type of tooth movement can also be controlled by varying the moment-to-force ratio to the CR by adding the moment to the bracket according to the principles of equivalent force systems (Figure 7.4(2)).

Holographic analysis and radiographic and clinical examinations have been used to estimate the position of the CR (Burstone and Pryputniewicz 1980). Local constraints from soft tissue function and differences in the quality of the alveolar bone do, however, also influence the resistance to tooth movement, and differences in force level may consequently affect the localisation of the CR (Cattaneo 2003).

While the type of tooth movement generally reflects the force system, the rate of tooth movement seems to be under genetic control; variation in force levels does not seem to influence the rate of dental movement (Pilon et al. 1996; van Leeuwen et al. 1999; Ren et al. 2004) (Figure 7.8). The optimal force system cannot be stated, but, with the

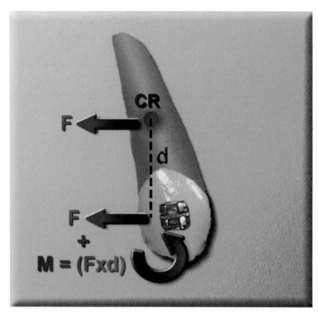

Fig. 7.7 Translation can be achieved by a force passing through the centre of resistance (CR) in the direction of the desired translation or by adding a force to the bracket in addition to a moment neutralising the moment generated by the force acting at a distance from the CR. This moment-to-force ratio is called the replacement force system.

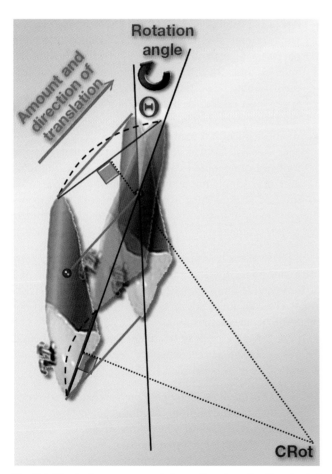

Fig. 7.6 The incisor movement from the clear to the shaded image is a translation (given by the distance and the direction) combined with rotation expressed as an angle and a line of direction. The total movement, however, can also be expressed by the localisation of the centre of rotation for the total movement and the degree of rotation. The movement will be the result of a force in the same direction as the displacement of the centre of resistance (CR) and applied above the CR. As the distance from the line of action to the CR will increase once rotation starts, the relative component of the movement made up of rotation increases.

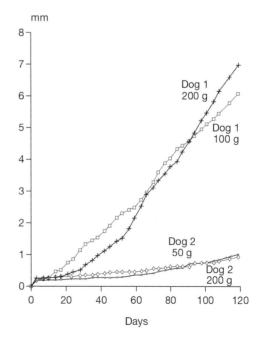

Fig. 7.8 The rate of tooth movement in two dogs: the rate is determined more by the bone turnover of the individual dog than the force level. (With permission from Pilon et al. (1996).)

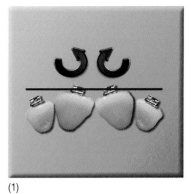
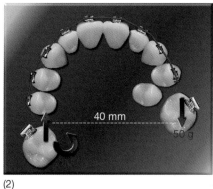

(1)   (2)

Fig. 7.9 (1) No anchorage is needed for correction of the depicted malocclusion, as the two units are displaced symmetrically against each other. (2) A slightly more complicated example of tooth movement where no anchorage problems exist. The patient requires distal rotation and mesialisation of 17 and distal rotation and distalisation of 27. This can be done with a transpalatal arch inserted into the lingual sheath of 17 delivering the desirable distally directed force to 27 at the level of the centre of resistance in the horizontal plane of space. The force system will not deliver any undesirable forces and is thus in a balance.

introduction of superelastic wires, a trend towards lower force levels has been noted. However, the initial force level is still high (Fuck and Drescher 2006).

Despite the apparent need for control of the force system, it is more the exception than the rule that force systems are seriously considered when inserting an orthodontic appliance. Despite this, there is a high success rate, which can be ascribed to the interaction of the forces generated by orthodontic appliances with growth, the occlusal forces and the balance between the external and the internal muscle matrices. In the adult patient, the absence of growth in the vertical dimension increases the risk of undesirable movements and iatrogenic damage. Careful planning of the applied force system is therefore recommended.

Anchorage evaluation

When the desired tooth movements have been identified and the necessary force systems for delivering these defined, the reactive forces acting on the anchorage unit should be evaluated. Some cases do not present any anchorage problems, as all delivered forces are desirable, while other cases are considered impossible to treat without the use of skeletal anchorage, as all teeth must be moved in the same direction. Not only the forces acting on the teeth to be moved but also those transferred to the anchorage unit should be assessed (Figure 7.9) (see Chapter 8).

Sequencing the treatment into phases

The division of treatment into phases is often related to the sequence of archwires and thus more related to the force level and the properties of the wire than to the exact tooth movement to be performed in the individual steps. However, there may be other reasons for which it is necessary to perform the treatment in phases for all of the dental arches (Burstone and Marcotte 2000):

- Anchorage cannot be maintained if all needed force systems are applied simultaneously. For example, it is often necessary to maintain the occlusion while moving the anterior units. In this case, levelling of the buccal segments should be postponed.
- Space must be created before certain tooth movements can be performed (Figure 7.10).
- Biomechanically, it may be difficult to design an appliance needed for a specific tooth movement and the tooth movement has to be performed in steps. The anatomy may simply not allow the optimal appliance to be inserted (Figure 7.11). If the desired tooth movements are divided into two stages, the goal could be achieved with less difficulty.

Each phase of the treatment may require different mechanics. In one phase, there may be a single reactive unit and one or more active units. Only in cases with absolute consistency, when all units are moved in the desired direction, there will be no reactive units.

The following aspects of treatment should be considered before establishing the sequence in which the tooth movements will be performed.

1) *Setting of the mandibular position*: This has already been discussed in the beginning of this chapter.
2) *Anchorage*: Phases in which little or no anchorage is needed should be first performed.
3) *Generation of space*: Space conditions often determine the sequence of treatment. Since both sagittal and vertical movements require space, transverse corrections should generally be performed at the beginning of treatment, whereby the displacement creates space for a subsequent resolution of crowding in the anterior area.

In the patient in Figure 7.10, widening of the intercanine distance by distal rotation of the molars was a precondition for the proclination and intrusion of the upper incisors.

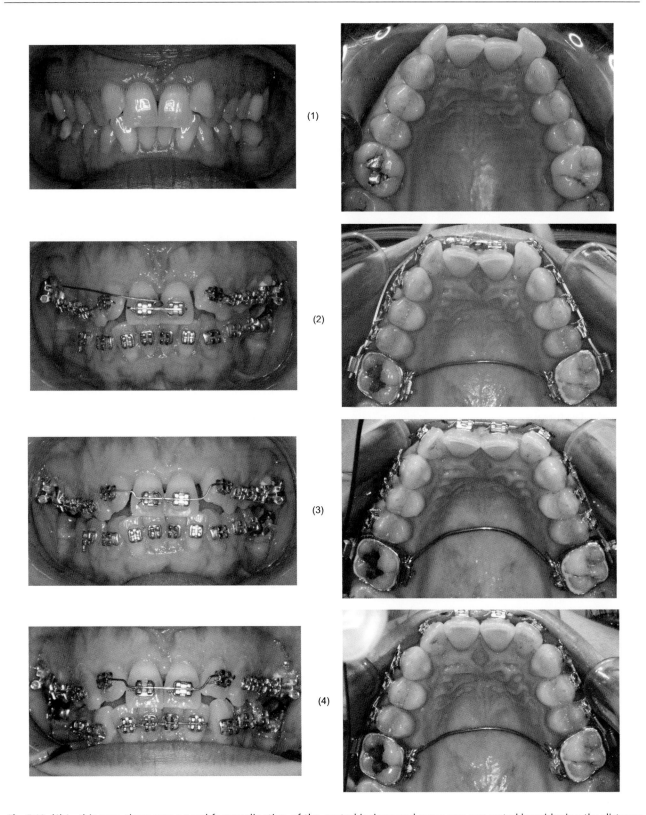

Fig. 7.10 (1) In this case, there was a need for proclination of the central incisors and space was generated by widening the distance between the two lateral incisors. This was done by segments extending from the molars that were distally rotated a transpalatal arch. (2) Once the space was generated, a cantilever was used to procline the central incisors. (3) In a later stage, a beta-titanium 0.016 × 0.022-inch segment was used to start the alignment of the four incisors. (4) An initial alignment was achieved. Note the change of the upper arch shape due to the expansion in the canine region.

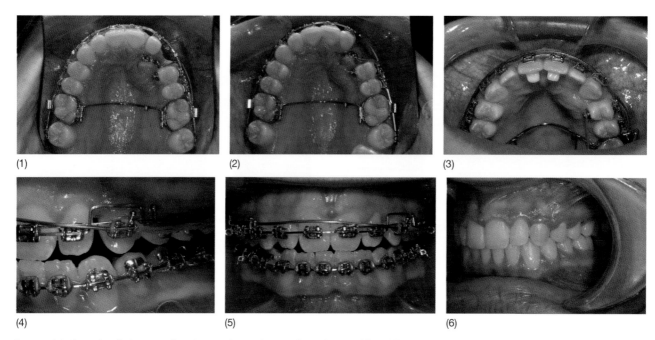

Fig. 7.11 (1) The palatally impacted canine was brought into the palate and freed from contact with the lateral incisor with a cantilever extending from the molar. (2) In the next phase, the canine was brought into the arch by using an overlay nickel–titanium (Ni–Ti) arch. (3) The bite opening necessary to allow the canine to be moved into the arch was obtained by using bonding pads on the lingual surface of the central incisors. (4) and (5) Buccal root torque with low-load deflection rate and a high moment-to-force ratio was obtained with a 0.17 × 0.25-inch titanium molybdenum (TMA) full arch extending from molar to molar and twisted 180° with respect to the canine bracket. Anchorage for the buccal root torque was obtained by using a stainless-steel 0.17 × 0.25-inch wire bypassing the canine. Since a buccal root torque will implicitly deliver intrusion, this was prevented by the extruding round bypass arch extending from central incisor to the second premolar. (6) Post-treatment view.

Appliance selection and design

Removable appliances

In adult patients, appliances aim to deliver tooth movements and if relevant modelling of the alveolar process. Both removable and fixed appliances have their advantages and disadvantages.

One type of removable appliance comprises acrylic plates with active units, including expansion screws and finger springs. A different approach to removable appliances is a series of thermoplastic splints (aligners) developed to achieve pre-determined sequential tooth movements. Conventional plates can only be used for uncontrolled tipping, as the forces are transferred through a one-point contact, and thus are rarely used in adult patients. Thermoplastic splints can be used for more controlled tooth movements and are aimed primarily for use in adult patients (Bollen et al. 2003; Clements et al. 2003) as they have more than one point of contact per tooth and can provide different M/F ratios (Gaoa and Wichelhaus 2017). Many companies are now marketing series of aligners for the correction of various types of malocclusions. See Chapter 17.

Fixed appliances

When using fixed appliances, the forces are transferred to the teeth via brackets. From a biomechanical point of view,

it is important to distinguish between brackets that allow three-dimensional control and attachments that only have one point (single brackets, buttons, cleats, and hooks). Fixed appliances can be bonded both buccally and lingually, and the bracket design has a significant impact on the appliance, selection of archwires, and auxiliaries used.

Selection of brackets and wires

Brackets vary for both material and design. The first brackets introduced by Angle had only one-point contact (Melsen 2020), but later Angle described the rectangular bracket which was a standard edgewise bracket without any build-in corrections. All corrections were bent into the wire.

The prescription brackets introduced by Andrews have built-in first-, second- and third-order control, following the principles of the pre-adjusted appliances (1976a, 1976b). The ideal prescription became, and still is, a hot topic of discussion. Planché (1997) published a review of the most common prescriptions. Besides, different prescriptions have been recommended for different ethnic groups and different types of malocclusions (Figure 7.12). Moreover, it should not be forgotten that the positioning of the bracket will have a crucial influence of the expression of the torque values. Miethke and Melsen (1999) demonstrated that a vertical displacement of a canine bracket of 0.4 mm would generate

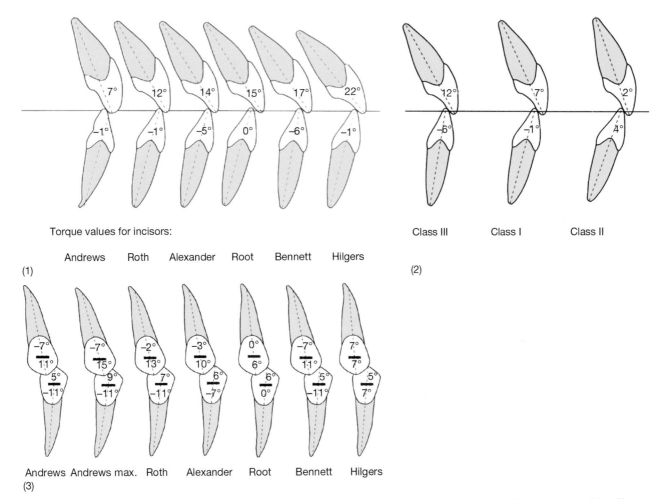

Torque values for incisors:

Andrews   Roth   Alexander   Root   Bennett   Hilgers

(1)

Class III   Class I   Class II

(2)

Andrews Andrews max. Roth   Alexander   Root   Bennett   Hilgers

(3)

Fig. 7.12 (1) Comparison of the recommended bracket prescriptions regarding torque according to different authors. (2) Different torque values recommended for different malocclusions. (3) Different built-in angulation (second order) recommended by different authors (From Planché (1997) with permission from EDP Sciences; http://odf.edpsciences.org).

a change in torque up to 11°. The positioning of the brackets is thus very critical and even when positioned optimally the torque will depend on the play between wire and bracket.

The latest approach regarding brackets is represented by 'Insignia®', where the company provides the doctor with a setup and trays for indirect bonding and a recommended sequence of wires.

The slot dimension of the bracket was initially limited to 0.022 × 0.028 inches and 0.018 × 0.025 inches, but other dimensions have a selection of brackets that have been also been presented.

The dimensions of the archwire significantly influence the force levels delivered to the teeth. The rationale behind the reduction of the slot size from the original 0.022 inches to 0.018 inches was that three-dimensional control could be achieved with a wire of a smaller dimension (Figure 7.13).

These alterations were done when the available alloys were limited to steel and chrome cobalt alloys. With the introduction of high-tech memory alloys, the lower force level was no longer merely dependent on the dimensions of the wire. The preference of the 'bracket 22' has the advantage that a larger slot dimension allows for a more rigid wire to be used in the reactive units. Recently, the combination of aligners and fixed appliances has been used to enhance a stiffer connection of the teeth belonging to the anchorage unit.

As the torque control was easier obtained with a '018' bracket system, Gianelly et al. (1985) recommended the bi-dimensional technique using 0.018-inch slots anteriorly and 0.022 laterally to obtain better torque control anteriorly and less friction laterally.

In relation to friction related to sliding mechanics, not only the dimension and the material of the brackets are of importance but also the method of ligation (Nicolls 1968; Farrant 1977; Frank and Nikolai 1980; Schumacher et al. 1990; Iwasaki et al. 2003). Conventional polyurethane modules increase friction when compared with stainless-steel ligatures.

The sales campaigns for brackets have increased in the later years. Especially, the self-ligation brackets have been in

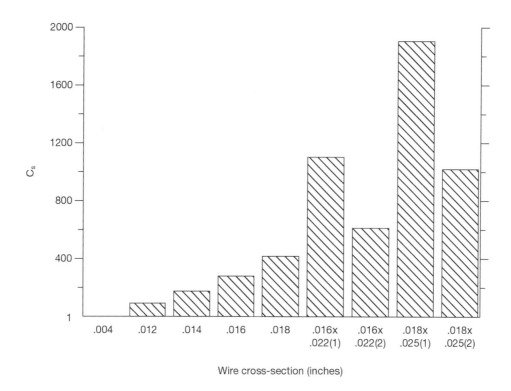

Fig. 7.13 Relationship between wire dimension and stiffness (relative force level). (Redrawn from Burstone (1982). Reproduced with permission from Elsevier.)

focus and the names have indicated what the companies wanted to sell: 'Fast Braces®, Speed Braces®, High-Speed Braces®, CFast Braces®, Quick Braces®, Bioquick®', etc. During the last decennia, the interest in self-ligating brackets has been increasing.

Originally, the aim of the first self-ligating bracket, the Russell attachment, was a reduction in ligating time and improvement in operator efficiency (Stolzenberg 1935, 1946), but a side effect was less resistance to sliding. However, interest in this bracket was temporary. A newer and more successful attempt to avoid ligation was the Speed® bracket, in which ligation was replaced with a cap that was passive in relation to wires of small dimensions, but which became an active spring in relation to rectangular archwires (Hanson 1980, 1986, 2002; Berger 1990, 1999; Berger and Byloff 2001). A similar principle is used in the In-Ovation® bracket (Voudouris 1997a, 1997b). In other self-ligating systems, the slot is turned into a tube with a passive lid, for example, the Damon® bracket (Ormco/Sybron) (Damon 1998a, 1998b) and the SmartClip™ System from Unitek. Thus, most manufacturers now produce self-ligating brackets of varying designs, and the reduction in chairside assistance, thus improving operator efficiency, is being used in the marketing of all products (Hanson 1986, 2002; Berger 1990; Shivapuja and Berger 1994; Damon 1998b; Turnbull and Birnie 2007).

The focus has meanwhile been on additional advantages such as improved control over tooth movements; constant low friction; less anchorage demand; shorter treatment time; longer intervals between appointments; more comfortable for the patient; easier hygiene; reduced chair time and a better work environment for the staff (Gottlieb et al. 1972; Hanson 1980; Shivapuja and Berger 1994; Voudouris 1997b; Damon 1998b; Pizzoni et al. 1998; Berger and Byloff 2001; Thorstenson and Kusy 2002a; Cacciafesta et al. 2003; Hain et al. 2003; Redlich et al. 2003; Thorstenson and Kusy 2003b; Henao and Kusy 2004, 2005; Kusy 2005). Most of these attributes are still controversial and to some degree related to the bracket design. The passive self-ligating brackets have the advantage of maximum initial friction reduction (Damon 1998b; Harradine 2003), while brackets with an active clip may allow greater and more precise control of wire insertion (Figure 7.13). The shorter gingival wall of the slot of inactive brackets such as Speed and In-Ovation may, on the other hand, reduce the length of the moment arm and consequently reduce the expression of torque (Harradine and Birnie 1996; Harradine 2001, 2003).

The modifications in bracket material and shape, which according to the manufacturers significantly facilitate sliding mechanics, are not supported by valid research. Several authors have claimed that low friction is a major factor in more efficient treatment (Shivapuja and Berger 1994; Harradine and Birnie 1996; Read-Ward et al. 1997; Hemingway et al. 2001; Cacciafesta et al. 2003; Hain et al. 2003; Harradine 2003; Katsaros and Dijkman 2003).

As binding is more important than friction (Harradine 2001), the effect of archwire activation and bracket pre-angulation are sufficient to greatly reduce the disparity in friction levels between the conventional pre-adjusted and self-ligating brackets (Thorstenson and Kusy 2002a). Braun et al. (1999), on the other hand, demonstrated that resistance to sliding was reduced significantly when the dynamics of the oral environment were simulated.

Some authors claim that the use of self-ligating brackets reduces treatment time (Voudouris 1997a; Damon 1998a, 1998b; Eberting et al. 2001; Harradine 2001). Damon claimed to have a reduction in the average treatment time in comparison with the traditional continuous steel archwire system, but the reduced treatment time was not confirmed by Miles and colleagues (Miles et al. 2006; Miles 2007). Since none of the studies fulfill the requirements of a well-designed clinical trial, the comparison is not conclusive. It can only be inferred that self-ligating bracket systems demonstrate considerably lower static frictional resistance than a conventional steel-ligated bracket in the case of zero angulation. The reduction in friction characterising self-ligating brackets is most pronounced when wires of smaller dimensions are used and is not advantageous during the final phase of treatment with full-size archwires, and reduced resistance to sliding results in reduced three-dimensional (3D) control (Thorstenson and Kusy 2002b). An example of an adult case treated with a self-ligating bracket system is shown in Case 5 (see www.wiley.com/go/melsen).

An important issue concerning brackets is the precision, that is, the play between wire and bracket. Dalstra et al. (2015) compared the precision of several conventional and self-ligating brackets and found a play of 28° where a theoretical play of 9° could be expected (Figure 7.14).

Sliding mechanics

In relation to sliding mechanics, teeth move along the arch-wire as beads along a string. The movement will always be tipping followed by an uprighting. Appliances in which tooth movement is generated using loops or springs placed between the units do not necessitate displacement of the teeth with respect to the wire, and resistance to sliding plays no role in these mechanics. This is discussed later in this chapter.

Resistance to sliding

The factors determining the resistance to the tooth movement along the archwire include classical or Coulomb friction, binding and notching. Friction is defined as the force that resists the relative motion or tendency to such motion of two bodies in contact (Kajdas 1990).

A distinction is also made between static frictional force, the smallest force required to start the motion, and kinetic frictional force, the force that resists sliding motion. Static friction is always higher than the kinetic force, which keeps the body in motion (Resnick and Halliday 1977). The former is considered of more importance in tooth movement, for when a tooth slides along an archwire, the movement occurs as a series of short jumps, and the resistance from static friction has to be overcome each time the tooth moves a little. Friction depends on the bracket and wire material, and the type of ligature delivering a normal force to the wire against the base of the slot.

As soon as the angle between the wire and the bracket slot exceeds the critical contact angle, the resistance to sliding will become dependent on the binding. Thorstenson and Kusy (2002a, 2002b, 2003a, 2003b) examined the effects of varying active tip (angulation) on the resistance to sliding and found that angulation beyond which the archwire first contacts the diagonally opposite corners of the bracket slot causes a similar rise in the resistance to sliding in self-ligated and conventional brackets (Kusy 2004). Although the critical binding angle is a product of the bracket size and the wire dimensions, the flexibility of the wire also plays a role. Stiffer wires result in higher resistance to sliding than flexible wires with the same dimensions. There will, on the other hand, be larger tipping before uprighting when a flexible wire is used. When using a stiff wire as recommended by McLaughlin (2001) concerning the MBT technique, the

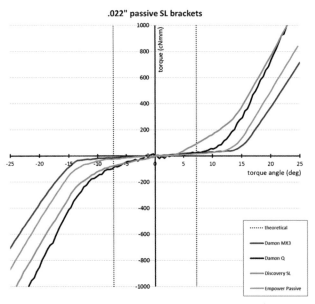

Fig. 7.14 Different self-ligating brackets: (1) Speed brackets; (2) The active clip; (3) In-Ovation brackets; (4) Damon® brackets and the (5) Smart-Clip bracket. When comparing the torque control of 5 different self-ligating brackets, it was found that the passive 'Damon bracket' exhibited almost 30° of play before expressing torque. The theoretical play was 16.

tipping is very small and the movement may simulate a translation on the radiographs.

Apart from the angle between the wire and the bracket, in other words, the type of the attempted tooth movement (Articolo and Kusy 1999; Thorstenson and Kusy 2002b, 2003a; Kusy 2004), notching may also influence the displacement of the bracket in relation to the wire. The occurrence of notching, which is the plastic deformation of the surface of the archwire, depends on the material of both the archwire and bracket and is related to the force system created between the archwire and the bracket. Notching is mostly seen on the lingual side of the archwire in the incisor and canine regions (Articolo et al. 2000), and it is a factor to be removed by changing the wire if the movement has to be continued, The dental movement that is performed with sliding mechanics when a force is applied at bracket level can be described as a sequence of crown inclination towards the space to be closed followed by a progressive root uprighting (often incomplete) generated by the action of the wire on the bracket. This sequence is repeated in several cycles to complete the space closure, and the length of this cycle is mostly related to the wire stiffness where stiffer archwires produce shorter and more frequent cycles because the maximum allowed inclination is more limited. In this way, the movement is perceived by the clinician as similar to a translation. However, this behaviour cannot be considered ideal both for clinical and biological reasons.

The distance between the applied force and the CR determines the frequency of the cycle, influencing the amount of CR displacement that is obtained by each cycle. If the force is placed more apical and closer to the CR, cycles tend to be longer with a limitation of the allowed angle of inclination while the amount of translation for each cycle is increased as described by Fiorelli and Melsen (1992–2022), and this can be considered an improvement in the mechanic efficiency of the system with a reduction of the jiggling effect (Figure 7.15).

Statically determinate and indeterminate force systems

Fixed appliances can also be classified as statically determinate and indeterminate systems. One-couple and two-couple mechanics show another way of denoting these systems (Davidovitch and Rebellato 1995; Isaacson and Rebellato 1995; Shroff et al. 1995).

In statically determinate systems acting between two units, the wire is only inserted into the bracket or the tube of one tooth and has a one-point contact with the other unit. Thus, a force and a moment act on the first unit, and at the latter only a force. Figure 7.16 illustrates how the point of force application and the configuration of cantilevers can influence the force systems developed (Fiorelli and Melsen 1992–2022; Fiorelli and Merlo 2015).

When a continuous arch is inserted into two or more brackets, as in sliding mechanics, moments and forces are developed in all brackets. The system is defined as statically indeterminate. As every tooth has 6° of freedom, 3 forces (1 for each plane of space) and 3 moments (1 in each plane of space), the result of a straight wire inserted into 2 brackets will potentially have 36 different outcomes. When 3 teeth are connected by a piece of straight wire, there are $6^3 = 216$ possible outcomes, and prediction of the tooth movements will become impossible.

Burstone and Koenig (1974) described the relationship between two teeth as 'segments' in one plane of space. This

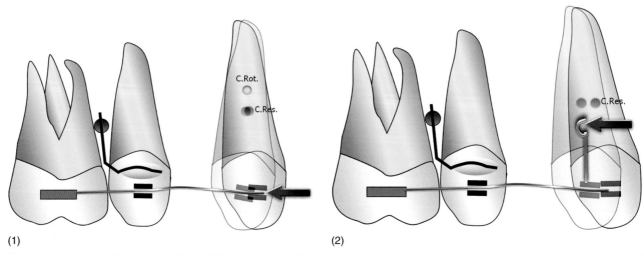

(1)   (2)

Fig. 7.15 Maximum inclination possible in sliding mechanics using stainless-steel 0.016-inch archwire with the posterior unit reinforced by a TAD for maximum anchorage. (1) If the distal force is applied at bracket level, the canine tips around a centre of rotation a few millimetres above the CR. During each cycle of distal crown inclination/uprighting, there is a minimal displacement of the centre of resistance (CR). (2) If the force is applied 3 mm below the CR of the canine, the centre of rotation is located several millimetres above the dental apex. Cycles are more extended, with less inclination allowed, and with a much larger CR displacement for each cycle. From Fiorelli and Melsen (1992–2022), 'Biomechanics in Orthodontics', release 4.

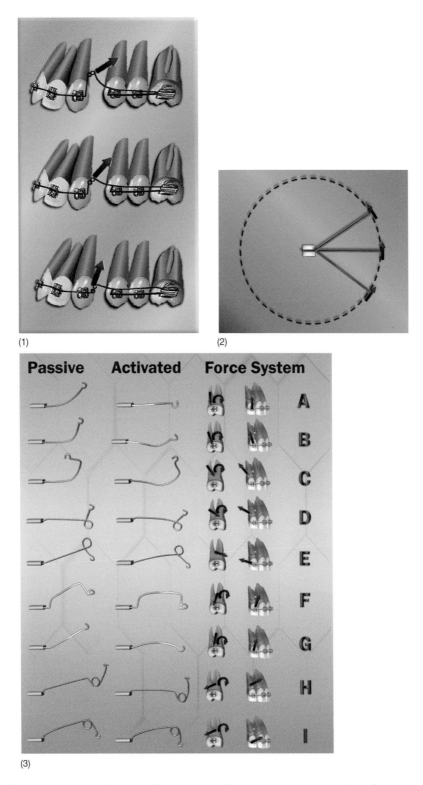

Fig. 7.16 Examples of statically determinate appliances acting between the posterior segment where the wire is inserted into the bracket and the anterior segment where the wire has only a point contact. (1) Changing the height of the anterior attachment of a cantilever changes the structural axis orientation and therefore the produced angulation of the force. (2) The structural axis is a line connecting the two points of connections between the wire and the dental units. The line of action of the force created by the cantilever with no incorporated loops is approximately perpendicular to this axis. (3) Different configurations of the cantilever determine different angulations of the force vector, which together with the point of force application determine the line of action of the force acting on the anterior unit. In these examples, several different cantilevers are engaged in a posterior tube and delivering anteriorly an intrusive vertical force combined by either protrusion or retraction. The force systems are represented as a single force anteriorly, while distal tipping and extrusion are generated to the molar posteriorly.

CLASS:	I	II	III	IV	V	VI
$\dfrac{\theta_A}{\theta_B}$	1.0	0.5	0	−0.5	−0.75	−1.0
LOWER LEFT QUADRANT						

Fig. 7.17 Classification of the relationship between two teeth or units of teeth. The six basic geometries are based on the ratio between the angle of the bracket slots to a line connecting the midpoints of the brackets. The geometry is independent of the inter-bracket distance. Force systems developed to the bracket in different geometries when a 0.016-inch stainless-steel wire is applied (see also Table 7.1). Only the initial force is described and the effect within the bracket is disregarded. (With permission from Burstone and Koenig (1974). Reproduced with permission from Elsevier.)

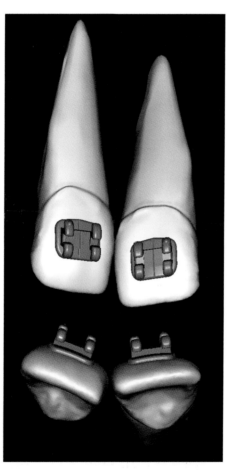

Fig. 7.18 This image illustrates how for the same two teeth two different geometries in the occlusal and the frontal plane exist: a low (I–II) geometry on the frontal plane and high geometry (IV–VI) when seen occlusally.

paper became one of the bases for the segmented approach to orthodontics, which includes also a large use of statically determinate appliances, and a milestone in orthodontic

biomechanics. These authors analysed that the force systems developed when a straight wire was inserted into brackets bonded to two teeth with different second-order angulations. Based on the ratio between the angles of the anterior and posterior brackets and the inter-bracket axis, they defined six basic two-unit geometries (Figure 7.17 and Table 7.1). The same geometries can be defined for every 2-bracket system in two planes: frontal/sagittal and occlusal (Figure 7.18). The force systems are based on mathematical calculations, and neither friction nor the impact of occlusal forces was taken into consideration. The displayed forces and moments, nevertheless, would indicate the direction of the initially generated tooth movements when a straight wire is placed between two teeth with different inclinations. The authors only analysed what happens in the case of two teeth, as the addition of more units to the wire would interfere with the force system. Later, the same authors repeated the analysis considering the friction (Koenig and Burstone 1989), whereby the results became more clinically relevant.

Another important piece of information that can be derived from the work of Burstone and Koenig is the concept of geometry-related stiffness. In their paper, they described a constant value K, which represents the stiffness related to the wire and the geometry. In the paper, this value is reported for all geometries in combination with a stainless steel wire of 0.016 inches, and its value goes from 2967 for geometry I to 987 in geometry VI. This means that in conditions where the same inter-bracket distance exists, and where the same wire is used, rigidity (moment/degrees) decreases from geometry I to geometry VI becoming 1/3. For this reason, alignment in low geometries is generally more difficult to achieve especially where the inter-bracket distance is reduced (i.e., between the lower front teeth).

The force systems in the work of Burstone and Koenig were still expressed to the bracket, although prediction of tooth movement requires knowledge of the force system

Table 7.1 Force systems by class.

Class	I	II	III	IV	V	VI
$\dfrac{q_A}{q_B}$	1.0	0.5	0	−0.5	−0.75	−1.0
$\dfrac{M_A}{M_B}$	1.0	0.8	0.5	0	−0.4	−1.0
Force system on wire at yield L = 7 mm	531.4 ⇧⇩ 531.4 1860 ∫∫ 1860	477.4 ⇧⇩ 477.4 1488 ∫∫ 1860	398.0 ⇧⇩ 398.0 930 ∫∫ 1860	265.4 ⇧⇩ 265.7 ∫ 1860	160.0 ⇧⇩ 160.0 740 ∫∫ 1860	160.0 1860 ∫∫ 1860
Force system on wire at yield L = 21 mm	177.0 ⇧⇩ 177.0 1860 ∫∫ 1860	160.0 ⇧⇩ 160.0 1488 ∫∫ 1860	133.0 ⇧⇩ 133.0 930 ∫∫ 1860	88.6 ⇧⇩ 88.6 ∫ 1860	53.3 ⇧⇩ 53.3 740 ∫∫ 1860	53.3 1860 ∫∫ 1860

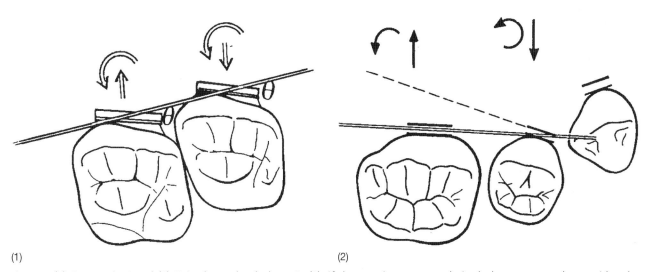

(1)   (2)

Fig. 7.19 (1) Geometries I and (2) III in the occlusal plane. In (1), if the rotations are not desired, the system can be considered as inconsistent, while in (2), if the molar is to be considered the reactive unit, we have a relatively consistent force system.

with respect to the CR. Halazonetis (1998) provided this information when describing the force systems from an ideal arch. He also described how the level of the delivered force systems to the bracket will diminish and how the localisation of the CR is displaced when the teeth are moving.

In a statically indeterminate system, the delivered force system to the individual teeth is practically unknown. The clinician knows that the teeth will align in relation to a given arch, but the localisation of this arch in space is not known; however, due to the interaction of growth, occlusal forces and the soft tissue matrix, the results will often be satisfactory.

Consistency and inconsistency

Before deciding to use a statically indeterminate appliance in a patient with a severe malocclusion, the mutual position of the teeth should be analysed. The mutual relationship between two teeth or two groups of teeth may be such that the forces and moments developed by a straight wire are absolutely consistent, as they are desirable for both units, which can be all considered as active (Figure 7.9(1)). A force system can be characterised as relatively consistent if the directions of both the force and the moment are desirable for the active unit, whereas an undesirable force system develops with respect to the anchorage unit (Figure 7.19(2)). This should be taken into consideration when planning anchorage. A force system is said to be inconsistent if the direction of the force is desirable, but the moment delivered is undesirable or vice versa (Figure 7.19(1)).

Whereas forces acting on the active and reactive units are always equal and opposite, the moments delivered to the two units may differ. The equilibrium is then maintained through the development of a couple, a pair of forces acting on the two units. In the case of lingual root torque to the anterior teeth, the equilibrium will be maintained by the application of intrusive forces to the anterior segment and extrusive forces to the posterior unit (Figure 7.20). In the case of inconsistency, undesirable forces are controlled in various ways: the vertical forces are to some degree controlled by the occlusal forces, and transverse and sagittal forces are neutralised by intermaxillary elastics, which, however, may generate other side effects (Figure 7.21).

In praxis, it is difficult to predict the force system developed by a statically indeterminate system, and this is impossible to describe for a continuous archwire. On the contrary, a statically determinate force system is easily assessed by measuring the distance between the two units and the force needed to tie the cantilever or the coil spring to the unit to which the wire is tied but not inserted into the bracket or the tube (Figure 7.20). From a clinical perspective, it is possible to overcome an inconsistent situation by the application of a force to the opposite side of the clinical crown (Figures 7.22 and 7.23).

Continuous archwires

In adult patients in whom no major changes in the occlusal plane are planned and where no asymmetries are present, most orthodontists would choose a continuous archwire approach. The dominant trend is in the direction of pre-adjusted brackets with self-ligation (Maijer and Smith 1990; Shivapuja and Berger 1994; Damon 1998a, 1998b; Berger and Byloff 2001; Henao and Kusy 2004, 2005) and Ni–Ti wires delivering a low force, which may also be temperature-dependent (Segner and Ibe 1995). With the application of low forces, the occlusal forces are less influenced and the

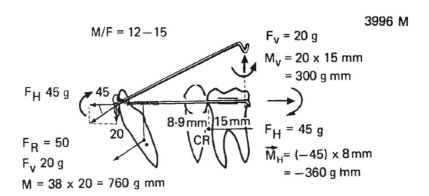

Fig. 7.20 Appliance design and force diagram used for combined labial and apical translation of the lower incisors. The appliance consists of a torque arch delivering labial root torque and intrusion to the incisors. This rectangular arch is inserted into the brackets of the four incisors and hooked onto the round continuous arch extending from molar to molar. The sagittal force is delivered from an open coil spring between the premolars and the incisors. The main arch is not inserted in the brackets of the incisors, but is placed as an overlay. The delivered force system is indicated on the drawing. This is also an example of two-vector mechanics, explained later in this chapter.

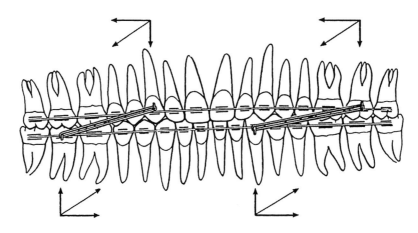

Fig. 7.21 Class II and Class III elastics as recommended for the correction of midline discrepancy and Class II subdivision. It is obvious that this appliance will create a cant of the occlusal plane.

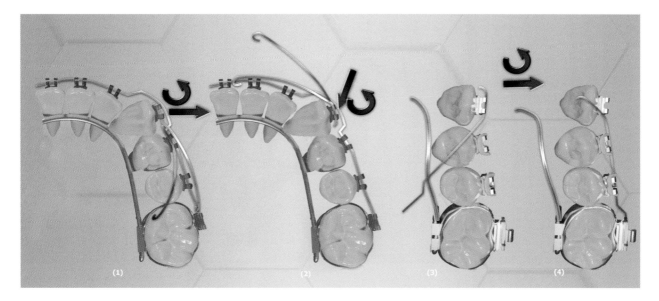

Fig. 7.22 (1)–(4) Illustration of how a cantilever can be used for correction of a distally rotated canine. (1) If a statically determinate cantilever is extending distally, it will also generate a labial displacement which, however, can be avoided by the bypassing full arch. (2) If the cantilever is extending mesially, it will deliver a distal and lingual force to the canine. As the cantilever is extending anteriorly and the side effect would be a proclination of the incisors, this is here prevented by the full arch. (3) and (4) If the wire is used in a statically indeterminate way and bent passively between the brackets of the premolars and the molar tube, the displacement will be determined by the geometry generated between the first premolar and the canine. If the bend added to the wire to produce a mesial rotation is close to the canine, a labial displacement of this tooth will often be the result.

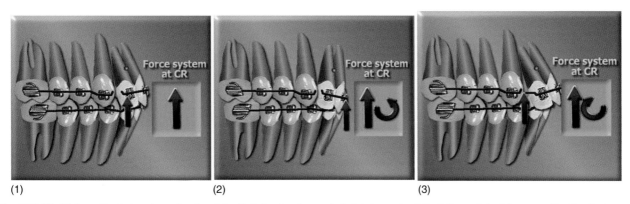

(1)   (2)   (3)

Fig. 7.23 (1)–(3) In patients in whom the front teeth intrusion is needed, it is important that the point of force application is chosen so that the correct combination of intrusion and inclination correction is obtained.

undesirable vertical effects can to some degree be neutralised by these forces. Control of the delivered force system seems to allow for expansion of the arches without the creation of dehiscences (Handelman 1997; Dalstra and Melsen 2004; Bassarelli et al. 2005).

If sliding mechanics is used in extraction cases, the wire on which the brackets slide should have maximum stiffness to avoid the side effects generated by its bending. In order to minimise friction and binding, the line of action of the force should therefore pass close to the CR. This may be facilitated by applying the forces to power-arms, or as Burstone suggested, rigid extensions.

On one hand, the use of sliding mechanics is preferred, as it is simple, and a predefined regimen can be followed. The disadvantage, on the other hand, is that the orthodontist only has limited control over the developed force system, as it is a product of the angle between the wire and the bracket. The indications for the sliding mechanics can be summarised as:

- Growing patients with skeletal discrepancies in whom levelling and coordination of the arches may help or prepare for an occlusal correction.
- Patients with symmetrical malocclusions requiring alignment and vertical development.

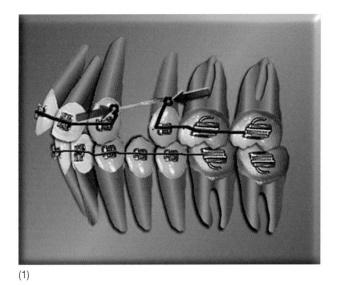
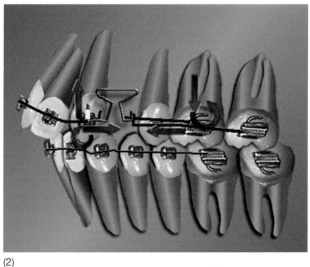

(1)   (2)

Fig. 7.24 Combined intrusion and retraction can be obtained (1) by changing the point of force application to obtain the desired line of action of the force or (2) by a composite T-loop activated to deliver the desired force vector.

- Patients in whom the mutual position of the teeth presents a consistent configuration and a straight wire to level is therefore beneficial.
- Patients in whom no change in occlusion is needed, but where the problem can be resolved by a symmetrical change in the shape of the upper and lower arches.
- Patients who need arch coordination before surgery.

The side effects generated by a continuous archwire can be reduced by a careful analysis of the initial relationships between the teeth. Initially, the wire should only be inserted into the brackets of the teeth that are in a consistent mutual position. Avoiding bonding or bypassing teeth that may be subject to undesirable force systems is advantageous, especially in adult patients (Figure 7.24). Postponement of bonding of the anterior teeth may be biomechanically advantageous and also appreciated by the patient from an aesthetic point of view. Continuous arches can also be combined with overlay arches or the addition of cantilevers or segments with loops (Figure 7.25).

Segmented mechanics

Although the pre-adjusted 'straight-wire' appliance is the main appliance system used nowadays, the types of patients listed in the following text may require segmented appliances to achieve the treatment goal:

- Patients where a straight wire would deliver undesirable forces to one or more of the teeth to be corrected; that is, an inconsistent configuration.
- Patients requiring asymmetrical tooth movements.
- Patients requiring absolute anchorage.
- Patients requiring absolute vertical control.
- Patients requiring true intrusion.

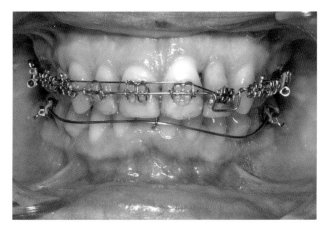

Fig. 7.25 Overlay mechanics used to obtain low forces for the intrusion of the elongated lateral incisor. Note that the proclination of the lower incisors is initiated before the brackets were placed. The base arch is tied to a lingually bonded wire.

- Patients with reduced periodontal support, where the force system should be adjusted in line with the apical displacement of the CR (Case 6, see www.wiley.com/go/melsen).

The advantages of the segmented arch approach in such patients are:

- The tooth movements are predictable.
- The force system is known.
- Possible differentiation between active and passive units.
- Possible use of variable-modulus orthodontics.
- Ability to control the occlusal plane.
- Minimal round-tripping.

- Allows for the use of both stable and replaceable segments.
- Long intervals possible between visits.
- The construction is forgiving (not requiring high precision).
- Displacement of single teeth is not geometry-dependent (Cases 7–9, see www.wiley.com/go/melsen).

However, there are also certain disadvantages related to segmented mechanics:

- It requires knowledge of biomechanics.
- It requires that the clinician has well-defined treatment goals in all three dimensions of space.
- It requires custom-made appliance construction.
- The active appliance should be monitored for both force magnitude and localisation of its line of action.
- The insertion of the appliance may be time-consuming.

If it is decided that the treatment should be carried out with segmented appliances, all treatments are carried out between two teeth, 'segments'. The first step is to sequence the treatment into phases and to design the appliance needed for the first phase. If alignment within segments has to be done, the necessary line of action with respect to the CR of the tooth/unit of teeth to be moved has to be defined and it has to be decided whether this line of action can be achieved directly, by means of rigid extensions establishing the necessary points of force application or whether loops or cantilevers are necessary. As the force system is generally applied to the bracket, the localisation of the effective line of action of the force vector can be expressed as the moment-to-force ratio to the bracket. It is important that the movement of the active unit and thus the localisation of the line of action are considered in all three planes of space.

Although the correlation between the localisation of the force vector and the dental movement is very high, the prediction of the treatment result depends on the validity of estimates of the position of the CR and the exact localisation is changing during the ongoing tooth movement. It is therefore necessary to monitor the dental movement in the initial stages and to adjust the force system and the appliance if needed.

Although, in theory, any force system can be produced between the bracket and a continuous wire if the correct angulation is generated between the wire and bracket of the tooth to be moved, the clinician has usually poor control of the force system. Due to the inherent characteristics of the continuous arch, the force system changes rapidly, as any change in position of the tooth will contribute to a change in geometry. Concerning levelling with continuous arches as well as intra-segmental levelling, it is important to avoid unnecessary side effects from the mutual configuration of the teeth, which should be analysed before levelling indiscriminately. The side effects can thereby be predicted before the levelling arches are inserted. Levelling of the

anterior unit may result in undesirable vertical displacements (Figure 7.26), whereas levelling of the posterior segments usually generates fewer side effects, as the occlusal forces interact with the force system.

Both during levelling and especially finishing, the addition of minor bends is frequently used. Burstone and Koenig (1988) and Ronay et al. (1989) analysed the effect of creative bending, used for minor corrections between two units, and demonstrated that a minimum change in the position of the bend and variation in the inter-bracket inclination significantly influenced the developed force system. In principle, any moment-to-force ratio can be developed, but the constancy of these force systems is very low and the tooth movement can even reverse if one unit is displaced more rapidly than the other (Figure 7.27).

Intrasegmental alignment with segments of an ideal arch

Even if the force system of a statically indeterminate system is not fully known in the clinical practice, it is possible to use the concepts of the six geometries to obtain reasonably predictable and controlled movements, limiting inconsistencies and round-tripping during intrasegmental alignment if the wire is activated only between two brackets.

In intrasegmental alignment it is important to assess whether both units can be considered active or if there is a need of having a reactive and an active unit. In the first case, both units will be left free to move. If only one of the units, generally one tooth, has to be moved, the other one has to be consolidated. Consolidation is often done to a molar by bending the wire segment, so that it is passively connected to the molar that is in the desired position. In other cases, the reactive unit is consolidated through a lingual or palatal arch to the contralateral teeth, or it is estimated that at least to teeth connected by a passive wire can be maintained by

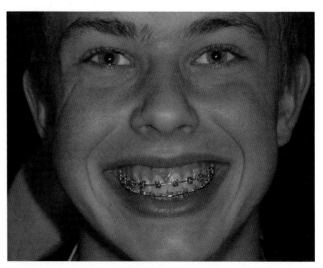

Fig. 7.26 Side effect of indiscriminate levelling of the upper arch: development of a canted plane of occlusion.

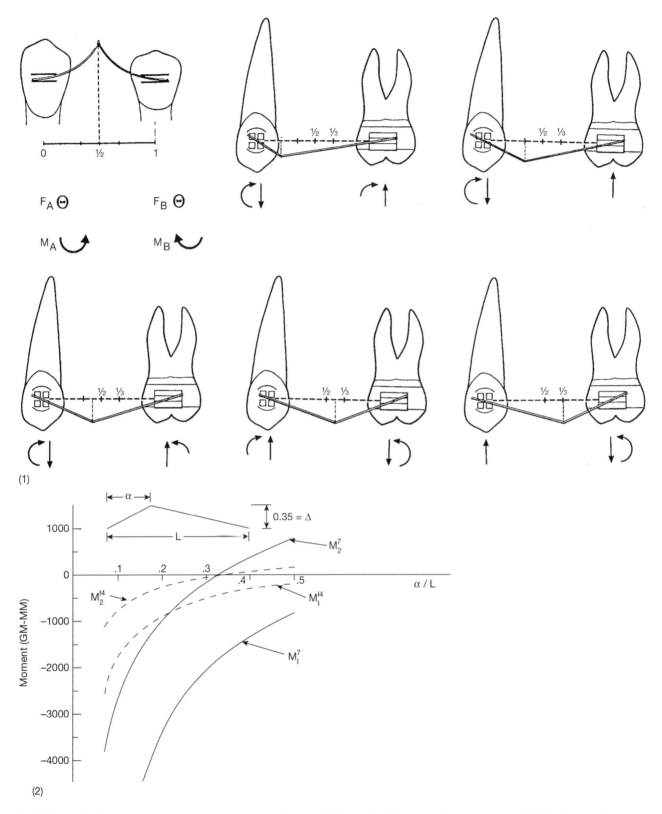

Fig. 7.27 So-called creative bend often used during levelling or finishing: the V-bend and the step bend. (1) With the positioning of the V-bend, any geometry apart from geometry I can be generated. (2) Illustration of the force systems generated when the 'V' is displaced. Observe how the force system is reversed with a displacement of the 'V'. (3) The step bend, which will develop the force system typical of geometry I: two identical moments in the same direction and two equal and opposite forces. (4) and (5) The position of the step bend does not influence the generated force system. (With permission from Burstone and Koenig (1988). Reproduced with permission from Elsevier.)

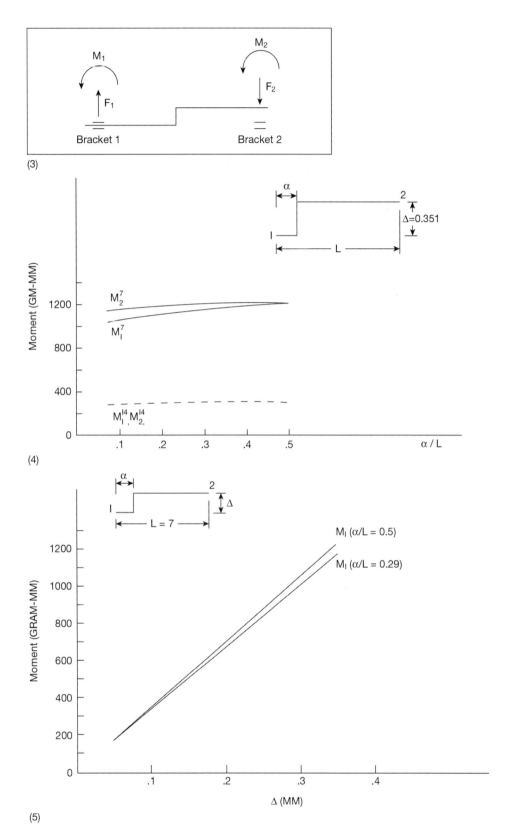

(3)

(4)

(5)

Fig. 7.27 (*Continued*)

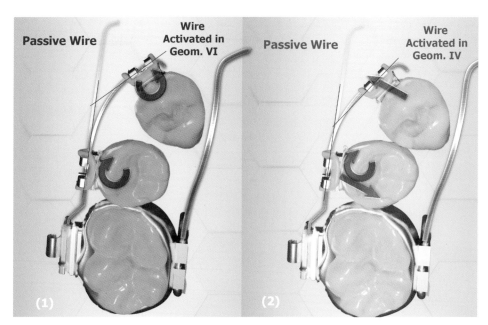

Fig. 7.28 (1) and (2) A SIA is active between the two premolar brackets to align tooth 3.4. In different stages of the movement, the bracket position geometries in the range VI to IV, with an alternate of the predominance of the moment or the force. However, even if not stable, the system can be considered consistent, since both the force and the moment applied to the active unit have always the right direction. The reactive unit (3.5), on the other hand, is limited in its movement by the connection with the molar, obtained by bending the segment passively in that area.

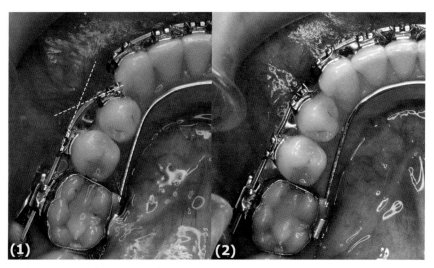

Fig. 7.29 (1) and (2) Clinical example of alignment with SIA in beta-titanium 0.017 × 0.025 inches. The geometry between teeth 3.5 and 3.4 swings between IV and VI and the first premolar is progressively moved buccally and rotated.

occlusal forces. If there is no other possibility to stabilise the reactive unit skeletal anchorage (TADs) can be used indirectly to reinforce it.

The use of segments of an ideal arch (SIA) is only indicated when the relationship between the active and the reactive unit represents high geometries (VI to IV) according to Burstone and Koenig (1974) and illustrated in Figure 7.17. This configuration selection depends on two factors: (1) high geometries have an inherent lower rigidity

than low geometries. (2) The change of spatial relationships between the brackets, when starting from a low geometry (III to I) and when only one active unit exists, begins with a rotation or inclination of the active unit in the opposite direction of the one desired for alignment. Such a system is inconsistent with the goal and generates a jiggling movement. If the relation between the brackets is corresponding to a low geometry, a rectangular loop configuration would solve the problems mentioned in the earlier text. If, on the other hand, an SIA is activated at its terminal part in a high geometry, the force system will swing between the one of the geometry VI (Figure 7.28(1), only moments acting) and the one of the geometry IV (Figure 7.28(2), single force to the active unit). Even if the force system will not be as stable as it could be with statically determinate mechanics, the direction of both force and moment will be consistent with the treatment goal throughout the whole movement (Figure 7.29).

Loops

In the case of major positional problems such as tipping or rotations, it may be advantageous in low geometry conditions to resolve these using loops even despite the availability of memory alloy archwires. With loops, the force system can be previewed and clear differentiation between the active and the passive units is possible. An alternative would be an overlay mechanism (Verna et al. 2004). Burstone recommended the application of free-end loops of various designs (Figure 7.30). The effect of vertical activation of the T-loop, the L-loop and the rectangular loop between two segments was studied by Vanderby et al. (1977) in the sagittal plane and by Menghi et al. (1999) in all three planes of space (Figure 7.31). In relation to intra-arch correction, the free-end loop can be welded to a bypass, a lateral or an anterior segment (Figure 7.31(3)).

Depending on the wire distribution, four different types of the loop have been described:

- The *vertical loop* and *T-loop* are symmetrical; therefore, the differences between the force systems developed on the two teeth adjacent to the loop do not differ significantly from that of the straight wire. The simplest loop is the vertical loop. The addition of a vertical loop is not used to change the force system on the two sides of the loop, but can be used to create a hinge in the archwire. Vertical loops were previously used to lower the load deflection rate of the wire. Presently, T-loops are mostly used for controlled space closure.
- *Asymmetrical loops* deliver a force system that is significantly different on the two sides of the loop. In the correction of malposition of single teeth, the L-loop is well suited, as it is possible to generate any combination of forces and moments to one unit of two teeth (Figure 7.30(2)). As a simple rule, the smaller moment is applied to the tooth engaged at the end towards which the loop is pointing, and the difference in the moment-to-force ratio is increasing with the increase in length of the 'boot'. In the correction of a malpositioned tooth, it is therefore important to note in which direction the L is pointing. The L-loop can be very useful in the uprighting of lower molars.
- The *rectangular loop* is the most frequently applied loop for corrections of malpositions of single teeth (Patel

et al. 1999). This loop delivers the largest deviation from the force system delivered by a straight wire and can be used for moving teeth in all three planes of space (Figure 7.30(3–4)).

When the amount of wire or the stiffness of the wire on either side of the bracket is varied through the displacement of the point of force application on the horizontal extension, the direction of the moment will be altered. The point at which no moment will be generated when the loop is engaged into the bracket is defined as the point of dissociation. At this point, no dependency exists between the moment and the forces (Figure 7.31). The moments delivered at either side of the point of dissociation are opposite and increase with increasing distance from the point of dissociation.

At the point of dissociation, the rectangular loop delivers a constant moment-to-force ratio and the loop can be activated for the delivery of forces or moments alone. This loop configuration can thus be used to overcome the problem of inconsistency, where either the force or the moment is in an undesirable direction. Depending on the point of force application, a clockwise or an anticlockwise moment can be generated. The same point of dissociation exists for the vertical and horizontal activation. As the load deflection rate is lowest when the point of force application is at the end of the horizontal beam, it is important to preview the combination of the desired forces and moments when choosing the orientation of the loop (Figure 7.31).

The force systems delivered by the loop are dependent not only on the configuration and difference in height and length, but also on the stiffness of the various parts of the loop. Since beta-titanium wires of different dimensions can easily be joined by welding, the rectangular loop can be made as a composite of 0.025 × 0.017- and 0.018-inch beta-titanium, whereby the point of dissociation can be displaced as seen in Figure 7.31. This makes it possible to apply a comfortable and biomechanical correct loop (Cases 7–9, see www.wiley.com/go/melsen).

The use of rigid extensions (power-arms)

Usually, forces are applied to teeth from the buccal or lingual aspect and the line of action of the force passes at the bracket level if loops are not inserted. It is, however, possible to shift the point of force application more apically by applying the forces to hooks or rigid extensions, in orthodontic jargon 'power-arms' (Figures 7.32–7.34).

Power-arms can be both fixed and welded, or removable and inserted into brackets. The variation in the point of force application is limited only by the anatomy and the consideration for the patient's comfort. On the buccal side, a power-arm can only have limited height and the desired line of action of the force can therefore not always be generated. However, palatally, it is possible to apply a force even above the CR. Varying the level of the points of force application

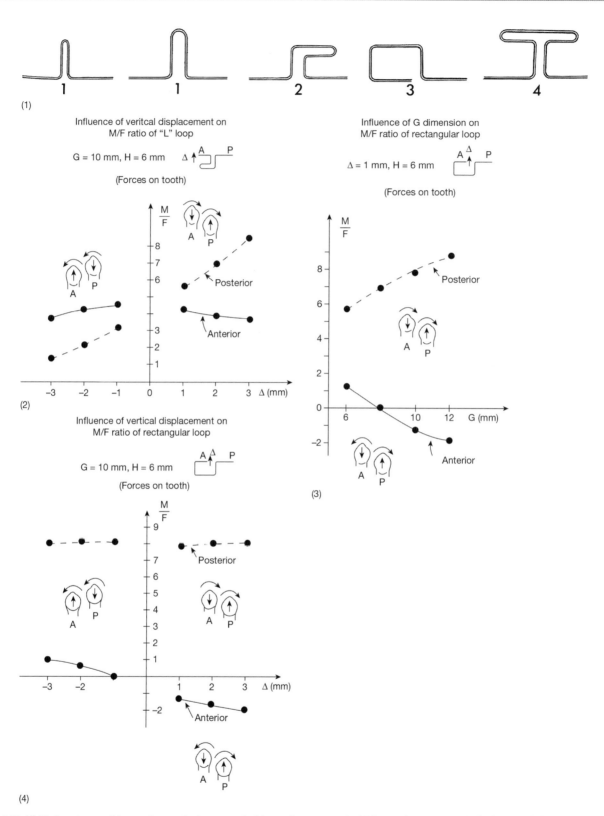

Fig. 7.30 (1) Various types of loops: the vertical symmetrical loop, the symmetrical T-loop, the asymmetrical L-loop and the asymmetrical rectangular loop. (2) The force system developed by the L-loop inserted by two brackets on different vertical levels. Note that the moments are smallest in the direction of the 'boot', where the amount of wire is higher. (3) Graph illustrating how the horizontal dimension of a rectangular loop influences the distribution of the force systems developed with respect to the two brackets. The force system to the bracket within the loop is very constant and the moment approximates zero when the horizontal length of the rectangular loop is close to the inter-bracket distance; the force systems delivered to the two brackets are very different but constant. (4) When the horizontal length is 10 mm, the M/F ratio is high and almost constant for the posterior unit. (With permission from Vanderby et al. (1977).)

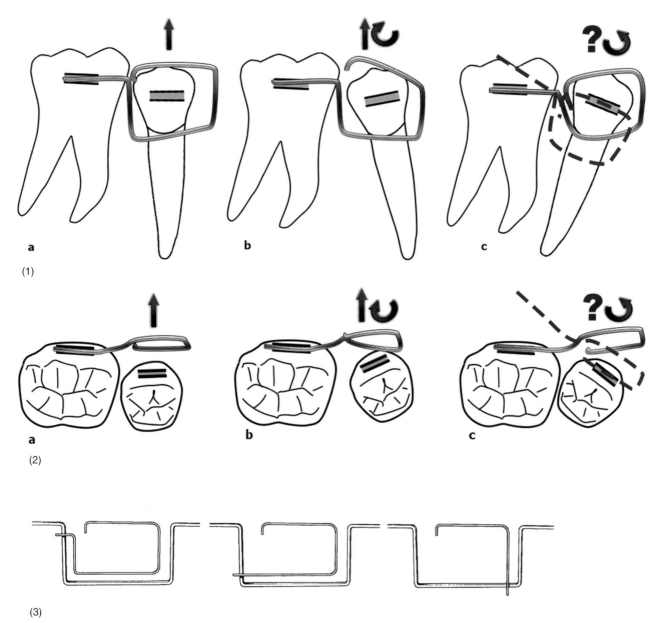

Fig. 7.31 (1) and (2): (a) Rectangular loops activated at the point of dissociation delivering no moment to the premolar. In this case, the terminal part of the loop does not change its angulation during the activation. (b) and (c) illustrate the combination of moments and forces generated in the two planes of space when a rectangular loop extends from the molar, in this case the passive unit, to the premolar. The force systems are used to displace the premolar with extrusion, or buccally. (b) The desired combination of moment and force is seen, while the largest deflection takes place at the end of the wire. (c) The loop is stiffer since the largest deflection is not at the end of the wire, furthermore the vertical force is not easily understandable, because it depends on the ratio between the two angles of insertion, as it is shown by the dashed line. This use of the rectangular loop is not recommendable. (3) When the combination of the moment is not desirable, the loop has to extend from the other side, the anterior side. This can be done by welding a 0.018 loop to a bypass of, for example, a 0.017 × 0.025-inch TMA wire with the variations illustrated here.

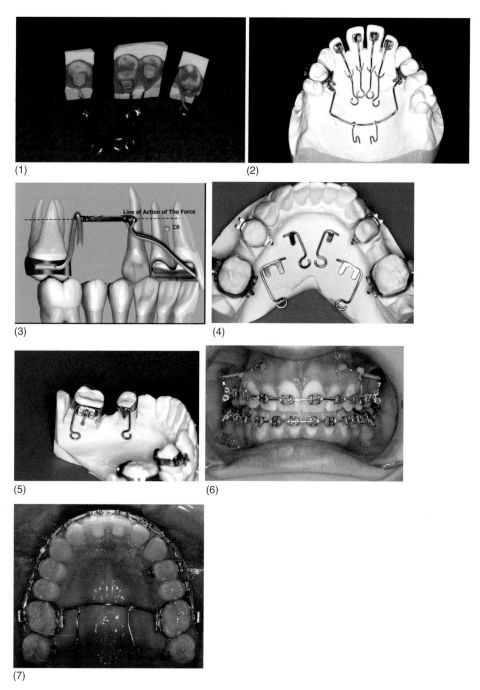

Fig. 7.32 Various types of rigid extensions. (1) Transfer trays for indirect bonding of lingual power-arms welded to base plates. (2) Rigid extensions bonded to the lingual pad on the upper incisors and welded to the transpalatal arch. These extensions would allow the generation of a force at the apical level of the incisors. The premolars are consolidated with a TAD on the buccal side. (3) Line of action of the force between two extensions on the palatal aspect. Due to its inclination and position, it can be located above the estimated CR position of the anterior teeth. (4) and (5) Removable lingual extensions: Wilson's 3D molar attachments (Rocky Mountain) with vertical inserts. Extensions with a double flat male part were used on the molars. In relation to the premolars, the attachments were cut into halves. To reinforce the welding, laser soldering was used. This system is easy to use and allows for precision, stability and reproducibility. (6) Extensions attached to a bracket on upper molars in order to translate the molars mesially against skeletal anchorage. (7) Rigid extensions welded to a transpalatal arch in order to intrude and tip the second molars lingually.

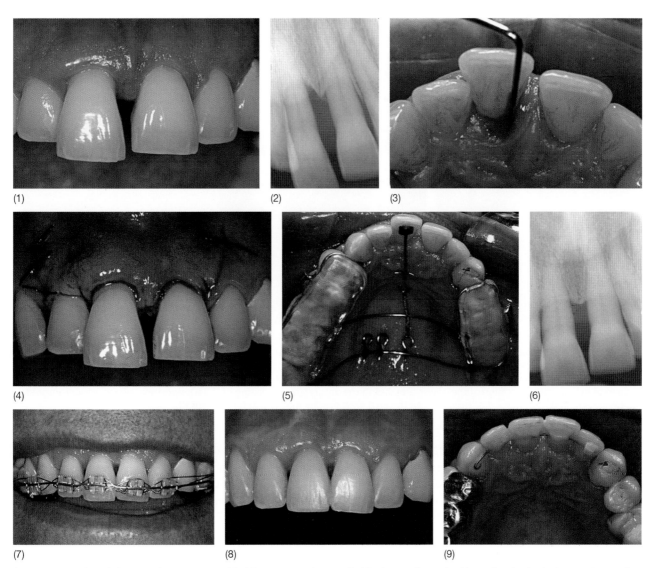

Fig. 7.33 Examples of the use of power-arms. (1)–(4) Patient with extruded incisor and marginal bone loss in the incisor region. Before orthodontic treatment, the patient had modified Widman flap surgery for pocket reduction and apical repositioning of the gingival level. (5)–(9) A combined intrusive and retraction force was generated by a coil spring extending from a power-arm on the lingual surface of the incisor to the transpalatal arch.

allows the clinician to choose the direction and inclination of the line of action of the force to the CR and thereby to control the tooth movement (Figures 7.32–7.35).

A single force at the bracket level produces uncontrolled tipping. To avoid deformation of the wires when loading the teeth at bracket level, the wires on which the brackets are sliding should have the maximum stiffness. The unavoidable friction could be minimised by applying the forces to power-arms, so the line of action passes close to the CR. Any force passing outside the CR of a tooth generates a rotational moment (the moment of the force), having the direction of the force and the magnitude of the intensity of the force multiplied by the perpendicular distance with the CR. The application of a single force to a known point makes it easy

to visualise the moment-to-force ratio at the CR and thereby to predict the tooth movement.

Varying the point of force application is a simple way to monitor tooth movement. In adult patients, it is often desirable to generate modelling of the alveolar process by moving teeth 'with bone' outside the existing alveolar envelope and it is crucial not to overload the periodontium. The stress/strain distribution along the root should therefore be under maximum control. Translation and root movement, with three-dimensional control of the movement, are difficult movements to achieve, but can be carried out if forces are applied to power-arms at the level of the CR (Fontenelle 1991; Park et al. 2000) (Figures 7.35 and 7.36), or exactly at the needed distance from it.

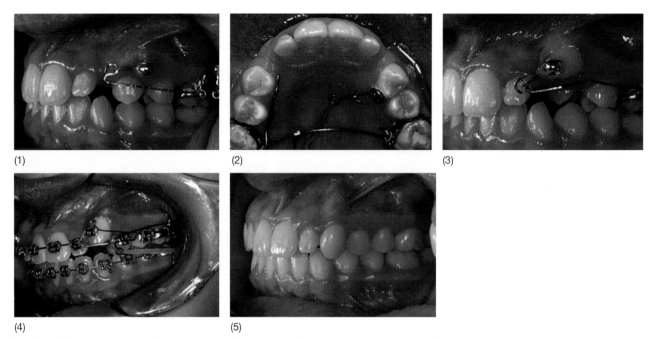

(1)   (2)   (3)

(4)   (5)

Fig. 7.34 (1) Powers-arms used for correction of a transposed canine. A power-arm extending from the molar was used to generate a mesial force on the transposed canine against a distal force to the molar. (2) Tooth 24 was displaced distally and lingually by a force extending from the power-arm on 24 allowing for the lingual movement of the root necessary for the correction of the transposition. (3) Change in length and direction of the power-arm during the progressive correcting of the transposition. (4) Once the transposition had been corrected, the canine was brought into the arch with overlay mechanics. (5) Final result.

Already in 1982, Fontenelle (1982) had suggested displacement of the point of application and applied the forces to transpalatal arches made of cast precious metal extended across the palatal vault. He also described the so-called 'hinge mechanics', as the arches could rotate at one end (Figure 7.36). They served as guiding mechanics, keeping both tipping and rotation under control. The combination of transpalatal arches and power-arms was also used by Weiland and Bantleon (Weiland et al. 1992a, 1992b, 1996) who developed a simple alternative combining active mechanics and a guiding wire.

With power-arms, only forces and no couples are applied, and the tooth movement can be accomplished without the significant loss of force normally caused by friction. The limiting factor of this technique is the anatomy. An obstacle has been the tissue impingement often occurring when bonding the power-arm directly to the clinical crown. However, these practical problems can to some degree be overcome with an indirect bonding system.

Easy or difficult tooth movement

The difficulty of treatment is a direct reflection of how difficult it is to obtain the correct line of action of the required force. Tooth movements which can be achieved by applying forces to brackets or power-arms are considered easy, whereas those that can only be performed with a force with a line of action outside the dental sphere are considered difficult (Figure 7.37(1)) (Case 10, see www.wiley.com/go/melsen).

Some types of tooth movement are universally considered more difficult than others. Space closure is easier with tipping than with translation. Molar uprighting combined with extrusion is easy, whereas uprighting combined with intrusion is difficult to achieve (Melsen et al. 1996). Intrusion with proclination is easy, whereas intrusion combined with lingual root movement is difficult (Fiorelli et al. 2003). The differences are not caused by any difference in tissue reactions to the different types of movement, but rather due to the localisation of the required force (Figure 7.37).

A custom-made appliance is designed to deliver the desired force vector. The design of the appliance can be developed based on mathematical calculations. The force magnitude is determined by the wire properties, the alloys, the dimensions, the length, the configuration and the amount of activation. The line of action is determined by the point of force application and the configuration, that is, the bending of the wire (Burstone 1962, 1966, 1975, 1982; Burstone and Koenig 1976; Fontenelle 1991; Dalstra and Melsen 1999; Fiorelli and Merlo 2015; Fiorelli and Melsen 1992–2022).

With this in mind, it is interesting to note that all the movements that are considered difficult are those that can be produced only by a force vector whose line of action passes outside the dental sphere and cannot be reproduced by the active elements of the appliances such as elastics or coil springs. In the case of a difficult tooth movement, the correct resultant force cannot be found by the trial and error

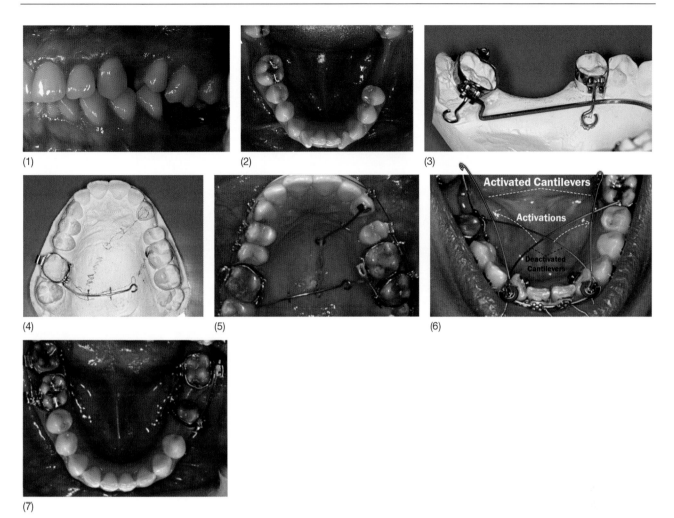

Fig. 7.35 Patient presenting with missing 24, 35, 36, over-erupted 26 and distally inclined 23. The whole dentition has to be moved to the right, as the patient's dental midlines were displaced to the left. (1) and (2) Start of treatment. (3)–(5) The power-arms used. (6) The cantilever is used for derotation of the lower lateral incisors. (7) Result of cantilever treatment. The treatment goal was to prepare the patient for reconstruction. (3) The mesially inclined second molar was displaced mesially with the root first. This was done with 35 as anchorage. (4) and (5) In the upper arch, the midline had to be displaced to the left by moving the 23 distally with the root first. (5)–(7) In the lower arch, the distally rotated lateral incisors were corrected by two cantilevers extending to the molar region.

method and it is often necessary to apply a combination of vectors obtained by using often two cantilevers.

Cantilevers

Cantilevers generate statically determinate force (or one-couple) systems. An important characteristic of the force delivered by cantilevers is a high degree of constancy of both the force and of the moment-to-force ratio during deactivation. The constancy of the force depends on the length, dimensions and characteristics of the wire material. With the increasing length of the cantilever, the wire dimensions and stiffness can be also increased. In cases where it is not possible to construct a cantilever of sufficient length to obtain the required force level, a composite cantilever can be constructed. The part of the cantilever inserted into a bracket or tube has to have a dimension not allowing any

rolling. The part that can be welded on has a smaller dimension and is attached with a one-point contact. A usual combination would be 0.017 × 0.025 inches for insertion into the bracket or tube to which a 0.018-inch wire is welded.

This combination would allow for a lower force level and a lower load deflection rate; furthermore, the welding can determine a different structural axis for the cantilever, thus changing the angle of the force.

Cantilevers offer a wide range of possibilities and can be inserted with full engagement both in the active and the reactive units. The wire is generally inserted into the reactive unit if the desired M/F ratio at the active unit is low, and in the active unit if a large M/F is desired. If extrusion or intrusion is needed in the anterior unit, the base arch or the cantilever is inserted into the molar tube and the effect on the molar can be avoided by consolidating the posterior

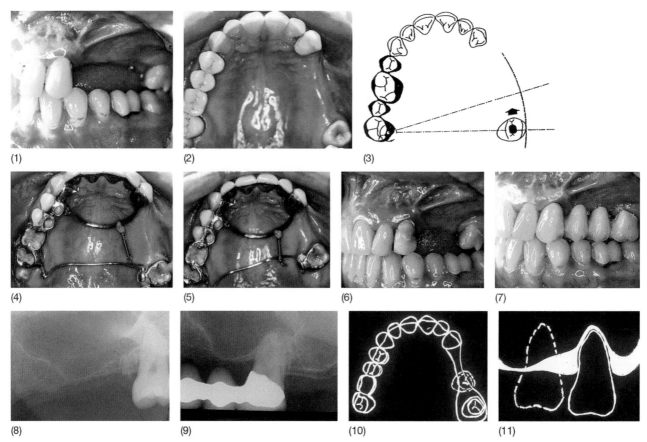

(1)   (2)   (3)

(4)   (5)   (6)   (7)

(8)   (9)   (10)   (11)

Fig. 7.36 Hinge mechanics. (1) and (2) A patient missing all teeth between 23 and 28. The span was too long for replacement with a bridge and implants were not recommendable either, because of atrophy of alveolar bone and the extension of the maxillary sinus, leaving the paper-thin bone in the area. (3) Illustration of the principle of hinge mechanics. (4) The anchorage unit was composed of all teeth, apart from the third molar that was to be moved. These teeth were consolidated by a cast splint. The cast retention also comprised a transpalatal bar extending from 14 to 24 and an extension palatally from 16. This extension was furnished with a vertical tube that served as the centre of rotation for the transpalatal arch, serving as guiding mechanics for the mesialisation of 28. The active unit was a coil spring at the level of the centre of resistance from the anterior to the posterior transpalatal arch. The width of the arch was maintained by the guiding mechanics. (5) and (6) The situation at the end of treatment. (7) After insertion of a bridge between 23 with 28. (8)–(11) Illustration of the tooth movement that took place through the maxillary sinus and widening alveolar process. (Case treated by A. Fontenelle.)

teeth into a single unit. In this way, the occlusion also becomes part of the anchorage. An exception may be in patients in whom distal tipping of the upper molars is required. A temporary bite opening bonded lingually to the upper incisors may be needed. Inserted into the molar tube, the cantilever can be used for tipping, rotation and extrusion of the molar, but there is no anchorage, since both posterior and anterior units are active (Figure 7.38).

In cases where the major moment is to be applied to one or more teeth, for example, lingual root torque of upper incisors, the torque arch is inserted into the brackets of the four anterior teeth and tied to the posterior unit. This appliance, however, will also extrude the incisors (Figure 7.39). Cantilevers can also be used for applying buccal root torque to a single tooth. When molar uprighting is required, the cantilever is inserted into the molar tube and tied to the anterior segment. With the same insertion and a lingual arch

to consolidate the molars, the cantilever can be used for buccolingual correction of the canine (or/and the premolars). In the case where, for example, canines have to be uprighted or rotated, the cantilever should be inserted into the active unit, the canine, and tied to the anchorage unit both anteriorly and posteriorly: the 'windmill' (Figure 7.40).

The localisation of the point of force application of the one-point contact to the CR of the unit to which the wire is tied determines the moment generated to that unit. The orthodontist has the freedom to alter the localisation of the point of force application utilising a power-arm, which can change the point of force application both horizontally and vertically (Figure 7.32).

When the cantilever is activated, the direction of the force it delivers is usually perpendicular to the structural axis (Figure 7.16). Minor deviations can be obtained if the configuration of the cantilever is altered, while more

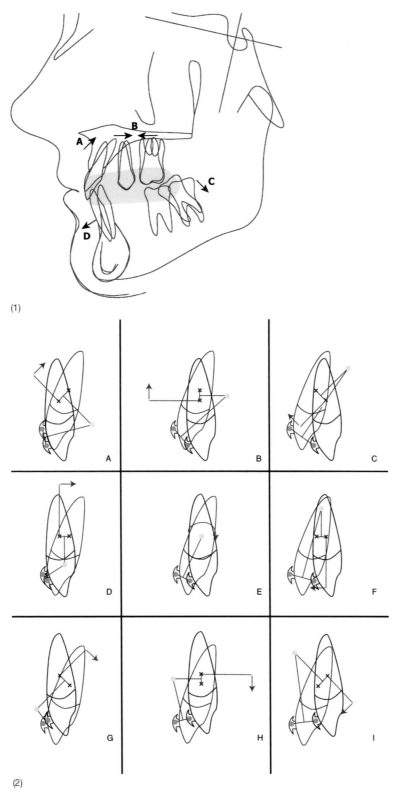

Fig. 7.37 (1) Force vectors necessary for so-called difficult movements. Arrow A generates the combination of lingual root torque and intrusion. B delivers root approximation of the posterior teeth, C results in a combination of uprighting and intrusion of the lower molars and D produces a combined intrusion and labial translation (with permission from Fiorelli et al. 2003). (2) Different solutions for the correction of steep incisors. In the upper panel, the correction is combined with intrusion, in the middle panel, the centre of resistance is not displaced vertically and in the lower panel, the correction is combined with extrusion. The necessary force vectors are indicated and it can be seen that A, B and D are difficult movements, as the necessary force vector is never within the confines of the dental system. In these cases, only two-vector mechanics can be used (Melsen and Fiorelli 2000. Courtesy of Quintessence).

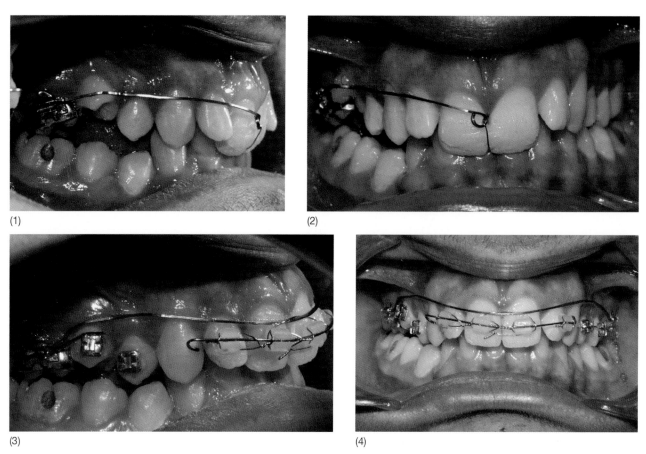

(1)

(2)

(3)

(4)

Fig. 7.38 (1) and (2) Cantilever extending from the right upper molar to the two central incisors. The effect will be extrusion and distal tipping of the molar and intrusion and proclination of 11 and 21. (3) The cantilever extending from 16 is generating an extrusion of 15. (4) The base arch will intrude and procline the anterior segment.

important changes can be obtained by adding loops (major configurations). Changes in the design of the cantilever will generate changes in the direction of the line of action, so that it can lead to an increase or decrease in the arch length. The five main types of configurations described by Dalstra and Melsen in 1999 are: (G) the tip-back, (A) the circular or harmonic curvature, (B) the logarithmic curvature, (F) the utility shape and (C) the cantilever produced by using two wires with two different dimensions and two helices. Fiorelli and Melsen (1992–2022) and Fiorelli and Merlo (2015) also described other configurations (D, E, H and I) where loops contribute to changing the force line of action in a more significant way. The configuration is especially important concerning the correction of a deep bite by intrusion. In these cases, it should be decided whether the arch length at the end of treatment should be increased or reduced. An increase in length can be achieved by using several different configurations: the utility shape will generate the largest increase followed by the tip-back. If the curvature is equally distributed over the wire, it generates a vertical force, whereas a logarithmic curve will deliver a force that produces a slight contraction and shortening of the arch

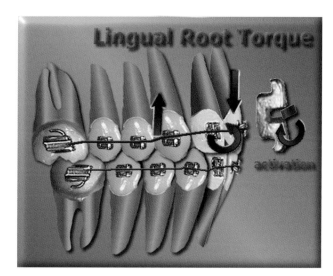

Fig. 7.39 Force system delivered from an arch inserted for lingual root torque.

length. If proclination is included in the first part of the treatment and later retraction is planned, the total tissue reaction will need to be reversed, which can be both

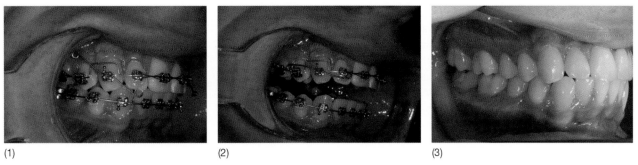

(1)   (2)   (3)

Fig. 7.40 (1) 'Windmill' before activation. (2) Activated 'windmill'. (3) The result. This kind of cantilever can be assimilated to two-vector mechanics. Differential activations of the 2 arms can lead to different effects.

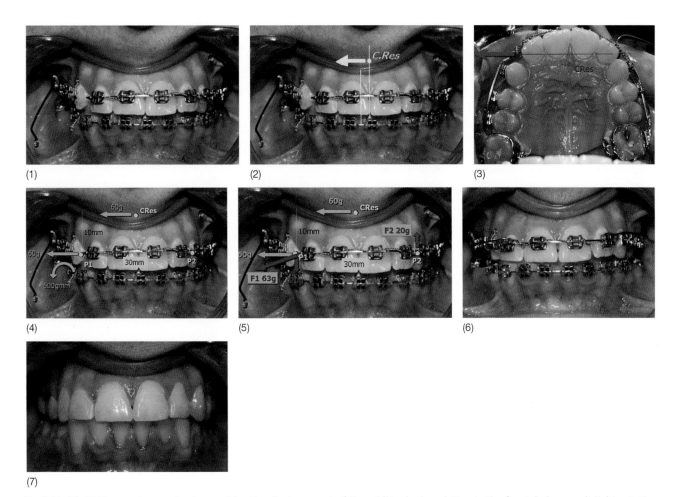

(1)   (2)   (3)

(4)   (5)   (6)

(7)

Fig. 7.41 (1)–(7) Two-vector mechanics used for the displacement of the midline by translation in the frontal plane and slight rotation in the horizontal plane of space (see text for details). Cres: Centre of resistance.

detrimental for the tissues and time-consuming; it is therefore important to select the correct configuration of the cantilever from the start.

If the cantilever is produced using wires with different dimensions, with the heavier wire in the posterior segment and the lighter wire in the anterior, the structural axis can be changed. The centre will now be the point where the light wire is added.

Two-vector mechanics

If the desired line of action is remote and cannot be reproduced by a simple cantilever, the combination of two cantilevers may be the solution (Fiorelli et al. 2003). The design of this type of mechanics is based on fairly simple mathematics that can also be carried out with software, which is supplied as part of the occlusogram software T3DO (IOSS GmbH – www.ioss-ortho.com).

One example of tooth movement that could not be achieved with conventional appliances but was performed with two-cantilever mechanics is shown in Figure 7.41.

In the patient in Figure 7.41, the treatment goal was to move the upper incisors towards the right by translation. These teeth are well-aligned and, therefore, it is advisable to perform any movement of these teeth as a group. Since no rotational movement of the group in the frontal plane or any kind of vertical displacement is needed, the vector that will produce the desired movement passes through the group CR in a purely transverse direction. As a slight rotation has to be generated in the occlusal plane, the force has to pass 2–3 mm in front of the estimated position of CR. This will lead to anticlockwise rotation of the incisor group needed to close the space anterior to 13. The group of incisors was consolidated with a stiff stainless-steel wire to obtain the movement of the group as a whole.

The required resultant vector was generated by applying two vectors, at point P1 and point P2 (Figure 7.41(5)). The vector at point P1 delivered the necessary horizontal force. This force will, as it is applied 10 mm below the CR, generate tipping. The tipping was neutralised by the addition of a force couple, an extrusive force of 20 cN to P1 and an intrusive force of 20 cN at P2. The activation was checked by means of a force gauge. The appliance was left in for 10 weeks and the desired movements occurred.

Conclusion

In the treatment of adult patients, the main challenge is to design an appliance that minimises round-tripping and thereby reduces the treatment time.

This can only be done after defining the treatment goal after which the least complicated appliance should be chosen. This is often a statically determinate appliance, as the preconditions for straight wire are rarely fulfilled by deteriorated dentitions. Most dental movements that are considered challenging by the orthodontist involve the need to generating a force vector that is beyond the scope of a conventional orthodontic appliance. The application of two-cantilever mechanics and the use of power-arms offer solutions to several typical problems. Visit the supporting companion website for this book (www.wiley.com/go/melsen) for examples of adult cases treated by our colleagues.

References

Andrews LF (1976a) The straight-wire appliance, origin, controversy, commentary. *J Clin Orthod* 10, 99–114.

Andrews LF (1976b) The straight-wire appliance. Explained and compared. *J Clin Orthod* 10, 174–195.

Articolo LC, Kusy K, Saunders CR and Kusy RP (2000) Influence of ceramic and stainless steel brackets on the notching of archwires during clinical treatment. *Eur J Orthod* 22, 409–425.

Articolo LC and Kusy RP (1999) Influence of angulation on the resistance to sliding in fixed appliances. *Am J Orthod Dentofacial Orthop* 115, 39–51.

Bassarelli T, Dalstra M and Melsen B (2005) Changes in clinical crown height as a result of transverse expansion of the maxilla in adults. *Eur J Orthod* 27, 121–128.

Berger J (1999) The engaging concept of self-ligation. *Ont Dent* 76, 26–33.

Berger J and Byloff FK (2001) The clinical efficiency of self-ligated brackets. *J Clin Orthod* 35, 304–308.

Berger JL (1990) The influence of the SPEED bracket's self-ligating design on force levels in tooth movement: a comparative in vitro study. *Am J Orthod Dentofacial Orthop* 97, 219–228.

Bollen AM, Huang G, King G, Hujoel P and Ma T (2003) Activation time and material stiffness of sequential removable orthodontic appliances. Part 1: ability to complete treatment. *Am J Orthod Dentofacial Orthop* 124, 496–501.

Braun S, Bluestein M, Moore BK and Benson G (1999) Friction in perspective. *Am J Orthod Dentofacial Orthop* 115, 619–627.

Burstone CJ (1962) Rationale of the segmented arch. *American Journal of Orthodontics* 48, 805–822.

Burstone CJ (1966) The mechanics of the segmented arch techniques. *Angle Orthod* 36, 99–120.

Burstone CJ (1975) Application of bio-engineering to clinical orthodontics. In Graber T and Swain BF (eds) *Current Orthodontic Concepts and Techniques*, 2nd edn. Philadelphia, PA: WB Saunders.

Burstone CJ (1982) The segmented arch approach to space closure. *Am J Orthod* 82, 361–378.

Burstone CJ (1991) The biomechanical rationale of orthodontic therapy. In Melsen B (ed) *Current Controversies in Orthodontics*, pp. 147–180. Chicago, IL: Quintessence.

Burstone CJ and Koenig HA (1974) Force systems from an ideal arch. *Am J Orthod* 65, 270–289.

Burstone CJ and Koenig HA (1976) Optimizing anterior and canine retraction. *Am J Orthod* 70, 1–19.

Burstone CJ and Koenig HA (1988) Creative wire bending – the force system from step and V bends. *Am J Orthod Dentofacial Orthop* 93, 59–67.

Burstone CJ and Marcotte MR (2000) The treatment midline. In Bywaters LC (ed) *Problem Solving in Orthodontics*, pp. 145–178. Chicago, IL: Quintessence.

Burstone CJ and Pryputniewicz RJ (1980) Holographic determination of centers of rotation produced by orthodontic forces. *Am J Orthod* 77, 396–409.

Cacciafesta V, Sfondrini MF, Ricciardi A, Scribante A, Klersy C and Auricchio F (2003) Evaluation of friction of stainless steel and esthetic self-ligating brackets in various bracket-archwire combinations. *Am J Orthod Dentofacial Orthop* 124, 395–402.

Cattaneo PM (2003) *Orthodontic Aspects of Bone Mechanics and Bone Remodelling*. Denmark: University of Aarhus.

Christiansen RL and Burstone CJ (1969) Centers of rotation within the periodontal space. *Am J Orthod* 55, 353–369.

Clements KM, Bollen AM, Huang G, King G, Hujoel P and Ma T (2003) Activation time and material stiffness of sequential removable orthodontic appliances. Part 2: dental improvements. *Am J Orthod Dentofacial Orthop* 124, 502–508.

Dalstra M, Eriksen H, Bergamini C and Melsen BJ (2015) Actual versus theoretical torsional play in conventional and self-ligating bracket systems. *Orthod* 2015 Jun;42(2), 103–113. doi: 10.1179/1465313314Y.0000000126. Epub 2015 Jan 14.

Dalstra M and Melsen B (1999) Force systems developed by six different cantilever configurations. *Clin Orthod Res* 2(1), 3–9.

Dalstra M and Melsen B (2004) Does the transition temperature of Cu-NiTi archwires affect the amount of tooth movement during alignment? *Orthod Craniofac Res* 7, 21–25.

Dalstra M and Melsen B (2009) From alginate impressions to digital virtual models: accuracy and reproducibility. *J Orthod* 36(1), 36–41. discussion 14.

Damon DH (1998a) The Damon low-friction bracket: a biologically compatible straight-wire system. *J Clin Orthod* 32, 670–680.

Damon DH (1998b) The rationale, evolution and clinical application of the self-ligating bracket. *Clin Orthod Res* 1, 52–61.

Davidovitch M and Rebellato J (1995) Two-couple orthodontic appliance systems utility arches: a two-couple intrusion arch. *Semin Orthod* 1, 25–30.

Eberting JJ, Straja SR and Tuncay OC (2001) Treatment time, outcome, and patient satisfaction comparisons of Damon and conventional brackets. *Clin Orthod Res* 4, 228–234.

Farrant SD (1977) An evaluation of different methods of canine retraction. *Br J Orthod* 4, 5–15.

Fiorelli G and Melsen B (1992–2022) *Biomechanics in Orthodontics [Rel.4].* Wollerau: IOSS GmbH. www.ortho-biomechanics.com.

Fiorelli G and Melsen B (1999) The '3-D occlusogram' software. *Am J Orthod Dentofacial Orthop* 116, 363–368.

Fiorelli G, Melsen B and Modica C (2003) Two-vector mechanics. *Prog Orthod* 4, 62–73.

Fiorelli G and Merlo P (2015) Statically determinate appliances and creative mechanics. In Burstone C and Choy K (eds) *The Biomechanical Foundation of Clinical Orthodontics*. Quintessence Publishing.

Fiorelli G, Merlo P, Dalstra M and Melsen B (2018) Le repositionnement mandibulaire: une alternative à la chirurgie chez des patients adultes? Un suivi sur deux ans. *L'Orthodontie Française* 89(2), 123–135.

Fontenelle A (1982) A periodontal concept of induced tooth movement: clinical evidence. *Rev Orthop Dento Faciale* 16, 37–53.

Fontenelle A (1991) Lingual orthodontics in adults. In Melsen B (ed) *Current Controversies in Orthodontics*, pp. 219–268. Chicago, IL: Quintessence.

Frank CA and Nikolai RJ (1980) A comparative study of frictional resistances between orthodontic bracket and archwire. *Am J Orthod* 78, 593–609.

Freshwater M (2003) 3D digital dental models using laser technology. *J Clin Orthod* 37, 101–103.

Fuck LM and Drescher D (2006) Force systems in the initial phase of orthodontic treatment – a comparison of different leveling archwires. *J Orofac Orthop* 67, 6–18.

Gaoa L. and Wichelhaus A. (2017) Forces and moments delivered by the PET-G aligner to a maxillary central incisor for palatal tipping and intrusion. *Angle Orthod.* 87(4): 534–541.

Gianelly A, Bednar JR and Dietz VS (1985) A bidimensional edgewise technique. *J Clin Orthod* 19, 418–421.

Gottlieb EL, Wildman AJ, Hice TL, Lang HM, Lee IF and Strauch EC Jr (1972) The Edgelok bracket. *J Clin Orthod* 6, 613–623.

Hain M, Dhopatkar A and Rock P (2003) The effect of ligation method on friction in sliding mechanics. *Am J Orthod Dentofacial Orthop* 123, 416–422.

Halazonetis DJ (1998) Ideal arch force systems: a center-of-resistance perspective. *Am J Orthod Dentofacial Orthop* 114, 256–264.

Handelman CS (1997) Nonsurgical rapid maxillary alveolar expansion in adults: a clinical evaluation. *Angle Orthod* 67, 291–305.

Hanson GH (1980) The SPEED system: a report on the development of a new edgewise appliance. *Am J Orthod* 78, 243–265.

Hanson GH (1986) JCO/interviews Dr. G. Herbert Hanson on the SPEED bracket. *J Clin Orthod* 20, 183–189.

Hanson GH (2002) Superelastic nickel titanium spring clips for the SPEED appliance. *J Clin Orthod* 36, 520–523.

Harradine NW (2001) Self-ligating brackets and treatment efficiency. *Clin Orthod Res* 4, 220–227.

Harradine NW (2003) Self-ligating brackets: where are we now? *J Orthod* 30, 262–273.

Harradine NW and Birnie DJ (1996) The clinical use of Activa self-ligating brackets. *Am J Orthod Dentofacial Orthop* 109, 319–328.

Hemingway R, Williams RL, Hunt JA and Rudge SJ (2001) The influence of bracket type on the force delivery of Ni-Ti archwires. *Eur J Orthod* 23, 233–241.

Henao SP and Kusy RP (2004) Evaluation of the frictional resistance of conventional and self-ligating bracket designs using standardized arch-wires and dental typodonts. *Angle Orthod* 74, 202–211.

Henao SP and Kusy RP (2005) Frictional evaluations of dental typodont models using four self-ligating designs and a conventional design. *Angle Orthod* 75, 75–85.

Hocevar RA (1981) Understanding, planning, and managing tooth movement: orthodontic force system theory. *Am J Orthod* 80, 457–477.

Hocevar RA (1987) Moment/force ratios. *Am J Orthod Dentofacial Orthop* 91, 350–351.

Isaacson RJ and Rebellato J (1995) Two-couple orthodontic appliance systems: torquing arches. *Semin Orthod* 1, 31–36.

Iwasaki LR, Beatty MW, Randall CJ and Nickel JC (2003) Clinical ligation forces and intraoral friction during sliding on a stainless steel archwire. *Am J Orthod Dentofacial Orthop* 123, 408–415.

Joffe L (2003) Invisalign: early experiences. *J Orthod* 30, 348–352.

Joffe L (2004) OrthoCAD: digital models for a digital era. *J Orthod* 31, 344–347.

Kajdas C and Elsevier Science Publishers (eds) (1990) *Encyclopedia of Trybolog*. New York: Elsevier.

Katsaros C and Dijkman JF (2003) Self-ligating edgewise brackets. An overview. *Ned Tijdschr Tandheelkd* 110, 31–34.

Koenig HA and Burstone CJ (1989) Force systems from an ideal arch – large deflection considerations. *Angle Orthod* 59, 11–16.

Kusy RP (2004) Influence on binding of third-order torque to second-order angulation. *Am J Orthod Dentofacial Orthop* 125, 726–732.

Kusy RP (2005) Influence of force systems on archwire-bracket combinations. *Am J Orthod Dentofacial Orthop* 127, 333–342.

Kusy RP and Tulloch JF (1986) Analysis of moment/force ratios in the mechanics of tooth movement. *Am J Orthod Dentofacial Orthop* 90, 127–131.

Luther F (2007) TMD and occlusion part II. Damned if we don't? Functional occlusal problems: TMD epidemiology in a wider context. *Br Dent J* 2007; 202, E3.

Mah J and Sachdeva R (2001) Computer-assisted orthodontic treatment: the SureSmile process. *Am J Orthod Dentofacial Orthop* 120, 85–87.

Maijer R and Smith DC (1990) Time savings with self-ligating brackets. *J Clin Orthod* 24, 29–31.

McLaughlin RP, Bennett JC and Trevisi HJ (2001) *Systemized Orthodontic Treatment Mechanics*. Edinburgh: Mosby.

Melsen B (1991) Limitations in adult orthodontics. In Melsen B (ed) *Current Controversies in Orthodontics*, pp. 147–180. Chicago, IL: Quintessence.

Melsen B (2020) Where do we come from? Where are we going? *Journal of the World Federation of Orthodontics* 9, 574–578.

Melsen B, Fiorelli G. (2000) Lingually Inclined Incisors. *World J Orthod* 1, 71–78.

Melsen B, Fiorelli G and Bergamini A (1996) Uprighting of lower molars. *J Clin Orthod* 30, 640–645.

Miethke RR, Melsen B. (1999) Effect of variation in tooth morphology and bracket position on first and third order correction with preadjusted appliances. *Am J Orthod Dentofacial Orthop* 116(3), 329–335.

Menghi C, Planert J and Melsen B (1999) 3-D experimental identification of force systems from orthodontic loops activated for first order corrections. *Angle Orthod* 69, 49–57.

Miles PG (2007) Self-ligating vs conventional twin brackets during en-masse space closure with sliding mechanics. *Am J Orthod Dentofacial Orthop* 132, 223–225.

Miles PG, Weyant RJ and Rustveld L (2006) A clinical trial of Damon 2 vs conventional twin brackets during initial alignment. *Angle Orthod* 76(3), 480–485.

Nicolls J (1968) Frictional forces in fixed orthodontic appliances. *Dent Pract Dent Rec* 18, 362–366.

Park YC, Choy K, Lee JS and Kim TK (2000) Lever-arm mechanics in lingual orthodontics. *J Clin Orthod* 34, 601–605.

Patel S, Cacciafesta V and Bosch C (1999) Alignment of impacted canines with cantilevers and box loops. *J Clin Orthod* 33, 82–85.

Pilon JJ, Kuijpers-Jagtman AM and Maltha JC (1996) Magnitude of orthodontic forces and rate of bodily tooth movement. An experimental study. *Am J Orthod Dentofacial Orthop* 110, 16–23.

Pizzoni L, Ravnholt G and Melsen B (1998) Frictional forces related to self-ligating brackets. *Eur J Orthod* 20, 283–291.

Planché P (1997) L'evaluation des techniques prè-enfermées depuis Andrews. *Rev Orthop Denta Faciale* 31, 453–471.

Read-Ward GE, Jones SP and Davies EH (1997) A comparison of self-ligating and conventional orthodontic bracket systems. *Br J Orthod* 24, 309–317.

Redlich M, Mayer Y, Harari D and Lewinstein I (2003) In vitro study of frictional forces during sliding mechanics of 'reduced-friction' brackets. *Am J Orthod Dentofacial Orthop* 124, 69–73.

Ren Y, Maltha JC, Van't Hof MA and Kuijpers-Jagtman AM (2004) Optimum force magnitude for orthodontic tooth movement: a mathematic model. *Am J Orthod Dentofacial Orthop* 125, 71–77.

Resnick R and Halliday D (1977) *Physics, Part 1*. New York, NY: John Wiley & Sons.

Ronay F, Kleinert W, Melsen B and Burstone CJ (1989) Force system developed by V bends in an elastic orthodontic wire. *Am J Orthod Dentofacial Orthop* 96, 295–301.

Sachdeva RC (2001) SureSmile technology in a patient-centered orthodontic practice. *J Clin Orthod* 35, 245–253.

Santoro M, Galkin S, Teredesai M, Nicolay OF and Cangialosi TJ (2003) Comparison of measurements made on digital and plaster models. *Am J Orthod Dentofacial Orthop* 124, 101–105.

Santoro M, Nicolay OF and Cangialosi TJ (2001) Pseudoelasticity and thermoelasticity of nickel-titanium alloys: a clinically oriented review. Part II: deactivation forces. *Am J Orthod Dentofacial Orthop* 119, 594–603.

Schumacher HA, Bourauel C and Drescher D (1990) The effect of the ligature on the friction between bracket and arch. *Fortschr Kieferorthop* 51, 106–116.

Segner D and Ibe D (1995) Properties of superelastic wires and their relevance to orthodontic treatment. *Eur J Orthod* 17, 395–402.

Shivapuja PK and Berger J (1994) A comparative study of conventional ligation and self-ligation bracket systems. *Am J Orthod Dentofacial Orthop* 106, 472–480.

Shroff B, Lindauer SJ, Burstone CJ and Leiss JB (1995) Segmented approach to simultaneous intrusion and space closure: biomechanics of the three-piece base arch appliance. *Am J Orthod Dentofacial Orthop* 107, 136–143.

Stolzenberg J (1935) The Russell attachment and its improved advantages. *Int J Orthod Dent Child* 21, 837–840.

Stolzenberg J (1946) The efficiency of the Russel attachment. *Am J Orthod* 32, 572–582.

Thorstenson GA and Kusy RP (2002a) Comparison of resistance to sliding between different self-ligating brackets with second-order angulation in the dry and saliva states. *Am J Orthod Dentofacial Orthop* 121, 472–482.

Thorstenson GA and Kusy RP (2002b) Effect of archwire size and material on the resistance to sliding of self-ligating brackets with second-order angulation in the dry state. *Am J Orthod Dentofacial Orthop* 122, 295–305.

Thorstenson G and Kusy RP (2003a) Influence of stainless steel inserts on the resistance to sliding of esthetic brackets with second-order angulation in the dry and wet states. *Angle Orthod* 73, 167–175.

Thorstenson GA and Kusy RP (2003b) Effects of ligation type and method on the resistance to sliding of novel orthodontic brackets with second-order angulation in the dry and wet states. *Angle Orthod* 73, 418–430.

Turnbull NR and Birnie DJ (2007) Treatment efficiency of conventional vs self-ligating brackets: effects of archwire size and material. *Am J Orthod Dentofacial Orthop* 131, 395–399.

Türp JC and Schindler H (2012) The dental occlusion as a suspected cause for TMDs: epidemiological and etiological considerations. *J Oral Rehabil* 39, 502–512. 116.

Van Leeuwen EJ, Maltha JC and Kuijpers-Jagtman AM (1999) Tooth movement with light continuous and discontinuous forces in beagle dogs. *Eur J Oral Sci* 107, 468–474.

Vanderby R Jr., Burstone CJ, Solonche DJ and Ratches JA (1977) Experimentally determined force systems from vertically activated orthodontic loops. *Angle Orthod* 47, 272–279.

Verna C, Troiani S, Luzi C and Melsen B (2004) Passive and active overlay systems. *J Clin Orthod* 38, 673–676.

Vlaskalic V and Boyd RL (2002) Clinical evolution of the Invisalign appliance. *J Calif Dent Assoc* 30, 769–776.

Voudouris JC (1997a) Interactive edgewise mechanisms: form and function comparison with conventional edgewise brackets. *Am J Orthod Dentofacial Orthop* 111, 119–140.

Voudouris JC (1997b) Seven clinical principles of interactive twin mechanisms. *J Clin Orthod* 31, 55–65.

Weiland F, Bantleon HP and Droschl H (1992a) The orthodontic treatment of deep bite in adults–a comparison of the straight-wire appliance and the segmented arch technic. *Fortschr Kieferorthop* 53, 153–160.

Weiland FJ, Bantleon HP and Droschl H (1992b) Molar uprighting with crossed tip back springs. *J Clin Orthod* 26, 335–337.

Weiland FJ, Bantleon HP and Droschl H (1996) Evaluation of continuous arch and segmented arch leveling techniques in adult patients–a clinical study. *Am J Orthod Dentofacial Orthop* 110, 647–652.

Zilberman O, Huggare JA and Parikakis KA (2003) Evaluation of the validity of tooth size and arch width measurements using conventional and three-dimensional virtual orthodontic models. *Angle Orthod* 73, 301–306.

8

Anchorage Problems

Birte Melsen, Carlalberta Verna

Introduction

Anchorage in orthodontics is a critical issue independent of the technique or philosophy followed by a clinician. Inadequate anchorage can be the most limiting factor of the therapy and unwanted side effects are frequently seen due to insufficient anchorage. In relation to the treatment of adult patients, many of the traditional means of obtaining anchorage are only of limited use.

In young and growing individuals, tooth movement depends on the interaction between ongoing growth and changes produced by the orthodontic appliance. Expressions such as 'favourable or unfavourable growth pattern' are often found in the orthodontic literature, clearly reflecting the impact of growth on the orthodontic treatment result. In the case of the adult patient, there is no growth to interfere with the effect of the forces generated by the orthodontic appliance,

Adult Orthodontics, Second Edition. Edited by Birte Melsen and Cesare Luzi.
© 2022 John Wiley & Sons Ltd. Published 2022 by John Wiley & Sons Ltd.
Companion Website: http://www.wiley.com/go/melsen-adult-orthodontics

and the tooth movement reflects the applied force system more closely. However, the soft-tissue balance and muscle function still modify the effect of orthodontic treatment that aims to change the arch form or the facial height.

Definition

The first mention of orthodontic anchorage was in the 'Standard Dental Dictionary' where the word was explained as 'the base against which orthodontic force or reaction of orthodontic force is applied' (Ottofy 1923). This definition did not assign any value to the word, but it is clear from the definition of anchorage given by Daskalogiannakis (2000) that loss of anchorage is undesirable. In the 'Glossary of Orthodontic Terms', anchorage was defined as resistant to unwanted tooth movements of the reactive unit. Proffit offered a more detailed definition when he described anchorage as the resistance to reaction forces usually provided by other teeth or sometimes by the palate, head and neck or implants in bone (Proffit et al. 2019).

Classification of anchorage

Conventional orthodontic anchorage can be classified as intraoral or extraoral (Melsen and Verna 1999). The former can be divided into intramaxillary and intermaxillary.

- Intraoral intramaxillary anchorage can be further subdivided into dental and extradental. In the case of extradental, the reactive forces will not be distributed to other teeth but to other tissues, that is, the mucosa of the palate, such as in the Nance appliance, or to alternative devices, such as wires or metallic implants.
- Intermaxillary anchorage comprises Class II and Class III elastics in addition to different types of bite-jumping appliances such as the Herbst appliance, bite correctors and the various types of appliances transferring forces from one arch to the other. Occlusion itself is also a type of intermaxillary anchorage.
- Extraoral anchorage implies reactive forces transferred to the head, the neck or both at the same time or to the chin.

In the workup of the treatment goal, it should be determined which teeth will be moved, that is, belong to the active unit, and which will be considered anchorage, that is, belong to the reactive unit. In relation to space closure, anchorage has been defined as (Burstone 1982):

- Type A, when space is closed primarily by retraction of anterior teeth.
- Type B, when there is equal contribution of the anterior and posterior units to closure of space.
- Type C, when space closure is primarily by protraction of posterior units.

Type B anchorage can be considered the easiest to achieve, since movement of both units is desired, while Type A and, especially, Type C anchorage are more critical, since the movement of the active unit must take place without any movement of the anterior reactive unit.

Many different approaches have been applied in order to obtain differential tooth movement in spite of the fact that every orthodontic appliance stays in a state of equilibrium. When inserting a continuous levelling arch, the force distribution will be a product of the mutual position of the teeth in each arch (Burstone and Koenig 1974), and there is no differentiation between an active and a reactive unit. Differentiation can only be obtained by segmenting the appliance (Burstone 1962, 1966; Ricketts 1980; Mulligan 1998). The appliance connects the active part of the dentition, the part to be moved, and the reactive anchorage unit, which should remain unaltered, and is mostly designed to deliver a specific force system to the active units. The force system delivered to the reactive unit, on the other hand, will maintain the equilibrium of the system independent on the type of appliance. The total sum of moments and forces generated by the appliance is always zero according to the third law of Newton. However, the line of action of the force can pass at different distances from the centre of resistance, for which reason the moment-to-force ratio may differ with respect to the two units, giving rise to differential tooth movements. When the line of action is not parallel to the occlusal plane, the equilibrium will be maintained through the generation of a force rotating the unit, in this case influencing the occlusal plane (Figure 8.1) (Melsen and Bosch 1997).

In the following sections, the basic principles of anchorage will be presented and the scientific and mechanical background will be discussed.

Intramaxillary anchorage

The traditional concept of anchorage is based on the use of 'many teeth against fewer teeth' (Figure 8.2).

The principle behind this concept is that undesirable tooth movements of the anchorage unit will not occur because the forces acting on the anchorage unit are below the necessary threshold value required to generate movement. This hypothesis was supported by Quinn and Yoshikawa (1985), who found a linear relationship between force level per tooth and rate of tooth movement in six clinical studies, and by Freeman (1965), who, instead of using the number of teeth, assigned anchorage values based on the root surface area. However, neither the number of teeth nor root surface measurements can be used as expressions for resistance to movement, since the alveolar surface is only vaguely related to root surface, as recent data obtained by microcomputed tomography (CT) of alveolar bone (Dalstra et al. 2006) demonstrates a pronounced

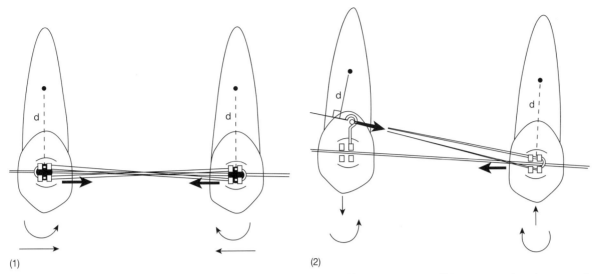

Fig. 8.1 (1) and (2) If the force vector is not parallel to the occlusal plane, different moments will be generated at the two units and the vertical forces will affect the occlusal plane.

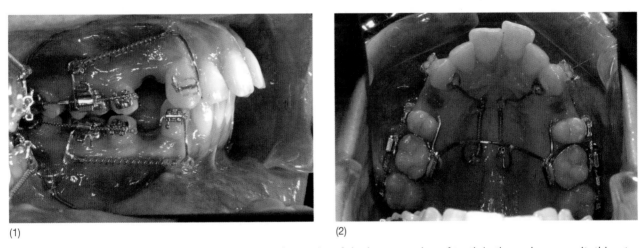

(1)   (2)

Fig. 8.2 Distalisation of canines against six posterior teeth. In spite of the larger number of teeth in the anchorage unit, this setup frequently leads to anchorage loss. Occlusal forces can prevent the loss of anchorage. (1) The canine being distalised against the posterior teeth with coil springs to the power arms. (2) Power arms are also placed lingually in order to avoid rotation.

variation in level, density and quality of alveolar bone (Figure 8.3).

A more plausible explanation in support of the 'more teeth against fewer teeth' theory is most likely grounded in the contribution of the occlusion to the anchorage.

The more teeth against fewer teeth hypothesis was never supported scientifically, as Weinstein in 1967 demonstrated that a few grams of force are sufficient for movement of a tooth. More recent studies focusing on the optimal force magnitude for orthodontic tooth movement have further shown that there is no scientific evidence regarding a threshold for force level that would switch on tooth movement (Ren et al. 2003). Minimal forces, leading to minute changes in the stress–strain distribution within the periodontal ligament (PDL), may be able to trigger the

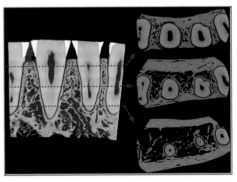

Fig. 8.3 Microradiograph of human alveolar bone. Note how the density is highest in the coronal part and lowest in the apical part of the root. (Courtesy M. Dalstra.)

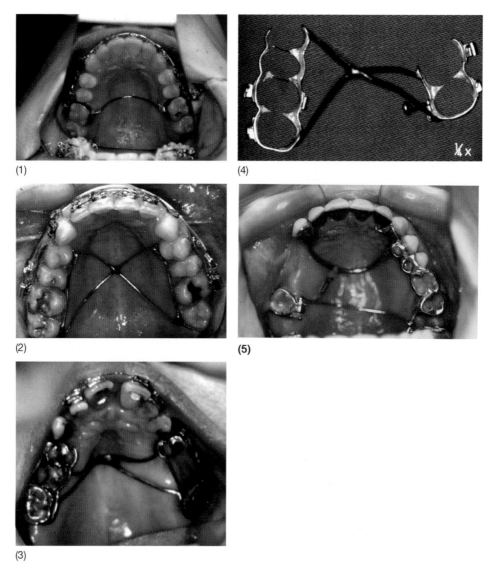

(1)

(2)

(3)

(4)

(5)

Fig. 8.4 (1) Transpalatal bar used to reinforce the anchorage unit. (2) Iron cross used to consolidate the posterior unit to improve anchorage. (3) Iron cross soldered to bands. (4) Iron cross soldered to custom-made cast bands for the posterior segments. (5) Cast anchorage units extending from 13 to 28; 17 is being mesialised with a coil spring extending from the anchorage unit to a transpalatal bar connected to the left side with a hinge. The transpalatal bar prevents rotation of the molar during the mesial movement. For more explanation on the 'hinge mechanics', see Figure 7.29 in Chapter 7.

necessary tissue reaction. This implies that the higher force levels commonly used in orthodontic treatments do not necessarily enhance tooth movement, but may have negative effects, such as hyalinisation, which can delay tooth movements (Reitan 1967).

Another common anchorage principle has been the use of 'rigid wires' such as transpalatal arches, lower lingual arches, cast structures or stiff stainless-steel wires to keep the teeth of the anchorage unit together (Figures 8.4).

The advantage of a rigid wire is in prevention of intra-segmental displacement. The combination of stiff passive wires and large segments allows for the maintenance of chewing function and thereby a positive interaction of occlusion with the forces attempting to displace the

anchorage. However, bending of a heavy stainless-steel wire passively is extremely difficult. It is therefore advantageous to bond the wire directly to the teeth of the reactive unit (Figure 8.5). The teeth of the reactive unit can also be consolidated with fibre-reinforced composites (Freudenthaler et al. 2001a, b) (Figure 8.6).

In the light of the recommendation to use rigid wires as anchorage, it may seem controversial that several authors (McLaughlin et al. 2001; Damon 2005) recommend that sliding of teeth (the active unit) should be done only on heavy wires. The reason for doing this, however, is to avoid the bending of the wire and thereby the undesirable tipping and anchorage loss that will occur when sliding along a flexible wire. The latter would lead to pronounced jiggling,

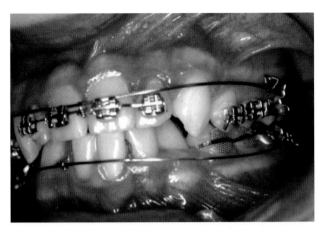

Fig. 8.5 Passive buccal segments constructed from 0.021 × 0.026-inch stainless-steel wires onto which small metal bases are welded. These passive segments in the mandible are bonded directly on the teeth that should remain mutually passive throughout the treatment.

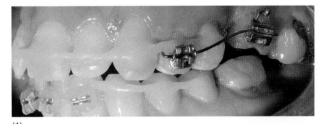

(1)

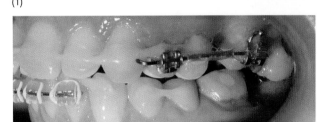

(2)

Fig. 8.6 (1) and (2) Consolidation of the reactive unit by fibre-reinforced composites. The active unit is the molar to be uprighted. (Courtesy of CJ Burstone and P Depasquale.)

which would increase the risk of root resorption. However, a stiff wire generates more friction and the lacebacks used in the MBT (McLaughlin, Bennet, Trisi) technique must be reactivated frequently (Figure 8.7).

The hypothesis that rigid wires render more anchorage than flexible wires can be explained by the influence of both friction and binding, both of which increase with increasing wire dimension (Drescher et al. 1989; Kusy and Whitley 1997). Friction is positively correlated with the size of the wire–bracket contact surface, whereas binding is a product of the wire–slot angle (Kusy and Whitley 1999; Thorstenson and Kusy 2002; Kusy 2004).

Another traditional concept, introduced by Tweed (1966) and still used by many clinicians, is that of 'anchorage preparation'. The basis behind the concept is that the direction of the force with respect to the root is related to the anchorage delivered by the teeth. During anchorage preparation, the lower molars and premolars are tipped distally by adding tipbacks to the lower buccal segments, usually 5° for each tooth with respect to the preceding tooth. Class II traction would thereby act almost perpendicularly to the distally tipped molars, which are therefore anticipated to generate better anchorage than if the teeth had been in their normal inclination. A description of the distribution of the resorptive and the appositional areas with and without anchorage preparation has been used to explain the rationale behind this hypothesis. Scientifically, the concept cannot be supported and the effect may in fact be the opposite to that intended. The tipback could lead to bite opening and posterior rotation of the mandible that could even accentuate the Class II malocclusion already present (Figure 8.8).

In addition, the beneficial effect of occlusion would be lost, since the dorsal tipping of the molars would reduce the

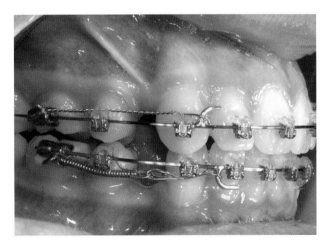

Fig. 8.7 Lacebacks for distal movement of canines following extraction of first premolars.

occlusal forces considerably. This theory is also in complete contradiction to the view that anchorage teeth should be kept stable and cellular activity around the reactive unit should be as low as possible in order to maximise the anchorage potential.

The difference in bone turnover between cortical and trabecular bones led Ricketts (1976a, 1976b) to introduce the concept of 'cortical anchorage'. The theory is based on the observation that when the roots of molars are moved against or into the buccal cortex before serving as anchorage, their anchorage potential increases due to the greater resistance of cortical bone. However, there is no evidence that roots cannot move through cortical bone, as alveolar bone dehiscences and fenestrations with root surface exposures have clearly demonstrated the opposite in an

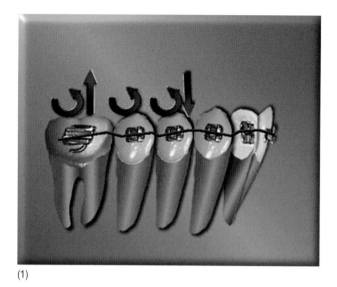

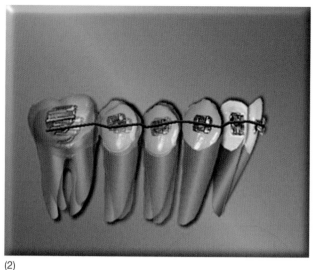

(1)   (2)

Fig. 8.8 Anchorage preparation by distal tipping of the molars, so that the force will be more perpendicular to the roots when Class II traction is used. (1) The force systems generated during anchorage preparation. (2) Tooth movement resulting from the anchorage preparation.

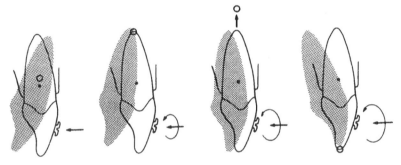

Fig. 8.9 Different types of tooth movement depending on the moment-to-force ratio delivered to the bracket.

animal model (Thilander et al. 1983). The key to the 'cortical anchorage' must therefore be the lag time between force application and tooth movement. This lag time is longer for cortical bone than for trabecular bone, since fewer osteoclasts and osteogenic cells are available to accomplish the remodelling process. The initial movement through cortical bone is thus delayed, but once started, the cortical bone perfectly allows the tooth to be moved through it.

Differential anchorage

'Differential anchorage', introduced by Burstone (1982) and Melsen et al. (1990), is based on the fact that tipping is an easier tooth movement to achieve than translation (bodily movement) and that the moment-to-force ratio delivered to the bracket determines the type of tooth movement (Figures 8.9 and 8.10). The limitation, though, is the inevitable generation of vertical forces during the deactivation phase, which can generate unwanted tooth movements, if not balanced by occlusion or adjunctive orthodontic mechanics (Figure 8.11). Both vertical forces and the large moment often delivered to the posterior unit may result in

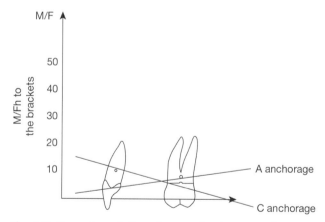

Fig. 8.10 Types A and C anchorage. In the case of Type A anchorage, the anterior teeth will be displaced and the posterior teeth serve as anchorage. The line of action of the necessary force system is indicated and passes below the centre of resistance (CR) with respect to the active unit, whereas it passes through the CR of the anchorage unit. The space closure will thus start with controlled tipping, intrusion of the anterior unit and translation and extrusion of the posterior anchorage unit. In the case of Type C anchorage, the line of action of the force will generate translation, extrusion of the anterior unit and tipping and intrusion of the posterior unit.

Tipping and intrusion

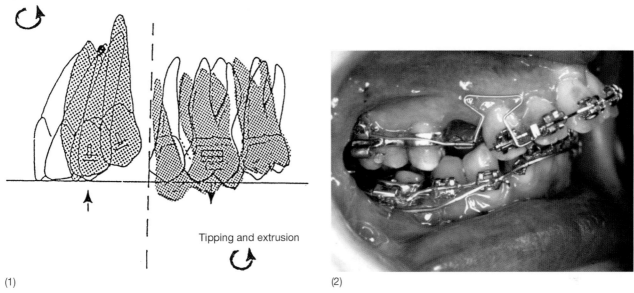

Tipping and extrusion

(1)　　　　　　　　　　　　　　　　　　(2)

Fig. 8.11 (1) Illustration of a side effect of differential anchorage generated by a T-loop delivering a large moment to the posterior unit. This has resulted in a distal tipping of the posterior unit and thus two occlusal planes, which can be avoided by keeping moment to the anchorage unit below the level where posterior tipping moments are generated. (2) Clinical example of a posterior unit that has tipped distally as a result of a too large moment delivered from the T-loop.

distal tipping of the posterior segment, leading to the development of two occlusal planes and a primary contact in the premolar region. Burstone and Koenig (1976) advocated the addition of a high-pull headgear with a short extraoral bow to control the distal tipping and the extrusion of the posterior segment. However, this solution is not ideal, as the extraoral traction is only used intermittently and with a different force magnitude than the mechanics applied for space closure.

Soft-tissue anchorage

With the aim of solving all the problems related to the patient's compliance, many clinicians started developing intraoral devices that could minimise cooperation and be completely under the orthodontist's control (Hilgers 1992; Jones and White 1992; Carano and Testa 1996; Fortini et al. 1999; Carano et al. 2002). A majority of these devices, generally used as molar distalisation appliances, consist of an active force-delivering unit and an anchorage unit, for example, a Nance button, an acrylic button held against the anterior part of the palate and connected by two stiff stainless-steel wires to molar or premolar bands (Figure 8.12). It has never been shown that the palatal mucosa can withstand the mesially directed molar relapse forces without being compressed and with problems such as inflammation, ischaemia and necrosis. Post-treatment evaluations of the efficiency of these compliance-free devices have demonstrated that the 'price' for a distal movement of molars is a significant anchorage loss with increased

anterior inclination of premolars and anterior teeth (Ngantung et al. 2001; Taner et al. 2003; Fortini et al. 2004), confirming the inability of these devices to deliver absolute anchorage.

Another way of using soft tissue as anchorage is to use lip bumpers. This is, however, mainly used in growing individuals.

Free anchorage

A completely different approach to anchorage is the application of the so-called 'free anchorage'. Free anchorage indicates that no 'price' has to be paid in terms of undesirable force on teeth belonging to the anchorage unit. The principle is that reactive forces are transferred to teeth which are to be extracted according to the treatment plan, and so there are no adverse effects on the teeth that will remain in the arches following treatment. By careful biomechanical planning, it is frequently possible to transfer the undesirable forces to teeth that have to be extracted later. The anchorage teeth may be within the same quadrant and will be displaced even out of the arch during the period when it is serving as anchorage. This principle is useful in cases of asymmetries where an extraction of a premolar within the same quadrant is foreseen. The patient in Figure 8.13 was referred from the gnathological department, as she had temporomandibular disorder (TMD) due to a laterally forced bite. Following treatment with a fully balanced splint, the symptoms disappeared, but a crossbite remained and only few occlusal

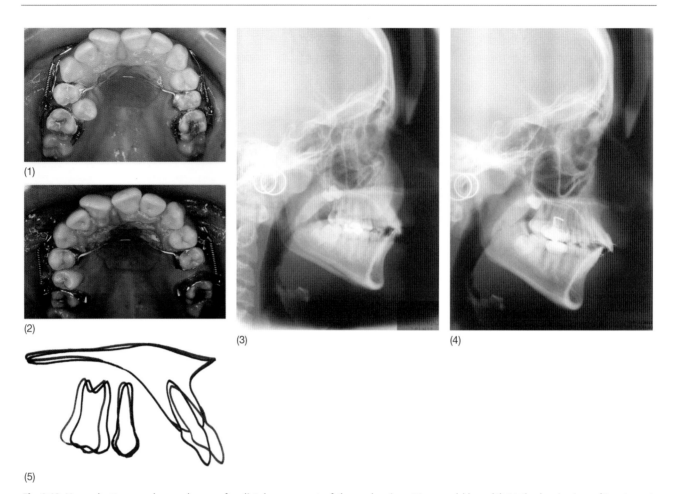

(1)

(2)

(3)

(4)

(5)

Fig. 8.12 Nance button used as anchorage for distal movement of the molars in a 14-year-old boy. (1) At the beginning of treatment, a sectional jig assembly was used to distalise both the first and second maxillary molars simultaneously. The anchorage comprised a Nance acrylic button on the palate (palatal anchorage) connected by stainless-steel wires to the premolar bands (dental anchorage). (2) The maxillary dental arch after 5 months of active treatment: distalisation of the first molars to a super Class I molar relationship has been achieved. (3) Pre-treatment cephalogram. (4) Cephalogram after 5 months of active treatment. (5) Superimposition of the maxilla (best fit on the palatal surface) of the pre- and post-treatment cephalometric tracings. The Nance button and anterior teeth mesial to premolars were not able to resist the mesially directed reciprocal forces and anchorage loss is evident, expressed mainly through mesial inclination of the premolars and mesial movement and proclination of the incisors. In addition, unwanted distal tipping of the first molars is also observed. (Courtesy of Moschos A. Papadopoulos.)

contacts were present laterally on the left side. In order to maintain the structural position of the mandible, intermaxillary elastics could not be used. In this case, the anchor tooth was the first right premolar planned for extraction. The patient had already had three premolars extracted in relation to orthodontic treatment and had an asymmetrical upper arch form. The asymmetry was caused by collapse of the maxilla on one side because of uncontrolled space closure following extraction of 24.

The 'free anchorage' principle has also been used in the correction of arch asymmetry with collapse of upper and lower arches on the same side (Figure 8.14).

In so-called non-extraction cases, it is often desirable to remove the third molar if no space is available for free eruption. The third molar, however, can also serve as free anchorage, as seen in the patient in Figure 8.15.

Another use of 'free anchorage' is via the use of ankylosed teeth. The use of ankylosed teeth was studied in rhesus monkeys in whom Guyman et al. (1980) ankylosed the lateral incisors. Parker et al. (1964) generated ankylosis by extracting the teeth and keeping them outside the socket for 60–75 minutes before reimplanting them. During that period, the pulp was extirpated and the roots were allowed to dry out. Eight weeks after reimplantation, the teeth showed signs of ankylosis and were loaded. During the loading, the teeth remained stable and histological examination carried out at the end of the experiment demonstrated replacement resorption of the root surfaces. Several authors have ankylosed deciduous canines and used them as abutments for maxillary protraction (Kokich et al. 1985; Omnell and Sheller 1994). Although ankylosed deciduous canines have proved to be efficient, the drawback

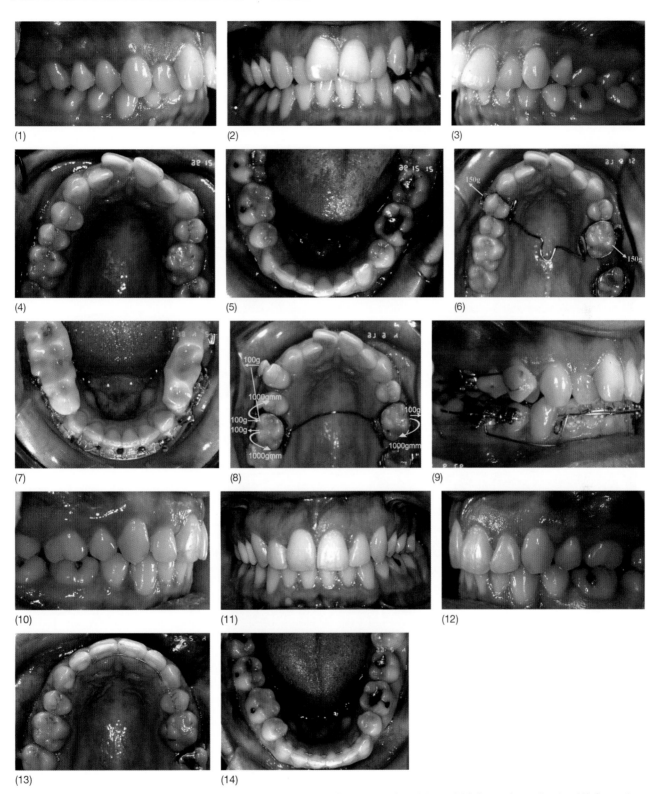

Fig. 8.13 (1)–(3) Intraoral frontal view taken with the mandible in the structural position, which has to be maintained if the patient is to be free of symptoms. No intermaxillary elastics could thus be used. (4) and (5) Occlusal photographs of the upper and lower arches. Note the asymmetry of the upper arch created during space closure following extraction of 24. (6) 14 was used as anchorage. The first appliance was a transpalatal arch that moved 14 buccally and 26 buccally and distally whereby the crossbite was corrected. (7) The mandibular position was maintained by a bonded onlay on the lower teeth. (8) Second appliance. A transpalatal arch with built-in expansion was inserted. The expansion on the left side was desirable. The expansion on the right side was transferred to 14 by means of a cantilever. (9) As a result of the correction of the crossbite on the left side, 14 was now in scissors bite and could be extracted. (10)–(14) Post-treatment photographs. The crossbite had been corrected by unilateral expansion against the premolar that was later extracted.

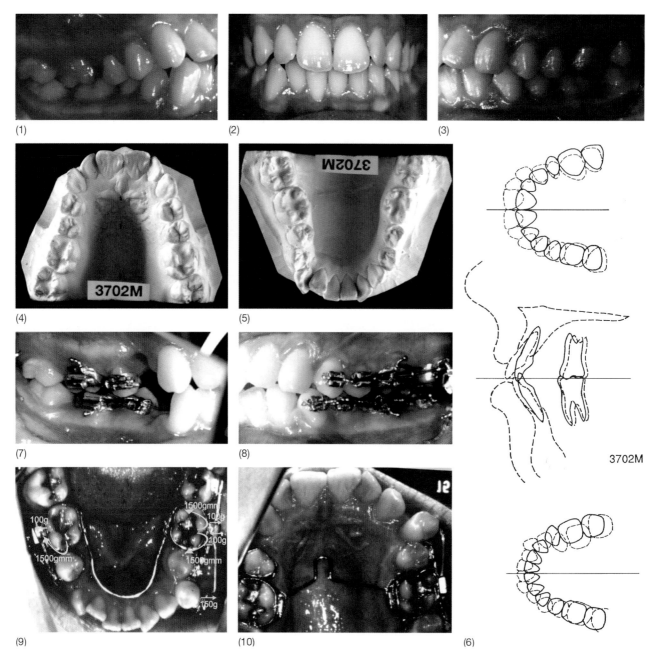

(1)   (2)   (3)
(4)   (5)
(7)   (8)
3702M
(9)   (10)   (6)

Fig. 8.14 (1)–(3) Intraoral photographs before treatment. The patient presented with bimaxillary protrusion, and four premolar extraction treatment was indicated. (4) and (5) Occlusal photographs of the study casts demonstrating that both upper and lower arches were saddle-shaped on the right side. (6) Virtual treatment objective (VTO) indicating the need for unilateral expansion on the right side to achieve symmetrical arch forms. (7) and (8) Two premolars, one upper and one lower, were extracted on the right side. (9) The force system applied. It can be seen that the expansion force on the left side is being transferred to the premolar. Bilateral expansion combined with distal rotation was delivered by a transpalatal arch in the upper arch and by a lower lingual arch in the lower arch. On the right side, the effect was desirable; on the left side, a cantilever was inserted and activated to deliver a buccally directed force to the left premolar. The reaction from this cantilever neutralised the expansion and rotational force acting on the molar. The appliance delivering the unilateral expansion is shown. (10)–(12) Following the unilateral expansion, note the expansion at the premolars to be extracted. (13)–(15) Once the desirable expansion was obtained, the premolars that had served as anchorage were displaced buccally and could be extracted. Unilateral expansion of both arches was achieved without any side effects and the case could be finished. (16)–(20) Intraoral photographs following treatment.

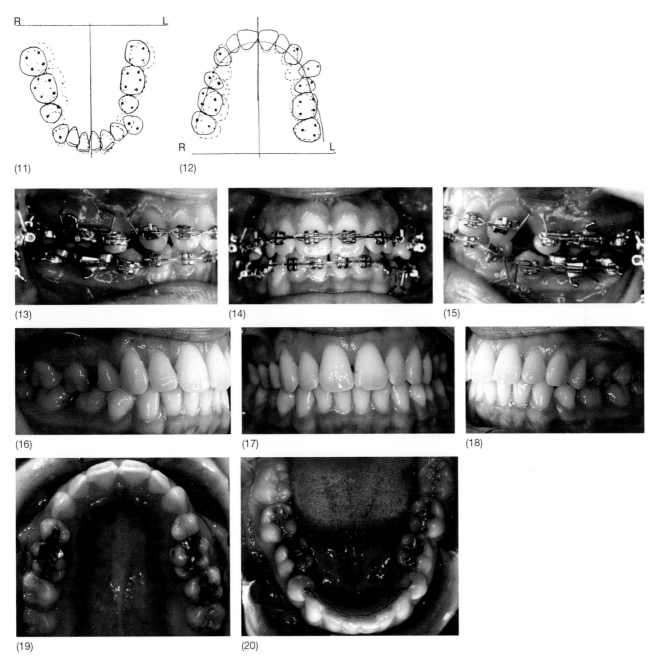

(11)   (12)

(13)   (14)   (15)

(16)   (17)   (18)

(19)   (20)

Fig. 8.14 (*Continued*)

is that the age group in which this can be applied is rather limited. However, if a tooth ankyloses either spontaneously, as often seen in temporarily ankylosed second deciduous molars or secondary to trauma, it can deliver anchorage for movement of teeth within the same arch in any direction. Kofod et al. (2005) used an upper incisor that had been ankylosed as a result of earlier trauma as anchorage for the correction of distal occlusion before the tooth, and its surrounding bone was extruded by a distraction osteogenesis to the normal occlusal level (Figure 8.16).

Intermaxillary anchorage

Intermaxillary elastics were introduced in 1904 by Baker and are widely used today in association with fixed appliances. Their use for anchorage purposes (Kanter 1956) derives from the need to move the teeth in one jaw in one direction while moving the teeth in the other jaw in the opposite direction. The side effects generated by intermaxillary traction are due to the vertical force components, causing extrusion and changes to the inclination of the occlusal

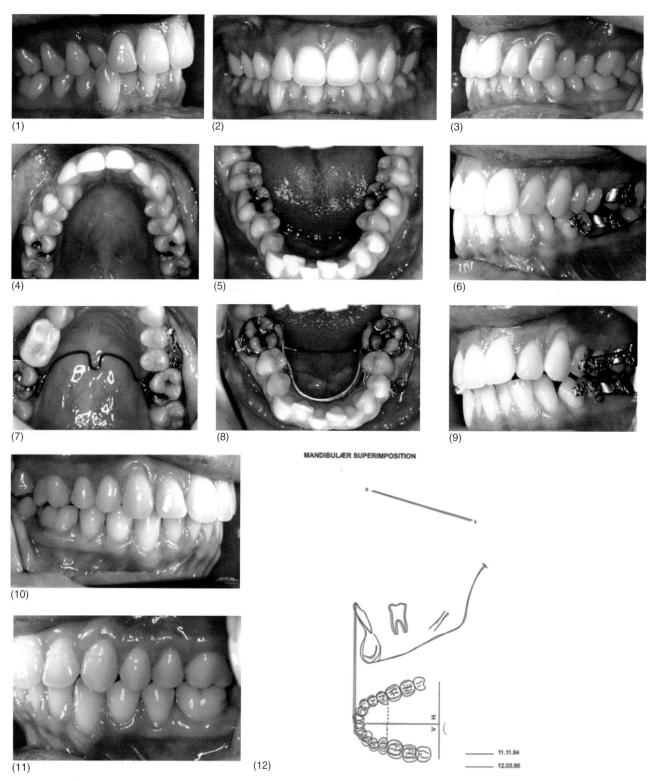

Fig. 8.15 (1)–(5) Patient with a chief complaint of a crossbite in the canine region and lower arch crowding. The analysis of the arches revealed an asymmetry of the lower arch. (6) The expansion of the left side of the lower arch was done by a cantilever extending from the third molar that later had to be extracted. (7) A change in mandibular position was prevented with a composite onlay bonded occlusally on the right side. (8) and (9) A lower lingual arch was inserted to maintain the width while aligning. (10) and (11) After treatment. (12) Three-dimensional analysis demonstrating that the left side of the lower arch has been expanded with the third molar as anchorage.

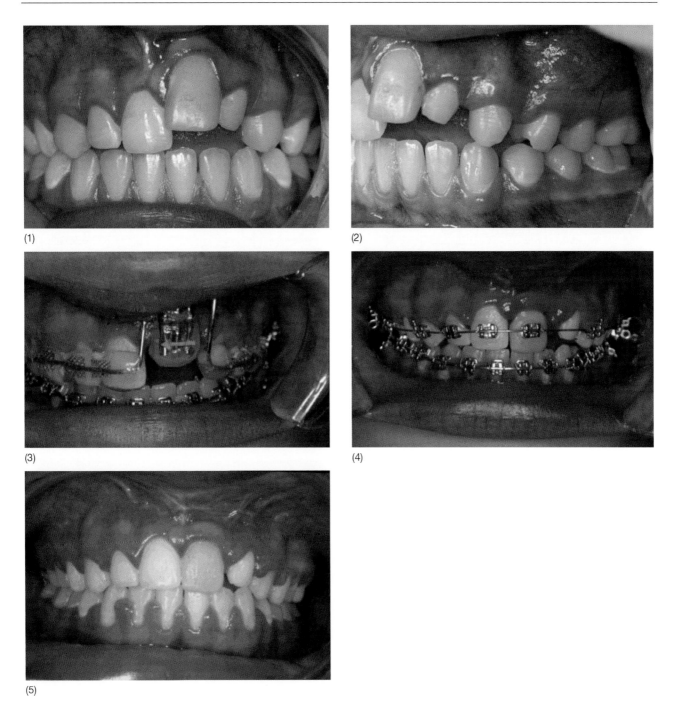

Fig. 8.16 (1) Intraoral photographs before treatment. The left upper incisor had luxated and was reimplanted several years earlier and was ankylosed. (2) This tooth was used as anchorage during the correction of the distal relationship in both posterior segments. (3) and (4) Following the correction of the sagittal problem, the ankylosed tooth and the adjacent bone were extruded by distraction osteotomy. (5) View immediately after the distraction of the ankylosed tooth (Kofod et al. (2005). (Reproduced with permission from Elsevier.)

plane (Figure 8.17). Other disadvantages are the intermittent nature of the forces, the dependence on the patient's compliance and the unavoidable changes in the inclination of the incisors.

Bite-jumping devices, such as the Herbst appliance and Jasper jumpers, are compliance-free and are often used to support Type A anchorage in the treatment of Class II malocclusions, but they can also be used to support the treatment of difficult situations such as Type C anchorage (Figure 8.18) (Fiorentino and Melsen 1996). As in the case of intermaxillary elastics, vertical forces are developed with bite-jumping devices, but there are intrusive force components acting on the upper molars and on the lower anterior region.

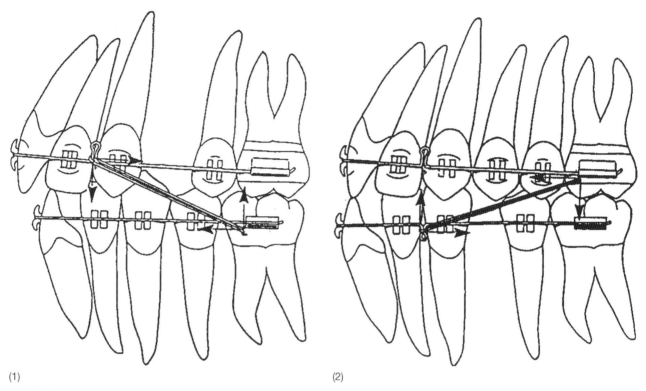

(1) (2)

Fig. 8.17 (1) and (2) Forces generated when Class II or Class III traction is used.

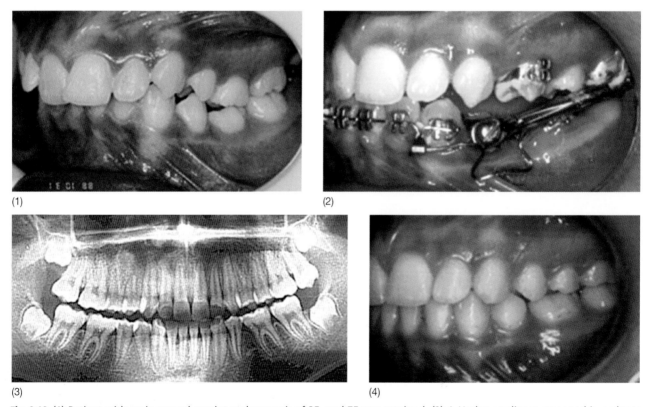

(1) (2)

(3) (4)

Fig. 8.18 (1) Patient with an increased overjet and agenesis of 35, and 75 was retained. (2) A Herbst appliance was used in order to correct the sagittal discrepancy; since the patient had agenesis of 35, the Herbst appliance was retained in the mouth on the left side and used as anchorage for the forward displacement of the molars to close the spaces. (3) Panoramic radiograph demonstrating the mesial movement of the lower left molars. (4) Post-treatment view. (With permission of Fiorentino and Melsen (1996).)

Occlusion

Among the intermaxillary anchorage approaches, occlusion probably plays the most important role. In order to maintain normal function, it is crucial that the proprioceptive input from the periodontium via the occlusion remains undisturbed. Only limited attention has been paid to the role of occlusal contacts in the stability of anchorage units. The proprioceptive input from occlusion is constantly changing during orthodontic treatment. Fewer occlusal contacts might be responsible for a reduction in the occlusal forces (Bakke et al. 1992). Since it has been argued that masseter-muscle activity is reduced during orthodontic treatment (Miyamoto et al. 1996), chewing exercises can be considered an important factor to enhance maximal intercuspation and occlusal forces, especially in non-growing individuals (Miyamoto et al. 1999). Moreover, the masticatory muscle function seems to increase the density of cortical bone (Bresin et al. 1999).

Occlusal forces can be maintained by consolidation of the posterior teeth into 'one big tooth' with a full-size stiff archwire and can further be enhanced by addition of a conventional transpalatal arch or an iron cross in the maxilla and a lingual arch in the lower arch. In addition to the consolidation, whether achieved with wires or fibre-reinforced composites, the stimulus from the occlusion can be increased by an occlusal build-up to maximise the occlusal contacts (Figures 8.13 and 8.15).

In adult patients, consolidation of the posterior segments is sometimes already present when the patient is first seen, for example, if a repositioning splint has been cemented for the maintenance of the mandibular position in patients with TMD (Melsen and Verna 1999) or patients where repositioning of the mandible was part of the plan (Figure 7.1 in Chapter 7). The advantage of occlusal coverage is that the splints can also include edentulous areas and thereby enhance the occlusal feedback even from the teeth without contacts in the opposing arch. In some adult patients, the occlusal splint is the only possible solution, such as in patients with several missing teeth or satisfactory restorative dentistry consolidating the posterior teeth (Figure 8.18).

In some adult patients, the occlusal splint is the only possible solution. This is the case in patients with satisfactory dental restorations consolidating the lateral segments (Figure 8.19).

The inclination of the occlusal plane seems to play an important role. When the inclination of the occlusal plane is steep, the occlusal forces are reduced and loss of anchorage occurs more easily (Mavreas 1991). Maintenance of occlusion also prevents vertical loss of anchorage and no sagittal anchorage loss can occur without being accompanied by posterior rotation of the mandible. The first to perceive changes in the occlusion is the patient, sensing even minor occlusal changes. When a patient reports an altered sensation, it may be time to

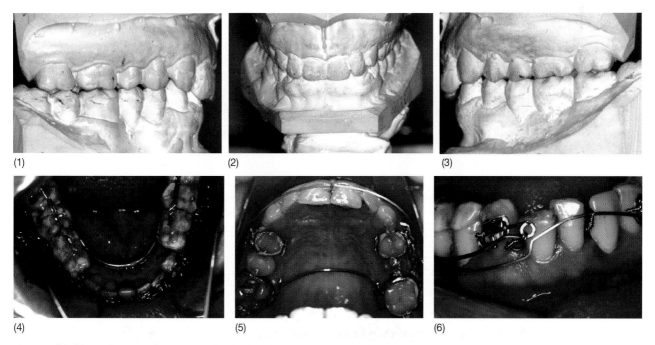

(1)   (2)   (3)

(4)   (5)   (6)

Fig. 8.19 (1)–(3) Study casts of a patient who had undergone major prosthetic rehabilitation with two bridges on both sides of the mandibular arch. Two thin fully balanced splints connected with a lingual wire were used as anchorage for intrusion and proclination of the lower incisors. (4) and (5) The anchorage unit consists of two lateral splints covering the posterior bridges. The incisors were proclined, but instead of using brackets, the incisors were consolidated with a wire bonded lingually. The retroclined incisors were proclined and intruded. (6) The space created between the bridges and the incisors was closed by a mesial tipping of the canines. (7)–(9) Post-treatment photographs.

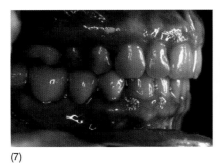
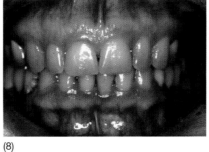
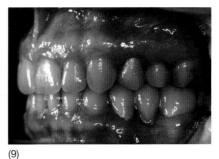

(7)   (8)   (9)

Fig. 8.19 (*Continued*)

change the force system or lower the force level. Patients should be encouraged to chew and exercise to stimulate and thereby enhance the proprioceptive input from occlusion (Spyropoulos 1985).

Differential timing of force application

In addition to the above-mentioned principles, the timing of the force delivery has been mentioned among the principles underlying use of anchorage. Proffit et al. (2019) wrote, 'clinical experience suggests that there is a threshold for force duration in humans in the 4–8 hours range, and that increasingly effective tooth movement is produced if the force is maintained for longer durations'.

In case of Type A anchorage, the anchorage would be assured by the alternation of the use of inter- and intramaxillary elastics, in order to avoid loading of the anchorage teeth for more than 8 hours, which seems to be the time after which the tooth movement is observed (Proffit and Fields 2000). If this empirical view is valid, it can be borne in mind when planning the anchorage. According to this theory, teeth loaded for only 8 or fewer hours would not be displaced. The biological reasoning behind this statement is difficult to understand, as loading of bone in order to maintain a certain level of modelling can be limited to a few hours a day. In addition, Hayashi et al. (2004) demonstrated in an animal study that intermittent force with the duration of 8 hours induced about 37% less movement than continuous forces, but even this tooth movement exceeds that acceptable for an anchorage unit. However, the regimen of loading seems to have a larger influence than the force magnitude (van Leeuwen et al. 1999).

An optimal way of maintaining anchorage is not to disturb cellular quiescence in the anchorage unit at all. The use of absolute anchorage is based on this principle.

Conclusion

The above-discussed anchorage approaches are all focusing on avoidance of undesired tooth movements of reactive unit. The following will focus on 'extradental anchorage'.

Extraoral anchorage

Extraoral devices such as headgears have been used since 1866. Kingsley was the first author to report the use of headgear anchorage to correct protruded upper anterior teeth (Weinberger 1926). The effect was described as both dental and orthopaedic changes, but both effects were temporary and rebound was seen post treatment of both the dental and the skeletal effects (Melsen 1978; Melsen and Dalstra 2003). In addition, Alwali et al. (2000) demonstrated severe root resorption related to the use of headgear. It is, nevertheless, still used frequently in treatment of children (Marcotte 1990; Pavlick 1998; Ferro et al. 2000; Kalunki et al. 2020).

Extraoral anchorage is not of practical use in adult patients. The molars are generally positioned below the key ridge (Atkinson 1951) and a finite element analysis (FEA) has demonstrated that distal movement leads to reduction in the efficiency by which occlusal forces are transferred to the cranial base (Cattaneo et al. 2003).

Skeletal anchorage

Frequently, especially when treating adults, the orthodontist faces the problem of lack of anchorage teeth or situations in which changes in the reactive unit are not acceptable. The development of skeletal anchorage has solved these problems. The first attempt to gain anchorage in basal bone goes back to 1945, when Gainsforth and Higley inserted and immediately loaded 13-mm long vitallium screws in the mandibular ramus of mongrel dogs. All the screws were loaded with forces in the range of 140–200 g and became loose between 16 and 31 days after insertion. Although unsuccessful, this experiment provided the impetus for future research in the field. In 1983, Creekmore and Eklund published a case report in which the upper incisors of a 25-year-old woman were intruded and proclined against a metallic screw inserted below the anterior nasal spine. However, at that time, this report did not attract much attention and it was primarily prosthodontic implants that were recommended as skeletal anchorage.

Prosthodontic implants

Dental implants are increasingly used as part of oral rehabilitation and can serve as anchorage before being used for restorative purposes. The first studies were conducted by Gray et al. (1983), who evaluated the stability of implants inserted in the rabbit femur and submitted to forces ranging from 60 g to 180 g after 4 weeks of healing. They found that the implants remained stable independent of the force level and concluded that implants constituted a useful adjunct to modern orthodontics (Figure 8.19). A number of authors have used dental implants as anchorage and special superstructures have been developed to make the use of the implants easier (Gray et al. 1983; Kokich et al. 1985; Douglass and Killiany 1987; Odman et al. 1988; Matthews 1993; Shroff et al. 1996; Goodacre et al. 1997; Favero et al. 2002; Ong and Wang 2002).

In the case where prosthodontic implants are used as anchorage, it is crucial that their exact position is determined as part of the treatment planning. If the final occlusal relationships and the intra-arch tooth positioning are not determined before the insertion of the implant, this may cause unresolvable problems at the end of treatment, as in the case shown in Figure 8.20. In this case, implants had been inserted before orthodontic treatment planning. The sagittal and vertical discrepancies in addition to the asymmetrical occlusal plane had not been taken into consideration before inserting the implants and the final rehabilitation was unsatisfactory due to the wrong position of the implants. A position more anteriorly or more posteriorly would have been beneficial for the outcome.

Figure 8.21 shows an example of a well-planned treatment where a lower implant was used as anchorage for the mesial displacement of a third molar.

If the patient required implants as part of prosthetic rehabilitation, it would be advisable to start treatment by inserting the prosthodontic implants and use them as anchorage for orthodontic treatment after the lag time. However, this routine cannot always be applied. Some patients will not require implants, others may need bone transplantation or/and sinus lift before insertion of implants and the time lag before implants can be used, as anchorage will allow further deterioration of the malocclusion. Conversely, the area where the implant should be inserted often has to be prepared by orthodontic tooth movement.

Temporary anchorage devices

A different type of skeletal anchorage is the use of TADs (Leo et al. 2016; Jones et al. 2020) which have proven extremely useful especially in adult patients. The TADs can be classified into different types.

According to the surface preparation of the intraosseous part of the implant, one group of anchorage systems is based on dental implants, while the other is derived from surgical screws and wires (Box 8.1). The intraosseous surface of the first group is either sandblasted or coated in a special way to enhance their osseointegration, which was defined by Branemark et al. (1977) as a 'direct structural and functional connection between living bone and the surface of a

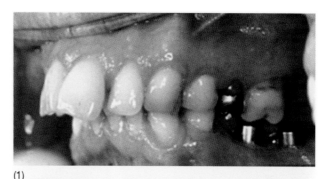

(1)

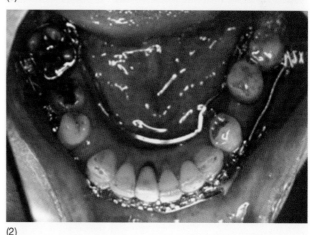

(2)

Fig. 8.20 (1) This patient had two implants inserted before starting orthodontic treatment. (2) Following orthodontic treatment, the distance from the implants to the anterior segment was either too large or too small for a suitable prosthesis.

Box 8.1   Classification of extradental intraoral skeletal anchorage

Originating from – dental implants – lag time
- Prosthodontic implants
- Palatal implants
- Onplants
- Retromolar implants
- Orthodontic implants

Originating from surgical screws – Temporary anchorage Devices (TAD) – immediate loading
- Miniplates one-point contact
- Mini-implant one-point contact
- Mini-implant two-dimensional (2D) control
- Mini-implant three-dimensional (3D) control

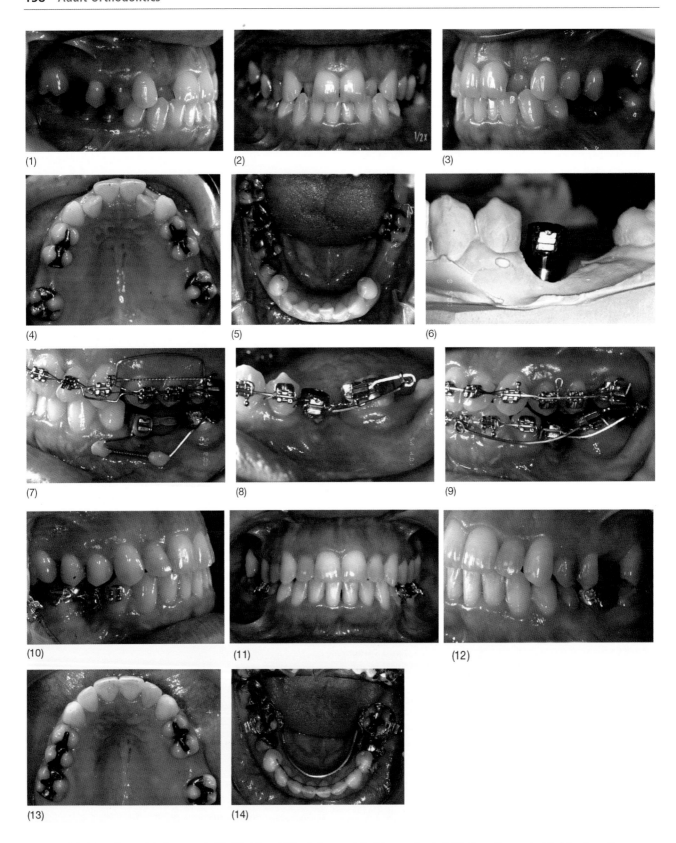

Fig. 8.21 (1)–(5) Patient with four teeth 16, 26, 36 and 35 missing and desiring oral rehabilitation. It was decided to close the spaces corresponding to 26 and 36. The space for 16 was kept open, as a closure of that space would have left 47 out of occlusion. (6) An implant to replace 35 was inserted, and following a suitable period of healing, the implant served as anchorage for uprighting and the mesial movement of 37. (7) A bracket was laser-welded to a suprastructure added to the implant, and a coil extending between the power arm on the implant and on the molar was used to mesialise 37. Another power arm on the lingual side prevented rotation. After mesialisation, combined uprighting and intrusion was required and done using two-cantilever mechanics. (8) A cantilever extending from the implant delivered intrusive forces to the tipped and extruded molar. (9) A second cantilever extending from the tube of the molar generated the uprighting moment. (10)–(14) Post-treatment photographs.

load-carrying implant', a bone-to-implant contact on a microscopic level. In relation to these skeletal anchorage systems, a healing period after insertion is recommended before the application of occlusal or orthodontic loads. The palatal implants, onplants and retromolar implants belong to this group. The other group of temporary anchorage systems is derived from the surgical world and the applied screws have a smooth surface. Miniplates and a large number of temporary anchorage systems belong to this category.

Palatal implants

An implant system specifically designed for palatal and ret-romolar anchorage (Straumann Orthosystem®, Institut Straumann AG, Basel/Switzerland) was developed (Wehrbein 1994; Wehrbein et al. 1996) (Figure 8.22). In a clinical report, titanium sandblasted and acid-etched implants with a diameter of 3.3 mm and a length of 4 or 6 mm were used in six adult patients as indirect anchorage while retracting anterior teeth. A histological analysis showed a good bone-implant contact at the interface between bone and the surface of the implant, indicating that orthodontic implants were well integrated into the host bone following long periods of orthodontic loading (Wehrbein et al. 1998).

Since then the Straumann palatal implant provides anchorage control for orthodontic corrections. The implant is inserted in the palate for the duration of the treatment, and is suitable for both adolescents (age 12 and older) and adults.

The second generation palatal implants are length-reduced screws with an endosteal part of the implant that is 4.2 mm long, and the neck 1.8 mm high. They are made of pure titanium, and available in two different endosteal diameters (4.1 mm and 4.8 mm). Animal studies have shown that despite their short length they undergo sufficient osteointegration to provide a valid long-lasting anchorage support (Wehrbein et al. 1997).

Their short length makes them especially well-suited for regions with a low vertical bone supply, such as the palate, whose thickness is evaluated through a lateral cephalogram. The insertion and removal procedures of palatal implants are slightly more extensive than that of miniscrews.

The implants are loaded after a healing period of 12 weeks, although recent studies showed that the success rate of the palatal implant, that several authors have estimated to be 90%, for the first 6 months does not significantly change even when the implants are loaded immediately with a force of 4 N (Jung et al. 2011).

The palatal implants retain their positional stability under the application of orthodontic force and provide a wide variety of anchorage solutions (Wehrbein et al. 2009) (Figure 8.23).

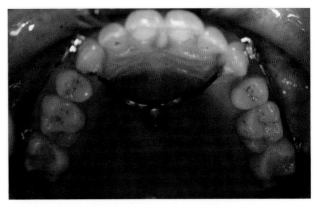

Fig. 8.22 Palatal implant used for distalisation of the posterior teeth after anchorage loss.

Palatal mini-implants with abutments, optimal insertion sites and possible mechanics

Temporary anchorage devices (TADs and especially mini-implants have become a common treatment modality in orthodontics within the last two decades. Still, today the alveolar process is the most preferred insertion site (Melsen and Costa 2000; Wilmes 2008). However, orthodontists are confronted with an average loss rate of 10–30% of buccal mini-implants as reported in the literature. The failure rate of mini-implants in the anterior palate is reported to be 1–5%, which is significantly lower than in other regions. In the anterior palate, a superior bone quantity and quality combined with thin attached mucosa and minimal risk of tooth-root injuries can be observed. The ideal zone with the lowest failure rates seems to be directly posterior from the palatal rugae. Regarding 16 and 17, distally from the rugae, an area with sufficient bone volume and a thin soft-tissue layer can be detected (Figure 8.24, T-zone). Mini-implants with interchangeable abutments (e.g., Benefit

System, PSM, Germany) were developed that allow integration into the orthodontic mechanics (Figure 8.25). For high demands on the anchorage quality, two or even three mini-implants are used and coupled with a miniplate (Beneplate19, 1.1 mm or 0.8 mm, Figure 8.26). These miniplates can be adapted to the mini-implants by bending of the miniplate body as well as the wire (Figure 8.27).

Implant placement and adaption of the mechanics

If the patient is apprehensive about use of a needle syringe, the miniscrews can be placed using only topical anaes-thetic (jelly). In adult patients, a pilot drilling (2–3 mm depth) should be performed due to very high bone densi-ties nearby the suture. In children and adolescents with relatively low bone mineralisation, pilot drilling is not

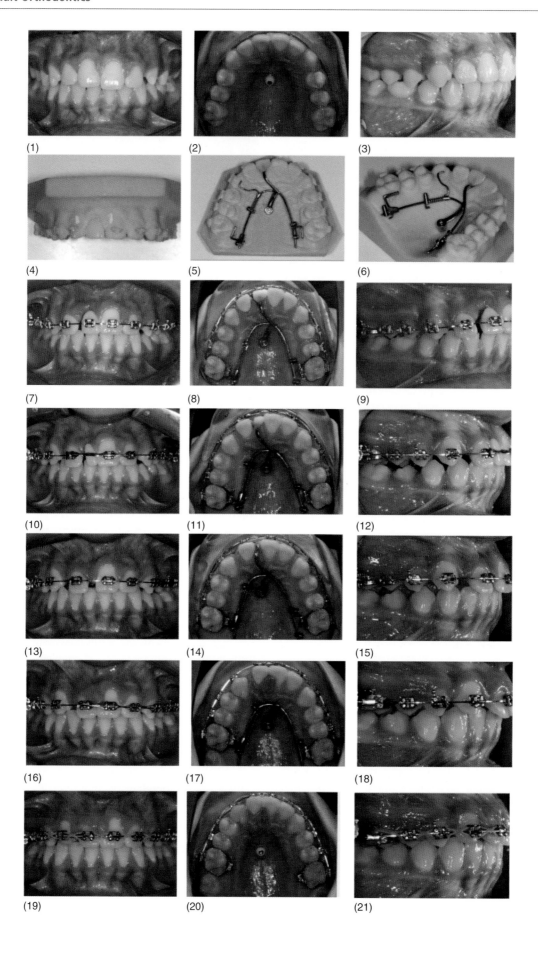

(1)

(2)

(3)

(4)

(5)

(6)

(7)

(8)

(9)

(10)

(11)

(12)

(13)

(14)

(15)

(16)

(17)

(18)

(19)

(20)

(21)

Fig. 8.23 (1)–(4) A 11-years-and-7-months-old boy, whose 11 underwent root replacement resorption and ankylosis following trauma. The extraction of 11 and the mesialisation of the 1st quadrant were planned. (5) and (6) After the insertion of the palatal implant (Straumann, Orthosystem®, Basel, Switzerland) and the following healing period, a digital impression through the CARES® Scanbody transfer system (Straumann, Basel, Straumann, Switzerland) was performed and the suprastructure produced. The suprastructure consisted both passive and active parts. The passive part included the tooth 26 that should not move and the pontic replacing the extracted tooth. The active part consisted a sliding mechanics through a closed coil spring. (7)–(12) The pontic was gradually reduced in size during the mesialisation, with no anchorage loss. (13)–(21) At the end of the mesialisation, the midlines were coincident, and there was a full distal occlusion in the right side and space for the build-up of 12 to camouflage the extracted 11 was left in place (treated by Dr Engeler and Dr Kanavakis at the Department of Pediatric Oral Health and Orthodontics at the University Center for Dental Medicine, Basel, Switzerland).

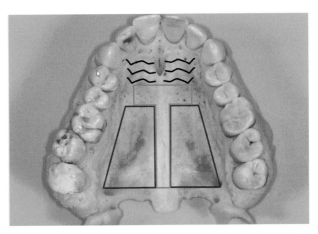

Fig. 8.24 Picture of a maxilla of a cadaver: recommended insertion site (T-zone) posterior from the rugae. The bone is very thin in the posterior and lateral areas. (Courtesy Benedict Wilmes.)

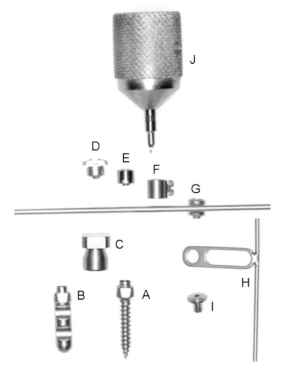

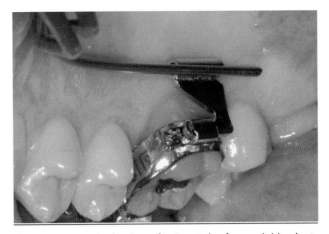

Fig. 8.25 Benefit/Beneplate System: (A) Mini-implant. (B) Laboratory analogue. (C) Impression cap. (D) Wire abutment with wire in place. (E) Bracket abutment. (F) Standard abutment. (G) Slot abutment. (H) Beneplate with wire in place. (I) Fixation screw. (J) Screwdriver for abutment fixation. (Courtesy Benedict Wilmes.)

Fig. 8.26 Intraoral adaption of a Benetube for a mini-implant-borne slider. (Courtesy Benedict Wilmes.)

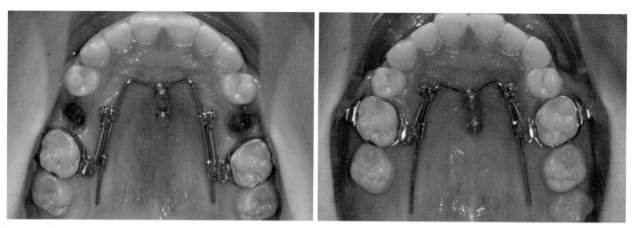

Fig. 8.27 Clinical example with missing upper second bicuspids: Mesialslider for bilateral upper mesialisation. (Courtesy Benedict Wilmes.)

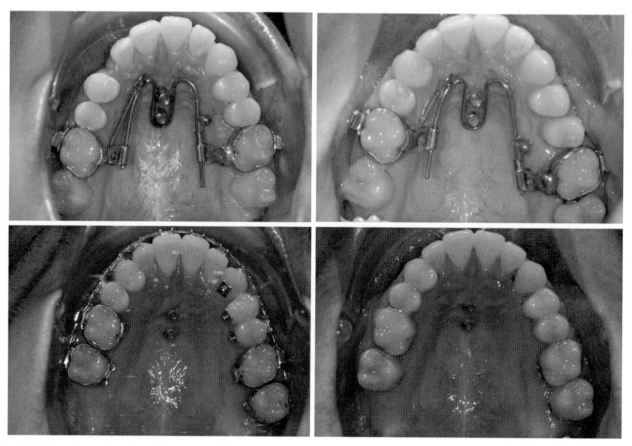

Fig. 8.28 Clinical example with missing upper right canine and midline shift: Mesial-Distalslider for unilateral upper mesialisation and contralateral distalisation. (Courtesy Benedict Wilmes.)

needed. Mini-implants with diameter of 2 mm or 2.3 mm and lengths of 9 mm (anterior) and 7 mm (posterior) are inserted, which provides a high stability to 20–23. In many cases, the appliance could be adapted intraorally, which, of course, implies some chair time (Figure 8.26).

The alternative is to adapt the mechanics in the laboratory by taking a silicon impression and transferring the intraoral setup to a plaster cast using the impression cap and the laboratory analogue (Wilmes and Drescher 2009) (Figure 8.25).

Clinical applications for palatal mini-implants

For upper molar distalisation purposes, the Beneslider sliding mechanics can be used and has proved to be a reliable distalisation device (Figure 8.27). To mesialise molars for space closure in the upper arch, a Mesialslider as a direct anchorage device can be used (Wilmes and Drescher 2008; Wilmes et al. 2009). The Mesialslider enables clinicians to mesialise upper molars unilaterally or bilaterally. Since the incisors are not fixed, a midline deviation can be corrected at the same time. The Mesialslider can be used to close all spaces in the upper arch from distal, for example, for missing premolars (Figure 8.27), incisors or canines (Figure 8.28). In many cases with unilaterally missing teeth, the midline is off. The favoured appliance to correct the midline, to close the space on one side and to distalise the contralateral segment is a combination of the Mesialslider and a Beneslider, the Mesial-Distalslider (Wilmes et al. 2013) (Figure 8.28). For the treatment of patients with a transversal and/or retrognathic maxilla, a rapid maxillary expansion (RME) device is used in Class III patients in combination with a face mask for protraction of the maxilla. To avoid complications caused by the tooth-borne character of conventional appliances, some authors reported about bone-borne RME devices. One very popular approach is the so-called Hybrid Hyrax which is half tooth-borne and half bone-borne (Wilmes et al. 2009, 2010).

Conclusion

To summarise, the use of palatal TADs with abutments is expanding the options in orthodontic and orthopaedic treatments significantly. Insertion and removal are minimally invasive procedures; orthodontists can place the screws by themselves and load them immediately. Usually, the screws can be removed without anaesthesia. The anterior palate is our preferred insertion region because of its superior bone quality and relatively low rates of miniscrew instability and failure. The attached mucosa has a better prognosis than other areas, and there is no risk of tooth damage. In the mandible, miniplates such as Bollard plates or the Mentoplate are recommendable for orthopaedic and orthodontic purposes.

Onplant

In 1995, Block and Hoffman designed the 'onplant', a thin titanium alloy disc to be inserted subperiostally. The surface facing bone was textured and coated with a 75-μm-thick layer of hydroxyapatite (HA) and the opposite side was prepared with a threaded hole into which various abutments could be inserted (Figure 8.29). Onplants can provide sufficient anchorage in the situations that require maximum anchorage. As with the palatal implant, the onplant is used for indirect anchorage. The palatal implant and the onplant

have the same disadvantages regarding cost and time lag between insertion and use. In addition, it was noticed that the osseointegration was depending on pressure delivered by a splint worn 24 hours a day the first month after insertion. This made the failure rate depend on patient compliance.

When using skeletal anchorage, it is not enough to take the stability into consideration, and when Blok and Ambruster (2001) tried to move molars distally against an onplant, they were trying to displace molars that were resting on the maxillary tuberosity against the pterygoid process. Even with skeletal anchorage, it is not possible to displace teeth if there is no space.

Retromolar implants

Palatal implants have mainly been recommended as replacements of other types of anchorage. The retromolar implant, on the other hand, has widened the range of the orthodontic treatment possibilities. Roberts et al. (1989, 1990) presented case reports in which a rigid endosseous retromolar implant was successfully used as indirect anchorage for intrusion and distal translation of the first and second molars into an atrophic first molar extraction site. Shortly after, Higuchi and Slack (1991) performed the first prospective clinical trial on seven adult patients to evaluate whether osseointegrated titanium implants placed in the third molar area could resist loading. After 4–6 months of healing, orthodontic forces with a magnitude of 150–400 g were applied to the abutments for a variable period within the total treatment time (17–30 months). The implants remained clinically and radiographically stable during the entire treatment period. The bone adjacent to the implants was studied histomorphometrically and the remodelling activity evaluated in multiple species (Garetto et al. 1995). A rise in the bone turnover was found independent of time and loading and it was concluded that successful long-term maintenance of rigidly fixed endosseous implants was related to a sustained elevation of remodelling activity.

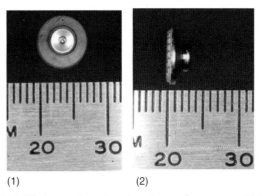

Fig. 8.29 (1) An onplant showing the surface onto which an extension can be added. (2) Lateral view of the onplant.

These results are in agreement with Trisi and Rebaudi (2002), who performed histological analysis of retrieved human retromolar implants, which had been submitted to orthodontic loading for different periods. The loading with orthodontic forces was, however, not the major determinant for the remodelling. Chen et al. (1995, 1999) performed a FEA with the objective of investigating the effect of varying bite force and orthodontic forces on the stress–strain distribution at the adjacent to the implants. They found that unloaded retromolar implants were surrounded by the same remodelling pattern as implants subjected to additional loading and concluded that the intense remodelling of interfacial bone is a response to the mismatch in the modules of elasticity between cortical bone and titanium. Addition of orthodontic forces in this investigation had little effect on the mechanical parameters around the implant.

Immediately loadable devices

The second type of skeletal anchorage system is basically derived from surgical screws, apart from the zygoma ligature. All these devices present a smooth surface and can undergo immediate loading (Costa et al. 1998; Umemori et al. 1999; Bernhart et al. 2001; Lee et al. 2001; Park et al. 2001; Bae et al. 2002; De et al. 2002; Sherwood et al. 2002; Sugawara et al. 2002; Keles et al. 2003; Kyung et al. 2003; Maino et al. 2003).

Zygoma ligature

The zygoma ligature was developed as cheap alternative to the implant in patients with increased overjet and insufficient teeth for conventional anchorage. In these patients, no implants were foreseen as part of reconstruction either because of lack of bone or more frequently for economical reasons. The zygoma ligature was first described by Melsen et al. (Melsen et al. 1998) as a solution to anchorage in patients with reduced number or no teeth in the posterior segments (Figure 8.30).

The surgery, necessary for insertion of the zygoma wire, was performed under local anaesthesia. An incision approximately 1 cm long was made on the superior aspect of the infrazygomatic crest and a horizontal bony canal was drilled through the infrazygomatic crest. A double-twisted 0.012-inch stainless-steel wire was pulled through the canal and twisted on the anterior aspect of the infrazygomatic crest. Once the incision was closed with a few sutures, the surgical wire was bend and adapted so that the correct point of force application could be established. The zygoma wires were used as anchorage for intrusion and retraction of flared and elongated maxillary incisors. The wires were loaded immediately with forces ranging

between 25 and 50 cN. The bone quality of the infrazygomatic crest is generally good, thus provided in most cases sufficient anchorage for the maintenance of the wire while loading (Cattaneo et al. 2003). As the force was concentrated to a minimum area, the wire would gradually be displaced within the zygomatic arch and thereby work its way out. This hypothesis was confirmed by the fact that 3 out of 15 cases were lost after a few months. In these cases, the surgeon had made the hole in the infrazygomatic ridges too close to the surface. In the remaining 12 cases, the wires were maintained during the necessary period varying between 3 and 6 months.

The drawbacks related to the zygoma ligature were the necessary surgical intervention and the limited variation in the lines of action of the possible forces.

Miniplates

The idea of using miniplates as orthodontic anchorage also originates from their use in orthognathic surgery. Miniplate placement on the intrazygomatic crest was described by Jenner and Fitzpatrick as early as 1985 and later applied by several authors (Jenner and Fitzpatrick 1985; Sugawara 1999; Umemori et al. 1999; Erverdi and Keles 2003; Sugawara and Nishimura 2005). Titanium miniplates fixed with monocortical bone screws at the buccal cortical bone of the apical regions of the first and second molars were used as anchorage for molar intrusion of 3–5 mm.

DeClerck et al. (2002) introduced a titanium miniplate with three holes for three self-tapping titanium miniscrews and an extension for the application of the orthodontic loading. The authors reported the use of this 'anchor system' in 27 patients for upper canine retraction without major complications or failures, apart from minor inflammation (Figure 8.31). The disadvantage of the miniplates is that they do require surgical intervention for both insertion and at removal. Another drawback is that the localisation of the point of force application is limited as in the case of the zygoma ligature.

Mini-implants

The single screw represents the largest group of the skeletal anchorage systems. A rapidly increasing number of different mini-implants are on the market (Papadopoulos and Tarawneh 2007; Leo et al. 2016; Ramírez-Ossa et al. 2020). The temporary implants vary in length, diameter, threading and design of the intraosseous and extraosseous parts. Generally, they appear in case reports supported by little if any mechanical, biomechanical or biological research. Several aspects have to be taken into consideration before deciding to use mini-implants anchorage (Box 8.2).

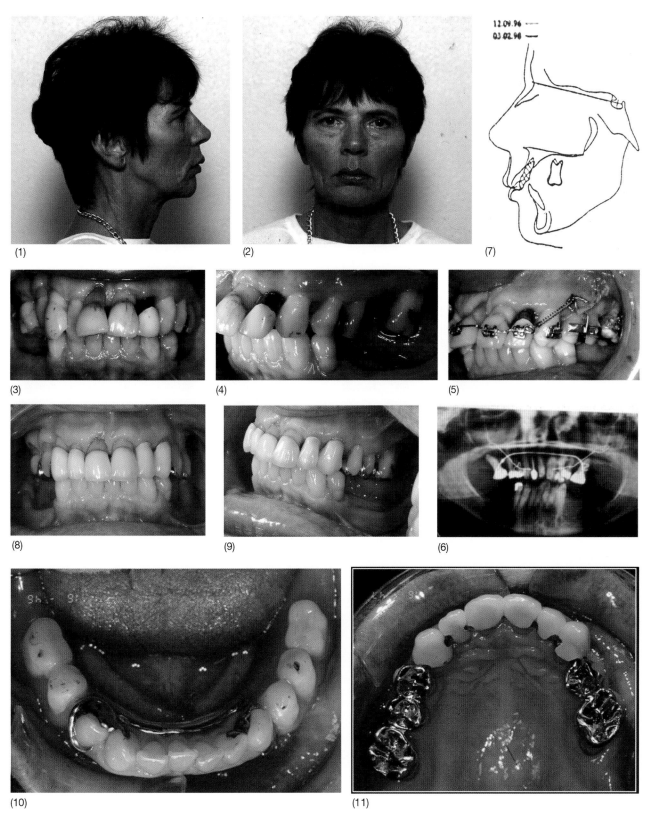

Fig. 8.30 (1–5) Pre-treatment photographs of a patient with large overjet and insufficient anchorage units for conventional anchorage. Note the underdeveloped masseter and temporalis muscles. (5) and (6) Zygoma ligature used as anchorage for the retraction and intrusion of the anterior teeth. (7) Cephalometric tracing illustrating the tooth movement. (8)–(12) Post-treatment photographs. Note the improved muscle balance of the face. Note that the upper front teeth are connected with a bar attached to the premolars and every tooth has individual crowns, so that if a problem arises in relation to one tooth, only one crown has to be removed and replaced by a pontic, which would be the case if the crowns had been connected.

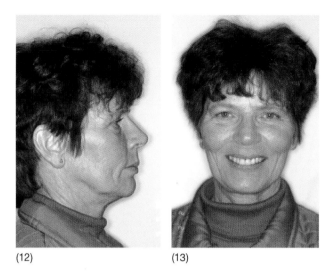

(12)   (13)

Fig. 8.30 (*Continued*)

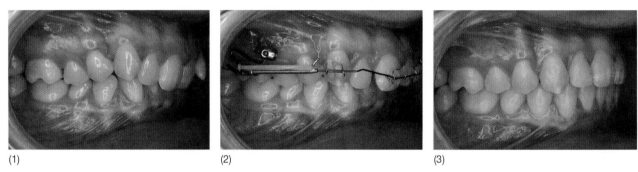

(1)   (2)   (3)

Fig. 8.31 Anchorage obtained with use of mini-implants. (1) Pre-treatment intraoral photographs. (2) Start of molar distalisation with a sliding hook pulling against a closed coil spring. Premolars and lateral incisors were not bonded. (3) Post-treatment intraoral photograph. It was important that this patient was treated without extractions and that both buccal segments were distalised along the skeletal anchorage. Miniscrews placed mesial of the upper first molars could interfere with the roots of the teeth during distalisation. No Class II elastics were used. (Courtesy of Hugo de Clerk.)

Box 8.2 Important facts related to TADs

Material
Design of intraosseous part
Design of transmucosal part
Design of head
The screwdriver
The insertion site
Insertion
Antibiotics
Load-transfer indication
Complication
Alternative uses of screws
Iatrogenic effect
Failures

Material

Although the precise specification is not provided for many mini-implants, most of them are made of Type IV or Type V titanium alloys, which are also used for permanent implants. The biocompatibility of the Aarhus® mini-implant has been tested against the Leibinger® (Stryker Leibinger GmbH and

Co, Freiburg, Germany) surgical screws (Melsen 2005) (Figure 8.32).

A single product from Leone, the orthodontic mini-implant (OMI®, Leone, Florence, Italy), is made of surgical steel 1.4441, which is still used in traumatology, where they are removed after a short period, but use of this is prohibited in neurosurgery. The alloy used for the Aarhus® mini-implan is Ti6AL-4V ELI acc ASTM F 136-02a (MEDICON eG, Tuttlingen, Germany) (Figure 8.32). This alloy is non-toxic, strong with a low modulus of elasticity and antimagnetic

Design of the intraosseous parts

The design of the intraosseous part varies extensively among the different types of mini-implants.

The mini-screws vary with respect to length and dimension and length. The length will vary according to the insertion site whereas the diameter, vary betweem different manufactories (Lietz 2008) The thinnest screws have a diameter of 1mm which allows an insertion between roots with small distance but have a heigh risk of fracture (Hourfar et al. 2017) A small increase in diameter reduces the fracture risk significantly (Figure 8.33).

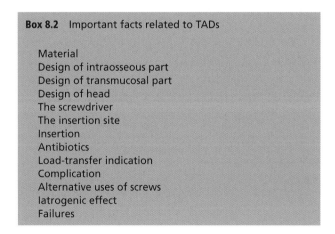

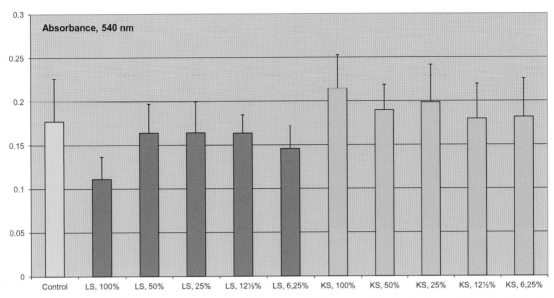

Fig. 8.32 Result of a biocompatibility test comparing the Leibinger surgical screws with the Aarhus mini-implant. (Courtesy Dorthe Arenholt Bindslev.)

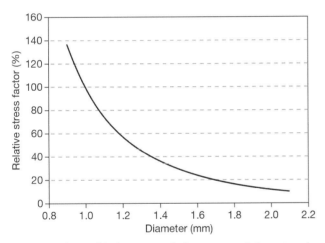

Fig. 8.33 Relationship between relative stress and diameter of a screw. (Courtesy of Michel Dalstra.)

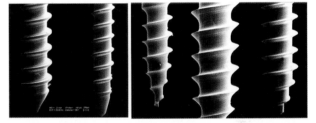

Fig. 8.34 (1) Two self-tapping TADs. To the left a Spider Screw®; to the right a tomas® pin. Note that the threadings are rounded and there is a slight difference in the diameter and in the threading angle. (2) Three non-sterile self-drilling TADs. From the left, the Aarhus mini-implant, the Dual-Top® and the LOMAS screw. It is obvious that the threading is asymmetrical. The threading is cut asymmetrically whereby the resistance towards extrusion force is increased. As the screws are delivered, minor particles may adhere to the surface, and the screws have to be cleaned and sterilised before use. (Courtesy of B Ludvig et al 2008.)

The design may be either cylindrical or conical. In vitro studies have demonstrated superior primary stability with cylindrical compared to conical screws (Sakoh et al. 2006; Lietz et al. 2007). A finite element analysis demonstrated that the maximal stress is concentrated at the tip of the screw during insertion and at the neck on removal (Dalstra et al. 2004). It is therefore advisable to choose a cylindrical design which is only conical at the apex and has a solid neck. Holes through the neck may weaken the screw and lead to fracture at removal.

The miniscrews can be characterised as self tapping or self drilling. The threading varies from self-tapping to self-drilling (Figure 8.34). The self tapping screws are inserted by pressure and require a predilling whereas the selfdrilling are inserted by a cutting aiming at a minimum af damage. This can be obtained by an asymmetric threading, where part of the cut is horizontal resisting pull-out forces. The optimal angle of the shreading was calculated to be 11 degrees and

the depth of the cut is, in relation to the 1.5 mm screw, 0.025 mm (Melsen et al. 2017).

The advantage of self-drilling threading is that predrilling is not necessary. The self-drilling screw are inserted manually, which is an advantage as a touching of a root will be detected immediately, which is not the case when the predrilling is done with a dental dril.

Most mini-implants are produced in a range of diameters between 1.1 mm and 2.5 mm. The slimmer screws are preferred for insertion between roots, as the risk of touching a root is smaller when the diameter is smaller. However, there is an increased risk of fracture of thinner mini-implants, as the mechanical strength is closely related to the diameter (Figure 8.33) (Dalstra et al. 2004). The cut can be symmetrical or asymmetrical. For primary stability, the asymmetrical cuts show more resistance in a pull-out test due to the stress–strain distribution during the pull (Figure 8.35).

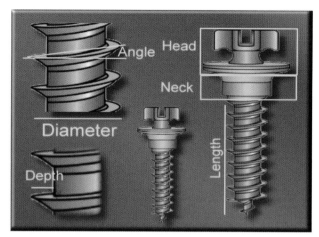

Fig. 8.35 Detailed image of the Aarhus mini-implant of which the intraosseous part was designed based on a finite element model. The material properties included the above-mentioned alloy and the properties of human cortical bone, and aiming at a minimal damage and a maximal retention. The transgingival mucosal part is smooth and has a diameter that is larger than the intraosseous part, allowing for the dentist to note when the neck has reached the periosteum. The coronal part of the collar is larger than the head, making it easier to keep the mucosa clean and healthy. The head has a cross slot, but when seen in two dimensions simulating a bracket.

Design of the transmucosal parts

The transmucosal part of the mini-implant should preferably be smooth to minimise the risk of plaque accumulation. Among available brands, several come in different neck lengths ranging from one to several millimetres, whereas others are offered with no or only one neck length (Figure 8.36).

Design of the head of the mini-implant

According to the morphology of the head, the mini-implant offers one-, two- or three-dimensional control of the extramucosal part and the skeletal anchorage screws can be divided into three groups (Figure 8.37).

The first group comprises screws allowing only a one-point contact and can therefore only be used as direct anchorage. The head can be a button or a hook with or without a hole perforating the neck, for example, AbsoAnchor® (Dentos Korea) (Kyung et al. 2003).

Two-dimensional control is obtained with a hole through the neck as in the Spider Screw® (HDC Company, Sarcedo, Italy), the LomMas Orthodontic Mini Anchorage System® (LomMas, Mondeal Medical Systems GmbH, Tuttlingen, Germany), the M.A.S. (Micerium S.p.aA. Avegno, Italy) (Lin and Liou 2003; Carano et al. 2004, 2005) and the Dual-Top® (Rocky Mountain Orthodontics, USA).

Three-dimensional control is offered by the mini-implants that have a bracket-like head. They can therefore be used as indirect anchorage. Examples of this group are the Aarhus® mini-implant, the Spider Screw® (Maino et al. 2003) and the Dual-Top® (Rocky Mountain Orthodontics, USA). The Aarhus® mini-implant (Figure 8.30) was first described by Costa et al. in 1998, but several variations have since appeared

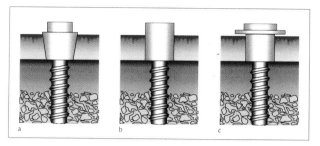

Fig. 8.36 The diameter of the transmucosal collar in relation to the diameter of the head. To avoid inflammation around the screw, it is recommended that diameter of the head should be (1) smaller than or (2) equal to the diameter of the head. The gingiva around the screw is difficult to clean, if the gingiva is covered by part of the miniscrew head (Lietz et al. 2008; Permission from Ludwig et al. 2008).

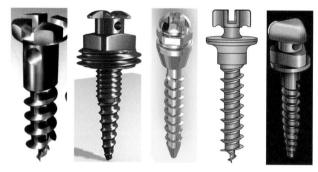

Fig. 8.37 Different TADs, different cuts, different necks and different heads.

on the market (Figure 8.37). Finally, there are TADs that have possibilities of adding different connectors to the intraosseous screw (Byloff and Darendeliler 1997; Wilmes et al. 2015).

The screwdriver

The screwdrivers may also vary from a screwdriver that surrounds the neck as an Allan wrench, which turns within a square or hexagonal hole in the head of the screw. The latter design weakens the neck and increases the risk of fracture, especially during removal and when combined with a hole through the neck. Allan systems have a screwdriver where a sleeve surrounds the entire head which then becomes locked not allowing for any micromovements with respect to the driver. Once the screw is captive from the sterile tray, it can be inserted without wobbling and the driver can be released easly so that no force is transferred to the mini-implants.

Insertion site

The type of insertion site depends on the designs of its different mini-implants (Kanomi 1997). Dry skulls have been studied with the purpose of evaluating the bone density and thickness in various regions where it would be desirable to place the orthodontic implant. Several authors have described the variation in thickness of the bone in the various areas of the facial skeleton (Costa et al. 1998, 2005;

Henriksen et al. 2003). Large variation was found in the thickness of the cortical bone from only a few hundred micrometres to several millimetres. The preferential areas in the maxilla are the the infrazygomatic crest, the palate, the subspinal area and the alveolar process. In the lower jaw, mini-implants can be placed in the retromolar area, in the alveolar process and in the symphysis if the not interfering with the attachment of the mentalis muscle (Figure 8.38). In a study performed with the use of the NewTom DVT9000, three- dimensional images of 50 maxillae were retrieved from a group of 200 patients in the age range of 20–40 years. According to this study, the sites that should be avoided are the maxillary tuberosity and the inter-radicular spaces, when too narrow above 8 mm from

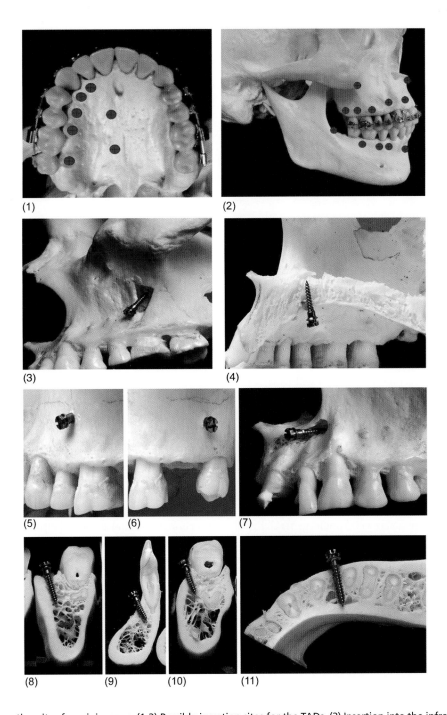

Fig. 8.38 Different insertion sites for mini-screws. (1-2) Possible insertion sites for the TADs. (3) Insertion into the infrazygomatic ridge, the possible perforation of the sinus has not given any undesirable effect. (4) Insertion in the palate. (5-6) Between roots. (7) Above the roots of the incisors. It is important not to perforate the nasal flor. (8-10) The insertion in symphysis may cause problems if the insertion are coinciding with the insertion of the mentalis muscle. An indirect use of the screw as anchorage would then be recommended and the screw could be placed distally to the canines and consolidated to the canines, that would then serve as anchorage. (11) The transcortical screw are mainly used in edentulous jaws and it is important that the screw is not perforating the bone lingually.

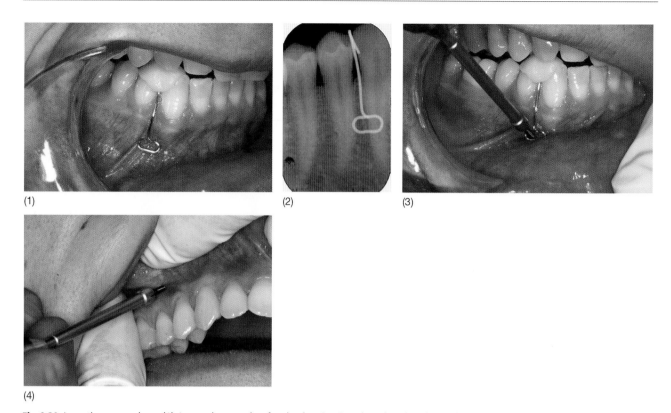

(1)   (2)   (3)

(4)

Fig. 8.39 Insertion procedure. (1) A template made of orthodontic wire placed at the planned insertion site. (2) A periapical radiograph taken to define the insertion site accurately. (3) and (4) The mucosa has to be kept tight when the screw is being inserted to avoid wrapping of the mucosa around the screw during insertion. Note that the direction of insertion is 45° to the long axis of the roots. Whenever possible, the insertion site should be located in attached gingiva.

the bony crest in both the premolar and the molar areas (Carano et al. 2005).

In the maxilla, the direction of insertion will usually be 45°–70° to the bone surface, whereas the insertion in the mandible may be even more perpendicular to the bone surface. For edentulous areas, a transcortical screw can be chosen, as the trabecular bone is usually scarce and a bicortical screw will give more stability.

Insertion

In the case of a self-cutting screw, it should generally not be necessary to predrill. The Aarhus® mini-implant, the LoMas Orthodontic Mini Anchorage System® screw and the Dual-Top Anchor System® are examples of self-drilling systems on the market. When no predrilling is necessary, it is recommended that the orthodontists insert the mini-implants themselves. In relation to the insertion the torque value has been considered an important factor (Di Leonardo et al. 2018).

The first step is to define the site of insertion. A template can be made with orthodontic wire and fixed to a tooth near the insertion site with light-cured composite. An ellipsoid shape on a periapical radiograph will reveal whether the X-ray was taken at an oblique angle. If the ellipsoid on the image has the same shape as the original,

the X-ray can be used to indicate the site of the implant insertion (Figure 8.39). Surgical guides (Morea et al. 2005) or special stents (Kitai et al. 2002) can be used, but are not necessary.

In relation to cross-infection, the procedure is comparable with that of extraction. The doctor, wearing a face mask and a surgical cap, performs surgical handwashing and puts on a pair of sterile gloves. When local anaesthetic has been given, the dental assistant washes the patient's lips and the insertion area with chlorhexidine 0.02%. The sterile kit is then opened, and the correct implant is selected. During insertion, the dental assistant helps keep the mucosa tight to avoid the mucosa getting caught in the threads of the implant (Figure 8.39(4)).

Predrilling a guiding hole of 1–2 mm sometimes may be necessary even when using self-drilling screws. This is the case when the cortex is thick and dense, as in the mandibular symphysis or in the retromolar area. Insertion directly in these areas without predrilling may lead to bending of the fine tip of the screw. The predrilling should only be 1–2 mm deep and should be done with a drill that is 0.2–0.3-mm thinner than the screw itself. The drill should be used at low speed with irrigation for cooling. In the case where predrilling is necessary, it should be done in an environment which allows for a surgical setting as for the insertion of a dental implant. If

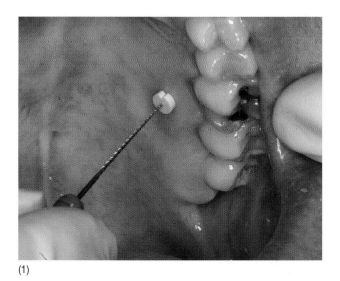

(1)

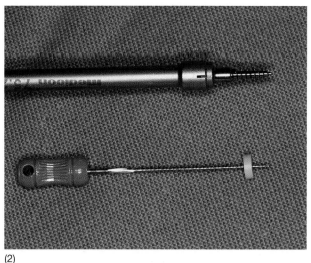

(2)

Fig. 8.40 (1) Endodontic file being used to assess the thickness of the mucosa. (2) Example of an endodontic file.

this is not the case, a surgeon or a periodontist should perform the insertion.

Not only the thickness of cortical bone but also of the mucosa is important, since it will determine the centre of rotation when the head of the mini-implant is loaded. The mucosal thickness should be measured with a probe or even better with an endodontic file on which a marker indicates the thickness (Figure 8.40). The mini-implant should then be inserted adjacently, not directly through the perforation done with the probe. This precaution is taken to reduce the risk of carrying epithelial cells into the bone.

Whenever possible, the mini-implants should be inserted through attached gingiva, as this leads to a minimum of local irritation (Figure 8.41). In the cases where this is not possible, one solution would be to allow the mini-implant to be covered with mucosa, with only a wire or a ligature emerging through the mucosa (Figure 8.41). In some cases, local irritation cannot be avoided. This applies especially to buccally placed mini-implants in the mandibular symphysis area. The lack of keratinised gingiva and the activity of the mentalis muscle may result in the growth of granulation tissue around the screw (Figure 8.41). When the oral hygiene is maintained, the loss of an implant or infection is rare.

The patient should be instructed to carefully cleanse around the screw. On the first day post insertion, swabbing with 0.02% chlorhexidine is recommended.

Antibiotics

Antibiotics have been recommended by several authors, but should not be given routinely. The risk of infection is obviously greater when drilling is performed, especially when the same insertion site is repeatedly entered. It is crucial to maintain sterility to avoid infection, so that antibiotics can be avoided.

Load transfer

The load transfer from the mini-implants to the surrounding bone under different loading conditions was described by Dalstra et al. (2004).

Based on a finite element analysis, these authors calculated the strain developed when loading of 50 cN was added perpendicular to the long axis of a mini-implant with a diameter of 2 mm. They evaluated the strain developed with different cortical thickness and different density of the trabecular bone and found that in the case of thin cortical bone and low-density trabecular bone, the strain values may exceed the value for microfractures and thereby lead to loosening (Frost 1992).

The 3D finite element models of mini-implants inserted into human autopsy material further demonstrated that the mini-screw is displaced in a tipping mode, indicating that the tip of the screw will be displaced in the opposite direction of the head of the screw, which causes tensile stresses in the direction of the force (Dalstra et al. 2004). In general, the stress levels are higher in the cortical shell than in the underlying trabecular core, but it is the opposite case for strain. Although a peak value for the strains in the trabecular bone of 2.465 microstrain was reached, the general order of magnitude for the bone strains was 10–100 microstrain, well within the physiological load (Figure 8.42). Whereas the thickness of the cortical bone is crucial for the transfer of load from the mini-implant to bone, the stiffness (or density) of the trabecular core only plays a minor role.

Based on these analyses, immediate loading with Ni–Ti coil springs delivering a known force of approximately 50 cN is recommended. This is preferred to the application of elastics, as the forces are less variable and the rate of decay is more gradual. Heavier forces can be applied once the density of the bone has increased. However, it is still advisable to start with low known forces.

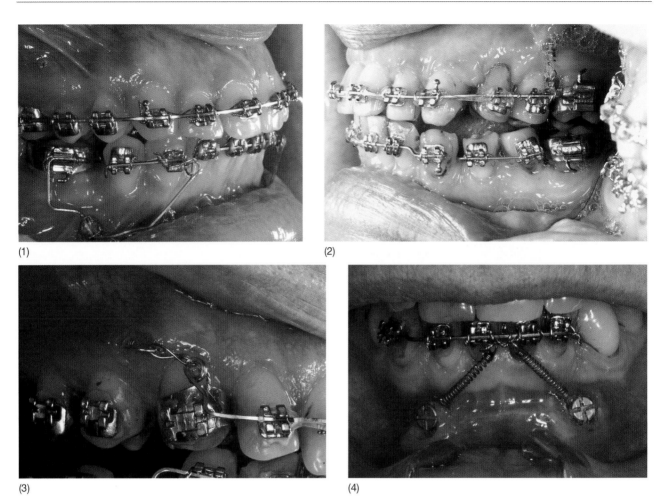

Fig. 8.41 (1) Mini-implant inserted into the mobile gingiva. The mini-implant is being used indirectly with a TMA™ wire passing through the slot of the head generating the forces for both proclination of the anterior teeth and uprighting of the molar. (2) Mini-implant inserted at the infrazygomatic crest and covered by mucosa. (3) Mini-implant inserted between the premolars. The point of force application is displaced distally by the insertion of a stainless-steel wire into the bracket of the mini-implant, thereby avoiding impingement of the mucosa. (4) Mini-implant inserted in non-keratinised mucosa of the symphysis showing reactive overgrowth of the mucosa.

Tissue reaction to loading

The tissue reaction related to immediate loading of the new generation of skeletal anchorage has been the subject of only a few studies to date (Melsen and Costa 2000; Ohmae et al. 2001; Deguchi et al. 2003; Luzi et al. 2005). On the basis of the experience gained from treating patients with zygoma ligatures as anchorage, it was anticipated that the retention of the osteosynthesis screws was purely mechanical (Costa et al. 1998; Melsen and Costa 2000). It was hypothesised that the concentrated pressure from the wire would generate a local necrosis. This would result in a gradual displacement of the wire through the bone. However, histological studies carried out on *Macaca fascicularis* (Melsen and Costa 2000) revealed that bone-to-screw contact and bone density adjacent to the screw increase when the loading was 25 or 50 cN. The observation time was 1 week to 6 months following insertion.

The increase in density continued over the 6-month observation period. The bone-to-screw contact also increased over time. There was no difference between the loading with

25 or 50 cN. Administration of fluorochrome bone labellings at two different time points before sacrifice allowed assessment of mineralising surface/bone surface (MS/BS) and mineral appositional rate (MAR μm/day). The bone close to the screw was predominantly woven bone and the turnover was significantly higher than in the alveolar bone in general (Figure 8.43) (Melsen 2005).

The tissue reaction adjacent to both smooth and osseointegrated implants seems to be independent of the orthodontic loading (Chen et al. 1999; Wehrbein et al. 1999; Ohmae et al. 2001; Trisi and Rebaudi 2002; Deguchi et al. 2003; Fritz et al. 2004). Finite element analyses have indicated that normal functional loads and the difference in stiffness of the implants from that of the surrounding bone result in variation in strain that is responsible for the elevated turnover rate of the bone adjacent to the implants (Chen et al. 1995, 1999). However, loading of mini-implants in the atrophic alveolar areas also results in a rebuild of the alveolar process in the direction of the force (Figure 8.43).

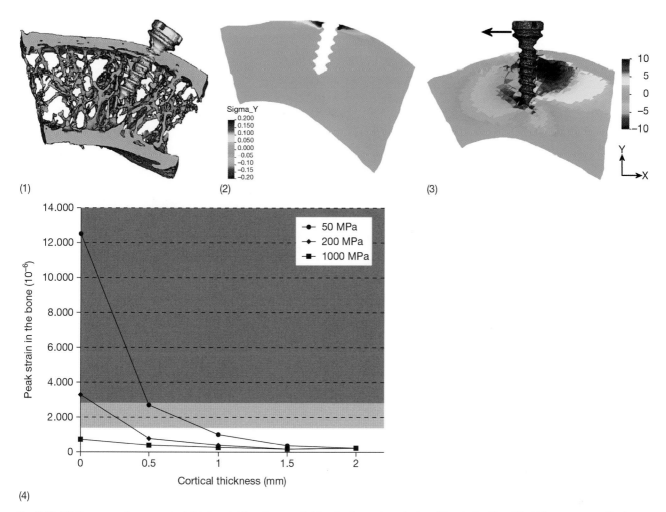

Fig. 8.42 (1) Human autopsy material into which a 2-mm mini-implant was inserted and loaded with a 50 cN force perpendicular to the long axis of the implant. The centre of rotation was localised to the internal border of the cortex. (2) Stress concentration in the cortical bone as a result of loading. (3) Strain concentration in the trabecular bone. (4) Peak strain occurring in the bone depends on the cortical thickness and the density of the trabecular bone. In the dark grey region of the graph, there is a large risk of losing the implant due to high overload of the bone. In the light grey area, the risk is reduced, and in the white area, the bone density will most likely increase as a result of loading. (Courtesy of Michel Dalstra.)

Loading

Based on the above-described animal experiments, the mini-implants can be loaded immediately if the force is controlled. Apart from the above-mentioned papers by Melsen et al. (Melsen and Costa 2000; Melsen 2004), Ohmae et al. (2001), Deguchi et al. (2003) and Luzi et al. (2009), none of the other publications indicated the magnitude of the added forces. The timing of the force application varies from minutes to 8 weeks. There seems to be no contraindication to immediate loading with a moderate force.

Orthodontic mechanics

The mechanics applied in relation to the use of skeletal anchorage should be carefully considered before inserting the implants. The line of action should be as perpendicular to the long axis of the screw as possible. Moments generating

shearing forces on the bone contacting the implants can result in loosening independent of the direction of the moments. When planning the mechanics, it is crucial that the implants do not impede the foreseen tooth movements. Examples of mechanics can be seen in the cases available on the supporting companion website for this book: www.wiley.com/go/melsen (cases 3–6).

Alternative application of TADs used as anchorage

When talking about anchorage, we are usually talking about anchorage for avoiding undesired tooth movements. Over the past decennium, the attention has been to the use of TAD handles for the displacement of alveolar segments. This approach was first introduced by Triaca et al. (2001), who displaced the mandibular incisor segment around a

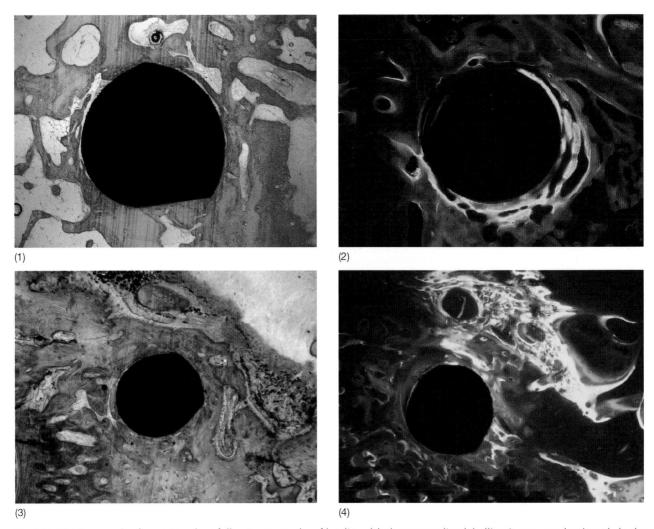

(1)

(2)

(3)

(4)

Fig. 8.43 (1) Micrograph of a mini-implant following 2 months of loading. (2) The tetracycline labelling is seen predominantly in the bone adjacent to the implant. (3) and (4) Following 3 months of loading, the bone is building up in the direction of loading.

special hinge mechanics. The incisors were thereby tipped forward and long-term follow-up revealed that a proclination of more than 10° resulted in gingival retractions (Joss et al. 2012; Antonarakis 2017). An alternative method whereby the anterior distraction was combined with an excision of a slice of alveolus below the apex of the incisors made it possible to translate the incisors anteriorly without tipping using the posterior segments as anchorage.

Indications

The indications for mini-implant anchorage are not well-defined, but the applications obtained from a literature review seem to indicate that the most frequent use has been for retraction of anterior teeth and intrusion of molars (Papadopoulos and Tarawneh 2007). Most of the published papers related to skeletal anchorage are case reports describing a new device used as an alternative to other approaches

to anchorage, frequently instead of headgear (Park et al. 2001; Kyung et al. 2003; Kaya et al. 2009; Buschang et al. 2011). In other cases, the mini-implants have been used as anchorage for tooth movements that could not otherwise have been performed.

At Aarhus University, mini-implants have been used since 1997 in the following situations:

1. Patients who do not have enough teeth for use in the application of conventional anchorage.
2. Patients in whom the forces acting on the reactive unit would generate adverse effects.
3. Patients requiring asymmetrical tooth movement in all planes of space.
4. In some cases as an alternative to orthognathic surgery.
5. As anchorage for tooth movement performed with the purpose of generating bone for an implant.

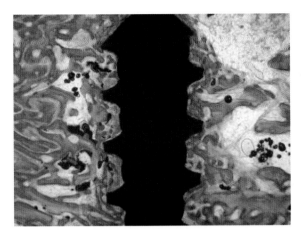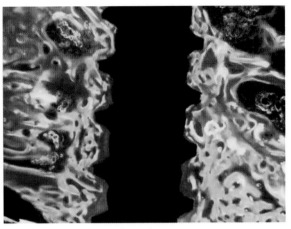

Fig. 8.44 Histological images of mini-implants inserted adjacent to the midpalatal suture seen to the left of the images. The intravital staining with tetracycline and calcin on the image to the right elucidates an active remodelling occurring close to the suture. In order to get a solid anchorage, two mini-implants connected by a plate are therefore recommended. (See the part on palatal implants by Wilmes).

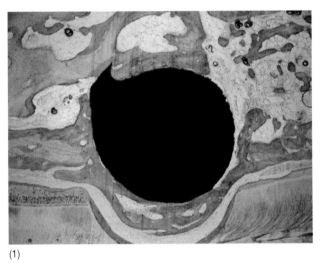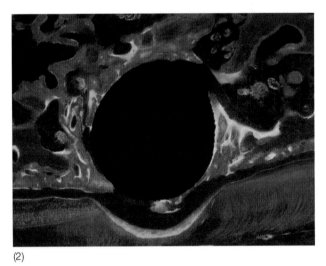

(1)   (2)

Fig. 8.45 (1) and (2) Healing of a root in which a defect was induced during the insertion of a mini-implant.

6. For bone movement.
7. As bone maintainer

Indications 2, 3 and 5 can also be considered as those with a lack of equilibrium in the appliance used.

Complications

The initial stability is crucial for the maintenance of anchorage. Failure rates between 10% and 25% have been reported and do not differ between miniplates and free-standing miniscrews (Cheng et al. 2004). In a prospective study, these authors found that the anatomical location and the peri-implant soft tissues were factors of importance with regard to prognosis. This also corroborates an ongoing study at Department of Orthodontics, Aarhus University, in which implants inserted through non-keratinised mucosa have been seen to be associated with a higher failure rate than

those inserted through the attached gingiva. According to Miyawaki et al. (2003), factors such as thin diameter screws, high mandibular plane angle and peri-implant inflammation should be considered as risk factors.

What happens if the screw touches a root?

With a hand-driven screwdriver, it will be obvious to the dentist when the mini-implant comes in contact with a root and a new insertion side can be chosen. The damage to the root will then only be minimum and frequently reversible. According to a histological study, in which notches were produced on purpose, repair of these lesions will take place spontaneously by the formation of cellular cementum (Figure 8.45). When a screw is inserted with a drill, even at low speed, the risk of not detecting a root is larger due to the lack of tactile sensation.

Failures

Failures can be classified as those related to the mini-implant, those related to the person inserting the implant and those related to the patient (Jung et al. 2012).

Problems related to the mini-implant and solutions

- Problem: Fracture either due to a too thin diameter or too low strength of the neck area, which will be subject to a larger stress at removal.
- Solution: Choose a system with a solid neck and a diameter corresponding to the bone quality.
- Problem: Infection around the mini-implant.
- Solution: Choose an implant system with variable neck length, so that the entire transmucosal part is smooth.

Instruct the patient regarding maintenance of satisfactory oral hygiene around the mini-implant.

Problems related to the insertion procedure

In the case of self-drilling screws, too high pressure and an oblique angle at the beginning of the insertion procedure can lead to fracture of the cutting tip of the screw. The solution will be to remove the part left in the bone and either wait for healing 3–4 month or choose a better position and use the TAD as indirect anchorage.

- Excessive tightening of the screw: Once the smooth part (the neck) has reached the periosteum, it is crucial to stop the turning of the screw that will otherwise loosen.
- In relation to screws with a bracket-like head, the ligature should be placed on the top of the screw in the slot perpendicular to the one in which the wire is resting. Turning the ligature around the screw, as is normally the case with a bracket head, will make it impossible for the patient to keep the screw area inflammation-free.
- Loosening due to 'wiggling' forces being used during removal of the screwdriver. When a screwdriver 'grabs' a screw, it is important that 'wiggling' forces are not applied when detaching the screwdriver from the screw. This can be avoided if a force parallel to the long axis and not at an angle to it is applied to remove the screw driver (Figure 8.46).

Problems related to the patient

- Too little bone: In patients in whom the thickness of the cortex is less than 0.5 mm and the density of the trabecular bone is low, primary stability cannot be obtained and the prognosis is poor.

- In patients with thick mucosa, the distance between the point of force application and the centre of resistance of the screw is greater, thus a large moment is generated when a force is applied.
- Bone remodelling: If a screw is inserted in an area with high bone remodelling, either in relation to the resorption of a deciduous tooth or healing after extraction, loosening can occur even after primary stability.
- Patient with systemic alterations of bone metabolism either due to disease, medication or heavy smoking.

The above-mentioned lists cover the majority of the failures observed over a period of 10 years of regular use of skeletal anchorage by the authors. The problems related to insertion usually resolve spontaneously as the clinician learns how to avoid the above-mentioned failures. Selection of suitable patients is also part of the learning curve and, independent of the type of instruction, in most cases, the failure rate ending up being around 5–10% of errors occurring with the use of mini-implants.

In case of failure during insertion, lack of stability or failure in the direction of insertion leading to contact with a root surface, a new screw should be inserted. Due to remodelling related to the healing of the defect, the new site should be at a distance of minimum 5 mm from the original one or the insertion should be postponed until healing of the bony defect has occurred. Healing for 6 weeks should be allowed before a mini-implant can be inserted in the same area.

Future of TADs

There is no doubt that the TADs make a significant contribution towards expanding the limits of what can be done orthodontically for patients with deteriorating dentitions. The examples on the supporting companion website for

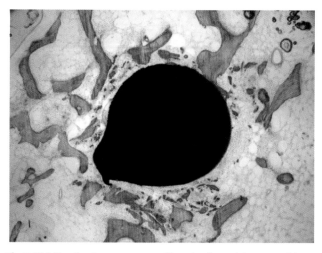

Fig. 8.46 Microfractures generated by wiggling of the screwdriver during insertion.

this book (www.wiley.com/go/melsen) show how these implants have been used to widen the spectrum of orthodontics and to improve the prognosis for patients who have lost both marginal bone and several teeth.

According to Gandedkar et al. (2019), the introduction of the TADs leads to a paradigm shift and a striking widening of the orthodontic possibilities within practically all types of orthodontic problems. The authors made a thorough literature review of factors determining the success rate of the TAD related to the patients, the type of TADs and the type of studies reported. There is however an impressive variation in the frequency TADs are used by different clinicians. Are the TADs replacing biomechanical thinking? Are tooth movements that cannot be maintained being done because the occlusion is not compatible with the normal function? The distalisation of the molars will always have a tendency to return towards the 'key ridge' and often only the immediate treatment results are demonstrated. The factor having the largest impact of whether to use a TAD or not is problem for the doctor. The TADs may also become a part of the outsourcing lowering the requirements to biomechanical knowledge, 'a crutch' and contributing to the trend to move the orthodontics out of the specialist's office. The TADs are here to stay, but they should be limited to indication where they widen the aspect of orthodontics and not be used as a chrutch replacing unsatisfactory biomechanical knowledge.

References

Armbrus PC, Block MS (2001) Onplant-supported orthodontic anchorage. *Atlas Oral Maxillofac Surg Clin North Am.* 9(1): 53–74.

Alwali S, Marklund M and Persson M (2000) Apical root resorption of upper first molars as related to anchorage system. *Swed Dent J* 24, 145–153.

Antonarakis GS, Joss CU, Triaca A, Kuipers-Jagtman AM and Kiliarides S (2017) Gingival recessions of lower incisors after proclination by orthodontics alone or in combination with anterior mandibular alveolar process distraction. *Clin Oral Investig.* 21(8): 2569–2579.

Atkinson SR. (1951) The mesio-buccal root of the maxillary first molar. *Am J Orthod.* 38: 642–652.

Bae SM, Park HS, Kyung HM and Sung JH (2002) Ultimate anchorage control. *Texas Dent J* 119, 580–591.

Baker HA (1904) Treatment of protruding and receding jaws by the use of intermaxillary elastics. *Int Dent J* 25, 344–356.

Bakke M, Michler L and Moller E (1992) Occlusal control of mandibular elevator muscles. *Scand J Dent Res* 100, 284–291.

Berens A, Wiechmann D and Dempf R (2006) Mini- and micro-screws for temporary skeletal anchorage in orthodontic therapy. *J Orofac Orthop* 67, 450–458.

Bernhart T, Freudenthaler J, Dortbudak O, Bantleon HP and Watzek G (2001) Short epithetic implants for orthodontic anchorage in the paramedian region of the palate. A clinical study. *Clin Oral Implants Res* 12, 624–631.

Block MS and Hoffman DR (1995) A new device for absolute anchorage for orthodontics. *Am J Orthod Dentofacial Orthop* 107, 251–258.

Branemark PI, Hansson BO, Adell R, Breine U, Lindstrom J, Hallen O and Ohman A (1977) Osseointegrated implants in the treatment of the edentulous jaw. Experience from a 10-year period. *Scand J Plast Reconstr Surg Suppl* 16, 1–132.

Bresin A, Kiliaridis S and Strid KG (1999) Effect of masticatory function on the internal bone structure in the mandible of the growing rat. *Eur J Oral Sci* 107, 35–44.

Burstone CJ (1962) Rationale of the segmented arch. *Am J Orthod* 48, 805–822.

Burstone CJ (1966) The mechanics of the segmented arch techniques. *Angle Orthod* 36, 99–120.

Burstone CJ (1982) The segmented arch approach to space closure. *Am J Orthod* 82, 361–378.

Burstone CJ and Koenig HA (1974) Force systems from an ideal arch. *Am J Orthod* 65, 270–289.

Burstone CJ and Koenig HA (1976) Optimizing anterior and canine retraction. *Am J Orthod* 70, 1–19.

Buschang PH, Carrillo R and Rossouw PE (2011) Orthopedic correction of growing hyperdivergent, retrognathic patients with miniscrew implants. *J Oral Maxillofac Surg* 69, 754–762.

Byloff FK and Darendeliler MA (1997) Distal molar movement using the pendulum appliance. Part 1: clinical and radiological evaluation. *Angle Orthod* 67(4), 249–260.

Carano A and Testa M (1996) The distal jet for upper molar distalization. *J Clin Orthod* 30, 374–380.

Carano A, Testa M and Bowman SJ (2002) The distal jet simplified and updated. *J Clin Orthod* 36, 586–590.

Carano A, Velo S, Incorvati C and Poggio P (2004) Clinical applications of the Mini-Screw-Anchorage-System (M.A.S.) in the maxillary alveolar bone. *Prog Orthod* 5, 212–235.

Carano A, Velo S, Leone P and Siciliani G (2005) Clinical applications of the Miniscrew Anchorage System. *J Clin Orthod* 39, 9–24.

Cattaneo PM, Dalstra M and Melsen B (2003) The transfer of occlusal forces through the maxillary molars: a finite element study. *Am J Orthod Dentofacial Orthop* 123, 367–373.

Chen J, Chen K, Garetto LP and Roberts WE (1995) Mechanical response to functional and therapeutic loading of a retromolar endosseous implant used for orthodontic anchorage to mesially translate mandibular molars. *Implant Dent* 4, 246–258.

Chen J, Esterle M and Roberts WE (1999) Mechanical response to functional loading around the threads of retromolar endosseous implants utilized for orthodontic anchorage: coordinated histomorphometric and finite element analysis. *Int J Oral Maxillofac Implants* 14, 282–289.

Cheng SJ, Tseng IY, Lee JJ and Kok SH (2004) A prospective study of the risk factors associated with failure of mini implants used for orthodontic anchorage. *Int J Oral Maxillofac Implants* 19, 100–106.

Costa A, Pasta G and Bergamaschi G (2005) Intraoral hard and soft tissue depths for temporary anchorage devices. *Semin Orthod* 11, 10–15.

Costa A, Raffainl M and Melsen B (1998) Miniscrews as orthodontic anchorage: a preliminary report. *Int J Adult Orthod Orthog Surg* 13, 201–209.

Creekmore TD and Eklund MK (1983) The possibility of skeletal anchorage. *J Clin Orthod* 17, 266–269.

Dalstra M, Cattaneo PM, Beckmann F and Melsen B (2006) Synchrotron radiation-based micro-tomography of alveolar support tissues. *Orthod Craniofac Res* 9(4), 199–205.

Dalstra M, Cattaneo PM and Melsen B (2004) Load transfer of miniscrews for orthodontic anchorage. *Orthodontics* 1, 53–62.

Damon DH (2005) Treatment of the face with biocompatible orthodontics. In Graber TM, Vanarsdall RL and Vig KWL (eds) *Orthodontics Current Principles and Techniques*, 4th edn, pp. 753–831. St Louis, MO: Elsevier/Mosby.

Daskalogiannakis J (2000) *Glossary of Orthodontic Terms.* Chicago, IL: Quintessence.

De CH, Geerinckx V and Siciliano S (2002) The zygoma anchorage system. *J Clin Orthod* 36, 455–459.

De Clerck H, Geerinckx V, and Siciliani S (2002) The Zygoma anchorage system. *J. Clin Orthod.* Aug; 36(8), 455–459

Deguchi T, Takano-Yamamoto T, Kanomi R, Hartsfield JK Jr, Roberts WE and Garetto LP (2003) The use of small titanium screws for orthodontic anchorage. *J Dent Res* 82, 377–381.

Di Leonardo B, Ludwig B, Lisson JA, Contardo L, Mura R and Hourfar J (2018) Insertion torque values and success rates for paramedian insertion of orthodontic mini-implants: a retrospective study. *J Orofac Orthop* 79, 109–115.

Douglass JB and Killiany DM (1987) Dental implants used as orthodontic anchorage. *J Oral Implant* 13, 28–38.

Drescher D, Bourauel C and Schumacher HA (1989) Frictional forces between bracket and arch wire. *Am J Orthod Dentofacial Orthop* 96, 397–404.

Erverdi N and Keles A (2003) Anchorage for closing open bites. *Am J Orthod Dentofacial Orthop* 123, 14A–15A.

Favero L, Brollo P and Bressan E (2002) Orthodontic anchorage with specific fixtures: related study analysis. *Am J Orthod Dentofacial Orthop* 122, 84–94.

Ferro F, Monsurro A and Perillo L (2000) Sagittal and vertical changes after treatment of Class II Division 1 malocclusion according to the Cetlin method. *Am J Orthod Dentofacial Orthop* 118, 150–158.

Fiorentino G and Melsen B (1996) Asymmetric mandibular space closure. *J Clin Orthod* 30, 519–523.

Fortini A, Lupoli M, Giuntoli F and Franchi L (2004) Dentoskeletal effects induced by rapid molar distalization with the first class appliance. *Am J Orthod Dentofacial Orthop* 125, 697–704.

Fortini A, Lupoli M and Parri M (1999) The first class appliance for rapid molar distalization. *J Clin Orthod* 33, 322–328.

Freeman DC (1965) *Root Surface Area Related to Anchorage in the Begg Tethnique.* Knoxville: Department of Orthodontics, University of Tennessee.

Freudenthaler JW, Haas R and Bantleon HP (2001a) Bicortical titanium screws for critical orthodontic anchorage in the mandible: a preliminary report on clinical applications. *Clin Oral Implants Res* 12, 358–363.

Freudenthaler JW, Tischler GK and Burstone CJ (2001b) Bond strength of fiber-reinforced composite bars for orthodontic attachment. *Am J Orthod Dentofacial Orthop* 120, 648–653.

Fritz U, Ehmer A and Diedrich P (2004) Clinical suitability of titanium microscrews for orthodontic anchorage-preliminary experiences. *J Orofac Orthop* 65, 410–418.

Frost HM (1992) Perspectives: bone's mechanical usage windows. *Bone Miner* 19, 257–271.

Gainsforth BL and Higley LB (1945) A study of orthodontic anchorage possibilities in basal bone. *Am J Orthod Oral Surg* 31, 406–416.

Gandedkar NH, Shrikantaiah S, Patil AK, Baseer MA, Chng CK, Ganeshkar SV and Kambalyal P (2019) Influence of conventional and skeletal anchorage system supported fixed functional appliance on maxillo-mandibular complex and temporomandibular joint: a preliminary comparative cone beam computed tomography study. *Int Orthod* 17, 256–268.

Garetto LP, Chen J, Parr JA and Roberts WE (1995) Remodeling dynamics of bone supporting rigidly fixed titanium implants: a histomorphometric comparison in four species including humans. *Implant Dent* 4, 235–243.

Goodacre CJ, Brown DT, Roberts WE and Jeiroudi MT (1997) Prosthodontic considerations when using implants for orthodontic anchorage. *J Prosthet Dent* 77, 162–170.

Gray JB, Steen ME, King GJ and Clark AE (1983) Studies on the efficacy of implants as orthodontic anchorage. *Am J Orthod* 83, 311–317.

Guyman GW, Kokich VG and Oswald RJ (1980) Ankylosed teeth as abutments for palatal expansion in the rhesus monkey. *Am J Orthod* 77, 486–499.

Hayashi H, Konoo T and Yamaguchi K (2004) Intermittent 8-hour activation in orthodontic molar movement. *Am J Orthod Dentofacial Orthop* 125, 302–309.

Henriksen B, Bavitz B, Kelly B and Harn SD (2003) Evaluation of bone thickness in the anterior hard palate relative to midsagittal orthodontic implants. *Int J Oral Maxillofac Implants* 18, 578–581.

Higuchi KW and Slack JM (1991) The use of titanium fixtures for intraoral anchorage to facilitate orthodontic tooth movement. *Int J Oral Maxillofac Implants* 6, 338–344.

Hilgers JJ (1992) The pendulum appliance for Class II non-compliance therapy. *J Clin Orthod* 26, 706–714.

Hourfar J, Bister D, Kanavakis G, Lisson JA and Ludwig B (2017) Influence of interradicular and palatal placement of orthodontic mini-implants on the success (survival) rate. *Head Face Med* 13, 14.

Jenner JD and Fitzpatrick BN (1985) Skeletal anchorage utilising bone plates. *Aust Orthod J* 9, 231–233.

Jones RD and White JM (1992) Rapid Class II molar correction with an open-coil jig. *J Clin Orthod* 26, 661–664.

Jones JP, Elnagar MH, and Perez DE (2020) Temporary Skeletal Anchorage Techniques. *Oral Maxillofac Surg Clin North Am;*32(1):27–37

Joss CU, Triaca A, Antonini M, Kiliarides S, and Kuipers-Jagtman AM, (2013) Skeletal and dental stability of segmental distraction of the anterior mandibular alveolar process. A 5.5 year follows up. *Int J Oral Maxillofac Surg.* Mar; 42(3), 337–344.

Jung BA, Harzer W, Wehrbein H et al (2011) Immediate versus conventional loading of palatal implants in humans: a first report of a multicenter RCT. *Clin Oral Invest* 15, 495–502.

Jung BA, Kunkel M, Göllner P, Liechti T, Wagner W and Wehrbein H (2012) Prognostic parameters contributing to palatal implant failures: a long-term survival analysis of 239 patients. *Clin Oral Implants Res* 23, 746–750.

Kanomi R (1997) Mini-implant for orthodontic anchorage. *J Clin Orthod* 31, 763–767.

Kanter F (1956) Mandibular anchoarage and extraoral force. *Am J Orthod* 42, 194–208.

Kaya B, Arman A, Uckan S and Uazici AC (2009) Comparison of the sygoma anchorage system with cervical headgear in buccal segment distalazation. *Eur J Orthod* 31(4), 317–424.

Keles A, Erverdi N and Sezen S (2003) Bodily distalization of molars with absolute anchorage. *Angle Orthod* 73, 471–482.

Kitai N, Yasuda Y and Takada K (2002) A stent fabricated on a selectively colored stereolithographic model for placement of orthodontic mini-implants. *Int J Adult Orthod Orthog Surg* 17, 264–266.

Kofod T, Wurtz V and Melsen B (2005) Treatment of an ankylosed central incisor by single tooth dento-osseous osteotomy and a simple distraction device. *Am J Orthod Dentofacial Orthop* 127, 72–80.

Kokich VG, Shapiro PA, Oswald R, Koskinen-Moffett L and Clarren SK (1985) Ankylosed teeth as abutments for maxillary protraction: a case report. *Am J Orthod* 88, 303–307.

Kusy RP (2004) Influence on binding of third-order torque to second-order angulation. *Am J Orthod Dentofacial Orthop* 125, 726–732.

Kusy RP and Whitley JQ (1997) Friction between different wire-bracket configurations and materials. *Semin Orthod* 3, 166–177.

Kusy RP and Whitley JQ (1999) Assessment of second-order clearances between orthodontic archwires and bracket slots via the critical contact angle for binding. *Angle Orthod* 69, 71–80.

Kyung HM, Park HS, Bae SM, Sung JH and Kim IB (2003) Development of orthodontic micro-implants for intraoral anchorage. *J Clin Orthod* 37, 321–328.

Lee JS, Park HS and Kyung HM (2001) Micro-implant anchorage for lingual treatment of a skeletal Class II malocclusion. *J Clin Orthod* 35, 643–647.

Leo M, Cerroni L, Pasquantonio G, Condò SG and Condò R (2016) Temporary anchorage devices (TADs) in orthodontics: review of the factors that influence the clinical success rate of the mini-implants. *Clin Ter* May-Jun;167(3).

Lietz T (2008) Mini-screws – Aspects of Assessment and Selection among different systems (Chapter 3, pp. 11–59). In Ludwig B, Baumgaertel S, Bowman J, editors, *Mini-Implants in Orthodontics*. Berlin, New York: Quintessenz.

Lim HJ, Choi YJ, Evans CA and Hwang HS (2011) Predictors of initial stability of orthodontic miniscrew implants. *Eur J Orthod* 33, 528–532.

Lin JC and Liou EJ (2003) A new bone screw for orthodontic anchorage. *J Clin Orthod* 37, 676–681.

Luzi C, Verna C and Melsen B (2005) *The Aarhus Anchorage System. Histological and Clinical Investigation.* Aarhus, Denmark: University of Aarhus.

Luzi C, Verna C and Melsen B (2009) Immediate loading of orthodontic mini-implants: a histomorphometric evaluation of tissue reaction. *Eur J Orthod* 31(1), 21–29. doi:10.1093/ejo/cjn087

Maino BG, Bednar J, Pagin P and Mura P (2003) The spider screw for skeletal anchorage. *J Clin Orthod* 37, 90–97.

Marcotte MR (1990) *Biomechanics in Orthodontics.* Toronto, Canada: BC Decker.

Matthews DC (1993) Osseointegrated implants: their application in orthodontics. *J Can Dent Assoc* 59, 454, 459–460, 463.

Mavreas D (1991) *Tomographic Assessment of Temporomandibular Joint Alterations following Orthognathic Surgery.* Aarhus, Denmark: University of Aarhus.

McLaughlin RP, Bennett JC and Trevisi HJ (2001) *Systemized Orthodontic Treatment Mechanics.* Edinburgh: Mosby.

Melsen B (1978) Effects of cervical anchorage during and after treatment: an implant study. *Am J Orthod* 73, 526–540.

Melsen B (2004) Is the intraoral-extradental anchorage changing the spectrum of orthodontics? In McNamara JA Jr (ed.) *Implants, Microimplants, Onplants and Transplants: New Answers to Old Questions in Orthodontics*, 1st edn, pp. 41–68. Ann Arbor: University of Michigan.

Melsen B (2005) Temporary skeletal anchorage – the Aarhus Anchorage System. In Cope JB (ed.) *Temporary Anchorage Devices in Orthodontics*. Dallas, TX: Under Dog Media, LP.

Melsen B and Bosch C (1997) Different approaches to anchorage; a survey and an evaluation. *Angle Orthod* 67, 23–30.

Melsen B and Costa A (2000) Immediate loading of implants used for orthodontic anchorage. *Clin Orthod Res* 3, 23–28.

Melsen B and Dalstra M (2003) Distal molar movement with Kloehn headgear: is it stable? *Am J Orthod Dentofacial Orthop* 123, 374–378.

Melsen B, Fotis V and Burstone CJ (1990) Vertical force considerations in differential space closure. *J Clin Orthod* 24, 678–683.

Melsen B, Petersen JK and Costa A (1998) Zygoma ligatures: an alternative form of maxillary anchorage. *J Clin Orthod* 32, 154–158.

Melsen B and Verna C (1999) A rational approach to orthodontic anchorage. *Prog Orthod* 1, 10–22.

Melsen B, Verna C, and Luci C (2017) *Mini-implants and their Clinical Applications*. The Aarhus experience. Edizioni Martina.

Miyamoto K, Ishizuka Y and Tanne K (1996) Changes in masseter muscle activity during orthodontic treatment evaluated by a 24-hour EMG system. *Angle Orthod* 66, 223–228.

Miyamoto K, Ishizuka Y, Ueda HM, Saifuddin M, Shikata N and Tanne K (1999) Masseter muscle activity during the whole day in children and young adults. *J Oral Rehabil* 26, 858–864.

Miyawaki S, Koyama I, Inoue M, Mishima K, Sugahara T and Takano-Yamamoto T (2003) Factors associated with the stability of titanium screws placed in the posterior region for orthodontic anchorage. *Am J Orthod Dentofacial Orthop* 124, 373–378.

Morea C, Dominguez GC, Wuo AV and Tortamano A (2005) Surgical guide for optimal positioning of mini-implants. *J Clin Orthod* 39, 317–321.

Mulligan TF (1998) *Common Sense Mechanics in Everyday Orthodontics*. Phoenix, AZ: CSM Publishing.

Ngantung V, Nanda RS and Bowman SJ (2001) Posttreatment evaluation of the distal jet appliance. *Am J Orthod Dentofacial Orthop* 120, 178–185.

Odman J, Lekholm U, Jemt T, Branemark PI and Thilander B (1988) Osseointegrated titanium implants – a new approach in orthodontic treatment. *Eur J Orthod* 10, 98–105.

Ohmae M, Saito S, Morohashi T, Seki K, Qu H, Kanomi R, Yamasaki KI, Okano T, Yamada S and Shibasaki Y (2001) A clinical and histological evaluation of titanium mini-implants as anchors for orthodontic intrusion in the beagle dog. *Am J Orthod Dentofacial Orthop* 119, 489–497.

Omnell ML and Sheller B (1994) Maxillary protraction to intentionally ankylosed deciduous canines in a patient with cleft palate. *Am J Orthod Dentofacial Orthop* 106, 201–205.

Ong MM and Wang HL (2002) Periodontic and orthodontic treatment in adults. *Am J Orthod Dentofacial Orthop* 122, 420–428.

Ottofy L (1923) *Standard Dental Dictionary*. Chicago, IL: Laird and Lee.

Papadopoulos MA and Tarawneh F (2007) The use of miniscrew implants for temporary skeletal anchorage in orthodontics: a comprehensive review. *Oral Surg Oral Med Oral Pathol Oral Radiol Endod* 103, e6–15.

Park HS, Bae SM, Kyung HM and Sung JH (2001) Micro-implant anchorage for treatment of skeletal Class I bialveolar protrusion. *J Clin Orthod* 35, 417–422.

Parker WS, Frishe HE and Grant TS (1964) The experimental production of dental ankylosis. *Angle Orthod* 34, 103–107.

Pavlick CT Jr (1998) Cervical headgear usage and the bioprogressive orthodontic philosophy. *Semin Orthod* 4, 219–230.

Proffit WR, Fields HW, Larson BE and Sarver DM (2019) The biologic basis of orthodontic therapy. In *Contemporary Orthodontics*. St. Louis, Mo: Elsevier/Mosby.

Proffit WR, Fields HW (2000) The biologic basis of orthodontic therapy. In *Contemporary Orthodontics*. St Louis: Mosby. Page 305

Quinn RS and Yoshikawa DK (1985) A reassessment of force magnitude in orthodontics. *Am J Orthod* 88, 252–260.

Ramírez-Ossa DM, Escobar-Correa N, Ramírez-Bustamante MA and Agudelo-Suárez AA (2020) An umbrella review of the effectiveness of temporary anchorage devices and the factors that contribute to their success or failure. *J Evid Based Dent Pract* Epub Jan 29EPub.

Reitan K (1967) Clinical and histologic observations on tooth movement during and after orthodontic treatment. *Am J Orthod* 53, 721–745.

Ren Y, Maltha JC and Kuijpers-Jagtman AM (2003) Optimum force magnitude for orthodontic tooth movement: a systematic literature review. *Angle Orthod* 73, 86–92.

Ricketts RM (1976a) Bioprogressive therapy as an answer to orthodontic needs. Part I. *Am J Orthod* 70, 241–268.

Ricketts RM (1976b) Bioprogressive therapy as an answer to orthodontic needs. Part II. *Am J Orthod* 70, 359–397.

Ricketts RM (1980) *Bioprogressive Therapy*. Denver, CO: Rocky Mountain Orthodontics.

Roberts WE, Helm FR, Marshall KJ and Gongloff RK (1989) Rigid endosseous implants for orthodontic and orthopedic anchorage. *Angle Orthod* 59, 247–256.

Roberts WE, Marshall KJ and Mozsary PG (1990) Rigid endosseous implant utilized as anchorage to protract molars and close an atrophic extraction site. *Angle Orthod* 60, 135–152.

Sakoh J, Wahlmann U, Stender E, Nat R, Al-Nawas B and Wagner W (2006) Primary stability of a conical implant and a hybrid, cylindric screw-type implant in vitro. *Int J Oral Maxillofac Implants* 21, 560–566.

Sherwood KH, Burch JG and Thompson WJ (2002) Closing anterior open bites by intruding molars with titanium miniplate anchorage. *Am J Orthod Dentofacial Orthop* 122, 593–600.

Shroff B, Siegel SM, Feldman S and Siegel SC (1996) Combined orthodontic and prosthetic therapy. Special considerations. *Dent Clin North Am* 40, 911–943.

Spyropoulos MN (1985) An early approach for the interception of skeletal open bite: a preliminary report. *J Pedod* 9, 200–209.

Sugawara J (1999) Dr. Junji Sugawara on the skeletal anchorage system. Interview by Dr. Larry W. White. *J Clin Orthod* 33, 689–696.

Sugawara J, Baik UB, Umemori M, Takahashi I, Nagasaka H, Kawamura H and Mitani H (2002) Treatment and posttreatment dentoalveolar changes following intrusion of mandibular molars with application of a skeletal anchorage system (SAS) for open bite correction. *Int J Adult Orthod Orthog Surg* 17, 243–253.

Sugawara J and Nishimura M (2005) Minibone plates: the skeletal anchorage system. *Semin Orthod* 11, 47–56.

Taner TU, Yukay F, Pehlivanoglu M and Cakirer B (2003) A comparative analysis of maxillary tooth movement produced by cervical headgear and pend-x appliance. *Angle Orthod* 73, 686–691.

Thilander B, Nyman S, Karring T and Magnusson I (1983) Bone regeneration in alveolar bone dehiscences related to orthodontic tooth movements. *Eur J Orthod* 5, 105–114.

Thorstenson GA and Kusy RP (2002) Effect of archwire size and material on the resistance to sliding of self-ligating brackets with second-order angulation in the dry state. *Am J Orthod Dentofacial Orthop* 122, 295–305.

Triaca A, Antonini M, Minoretti R, and Merz B (2001) Segmental distraction osteogenesis of the anterior alveolar process. *J Oral Maxillofac Surg*. Jan; 59(1), 26–34

Trisi P and Rebaudi A (2002) Progressive bone adaptation of titanium implants during and after orthodontic load in humans. *Int J Periodontics Restorative Dent* Feb; 22(1), 31–43

Tweed CH (1966) *Clinical Orthodontics*. St Louis, MO: Mosby.

Van Leeuwen EJ, Maltha JC, and Kuijpers-Jagtman AM. (1999) Tooth movements es with light continuous and discontinuous forces in beagle dogs. *Eur J Oral Sci* 107, 468–474.

Umemori M, Sugawara J, Mitani H, Nagasaka H, and Kawamura (1999) Skeletal anchorage system for open-bite correction. *Am J Orthod Dentofacial Orthop*. Feb; 115(2), 166–74.

Wehrbein H (1994) Endosseous titanium implants as orthodontic anchorage elements. Experimental studies and clinical application. *Fortschr Kieferorthop*. Oct; 55(5), 236–50.

Wehrbein H, Glatzmaier J, Mundwiller U and Diedrich P (1996) The Orthosystem—a new implant sytem for anchorage in the palate. *J Orofac Orthop* Jun; 57(3), 142–53

Wehrbein H, Glatzmaier J and Yildirim M (1997) Orthodontic anchorage capacity of short titanium screw implants in the maxilla. An experimental study in the dog. *Clin Oral Implants Res* Apr;8(2), 131–141.

Wehrbein H and Göllner P (2009) Do palatal implants remain positionally stable under orthodontic load? A clinical radiologic study. *Am J Orthod Dentofacial Orthop* Nov;136(5), 695–699.

Wehrbein H, Merz BR, Hämmerle CH and Lang NP (1998) Bone-to-implant contact of orthodontic implants in humans subjected to horizontal loading. *Clin Oral Implants Res* Oct;9(5), 348–353.

Weinberger BW (1926) *Orthodontics A historical review of its originand evolution*. St Louis, MO: Mosby.

Wilmes B (2008) Fields of application of mini-implants. In Ludwig B, Baumgaertel S and Bowman J (eds) *Innovative Anchorage Concepts. Mini-Implants in Orthodontics*. Berlin, New York: Quintessenz.

Wilmes B et al (2015) Mini-implant-anchored Mesialslider for simultaneous mesialisation and intrusion of upper molars in an anterior open bite case: a three-year follow-up. *Aust Orthod J* 31(1), 87–97.

Wilmes B and Drescher D (2008) A miniscrew system with interchangeable abutments. *J Clin Orthod* 42, 574–580;quiz 595.

Wilmes B, Drescher D and Nienkemper M (2009) A miniplate system for improved stability of skeletal anchorage. *J Clin Orthod* 43, 494–501.

Wilmes B, Nanda R, Nienkemper M, Ludwig B and Drescher D (2013) Correction of upper-arch asymmetries using the Mesial-Distalslider. *J Clin Orthod* 47, 648–655.

Wilmes B, Nienkemper M and Drescher D (2010) Application and effectiveness of a mini-implant- and tooth-borne rapid palatal expansion device: the hybrid hyrax. *World J Orthod* 11, 323–330.

9

Bonding Problems Related to Adult Reconstructed Dentitions

Vittorio Cacciafesta

Introduction

Aesthetics have become increasingly crucial when it comes to determining the success of dental treatment, and in recent years, the demand for a better look has grown exponentially. The number of adults seeking orthodontic care increased from 14% to 27% between 2010 and 2014, based on a survey conducted by the American Association of Orthodontists back in 2015, meaning that the number of orthodontic adult patients has almost doubled in 4 years and likely to continue growing as time passes (Alzainal et al. 2020). In clinical practice, management of adults may be somewhat different than for most adolescents. Adults are more likely than adolescents to have dentitions that have undergone some degree of mutilation over time, which may necessitate alterations in the treatment strategy and bonding procedure. Excessive wear and missing, compromised, and restored teeth are some of the differences observed. Contemporary fixed appliances are mostly variations of the edgewise appliance system developed by Angle in 1928. They consist of an archwire that is inserted into the slots of the brackets which are generally bonded directly or indirectly to the teeth or soldered to steel bands. Usually, brackets have a rectangular slot which can engage either round or rectangular archwires. The only current fixed appliance which does not use rectangular archwires in a rectangular slot is the Begg appliance, which is closer to the ribbon-arch appliance. With the advent of the acid-etching technique and different adhesives, orthodontic bonding procedure began to change (Buonocore 1955). Today many adhesive systems, types of labial and lingual brackets, light-curing devices and digital indirect procedures are currently available on the market and it is difficult for the practising orthodontist to stay properly oriented. However, some important factors make the bonding of brackets efficient and trouble-free. In the contemporary straight-wire appliances, the first-order (or in–out) bends, the second-order (or tip) bends, and the third-order (or torque) bends are built into the base of the bracket itself with the goal of minimising the number of actual bends in the archwire (Andrews 1989). While the appliance's slot will accommodate virtually any size or configuration of archwire, the proper selection and progression of archwires are most important in ensuring excellence in treatment results. Different brackets or tubes are made for each tooth, and various prescriptions are available to suit individual preferences, thus making the chairside clinical management considerably easier.

An ideal outcome of bracket bonding to any surface should result in an attachment that is strong enough to endure the forces of orthodontic treatment and mastication without dislodgement, while at the same time be safe enough to avoid damage to the surface during debonding following

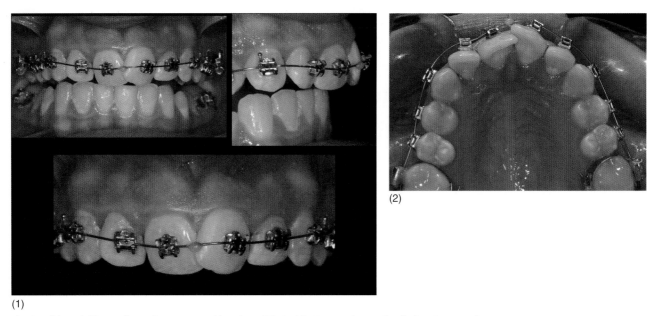

(2)

(1)

Fig. 9.1 (1) and (2) Bonding of upper metal brackets (BioQuick, Forestadent, Pforzheim, Germany).

the end of the treatment. The desired tensile bond strength of metal brackets to tooth structure required to carry out orthodontic treatment is said to be approximately 6–8 MPa (Reynolds 1975). Therefore, the bond strength of brackets to the surface should not exceed the upper limit. This can be a challenging task if the bracket is to be placed on the surface of restorative material.

Brackets

Bonded brackets became available in the mid-1970s. They have several advantages over conventional bands (Graber and Vanarsdall 1994):

a) They have no interproximal component; thus, no separation is required before bonding.
b) They are easier to be placed, to be repositioned, and to be removed.
c) They can be placed more precisely than bands.
d) They are more aesthetic and more hygienic.
e) They allow interproximal strippings or build-ups already during treatment.
f) They can also be applied to partially erupted or fractured teeth.

Metal brackets

Although less aesthetic than ceramic and polycarbonate brackets, metal appliances still represent the system of choice among full-bonded orthodontic appliances (Alzainal et al. 2020) (Figure 9.1(1),(2)). Bracket bases come in different shapes and forms. The design of the bracket base is a factor that influences bond strength to the attached surface. Their adhesion is based on mechanical retention by means of a mesh base or with grooves/undercuts (Figure 9.2(1)–(3)). It is

difficult to determine which base design is superior, as certain base designs performed particularly well with certain cements, but not as well with others (Knox et al. 2000). Those brackets have low levels of friction between archwire and slot, are more resistant to fracture, easier to debond, do not cause generally damages to enamel during debonding, and accumulate less plaque. However, they present some disadvantages, as corrosion phenomena, that can determine the appearance of black or green spots around the margins of the brackets (Ceen et al. 1980; Maijer et al. 1982). These stains may be due to the type of stainless-steel (SS) alloy used, the bracket base design and construction, particular oral environment, galvanic action, and thermal recycling (Hixson et al. 1982).

Aesthetic brackets

In order to improve the aesthetic appearance of the appliance, three possibilities have been attempted:

- Altering the appearance of or reducing the size of stainless-steel brackets.
- Repositioning the appliance on to the lingual surfaces of the teeth.
- Changing the material from which brackets are made.

Early attempts to coat metal brackets with a tooth-coloured coating were unsuccessful due to failure of the coating to adhere and its translucence. Smaller brackets offer only a limited aesthetic advantage over conventionally sized appliances. Lingual orthodontics satisfies aesthetic criteria by positioning the fixed appliance on the lingual surfaces of the teeth (Figure 9.3(1)–(3)). The same three-dimensional control of crown and root position should be obtained as on the labial surfaces. The principle of a rectangular wire in a rectangular slot remains, but the design of the brackets is quite different from that used when the

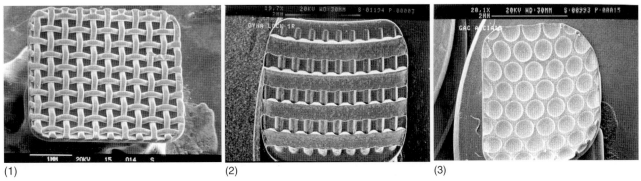

(1)   (2)   (3)

Fig. 9.2 Mechanical retention of metal brackets with (1) a mesh or (2) and (3) grooves/undercuts.

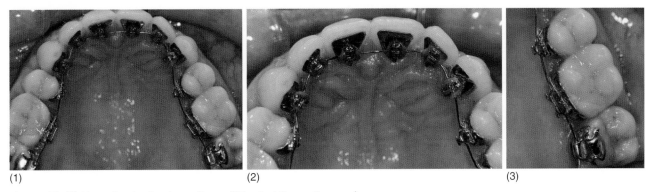

(1)   (2)   (3)

Fig. 9.3 (1)–(3) Lingual orthodontic appliance (Win, Bad Essen, Germany).

attachments are placed on the facial surface of the teeth. The major problem is the small interbracket span between lingual attachments; thus, the use of Ni–Ti wires is recommended for the initial phases of treatment, to reduce the number of appointments and archwire changes.

Polycarbonate brackets

Early attempts to produce brackets of different materials included the use of polycarbonate. These brackets, while aesthetically satisfactory in the early stages of treatment (Figure 9.4), deteriorate in appearance with time, are insufficiently strong to withstand long treatments, or to transmit torque, and lack strength to resist distortion and breakage (Miura et al. 1971; Reynolds 1975). Recently, some manufacturers have produced polycarbonate brackets with metal slots, in order to reduce the friction between archwires and the slot, and allow a better torque transmission, while preserving their aesthetic appeal (Figure 9.5(1),(2)) (Thorstenson et al. 2003). Polycarbonate brackets with metal slots show a lower degree of deformation under torque stress (Sadat-Khonsari et al. 2004). The bracket base shows a chemical retention (Figure 9.6).

Ceramic brackets

In 1986, ceramic brackets became available (Figure 9.7). The ceramic material used in almost all orthodontic brackets is alumina, either in its polycrystalline (Figure 9.8) or monocrystalline form. In theory, monocrystalline form should offer greater strength, which is true until the bracket

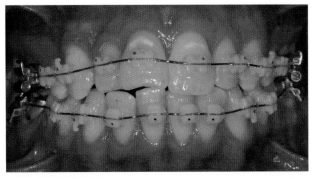

Fig. 9.4 Full-bonded polycarbonate brackets (Brillant, Forestadent, Pforzheim, Germany).

surface is scratched; at that point, the small surface crack tends to spread, and fracture resistance is reduced to or below the level of the polycrystalline form (Flores et al. 1990). The need to be able to use a material with aesthetic characteristics of ceramic and mechanical properties of the metallic brackets has led clinical and industrial research towards the realisation of zirconium brackets; these brackets show some interesting aesthetic and biomechanical qualities, such as hardness, resistance to abrasion, resistance to compression, reduced coefficient of friction during mechanical sliding, stability in a humid temperature and to the aggression of oral fluids (Condo et al. 2005). Ceramic brackets bond to enamel by indentations and/or undercuts in the base (mechanical retention) (Figure 9.9) and chemical bonding with a silane-coupling agent (Figure 9.10).

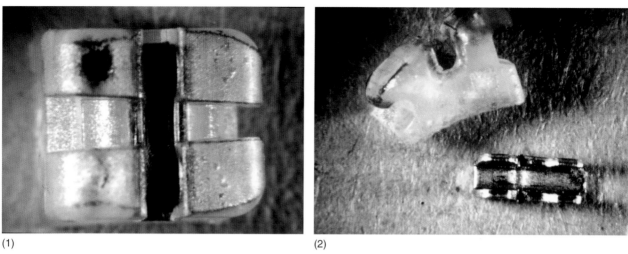

(1)   (2)

Fig. 9.5 (1) and (2) Polycarbonate brackets with metal slot (Spirit, Ormco, Glendora, California).

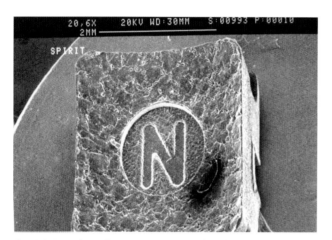

Fig. 9.6 Scanning electron microscope (SEM) of polycarbonate bracket base with chemical retention (Spirit, Ormco, Glendora, California).

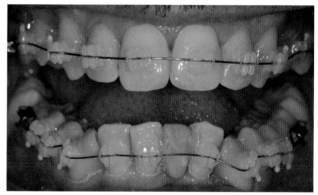

Fig. 9.7 Full-bonded ceramic brackets (Clarity Advanced, Unitek/3 M, Monrovia, California).

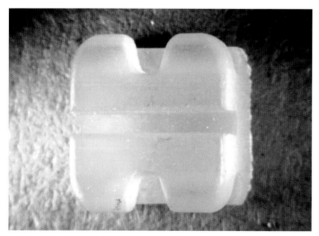

Fig. 9.8 Polycrystalline ceramic bracket (Transcend 6000, Unitek/3 M, Monrovia, California).

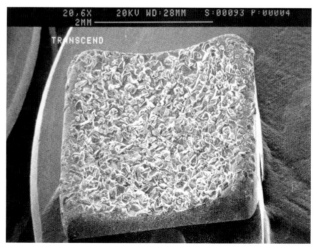

Fig. 9.9 Mechanical retention of a ceramic bracket base.

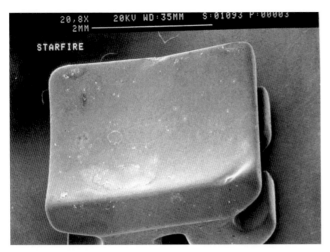

Fig. 9.10 Chemical retention of a ceramic bracket base.

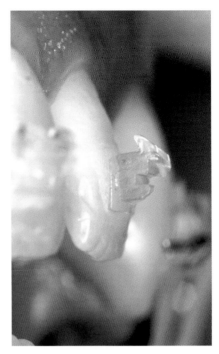

Fig. 9.11 Fracture of two tie-wings.

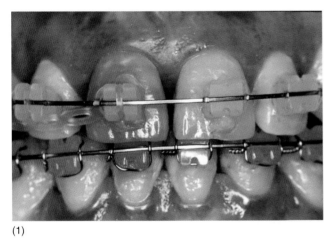

(1)

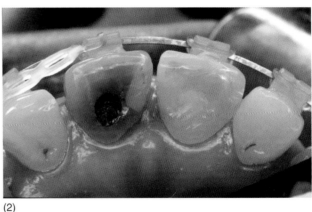

(2)

Fig. 9.12 (1) and (2) Enamel wear of maxillary incisors after occlusal contacts with opposing lower ceramic brackets.

Mechanical bonding is one way to make debonding of these attachments easier and safer. No-mix adhesives are not recommended for these types of attachments; most clinicians prefer light-cured adhesives (Odegaard et al. 1990; Swartz 1988). The advantage of using alumina for orthodontic brackets is that its appearance is very good, its chemical resistance is excellent, and it is both hard and, in certain respect, very strong. The disadvantages are that it lacks ductility, and is difficult and expensive to manufacture (Swartz 1988). The mechanical properties of ceramic brackets which give rise to potential clinical problems are low fracture toughness, lack of ductility and hardness. The low fracture toughness leads to a higher rate of bracket breakage than with stainless-steel brackets. Under stress,

metal brackets begin to deform under lower loads than those at which ceramic brackets fail, but the ceramic brackets break catastrophically at the point of failure, with no plastic deformation. Placement of additional torque in the archwires may cause tie-wing fractures (Scott 1988; Holt et al. 1991; Johnson et al. 2005) (Figure 9.11). When an archwire is ligated into position, tensile forces are placed under the tie-wing, one of the most common areas of ceramic bracket fracture. For this reason, it may be necessary to use torquing auxiliaries to complete the final positioning of incisor teeth when ceramic brackets are employed. Ceramic brackets are much harder than enamel and can abrade enamel rapidly if occlusal interferences are present (Swartz 1988; Viazis 1989) (Figure 9.12(1),(2)).

This risk is largely avoided if ceramic brackets are placed only on the upper arch and steel brackets on the lower arch; most patients accept this arrangement, which in most circumstances is preferred. Moreover, ceramic brackets produce more friction than stainless-steel brackets between orthodontic wire and slot, so it is difficult to determine optimal force levels and anchorage control (Angolkar et al. 1990; Kusy et al. 1990; Pratten et al. 1990). The surface is more porous and rough than that of steel brackets (Figure 9.13). Despite the smoother surface of the monocrystalline bracket, frictional resistance is similar to that of polycrystalline brackets. The bracket surface can abrade relatively the surface of the wire, especially beta-titanium wires, so that small pieces of the wire are pulled out and adhere to the bracket, explaining the high resistance to sliding (Angolkar et al. 1990). In decreasing order, the beta-titanium wires show the highest statistically significant frictional force value, followed by the nickel–titanium and the stainless-steel archwires. The static and kinetic frictional force values are directly proportional to the angulation increase between the bracket and the wire, and to the wire size (Cacciafesta et al. 2003; Nishio et al. 2004). More recently, ceramic brackets with metal slots have been introduced on the market (Figure 9.14(1),(2)). This new design should reduce friction during sliding mechanics (Thorstenson and Kusy 2003). Another disadvantage of ceramic brackets is the risk of wing fractures and enamel damage during debonding. The very high bond strength can cause enamel cracks when removing those brackets at the end of treatment (Winchester 1991; Jeiroudi 1991; Alzainal et al. 2020; Ferreira FG et Al, 2020) (Figure 9.15). Most of the brackets, debonded with pliers recommended by the manufacturers, failed at the bracket–adhesive interface; therefore, the safest method to remove ceramic brackets without the chance of enamel damage is to use the debonding technique specifically designed for each type (Theodorakopoulou et al. 2004; Ferreira et al.

2020). New Clarity brackets can be safely removed by collapsing the bracket in the middle part (Figure 9.16(1)–(4)). However, most clinicians still prefer the metal attachments for routine applications (Alzainal et al. 2020).

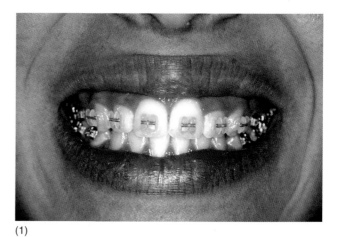

(1)

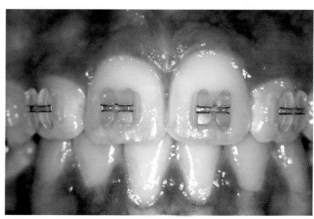

(2)

Fig. 9.14 (1) and (2) Ceramic brackets with metal slots (Clarity, Unitek/3 M, Monrovia, California).

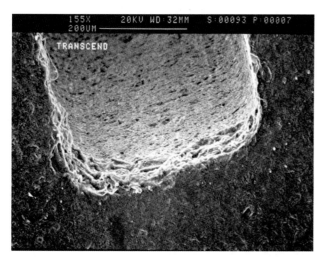

Fig. 9.13 SEM of the slot surface of a ceramic bracket.

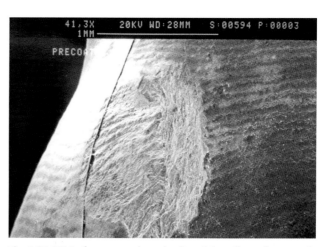

Fig. 9.15 SEM of an enamel crack after debonding of a ceramic bracket.

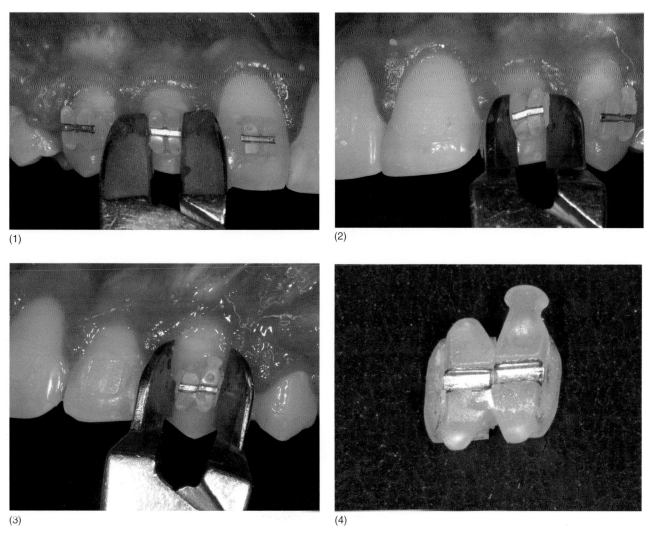

(1)   (2)

(3)   (4)

Fig. 9.16 (1)–(4) Debonding procedure with Clarity brackets; note that the bracket collapses in the middle part of the slot.

Self-ligating brackets

Although the first self-ligating bracket, the Russell attachment, was developed in the early 1930s (Stolzenberg 1935), the concept of self-ligating brackets fell more or less into obscurity until the early 1970s. During the last years, a lot of self-ligating systems have been introduced, including Edgelock (Wildman et al. 1972), Mobil-Lock, SPEED (Hanson 1994) (Figure 9.17), Activa (Figure 9.18), Damon SL II (Figure 9.19) and SL III (Damon 1998), Time (Heiser 1998), SmartClip (Figure 9.20) and BioQuick (Figure 9.21(1),(2)). These brackets are different in shape and function, but each, whether active or passive, uses the movable fourth wall (for example, a solid sliding cover or flexible spring clip or rigid arm or solid labial slider) of the bracket to convert the slot into a tube, thus eliminating the need for stainless-steel or elastomeric ligatures. Many studies have demonstrated a decrease in friction for these attachments, compared to conventional brackets (Read-Ward et al. 1997; Pizzoni et al. 1998; Cacciafesta et al. 2003).

However, less frictional resistance to sliding is a disadvantage for frictionless space closure; these attachments may not hold a wire in place well to prevent tipping when closing gaps. Self-ligating appliances permit the use of lighter forces, allow efficient initial alignment, require fewer instruments during archwire changes, save significant chair time in changing archwires (approximately 3–4 minutes per archwire change) and reduce significantly the risk of percutaneous injury to the index finger or thumb during archwire changes by orthodontists or orthodontic assistants or hygienists (Maijer et al. 1990; Forsberg et al. 1991; Bagramian et al. 1998; McNamara et al. 1999). However, based on current clinical evidence obtained from randomized clinical trials (RCTs), self-ligating brackets (SLBs) do not show clinical superiority compared to conventional brackets (CBs) in expanding transversal dimensions, space closure or orthodontic efficiency. Further high-level studies involving randomised, controlled, clinical trials are warranted to confirm these results (Dehbi H et al. 2017; Yang et al. 2018). Recently,

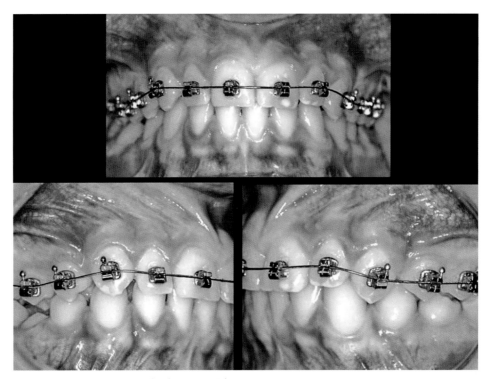

Fig. 9.17 SPEED brackets (Strite Industries, Cambridge, Ontario).

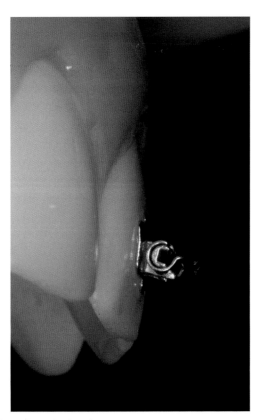

Fig. 9.18 Activa bracket.

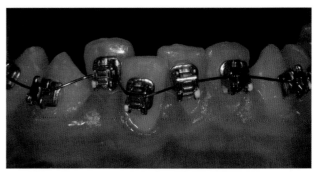

Fig. 9.19 Damon II brackets (Ormco, Glendora, California).

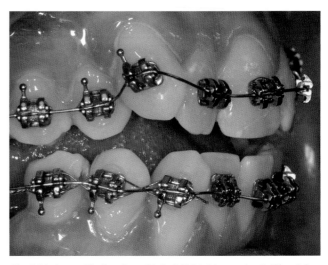

Fig. 9.20 SmartClip brackets (Unitek/3 M, Monrovia, California).

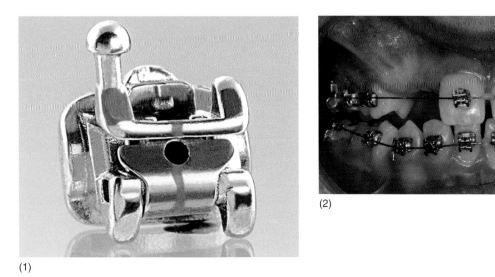

(1)

(2)

Fig. 9.21 (1) and (2) BioQuick brackets (Forestadent, Pforzheim, Germany).

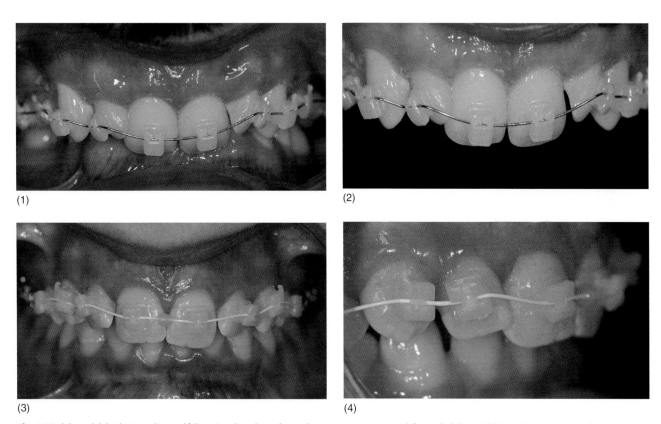

(1)

(2)

(3)

(4)

Fig. 9.22 (1) and (2) Clarity ultra self-ligating brackets (Unitek/3 M, Monrovia, California). (3) and (4) TruKlear brackets (Forestadent, Pforzheim, Germany).

ceramic self-ligating brackets have been introduced (Figure 9.22(1)–(4)).

The Basis of the Bonding Clinical Procedure

Successful bonding requires careful attention to three essential components: the tooth surface and its preparation, the design of the bracket base and the bonding agent. The

concepts related to bonding to enamel of adults as well as the variations in bonding required for gold crowns, porcelain crowns and resin or plastic materials utilised in dentistry are essential. The goal of tooth preparation is to create an optimum surface to attach brackets to the teeth utilising bonding materials. Well-bonded brackets remain in place despite everyday chewing and functioning. Broken brackets lead to clinical inefficiency, emergencies which negatively affect the schedule, as well as inconveniences to patients and parents. The aim of preparing teeth for bonding is to create a material surface which will couple chemically with bonding materials that are placed on the bracket bases. The common element in the composite materials used to adhere brackets to teeth is made of a resin chemical structure. This resin is present in the bracket-bonding composite and also in the unfilled resin known as the bonding agent, primer or bonding resin. Another goal is to create a thin surface layer of bonded resin on the tooth that is tightly bound and sealed. This can be achieved by pressing the bracket gently against the tooth to allow excess material to be extruded. This layer of material will in turn chemically bond to the material that is applied to the orthodontic bracket, since it is made of the same or a similar material. No matter whether the tooth surface is composed of gold, porcelain, plastic or enamel, the goal is the same, to end with a surface layer of bonding resin that will bond chemically to the material placed on the back of the bracket. The steps involved for an optimal performance in bonding of orthodontic attachments (on facial or lingual surfaces) are as follows:

- Cleaning.
- Enamel conditioning.
- Sealing.
- Bonding.
- Light curing (if necessary).

Armamentarium

A list of typical materials and instruments is presented. Different clinicians will vary their procedures and can subtract or add additional materials they find helpful in successful bonding:

1. Prophy paste and pumice without fluoride.
2. Prophy angle and slow-speed handpiece.
3. High-speed drill (when indicated for surface preparation).
4. Microetcher.
5. High-speed evacuation and tip.
6. Air–water syringe and tip
7. Mouth mirror.
8. Scaler or explorer.
9. Cheek retractors with tongue guard and saliva ejector assembly.
10. Bonding gauges.
11. Short and long cotton rolls.
12. Dry angles.
13. Individual brushes/applicators.
14. Liquid wells or disposable sheets for dispensing agents.
15. Acid etchant in syringe.
16. Bonding agent/primers.
17. Additional etchants and primers for bonding to dental restorations.

Cleaning

Before bonding brackets, it is essential to remove the organic pellicle that normally covers all teeth (Aboush et al. 1991). This is accomplished by cleaning the enamel surface using a mix of pumice and water, or prophylaxis paste, with a rubber cup or a polishing brush mounted on a low-speed rotary instrument (Figure 9.23(1)). The tooth is subsequently rinsed with water to remove any pumice debris, thoroughly dried with a stream of oil-free air. During this procedure, cheek and lip retractors, saliva ejectors and cotton or gauze rolls should be used (Figure 9.23(2)). Cheek retractors are available from a number of manufactures to retract the lips and cheeks. Retractors can free the hands from continually

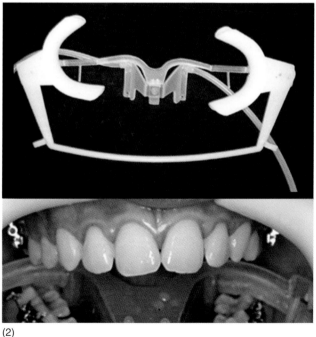

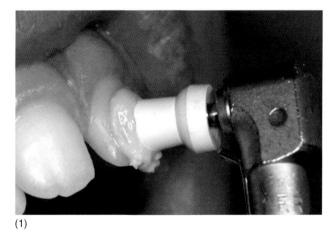

(1)   (2)

Fig. 9.23 (1) and (2) Initial prophylaxis with pumice.

holding a mirror to retract the cheek or lip. Some retractors are designed as scaled for the size of the patient and include optional tongue guards as well as saliva-ejection tubing. Dry angles can also assist with moisture control from the parotid salivary ducts. Auxiliary saliva ejectors can prove helpful for patients with excessive saliva production. High-speed evacuation is recommended to suction the majority of the saliva from the oral cavity as well as to remove etchant and water spray. To reduce etchant from dispersing throughout the mouth, first suction excess etchant and then rinse/suction.

Both in vitro (Lindauer et al. 1997) and clinical studies (Barry 1995; Ireland and Sherriff 2002) have demonstrated that prior pumicing of enamel has no significant effect on either bond strengths or failure rate of composites and glass ionomers. Thus, if there is a need to increase the bond strengths, it is recommended to use the microetcher with 50 μm aluminium oxide powder (sandblaster) on the enamel surface for 3 seconds (Alzainal et al. 2020) (Figure 9.24(1),(2)).

Enamel conditioning

The idea of using phosphoric acid on dental surfaces was first introduced by Buonocore (1955), who observed that adhesion to metal surfaces by paints improved when acids were used to etch the metal surface increasing the strength of the bond. An unprepared enamel surface is a poor surface to bond mechanically or chemically which leads to poor adherence of the brackets. Placing an acid on the enamel surface changes the surface of the enamel by dissolving some of the calcium salts increasing the number and size of microscopic depressions. The liquid resin found in orthodontic bonding agents penetrates into the depressions and over the projections left from the etching process. Once the bonding agent is cured typically with a light-curing unit, these finger-like projections of resin are tightly bound to the enamel surface. The surface of the enamel is now covered with a thin resin which chemically bonds to the more viscous (thicker) composite bonding materials placed on the back of the brackets. Since the mechanical lock of the resin

into the enamel is critical, proper preparation and protection of this prepared enamel surface are critical to successful bonding of brackets.

After moisture control, it is necessary to keep a completely dry working field (Figure 9.23(2)) and to create irregularities on the enamel surface. This is accomplished by covering the entire enamel surface with orthophosphoric acid for about 15–30 seconds (Alzainal et al. 2020) (Figure 9.25(1)). Longer etching periods provide no more but actually less retention because of the loss of surface structure. As the acid remains in contact with the tooth beyond the optimum time, more calcium salts are dissolved which end up filling the crevices with additional debris, thus reducing the places the liquid resin can flow into and shortening the resin tags which give the bond strength. For increasing the simplicity of etching procedure, acid gels should be preferable to acid solutions; gels provide better control for restricting the working field to avoid insulting the gingival margin and initiating bleeding, although there is no apparent difference in the degree of surface irregularity (Brannstrom et al. 1989). A small amount of the softer interprismatic enamel is removed and pores are opened up between the enamel prisms, so that the adhesive can penetrate into the tooth surface (Figure 9.25(2),(3)). The enamel surface must not be contaminated with saliva, which promotes immediate remineralisation, until bonding is completed; otherwise, reetching is required (Zachrisson 1985). After rinsing again the enamel in order to completely remove the etching, the tooth surface must be dried with a moisture-and-oil-free source to obtain uniform and frosty white appearance (Figure 9.25(4)). Recent advances indicate that microetching is also essential for successful treatment (Alzainal et al. 2020) (Figure 9.24(1),(2)). If gums are bleeding after the microetching procedure, it is advised to cover the bleeding gums with some protective light-curing fast dam to prevent any blood contamination of the enamel, and then complete the bonding (Figure 9.26(1)–(4)). A recent study has demonstrated that Er:YAG and Er,Cr:YSGG laser etching resulted in clinically acceptable shear bond strength (SBS);

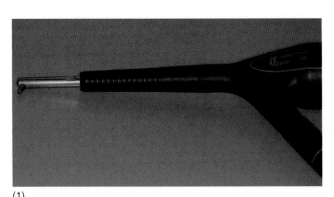

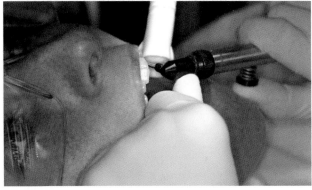

(1)   (2)

Fig. 9.24 (1) and (2) Use of sandblaster.

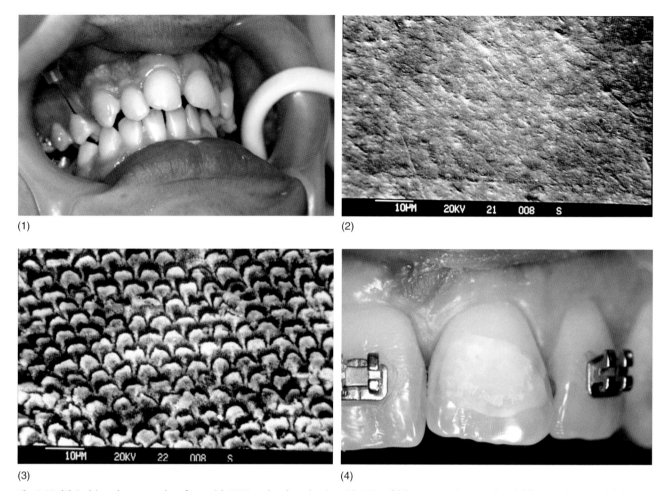

(1)　　　　　　　　　　　　　(2)

(3)　　　　　　　　　　　　　(4)

Fig. 9.25 (1) Etching the enamel surface with 37% orthophosphoric acid. SEM of (2) untreated enamel and (3) etched enamel. (4) Note the frosty appearance of etched enamel.

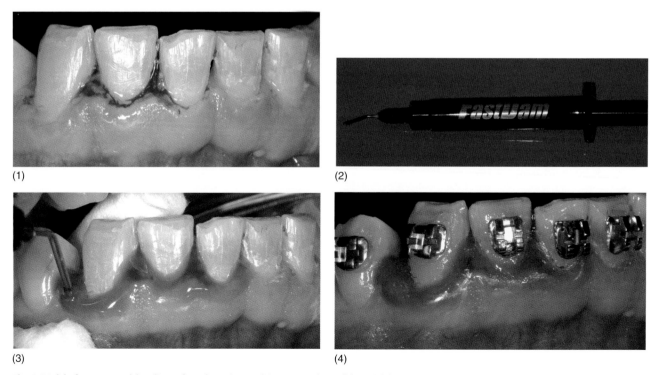

(1)　　　　　　　　　　　　　(2)

(3)　　　　　　　　　　　　　(4)

Fig. 9.26 (1) If gums are bleeding after the microetching procedure, (2) and (3) it is advised to cover the bleeding gums with some protective light-curing fast dam to prevent any blood contamination of the enamel, and (4) then complete the bonding (4).

therefore, apart from its other advantages over acid etching, it can be a good appropriate alternative for bonding of orthodontic brackets (Mollabashi et al. 2019).

Tooth bleaching with carbamide peroxide decreases the bond strengths, especially if the bracket bonding is performed shortly after bleaching (Azizi F et al. 2020).

Phosphoric acid precautions and patient safety

Phosphoric acid etchants are the moderate-strength acids. Etchant dangers should be understood by all dental staff members who use these materials as well as the precautions and means by which to mitigate the effects to the gums and mucosal tissues.

1. All dental staff should wear gloves when handling these materials.
2. Patient precautions should include methods to isolate skin, oral mucosa, and the eyes from accidental contact with etchant.
3. Avoid contact with the eyes with the use of safety glasses. Avoid passing items over the patient face.
4. The longer the etchant is in contact with tissue, the greater the damage from the acid.
5. Remain vigilant and watchful of where the acid etchant is placed and practise good isolation in the oral cavity to limit contact of the acid etchant with oral mucosa.
6. If the etchant comes in contact with the oral mucosa or the eyes, immediately rinse with water.

Sealing

A liquid resin is then applied with a small foam pellet or brush with a single gingivoincisal stroke on each etched tooth (Figure 9.27(1),(2)). The resin is able to penetrate into the irregularities created in the etched enamel surface, allowing the bonding material to mechanically interlock with the tooth surface. Kilponen L et al. (2019) investigated if primers can be used to modify bonding characteristics of orthodontic metal and ceramic brackets. They found out

that using silane as primer increased the bond strength of ceramic brackets significantly.

Self-etching primers (SEPs), both an etchant and a primer combined into a single product, have recently been introduced to simplify the orthodontic bonding process and to save chairside time during this procedure (Figure 9.28(1)–(6)) (Ajlouni et al. 2004; Bishara et al. 2005b; Bilen and Çokakoğlu S 2020; Ibrahim AI et al. 2020). It is indicated for use only with light-curing direct-bonding orthodontic adhesives. SEPs can be used safely instead of two-step total-etch adhesives during the bonding of metal and ceramic brackets due to less microleakage and adequate SBS values (Bilen and Çokakoğlu 2020; Ibrahim et al. 2020). Farhadian et al. (2019) indicated that although there is no significant difference in bond strength between SEPs and conventional acid etching for bonding orthodontic metal brackets, the amount of residual adhesive on the enamel surface is significantly less with SEPs than with conventional acid-etching procedure.

In a study, the mean clinical chairside time required for bracket bonding and the mean bond failure rate at 6 and 12 months of stainless-steel brackets bonded with a light-cured composite using a SEP or a two-stage etch and primer system were compared. The mean bracket-bonding time with the SEP per patient was significantly shorter than that of the two-stage bonding system (P < 0.001). The difference between the overall bond failure rate and the mean bond failure rate per patient for the two bonding systems was neither statistically nor clinically significant at 6 and 12 months (Aljubouri et al. 2004). Furthermore, with the self-etching primer, the median enamel loss is significantly lower than the conventional two-stage etching and priming process, such as adhesive remaining on the enamel after debonding. SEM observations show that the non-rinse conditioner produces a more conservative bonding pattern than conventional phosphoric acid (Hosein et al. 2004; Vicente et al. 2005). Today a new antibacterial and fluoride-releasing bonding system is available; it consists of a self-etching primer that contains an antibacterial monomer and

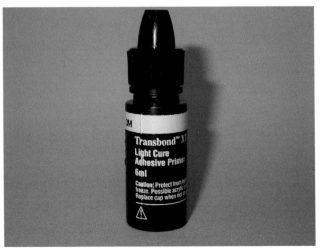

(1)

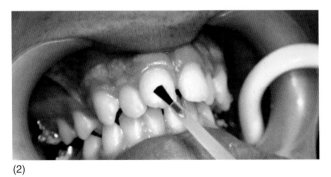

(2)

Fig. 9.27 (1) and (2) Sealing with a liquid primer (Transbond XT, Unitek/3 M, Monrovia, California).

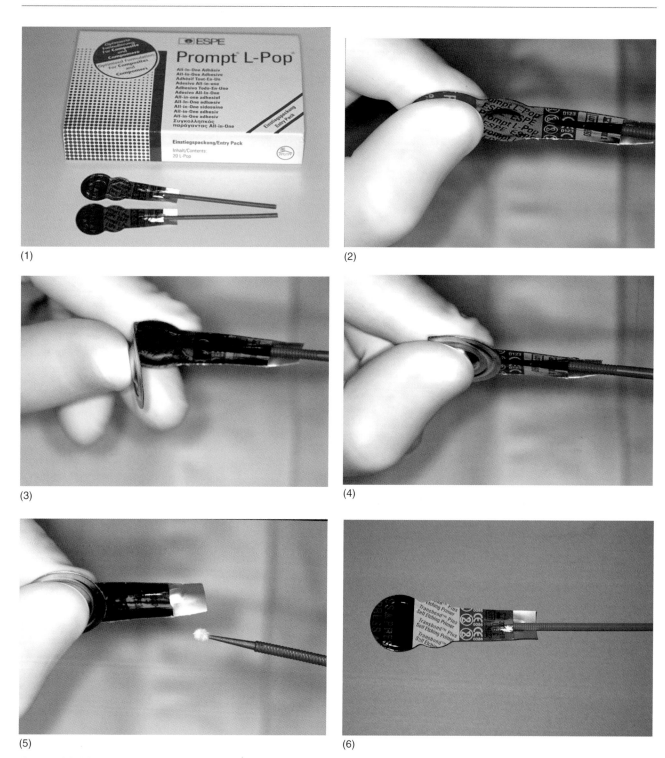

(1)

(2)

(3)

(4)

(5)

(6)

Fig. 9.28 (1)–(6) Use of self-etching primers (SEP).

a bonding agent that contains sodium fluoride (Bishara et al. 2005b). Bond failure is often attributed to moisture contamination and to overcome this problem hydrophilic materials have been developed; moisture-insensitive primers (MIP) are believed to offer better bond strength in moisture-contaminated environment (Figure 9.29)

(Rajagopal et al. 2004). MIP with chemically activated resin produces slightly higher bond strengths compared with the conventional primers under wet conditions (with water and saliva); however, moisture-insensitive primer in combination with light-activated resin produces comparable bond strengths on both the dry and wet etched enamel. The results suggest that moisture-insensitive primer be used only with light-activated composite resins (Grundht et al. 2001). On the other hand, blood contamination of enamel during the bonding procedure of conventional and hydrophilic primers significantly lowers their strength values and might produce a bond strength that is not clinically adequate (Cacciafesta et al. 2004c).

Bonding

After application of a thin layer of liquid resin to the tooth, a small quantity of adhesive is applied to the bracket base, which is then pressed against the enamel in its correct position with the help of gauges to assess its vertical position (Figure 9.30(1)–(4)). Depending on the type of bonding material, it can set either by a self-curing process or by light-curing. An adhesive should have sufficient viscosity, so that the bonded attachments do not drift out of position before the adhesive has set.

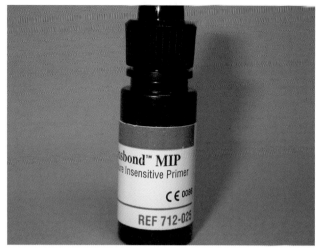

Fig. 9.29 Moisture-insensitive primer (MIP, Unitek/3 M, Monrovia, California).

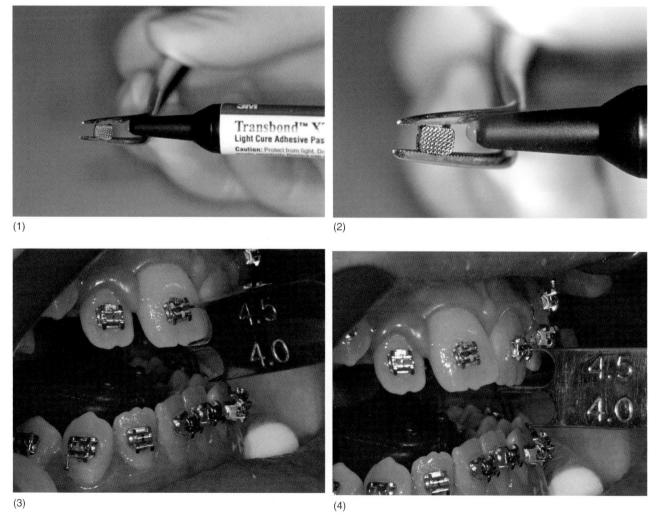

(1)   (2)

(3)   (4)

Fig. 9.30 (1)–(4) Application of the adhesive onto the bracket base and bonding to the tooth with gauges.

At present, there are many different types of adhesives for bonding:

- *Composite resins* (formulated from glass particles and dimethacrylate monomers) (Figure 9.31(1),(2)).

- *Glass ionomer cements or GICs* (supplied as a powder and a liquid that are either mixed by hand or are encapsulated for automatic mixing; the powder is a calcium fluoroaluminosilicate glass and the liquid is typically a solution of a polyacrylic acid copolymer in water).

- *Resin-modified glass ionomer cements or RMGICs* (combination of GICs and composite resins) (Craig 1997) (Figure 9.32(1),(2)).

Comparing the clinical performance of a glass ionomer cement with a composite resin when used for direct bracket bonding, the results demonstrate a significantly lower debonding index for the composite than for the GIC; GIC may be an alternative to composite for use with light archwires and with limited treatments (Oliveira et al. 2004).

On the contrary, the use of flowable composites is not advocated for orthodontic bracket bonding because of significantly lower SBS values achieved (Uysal et al. 2004). GICs have the ability to bond chemically to enamel, cementum, dentine, non-precious metals and plastics (Hotz et al. 1977). The potential advantages of GICs are adhesion in a wet field, a non-etching technique, and the release of fluoride ions over long periods into adjacent enamel. In addition, they have the capability of absorbing fluoride from sources, such as fluoride toothpastes, thus acting as a rechargeable, slow release fluoride device (Hatibovic-Kofman and Koch 1991). The biggest disadvantage of GICs is their weak bond strength, as shown by *in vivo* (Miguel et al. 1995; Miller et al. 1996) and *in vitro* (Rezk-Lega and Ogaard 1991) studies. In order to retain the positive characteristics of GICs, and also to improve bond strength, combinations of GICs and composite resins were developed as RMGICs. Light-cured RMGICs were

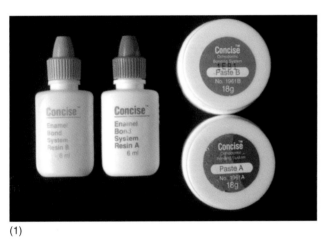

(1)

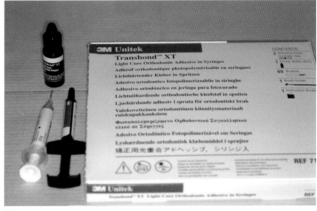

(2)

Fig. 9.31 (1) Self-curing and (2) light-curing composite resins.

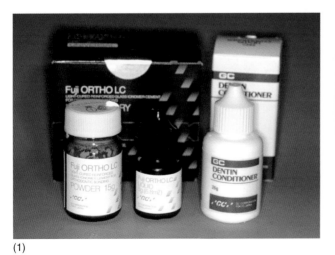

(1)

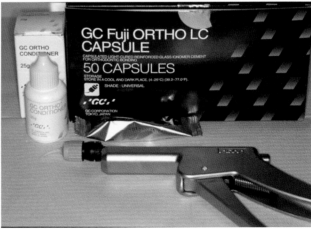

(2)

Fig. 9.32 Light-curing resin-modified glass ionomers as (1) powder/liquid and (2) in capsules.

formulated to overcome the problems of moisture sensitivity of composites and low early mechanical strength of glass ionomers, while maintaining the clinical advantages of conventional GICs. Several studies have reported less enamel demineralisation under orthodontic brackets retained with light-cured RMGICs (Vorhies et al. 1998; Wilson and Donly 2001). The bond strengths of the RMGIC are similar to or somewhat higher than those achieved with light-cured composite resin when lamps with short polymerisation times are used, but are lower when compared with a self-curing composite adhesive; after 24 hours the bond strengths of all adhesives show a significant increase (Wendl et al. 2004).

In an attempt to save chair time during bonding, orthodontists are using ceramic and metal brackets that have been precoated with the adhesive material (Figure 9.33(1),(2)). The adhesive used on the precoated brackets is similar in composition to that used for bonding uncoated brackets. The difference is essentially in the percentages of the various ingredients incorporated in the material. Precoated ceramic brackets that used a slightly modified adhesive have similar shear bond strengths as that provided by adhesive on uncoated brackets; precoated metal brackets that used the same adhesive have significantly lower shear bond strength than those obtained with adhesive on uncoated brackets. The differences in the bond strength between the ceramic and metal brackets are attributed to the combined effects of the changes in the composition of the adhesives used and in the retention mechanisms incorporated in the bracket bases of the different types of brackets. All bracket/adhesive combinations provide clinically acceptable shear bond forces (Bishara et al. 1997; Verstrynge et al. 2004).

The bracket-bonding procedure consists in transfer, positioning, fitting, removal of excess (Figure 9.34(1)–(4)),

and light-curing. When excess adhesive is carefully removed and good oral hygiene is maintained, the gingival condition is not adversely influenced by bonded appliances; on the other hand, when excess adhesive is close to the gingival margin, it will produce periodontal damages (gingival inflammation and hyperplastic gingival changes) and the possibility of decalcifications around the periphery of the bonding base (Zachrisson 1977a).

Indirect bonding

Proper bracket placement is crucial in orthodontic treatment and with a suitable archwire provides the desired mechanical effect. Imprecision in bracket location may lead to unwanted tooth movement: unplanned torque, rotation and vertical issues. The introduction of adhesion was a revolution in orthodontics and facilitated appliance-fixing procedures (Nawrocka and Lukomska-Szymanska 2020). There are two main techniques of bracket placement. Direct bonding is easier, faster (especially if only a few teeth are to be bonded) and less expensive than indirect bonding (IDB) technique. However, indirect bonding is becoming more and more popular nowadays thanks to the use of 3D intraoral scanners, digital set-up softwares and 3D printers (Layman 2019; Nawrocka and Lukomska-Szymanska 2020). Before digital workflows were introduced, the indirect bracket-placement process involved multiple messy and time-consuming steps. Indirect bonding was first described in 1972 by Silverman et al., and then in 1974 by Newman. Stone or resin models were fabricated, brackets were temporarily placed on the models with either a dissolvable material or a composite and a transfer tray was created (usually a quick-setting silicone rubber or thermoformed sheet) to transfer the positioning from the study casts to the teeth. All brackets are usually incorporated into the tray and are bonded simultaneously

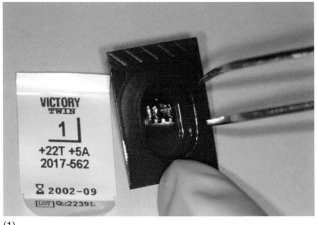 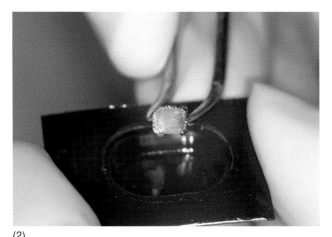

(1)   (2)

Fig. 9.33 (1) and (2) Metal brackets precoated with the adhesive (APC, Unitek/3 M, Monrovia, California).

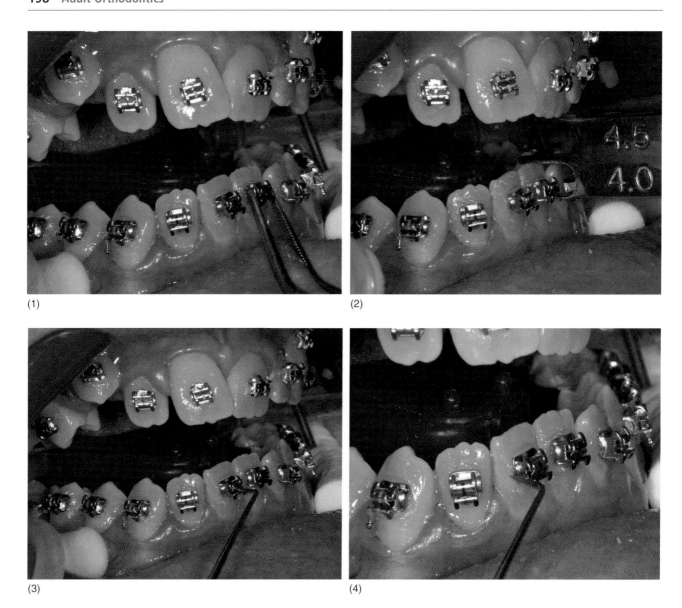

(1)

(2)

(3)

(4)

Fig. 9.34 Bracket-bonding procedure: (1) transfer, (2) positioning and vertical check, (3) fitting, (4) removal of excess.

(Figure 9.35(1)–(7)) (Zachrisson et al. 1978; Aguirre et al. 1982). The transfer tray must be strong and dimensionally accurate, but elastic enough to be placed without difficulty and removed without pulling the brackets off. Several indirect bonding techniques are available; in the past, the two most popular techniques were the silicone impression material and the double sealant. Several studies have reported that, in general, indirect bonding trays lead to higher bracket placement accuracy than the usually used direct bonding techniques (Thomas 1979; Hodge et al. 2004). This is attributed to the fact that in the first stage, the placement of the attachments is completed away from clinical influences and variables that complicate the direct method, such as moisture control, patient management or hurried schedules (Grunheid et al. 2016); however, the placement of the brackets on the dental cast also includes

potential constraints and variables, which can influence the reliability of the transfer to the patient's dentition. Possible influencing factors, which affect final bracket placement error during transfer, can be errors in tray fabrication, contaminants or soft-tissue interferences, bonding thickness, adhesive material between the brackets and teeth during clinical bonding as well as errors in clinical technique. Thus, differences in bracket transfer accuracy as a function of trays and tooth type were already reported (Castilla et al. 2014; Grunheid et al. 2016). Current studies on IDB tray-dependent bracket accuracy focus on vacuum-formed thermoplastic sheets, silicone materials, or a combination of both. Dorfer et al. compared bracket transfer accuracy between three different IDB techniques and found that bracket transfer accuracy was significantly better for trays made of addition silicone than single vacuum-formed trays

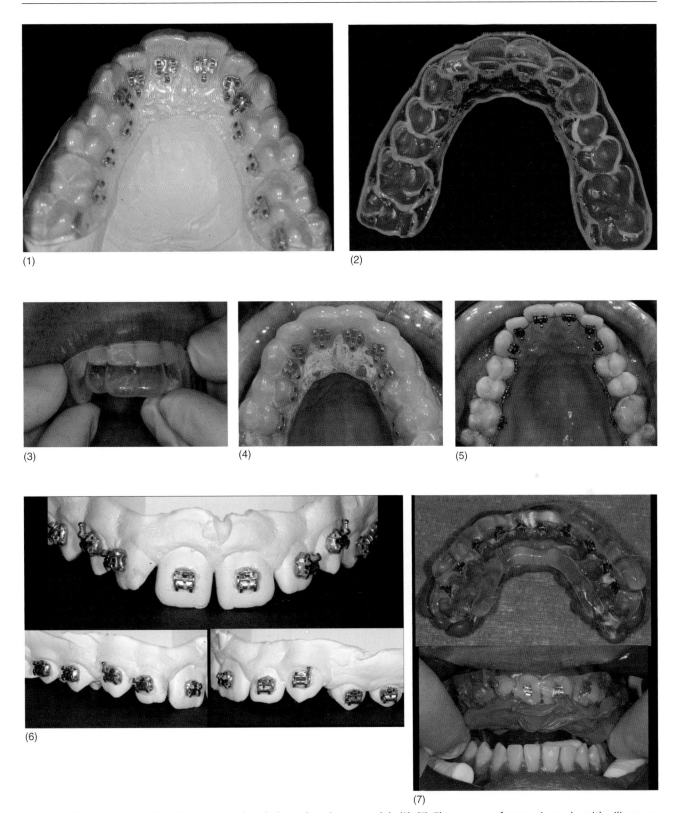

Fig. 9.35 (1) Indirect bonding: brackets are bonded on the plaster model. (2)–(7) Then, a transfer tray is made with silicone or thermoformed sheet, to bond indirectly all the brackets simultaneously.

(Dorfer et al. 2006). Castilla et al. also obtained similar results, wherein five transfer techniques were compared with each other and overall small differences in bracket position were observed; however, the silicone based trays had a highly consistent high transfer bracket accuracy, whereas methods that exclusively used vacuum formed trays were less consistent (Castilla et al. 2014).

Today, softwares can be used to precisely place brackets based on computer-aided measurements, greatly reducing lab time. Not only does this approach improve the daily schedule flow, but it compounds efficiency through increased accuracy, by reducing the number of repositioned brackets and wire bends needed during treatment (Layman 2019). There are no significant differences in shear bond strength of orthodontic brackets bonded to enamel, whether they are bonded with the direct or indirect techniques (Yi et al. 2003; Iglesias A, et al. 2020; Nawrocka and Lukomska-Szymanska 2020). Mean bracket placement errors are similar with both techniques: vertical errors (Figure 9.36(1)) are greater than those in the horizontal plane (Figure 9.36(2)), which in turn are greater than angular errors (Figure 9.36(3)), and errors are greater in the maxillary arch than in the mandibular arch (Hodge et al. 2004). In a recent study, Möhlhenrich et al. (2020) aimed at comparing bracket placement and excess bonding adhesive depending on different indirect bonding techniques and bracket geometries (with and without hooks). The double-PVS (polyvinyl siloxane) group revealed promising results with respect to transfer accuracy. Basically, hooks lead to lower precision and higher excess bonding adhesive. PVS trays for indirect bonding generate high bracket placement accuracy. PVS-putty is the easiest to handle with and also the cheapest, but leads to large excess bonding adhesive, especially in combination with hooked brackets or tubes.

At present, direct bonding is used routinely by most practitioners, but indirect bonding is definitely recommended for special circumstances, particularly for lingual attachments because they are more difficult to be bonded in direct visualisation (Alexander et al. 1982). Modern digital bracket placement for indirect bonding can be easily added to our daily workflow. Progressing from digital placement to conventional chairside delivery as described by Layman (2019), it will translate the treatment-planning data to the patient with minimal loss of detail. Czolgosz et al. (2021) in a randomised controlled trial found out that the clinical chair time was significantly shorter for computer-aided indirect bonding than for direct bonding. However, the total bonding time for computer-aided indirect bonding, including digital bracket placement, was longer than for direct bonding. There were significantly more immediate debondings with computer-aided indirect bonding than with direct bonding. Under these conditions, computer-aided indirect bonding was more expensive than direct bonding.

This computer-aided technique allows the practitioner to benefit from the chairside efficiencies of indirect bonding while drastically reducing lab time. Moreover, the ability to efficiently fabricate indirect bonding trays can expand practice capacity and create a real return on investment for our digital equipment (Layman 2019; Nawrocka and Lukomska-Szymanska 2020).

Light-curing

Different light-curing units are available: conventional halogen light (Figure 9.37(1)), light-emitting diode or LED (Figure 9.37(2),(3)), plasma arc light (Figure 9.37(4),(5)). When evaluating the effect of the light-tip distance (0, 3 and 6 mm) on each light-curing unit, the halogen light shows no significantly different shear bond strengths between the three distances; however, the LED light produces lower shear bond strengths at a greater light-tip distance, and the plasma arc lamp shows higher shear bond strengths at a greater light-tip distance (Cacciafesta et al. 2005b). Plasma arc lights can be considered an advantageous alternative to conventional halogen lights, because they enable the clinician to reduce the curing time of brackets without significantly affecting their bond failure rate (Ip et al. 2004; Neugebauer et al. 2004; Cacciafesta et al. 2004b, c). The new generation of LEDs is able to have similar curing times to plasma arc light with significant advantages in terms of reduced weight, improved portability, and possibility to be used as cordless units.

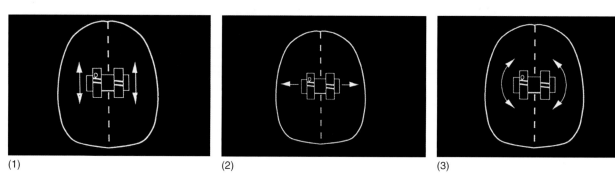

(1) (2) (3)

Fig. 9.36 Possible bonding errors: (1) vertical, (2) horizontal and (3) angular.

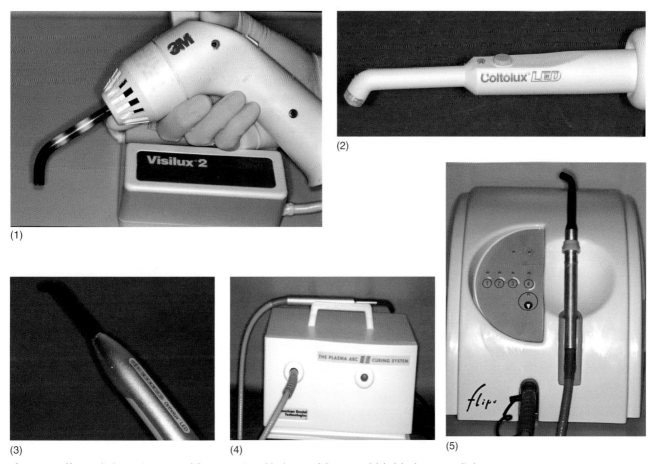

Fig. 9.37 Different light-curing units: (1) conventional halogen, (2) LED and (3)–(5) plasma arc light.

Bonding to crowns and restorations

Today's orthodontic practice includes a larger proportion of adult patients and it is possible that crowns, bridges (porcelain, gold, non-precious metals, etc.) or restorations (amalgam, composite, etc.) may be bonded (Buyukyilmaz et al. 1995; Zachrisson et al. 1995; Sinha et al. 1997; Andreasen et al. 1988; Smith et al. 1988; Alzainal et al. 2020). Recent advances in materials and techniques suggest that bonding of orthodontic attachments to surfaces other than enamel may now be possible. A bracket may be placed on single-unit crown of porcelain or gold, but banding becomes difficult or even impossible; thus, in such cases, bonding rather banding would be preferable. Bonding the bracket to the restoration provides a satisfactory alternative and the orthodontist must use methods that permit the attachment of brackets to porcelain and non-precious metal or gold. Depending on the materials and the technique employed, one can achieve satisfactory bonding. Microetching (for about 3 seconds with 100 μm aluminium oxide powder) is essential for bonding to large amalgams, gold or other non-precious metals; the abrasive particles create a retentive surface to which bonding with highly filled composite is greatly enhanced, at least 300%. A uniform coat of metal primer (Figure 9.38) will set

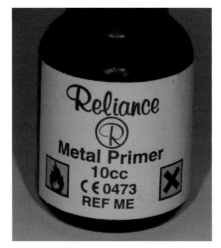

Fig. 9.38 Metal primer (Reliance, Itasca, Illinois).

up a chemical bond between all precious and non-precious metals and any adhesive on the area to be bonded (Gross et al. 1997; Alzainal et al. 2020). The surface characteristics of the amalgam appear to be more influential in the strength of the bond than does the nature of the adhesive (Sperber et al.

1999). With selected conditioners (Figure 9.39(1)), adhesives and pre-treatments of the surfaces (for example, microetching or roughening the surface of old restorations with sandpaper disks or a fine diamond bur), metal or plastic or ceramic brackets also may be bonded to acrylic and composite crowns or build-ups (Borzangy 2019) (Figure 9.39(2)–(5)). For bonding to porcelain surfaces, conventional acid-etching is ineffective for mechanical retention of brackets; the most commonly used etchant is 9.6% hydrofluoric acid (HF) in gel form for 2–4 minutes (Figure 9.40(1)) (Wood et al. 1986; Edris et al. 1990; Alzainal et al. 2020; Tahmasbi et al. 2020). Placement of a rubber dam and a barrier gel on the gingival is suggested; the material is severe tissue-irritant. The hydrofluoric acid will prepare all porcelain surfaces for the application of selected conditioner (Figure 9.40(2)) and adhesive (micro-mechanical bond) (Figure 9.40(3)–(7)). The use of a heavily filled resin adhesive after micro-etching, with the application of hydrofluoric

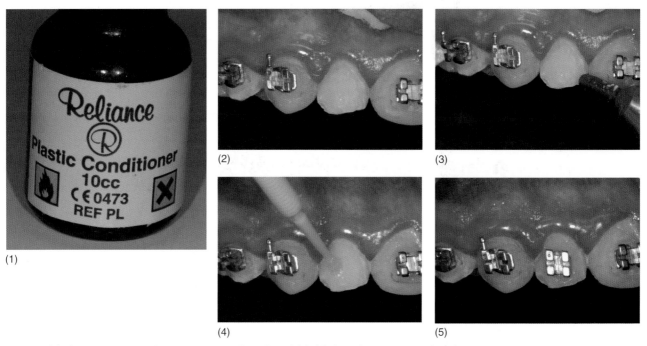

(1)

(2)

(3)

(4)

(5)

Fig. 9.39 (1) Plastic conditioner (Reliance, Itasca, Illinois), and (2)–(5) clinical procedure to bond composite restorations.

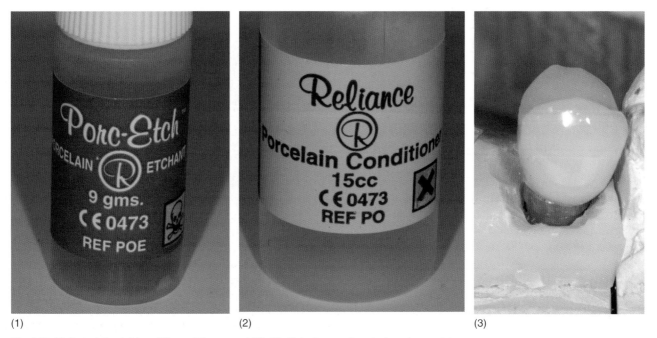

(1)

(2)

(3)

Fig. 9.40 (1) Porcelain etching, (2) conditioner and (3)–(7) clinical procedure to bond porcelain crown.

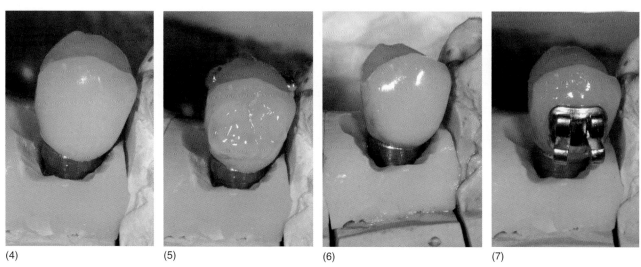

(4) (5) (6) (7)

Fig. 9.40 (*Continued*).

acid and silane primer (chemical bond), provides the highest shear bond strength, and this also produces the greatest damage to the porcelain surface such as a greater risk of porcelain fracture during debonding (Alzainal et al. 2020; Tahmasbi et al. 2020); on the other hand, the cyanoacrylate adhesive has the lowest shear bond strength, followed by the RMGIC and the conventional bonding using a 37% phosphoric acid (H_3PO_4) etch and composite adhesive (Wood et al. 1986; Zachrisson et al. 1996; Ajlouni et al. 2005; Bishara et al. 2005a, b, c; Fan et al. 2005; Larmour et al. 2005). Laser irradiation (by 2 watts for 20 seconds) might be an alternative conditioning method for pretreating ceramic surfaces; it provides a porous surface texture without cracks. Increased bond strength can be achieved by priming with silane after laser irradiation (Akova et al. 2005; Kara et al. 2020). Recently, Reliance has developed Assure Plus, an all surface bonding resin, which is able to bond to wet or dry normal/atypical enamel, dentine/cementum, composite, gold, amalgam, stainless steel, zirconia, acrylic/pontic teeth, porcelain, etc. (Figure 9.41).

Debonding

To remove the attachment (with ligature cutter, Weingart plier, special debonding plier [Figure 9.42(1)–(5)]) and all adhesive from the tooth (scraping with debonding plier, or with a scaler, or a tungsten carbide bur and contra-angle handpiece, followed by polishing with disks and pumicing [Figure 9.43(1),(2)]), a correct debonding procedure is of fundamental importance. The objective of this procedure is to restore the surfaces as closely as possible to their pretreatment condition without damages, such as enamel fractures, cracks, split lines, decalcifications or enamel loss (Zachrisson et al. 1979; Diedrich 1981; Thompson et al. 1981). The safest way to remove bonded steel brackets is to deliberately distort the bracket base to break the bond, but

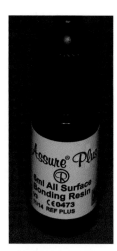

Fig. 9.41 Assure Plus (Reliance, Itasca, Illinois), an all-surface bonding resin.

this is not possible with ceramic brackets, which break before they bend. Electrothermal debonding can be used for enamel protection; the heat should soften the adhesive and make bracket removal easier (Rueggeberg et al. 1990). Orthodontist also can use laser energy to debond ceramic brackets; laser energy degrades the adhesive used to bond brackets (Azzeh et al, 2003; Bai et al, 2004; Hayakawa 2005). The bond strength of ceramic bracket is significantly reduced by laser irradiation. Consequently, lower forces can be used than when mechanical debonding is performed, reducing the risk of enamel damage. However, the heat produced by some lasers can damage the tooth pulp. Selecting the appropriate laser, adhesive and bracket combination can minimise risks and make debonding more efficient. At debonding, most enamel loss occurs after the use of high-speed tungsten carbide bur or the ultrasonic scaler, and least with the slow-speed tungsten carbide bur or debonding

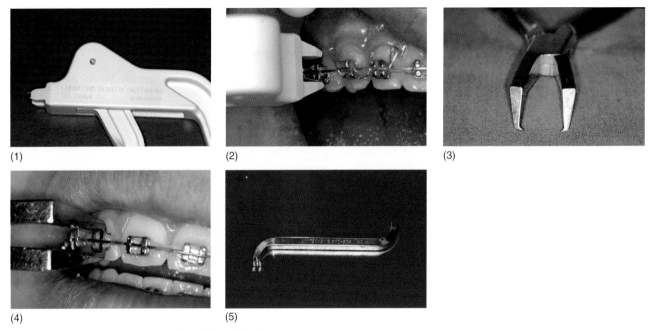

(1) (2) (3)

(4) (5)

Fig. 9.42 (1)–(5) Various devices used to debond brackets.

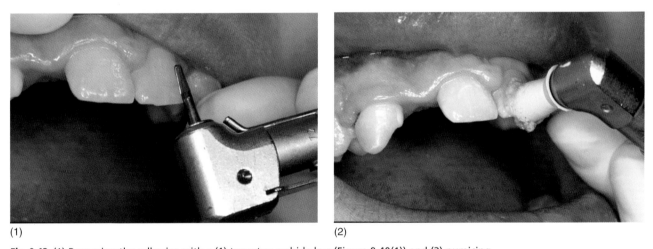

(1) (2)

Fig. 9.43 (1) Removing the adhesive with a (1) tungsten carbide bur (Figure 9.40(1)) and (2) pumicing.

pliers during enamel cleaning. To minimise the damage of the sound enamel surface during etching and debonding procedures, a mixture of phosphoric acid and an acidulated phosphate fluoride (APF) gel can be used as a phosphoric acid and etchant substitute without loss of the proper bracket bond strength (Kim et al. 2005).

Reconditioning of stainless-steel attachments

Stainless-steel brackets may be recycled; no statistically significant differences were found between the total bond failure rate of recycled and new stainless-steel brackets, the upper and lower arches and the anterior and posterior segments. Recycling metallic brackets can be of benefit to the profession, both economically and ecologically, as long as

the orthodontist is aware of various aspects of recycling methods, and the patients are informed about the type of bracket that will be used for their treatment (Cacciafesta et al. 2004a, b, c). In the orthodontic office, the debonded stainless-steel brackets may be reconditioned using different techniques: flamed and then sandblasted, flamed and ultrasonically cleaned, flamed and ultrasonically cleaned followed by silane treatment and only flamed or sandblasted or roughened with a greenstone. Sandblasting is the most effective in removing adhesive without significant change in bond strength compared with new attachments; on the other hand, silane application does not improve the bond strength values of flamed and ultrasonically cleaned brackets. Attachments that had only been flamed have the lowest bond strength, followed by those that had been roughened with a greenstone (Quick et al. 2005).

Banding

Until recently, the only practical way to place a fixed attachment was to put it on a band that could be cemented to a tooth. The pioneer orthodontists of the early 1900s used clamp bands, which were tightened around molar teeth by screw attachments. Preformed steel bands came into widespread use during the 1960s and are now available in anatomically correct shapes for all the teeth. Indications for the use of bands rather than a bonded attachment include (Graber and Vanarsdall 1994):

a) Teeth that will receive heavy intermittent forces against the attachments. A common example is an upper first molar to which an extraoral force will be applied by means of a headgear ([Figure 9.44(1)] or a rapid palatal expander [Figure 9.44(2)]).

b) Teeth that will need both labial and lingual attachments. A common example is again the upper or lower first molar to which a transpalatal arch or a lingual arch will be applied ([Figure 9.44(3)] or a Jasper Jumper [Figure 9.44(4)]).

c) Teeth with short clinical crowns.

d) Teeth incompatible with successful bonding, as for example teeth affected by fluorosis.

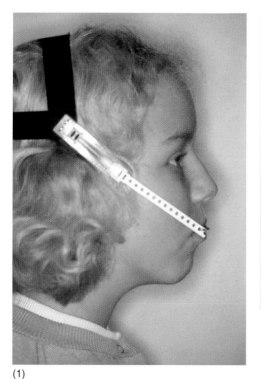

(1)

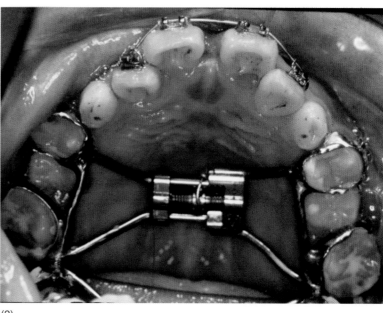

(2)

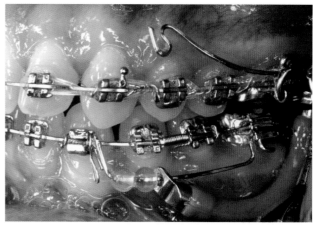

(3)   (4)

Fig. 9.44 (1)–(4) Examples of indications to the use of bands.

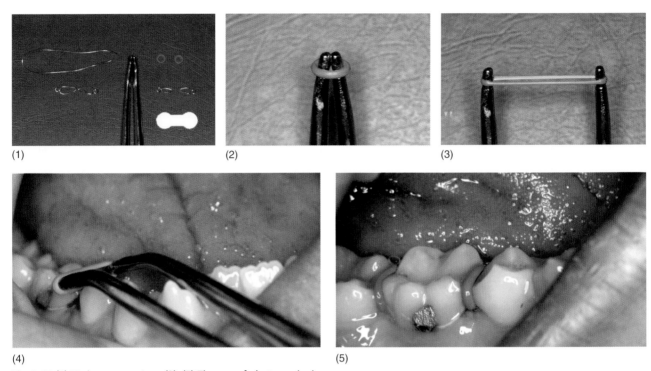

(1)   (2)   (3)

(4)   (5)

Fig. 9.45 (1) Various separators. (2)–(5) The use of elastomeric rings.

In contemporary practice, bonded attachments are always preferred for anterior teeth, bands may be used on premolars, usually on second premolars in adolescents, and they are preferred for molars. Incisor and canine bands are needed rarely in unusual circumstances. In order to properly seat a band, some tooth separators must usually be used before banding (Figure 9.45(1)). There are several methods that can be used to separate the teeth: the most commonly used are the elastomeric rings (Figure 9.45(2)–(5)), the steel-separating springs (Figure 9.46) and the soft brass wire (Figure 9.47(1)–(3)). Those devices must be left in place for maximum one week before the banding procedure can start. Separation can be painful, so it is important to use the easiest device to tolerate, both when it is placed and removed, from the patient. After removing separators, it is important to clean teeth to be banded with an oil-free pumice or paste in order to remove any plaque, and then to rinse with water. Heavy force and specific instruments are needed to seat a preformed band (Figure 9.48(1)); the band is pressed over the height of contour with finger pressure (Figure 9.48(2), followed by the use of a band seater from the distal side of the tooth (Figure 9.48(3)). Additionally, an instrument with a serrated tip which patients can bite (Figure 9.48(4)) can be employed; finally, open margins are burnished with a hand instrument (Figure 9.48(5)). It is important to follow the manufacturer's instructions because preformed bands are designed to be fitted in a certain sequence. For example, upper molar bands are designed to be placed initially by hand pressure on the distal and mesial surfaces, bringing the band down close to the height of the

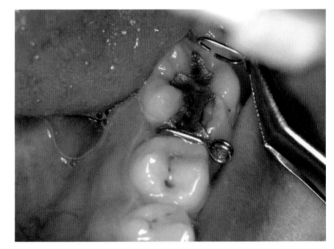

Fig. 9.46 Metal springs.

marginal ridges. Then, it is driven to place by pressure on the mesiobuccal and distolingual corners (Figure 9.49(1)). Lower molar bands are designed to be seated initially with hand pressure on the proximal surfaces, and then with heavy biting force along the buccal but not the lingual margins (Figure 9.49(2)). After final seating, the bands are usually cemented using glass ionomers (Figure 9.50(1)), RMGICs (Figure 9.50(2)) or compomers (polyacid-modified composite resins) (Figure 9.50(3)), which are able to release fluoride ions to the enamel surface in an attempt to reduce enamel surface decalcifications which can often

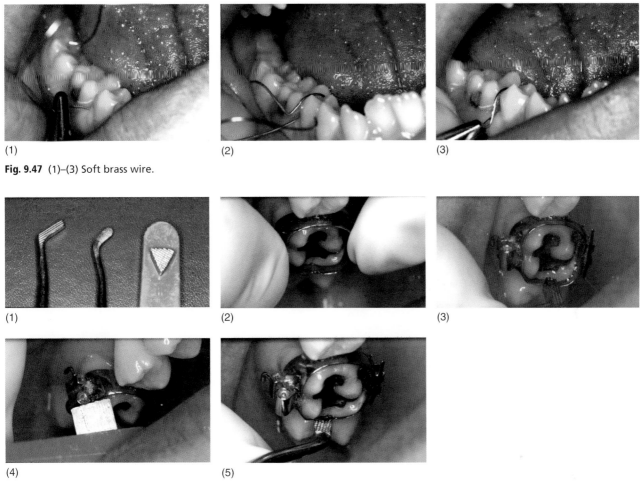

Fig. 9.47 (1)–(3) Soft brass wire.

Fig. 9.48 (1) Seating instruments and (2)–(5) clinical procedure.

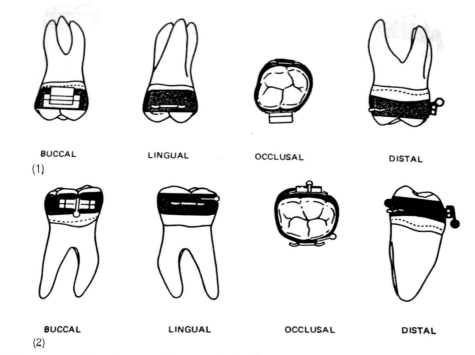

BUCCAL   LINGUAL   OCCLUSAL   DISTAL

(1)

BUCCAL   LINGUAL   OCCLUSAL   DISTAL

(2)

Fig. 9.49 (1) and (2) Correct position of upper and lower molar bands.

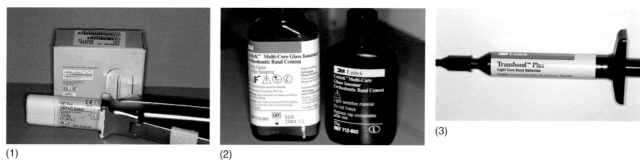

(1) (2) (3)

Fig. 9.50 (1)–(3) Various adhesives for band cementation.

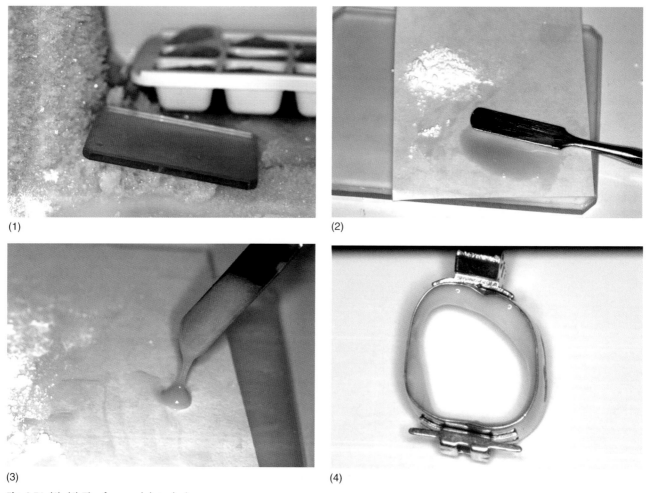

(1) (2)

(3) (4)

Fig. 9.51 (1)–(4) The frozen slab technique.

develop around the margins of the band or underneath (Wilson and Donley 2001). The inner surface of the bands can be microetched for a better adhesion to the tooth structure. Teeth to be banded must be isolated, and for lower bandings, cotton rolls are placed also between the tongue and molars. Cementation of bands is facilitated by using a cold mixing slab (the 'frozen slab technique'; Figure 9.51(1)–(3)) and a large cement spatula. The cement must cover all interior surfaces of the band (Figure 9.51(4)).

When the band is carried to place, its occlusal surface should be covered with a gloved finger over the top of the band, so that cement is expressed from its gingival margin. After removing excess material with a scaler, if necessary, light-cure the cement by placing the light guide 1–2 mm above the occlusal surface of the tooth banded and cure the material for 40 seconds. After the initial light-curing, the chemical curing will continue the hardening of the material where light does not penetrate.

Auxiliary Attachments and Aesthetic Buttons

Auxiliary attachments are an integral part of the fixed appliance. Headgear tubes, for example, are placed routinely on maxillary first molars. There are 45 or 51 mm round tubes used for the insertion of the inner bow of a face bow appliance or a heavy auxiliary labial archwire. They are placed occlusally relative to the main slot for ease of the access and better hygiene. The auxiliary tubes for molars are strongly recommended in all patients. A rectangular auxiliary tube should be present on the upper and lower first molars; it is placed gingivally to the plane of the main archwires and it allows the use of segmented arch technique.

In the appliance designed by Burstone for segmented arch technique, during closure of extraction spaces, auxiliary rectangular tubes on the canines are also used. Burstone canine bracket combines a rectangular bracket slot with a vertical tube used for attachment of retraction springs and for connecting the anterior and posterior segments. Into the labial attachments hooks are routinely incorporated; they are used as needed for Class II, Class III, criss-cross and intra-arch elastics.

Lingual arches should be used for anchorage control in space closure in extraction cases or in intrusion with segmented arch technique; for tooth movements, lingual attachments may be horizontal lingual sheaths or twin vertical tubes.

It is common practice to place lingual cleats, buttons, sheaths and eyelets to allow the use of cross-elastic, controlling rotations on premolars and canines during space closure or pulling down impacted canines.

Low-profile composite buttons are a very useful and aesthetic alternative to steel buttons or bulky, expensive ceramic brackets in managing vertical tooth positions, rotations and antero-posterior corrections with elastics in patients treated with removable aligners or lingual brackets (Figure 9.52), or to assist in making difficult tooth movements with aligners (Kravitz and Kusnoto 2007). The clinical procedure requires microetching, tooth isolation, etching and priming the tooth surface where the button is to

be placed. For directly having a separator to the tooth, apply a low-viscosity composite resin, allowing it to flow over the edges of the separator to create the ledge for the button. If a low-viscosity resin is not available, a primer can be applied to a standard composite resin to reduce its viscosity. After curing the resin for 20 seconds with the separator in place, gently peel away the separator. If necessary, shape and bevel the button with a diamond bur. An elastomeric O-ring can be used instead of a separator to further reduce the profile of the button. The O-ring should be cut in half to increase the width of the button base, since its small lumen would otherwise produce a base that might be too narrow to withstand heavy forces (Kravitz and Kusnoto 2007).

A similar technique can be used to quickly fabricate at the chairside the aesthetic attachments for orthodontic aligners (Figure 9.53(1),(2)). The choice of composite will also influence bonding success. Kravitz et al. (2018) recommend either Tetric EvoCeram (shade T), a dense restorative nanohybrid composite, or Transbond LR, a viscous lingual retainer paste that is readily available and somewhat easier to apply. Small slits are made in the template tray above the attachment moulds. The authors recommend using a

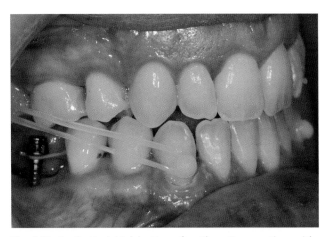

Fig. 9.52 Aesthetic labial buttons for Class III correction with lingual braces.

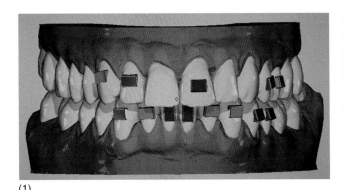

(1)

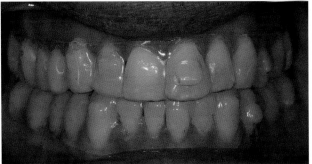

(2)

Fig. 9.53 (1) and (2) Buccal attachments for orthodontic aligners.

ligature cutter. The slits can be placed over all the attachment moulds or just the larger posterior ones. At the bonding appointment, the teeth are isolated with a cheek retractor and prepared with self-etching adhesive. After the initial cure, the light can be moved closer to the tray. Next, the template tray is gently lifted off the attachments, beginning at the slits. The authors prefer to use a heavier sickle scaler rather than a dental explorer, even though this will tear the tray (Kravitz et al. 2018). This technique can also be applied when a previously worn aligner is used to rebond attachments that break off during treatment.

Anchorage Needs and Reinforcement

For a correct biomechanical planning, it is mandatory to distinguish between an active unit (teeth to be moved) and a passive or reactive unit (teeth used as anchorage). In order to obtain a maximum anchorage, we can use extremely rigid and passive wires, sometimes directly bonded to the teeth, even in patients treated with lingual braces (Figure 9.54). A better aesthetic option is the use of fibre reinforced composites (FRCs), which are as rigid as metal, but tooth-coloured, thus almost invisible. The FRCs have been widely used in dentistry for fabrication of crowns, surface retained bridges, root canal restorations and periodontal and orthodontic splintings (Scribante et al. 2018). In orthodontics, Burstone and Kuhlberg (2000) and Freudenthaler et al. (2001) have advocated the use of FRCs for both passive and active applications. FRCs are able to connect different teeth into a rigid unit, thus reinforcing the anchorage. They can represent an excellent alternative for those patients who, for aesthetic reasons, do not want to show any metal in the mouth.

A classical indication to use FRCs is when molar uprighting is needed and anchorage reinforcement becomes a must buccally and lingually. Titanium molybdenum alloy (TMA) cantilevers can efficiently upright molars, and

FRCs can reinforce the anchorage reducing the visibility of the appliance (Figure 9.55(1),(2)).

The FRCs are very often used in lingual treatments especially on the buccal side (Cacciafesta et al. 2005a, b). The anchorage of posterior teeth can be reinforced with buccal FRCs, and contralateral teeth can be solidarised by conventional or custom-made transpalatal bars (Figure 9.56(1),(2)). An FRC bar (A&O, Stick Tech Ltd., Turku, Finland) was bonded on the labial side of first premolar to first molar on the left side, and from canine to first molar on the right side, to form a rigid anchorage unit between those teeth (Figure 9.56(1),(2)). No metal could be detected from outside the mouth. The exact length of the glass fibre was measured and the fibre was cut with scissors directly from the package. The buccal surfaces of the teeth were sandblasted with microetcher for 3 seconds each. After sandblasting, the surface was etched with 37% orthophosphoric acid for 30 seconds. After etching, the bonding agent was applied using a small brush and then the area was light-cured. After

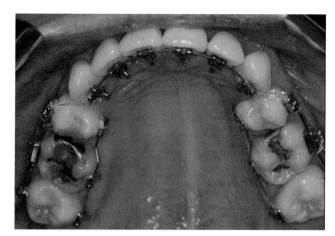

Fig. 9.54 Anchorage reinforcement with labial stiff SS rectangular sectionals in a lingual patient.

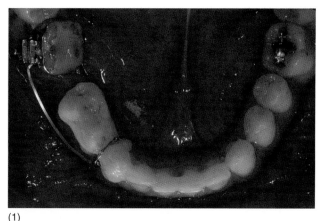

(1)

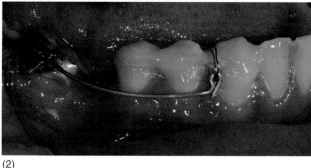

(2)

Fig. 9.55 (1) and (2) Molar uprighting by means of a TMA cantilever. FRCs can be employed to reinforce the anchorage buccally and lingually, thus reducing the visibility of the appliance.

this phase, a thin layer of flow composite was applied on the enamel surfaces. The glass fibre was consequently positioned on the composite flow and pressed with hand instruments. Each tooth was light-cured for 5 seconds. Then, the entire glass-fibre bundle was covered with another layer of flow composite and each site light-cured for 40 seconds.

In more severe cases, the Iron Cross developed by Prof Birte Melsen can be employed. This is a reinforcement of the transpalatal bar with a bonded splint, used for the stabilisation of the lateral segments across the palate. We use it to reinforce the impact of occlusion on anchorage, especially where you have loss of teeth in periodontally involved patients (Figure 9.57(1)–(3)).

Bonded Retainers

Retention is an integral phase after the completion of orthodontic treatment. It is the stage that enables the dentition to adapt the newly attained position and to maintain the stability and alignment of the teeth which otherwise will revert back to their pretreatment position, resulting in relapse. Post retention orthodontic treatment records reveal loss of stability and alignment specifically in the mandibular anterior region (Salehi et al. 2013). Therefore, permanent retention is highly recommended to ensure the stability and to maintain the long-term effects of the dentition achieved by the treatment. These consequences can be accomplished by a fixed lingual retainer inserted for an optimum time interval (Booth et al. 2008). Zachrisson in 1977 was the first one who boosted the usage of multistranded stainless-steel wire (MSW) as fixed lingual retainers instead of round SS wire (Zachrisson 1977b). Fixed lingual retainers are specifically inserted in cases of generalised spacing, midline diastemas or to maintain implant/pontic spaces. However, with the passage of time, these are preferred usually in all cases, as they offer numerous benefits; for instance, they are aesthetically pleasing, easily acceptable, provide greater stability, compliance-free and cause no soft-tissue irritation and speech problems, although they are technique-sensitive and time-consuming. Fracture and bond failure are also reported (Renkema et al. 2011). Bond failure may be of

cohesive or adhesive type. Cohesive failure is the type of failure at wire–adhesive interface which occurs due to inadequate composite resin, whereas adhesive failure which is between adhesive and enamel surface results from movement of wire during bonding or moisture contamination

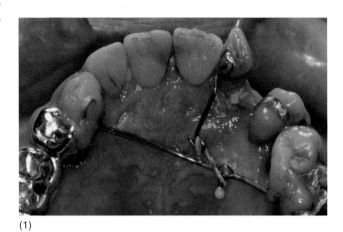

(1)

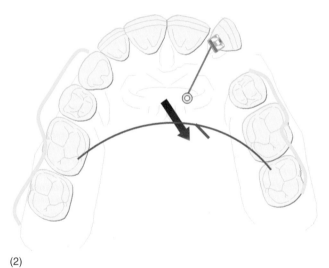

(2)

Fig. 9.56 (1) and (2) Anchorage reinforcement of posterior teeth with buccal FRCs for retraction and derotation of UL2. Contralateral teeth are solidarised by a custom-made transpalatal bar.

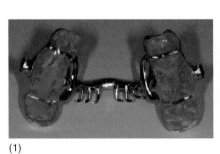

(1)

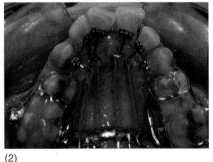

(2)

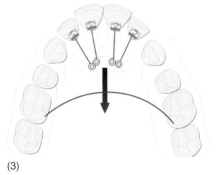

(3)

Fig. 9.57 (1)–(3) Anchorage reinforcement of posterior teeth with Iron Cross for retraction and intrusion of the upper incisors.

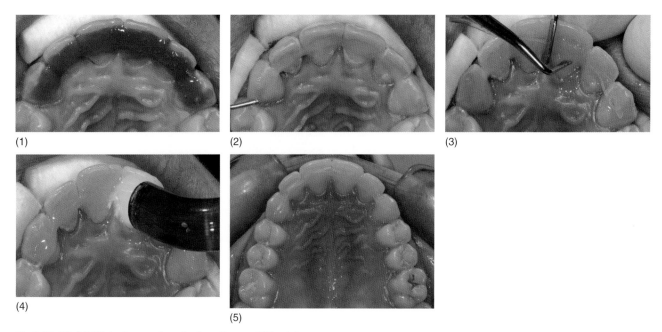

(1)   (2)   (3)

(4)

(5)

Fig. 9.58 (1)–(5) Clinical procedure for bonding an FRC retainer.

(Renkema et al. 2011). Various factors that determine the survival rate of retainers are site of placement, type of material used, total number of teeth bonded and type of composite resin used.

FRCs are metal-free materials. They provide an opportunity to minimise the volume of splints and increase aesthetics and can be used in nickel-allergy prone patients. In clinical orthodontics, they are used as retainers after active treatment in order to avoid relapse. However, although the modulus of the elasticity of FRCs is low, the rigidity of the material in the form of a relatively thick retainer with a surface cover of a flowable resin composite is known to have higher structural rigidity than stainless-steel splints. The clinical procedure for bonding FRC retainers requires that the lingual surfaces of the teeth are sandblasted with a microetcher 3 seconds per each tooth. After sandblasting, the tooth surfaces are etched with 37% phosphoric acid for 30 seconds (Figure 9.58(1)). After proper rinsing and drying, the enamel surface should have a white chalky appearance. After etching, the bonding agent is applied with a brush and cured. Subsequently, a thin layer of flowable composite is applied onto the lingual surfaces (Figure 9.58(2)). Note that the flowable composite should also cover the interproximal spaces and should not be cured at this time. The fibre bundle is then placed onto the flowable composite and pressed down with a hand instrument (Figure 9.58(3)). Each tooth is light-cured for 5 seconds, protecting the rest of the fibre bundle with a wide instrument. After curing each single tooth for 5 seconds, the whole retainer is covered with a layer of flowable composite and light-cured for 40 seconds per tooth (Figure 9.58(4)). Note that the flowable composite must cover the entire length of the fibre bundle, also in the

interproximal areas. After curing, the retainer is polished, and the occlusion is checked to ensure that the fibre bundle is not placed in occlusion (Figure 9.58(5)).

Nagani et al. (2020) compared MSW and FRC retainers in a randomised clinical trial. Their findings indicate that multistranded stainless steel wire retainer is a superior option to be used for fixed lingual retention in mandibular arch, as it exhibited lower bond failure as compared to fibre reinforced composite retainer. Different types of failure patterns have been observed, but adhesive failure is the most common type of bond failure observed with both groups of fixed lingual retainers.

References

Aboush YEY, Tareen A and Elderton RJ (1991) Resin-to-enamel bonds: effect of cleaning the enamel surface with prophylaxis pastes containing fluoride or oil. *Br Dent J* 171, 207.

Aguirre MJ, King GJ and Waldron JM (1982) Assessment of bracket placement and bond strength when comparing direct bonding to indirect bonding techniques. *Am J Orthod* 82, 269.

Ajlouni R, Bishara SE, Oonsombat C and Denehy GE (2004) Evaluation of modifying the bonding protocol of a new acid-etch primer on the shear bond strength of orthodontic brackets. *Angle Orthod* 74(3), 410–413.

Ajlouni R, Bishara SE, Oonsombat C, Soliman M and Laffoon J (2005) The effect of porcelain surface conditioning on bonding orthodontic brackets. *Angle Orthod* 75(5), 858–864.

Akova T, Yoldas O, Toroglu MS and Uysal H (2005) Porcelain surface treatment by laser for bracket-porcelain bonding. *Am J Orthod* 128(5), 630–637.

Alexander M, Alexander RG, Gorman JC, Hilgers JJ, Kurz C, Scholz RP, Smith JR (1982) Lingual orthodontics: A status report. *J Clin Orthod* 16, 225.

Aljubouri YD, Millet DT and Gilmor WH (2004) Six and 12 months' evaluation of self-etching primer versus two-stage etch and primer for orthodontic bonding: a randomized clinical trial. *Eur J Orthod* 26(6), 565–571.

Alzainal AH, Majud AS, Al-Ani AM and Mageet AO (2020) Orthodontic bonding: Review of the Literature. *Int J Dent* Jul 14;2020, 1–10

Andreasen GF and Stieg MA (1988) Bonding and debonding brackets to porcelain and gold. *Am J Orthod* 93(4), 341–345.

Andrews LF (1989) *Straight Wire: The Concept and Appliance*. San Diego: LA Wells.

Angolkar PV, Kapila S, Duncanson MG and Nanda RS (1990) Evaluation of friction between ceramic brackets and orthodontic wires of four alloys. *Am J Orthod Dentofacial Orthop* 98, 499–506.

Azizi F, Bahrami K, Imani MM, Golshah A and Safari-Faramani R (2020) Effect of bleaching with carbamide peroxide on shear bond strength of orthodontic brackets: a meta-analysis of in vitro studies. *Int Orthod* Jun;18(2), 214–224.

Azzeh E and Feldon PJ (2003) Laser debonding of ceramic brackets: a comprehensive review. *Am J Orthod* 123(1), 79–83.

Bagramian RA and McNamara JA Jr (1998) A prospective survey of percutaneous injuries in orthodontists. *Am J Orthod* 114, 654–658.

Bai D and Liu XL (2004) The effects of Nd: yAGlaser-aided debracket on the bonding strength of brackets and the temperature of pulp cavity. *Hua Xi Kou Qiang Yi Xue Za Zhi* 22(4), 287–289.

Barry GR (1995) A clinical investigation of the effects of omission of pumice prophylaxis on band and bond failure. *Br J Orthod* 22, 245–248.

Bilen HB and Çokakoğlu S (2020) Effects of one-step orthodontic adhesive on microleakage and bracket bond strength: an in vitro comparative study. *Int Orthod* Jun;18(2), 366–373.

Bishara SE, Ajlouni R, Oonsombat C and Laffoon J (2005a) Bonding orthodontic brackets to porcelain using different adhesive/enamel conditioners: a comparative study. *World J Orthod* 6(1), 17–24.

Bishara SE, Olsen M and Von Wald L (1997) Comparison of shear bond strength of precoated and uncoated brackets. *Am J Orthod* 112(6), 617–621.

Bishara SE, Oonsombat C, Soliman MM, Wrren JJ, Laffoon JF and Ajlouni R (2005b) Comparison of bonding time and shear bond strength between a conventional and a new integrated bonding system. *Angle Orthod* 75(5), 237–242.

Bishara SE, Soliman M, Laffoon J and Warren JJ (2005c) Effect of antimicrobial monomer-containing adhesive on shear strength of orthodontic brackets. *Angle Orthod* 75(3), 397–399.

Booth FA, Edelman JM and Proffit WR (2008) Twenty-year follow-up of patients with permanently bonded mandibular canine-to-canine retainers. *Am J Orthod Dentofac Orthop* 133(1), 70–76.

Borzangy S (2019) Impact of surface treatment methods on bond strength of orthodontic brackets to indirect composite provisional restorations. *J Contemp Dent Pract* Dec 1;20(12), 1412–1416.

Brannstrom M, Malmgren O and Nordenvall KJ (1989) Etching of young permanent teeth with an acid gel. *Am J Orthod* 82, 379.

Buonocore MG (1955) A simple method of increasing the adhesion of acrylic filling materials to enamel surface. *J Dent Res* 34, 849–853.

Burstone CJ and Kuhlberg AJ (2000) Fiber-Reinforced Composites in orthodontics. *J Clin Orthod* 34, 271–279.

Buyukyilmaz T, Zachrisson YO and Zachrisson BU (1995) Improving orthodontic bonding to gold alloy. *Am J Orthod* 108(5), 510–518.

Cacciafesta V, Sfondrini MF, Melsen B and Scribante A (2004a) A 12 month clinical study of bond failure of recycled versus new stainless steel orthodontic brackets. *Eur J Orthod* 26(4), 449–454.

Cacciafesta V, Sfondrini MF, Norcini A and Macchi A (2005a) Fiber reinforced composites in lingual orthodontics. *J Clin Orthod* 39, 710–714.

Cacciafesta V, Sfondrini MF and Scribante A (2004b) Plasma arc versus halogen light-curing of adhesive-precoated orthodontic brackets: a 12-month clinical study of bond failures. *Am J Orthod* 126(2), 194–199.

Cacciafesta V, Sfondrini MF, Scribante A, Boehme A and Jost-Brinkmann PG (2005b) Effect of light-tip distance on the shear bond strengths of composite resin. *Angle Orthod* 75(3), 386–391.

Cacciafesta V, Sfondrini MF, Scribante A, De Angelis M and Klersy C (2004c) Effects of blood contamination on the shear bond strengths of conventional and hydrophilic primers. *Am J Orthod* 126(2), 207–212.

Cacciafesta V, Sfondrini MF, Scribante A, Klersy C and Auricchio F (2003) Evaluation of friction of conventional and metal-insert ceramic brackets in various bracket-archwire combinations. *Am J Orthod* 124(4), 403–409.

Castilla AE, Crowe JJ, Moses JR, Wang M, Ferracane JL and Covell DA Jr (2014) Measurement and comparison of bracket transfer accuracy of five indirect bonding techniques. *Angle Orthod* 84(4), 607–614.

Ceen RF and Gwinnett AJ (1980) Indelible iatrogenic staining of enamel following debonding. *J Clin Orthod* 14, 713.

Condo R, Casaglia A and Cozza P (2005) SEM analysis of zirconium brackets using MIM technology. *Minerva Stomatologica* 54(4), 207–217.

Craig RG (1997) *Restorative Dental Materials*, 10e. St Louis, MO: Mosby.

Czolgosz I, Cattaneo PM and Cornelis MA (2021) Computer aided indirect bonding versus traditional direct bonding of orthodontic brackets: bonding time, immediate bonding failures, and cost-minimization. A randomized controlled trial. *Eur J Orthod* Apr 3; 43(2), 144–151.

Damon DH (1998) The Damon low-friction bracket: A biologically compatible Straight-Wire system. *J Clin Orthod* 32, 670–680.

Dehbi H, Azaroual MF, Zaoui F, Halimi A and Benyahia H (2017) Therapeutic efficacy of self-ligating brackets: a systematic review. *Int Orthod* Sep;15(3), 297–311.

Diedrich P (1981) Enamel alterations from bracket bonding and debonding: A study with the scanning electron microscopy. *Am J Orthod* 79, 500.

Dorfer S, König M and Jost-Brinkmann P-G (2006) Übertragungsgenauigkeit beim indirekten Platzieren von brackets. *Kieferorthopädie* 20, 91–104.

Edris AA, Jabr AA Cooley RL, Barghi N (1990) SEM evaluation of etch patterns by three etchants on three porcelains. *J Prosthet Dent* 64, 734.

Fan CH, Chen J, Liu XQ and Ma X (2005) Influence of different porcelain surface treatment method on the bonding of metal brackets to porcelain. *Hua Xi Kou Qiang Yi Xue Za Zhi* 23(4), 341–344.

Farhadian N, Miresmaeili A and Zandi VS (2019) Shear bond strength of brackets bonded with self-etching primers compared to conventional acid-etch technique: a randomized clinical trial. *Front Dent* Jul-Aug;16(4), 248–255.

Ferreira FG, Da Silva EM and de Vilella OV (2020) A novel method using confocal laser scanning microscopy for three-dimensional analysis of human dental enamel subjected to ceramic bracket debonding. *Microsc Microanal* Aug;26, 1–8.

Flores DA, Caruso IM, Scott GE and Jeroudi MT (1990) The fracture strength of ceramic brackets: a comparative study. *Angle Orthod* 60, 269–276.

Forsberg CM, Brattstrom V, Malmberg E, Nord CE (1991) Ligature wires and elastomeric rings: two methods of ligation and their association with microbial colonization of *Streptococcus mutans* and lactobacilli. *Eur J Orthod* 13, 416.

Freudenthaler JW, Tischler GK and Burstone CJ (2001) Bond strength of fiber-reinforced composite bars for orthodontic attachment. *Am J Orthod Dentofacial Orthop* 120, 648–653.

Graber TM and Vanarsdall RL (1994) *Orthodontics – Current Principles and Techniques*, 2e. St. Louis, MO: Mosby.

Grandhi RK, Combe EC and Speidel TM (2001) Shear bond strength of stainless orthodontic brackets with a moisture-insensitive primer. *Am J Orthod* 119(3), 251–255.

Gross MW, Foley TF and Mamandras AH (1997) Direct bonding to Adlloy-treated amalgam. *Am J Orthod* 112(3), 252–258.

Grunheid T, Lee MS and Larson BE (2016) Transfer accuracy of vinyl polysiloxane trays for indirect bonding. *Angle Orthod* 86(3), 468–474.

Hanson GH (1994) The SPEED System: a report on the development of a new edgewise appliance. *Am J Orthod* 105, 217–223.

Hatibovic-Kofman S and Koch G (1991) Fluoride release from glass ionomer cement *in vivo* and *in vitro*. *Swed Dent J* 15, 253–258.

Hayakawa K (2005) Nd: yAGlaser for debonding ceramic orthodontic brackets. *Am J Orthod* 128(5), 638–647.

Heiser W (1998) Time: a new orthodontic philosophy. *J Clin Orthod* 32, 44–53.

Hixson ME, Brantley WA, Pincsak JJ, Conover JP (1982) Changes in bracket slot tolerance following recycling of direct-bond metallic orthodontic appliances. *Am J Orthod* 81, 447.

Hodge TM, Dhopatkar AA, Rock WP and Spary DJ (2004) A randomized clinical trial comparing the accuracy of direct versus indirect bracket placement. *J Orthod* 31(2), 132–137.

Holt MH, Nanda RS and Duncason MG (1991) Fracture resistance of ceramic brackets during arch-wire torsion. *Am J Orthod* 99, 287–293.

Hosein I, Sherriff M and Ireland AJ (2004) Enamel loss during bonding, debonding, and cleanup with use of a self-etching primer. *Am J Orthod* 126(6), 717–724.

Hotz P, McClean JW, Sced I and Wilson AD (1977) The bonding of glass ionomer cements to metal and tooth substrates. *Br Dent J* 142, 41–47.

Ibrahim AI, Al-Hasani NR, Thompson VP and Deb S (2020) *In vitro* bond strengths post thermal and fatigue load cycling of sapphire brackets bonded with self-etch primer and evaluation of enamel damage. *J Clin Exp Dent* Jan 1;12(1), e22–e30.

Iglesias A, Flores T, Moyano J, Artés M, Gil FJ and Puigdollers A (2020) In vitro study of shear bond strength in direct and indirect bonding with three types of adhesive systems. *Materials (Basel)* Jun 10;13(11), 2644–2657.

Ip TB and Rock WP (2004) A comparison of three light curing units for bonding adhesive pre-coated brackets. *J Orthod* 31(3), 243–247.

Ireland AJ and Sherriff M (2002) The effect of pumicing on the in vivo use of a resin-modified glass poly(alkenoate) cement and a conventional no-mix composite for bonding orthodontic brackets. *J Orthod* 29, 217–220.

Jeiroudi MT (1991) Enamel fracture caused by ceramic brackets. *Am J Orthod* 99, 97–99.

Johnson G, Walker MP and Kula K (2005) Fracture strength of ceramic bracket tie wings subjected to tension. *Angle Orthod* 75(1), 95–100.

Kara M, Demir O and Doğru M (2020) Bond strength of metal and ceramic brackets on resin nanoceramic material with different surface treatments. *Turk J Orthod* Jun 1;33(2), 115–122.

Kilponen L, Varrela J and Vallittu PK (2019) Priming and bonding metal, ceramic and polycarbonate brackets. *Biomater Investig Dent* Nov 6;6(1), 61–72.

Kim MJ, Lim BS, Chang WG, Lee YK, Rhee SH and Yang HC (2005) Phosphoric acid incorporated with acidulated phosphate fluoride gel etchant effects on bracket bonding. *Angle Orthod* 75(4), 678–684.

Knox J, Hubsch P, Jones ML and Middleton J (2000) The influence of bracket base design on the strength of the bracket-cement interface. *Journal of Orthodontics* 27(3), 249–254.

Kravitz ND, Johnson BM and Kilic H (2018) A modified bonding technique for Invisalign attachments. *J Clin Orthod* LII(12), 715–716.

Kravitz ND and Kusnoto B (2007) A quick and inexpensive method for composite button fabrication. *J Clin Orthod* XLI(2), 65–66.

Kusy RP and Whitley JQ (1990) Coefficients of friction for arch wires in stainless steel and polycrystalline aluminia bracket slots. *Am J Orthod* 989, 300–312.

Larmour CJ, Bateman G and Stirrups DR (2005) An investigation into the bonding of orthodontic attachments to porcelain. *Eur J Orthod* 30.

Layman B (2019) Digital bracket placement for indirect bonding. *J Clin Orthod* 7, 387–396.

Lindauer SJ, Browning H, Shroff B, Marshall F, Anderson RH and Moon PC (1997) Effect of pumice prophylaxis on the bond strength of orthodontic brackets. *Am J Orthod Dentofacial Orthop* 111, 599–605.

Maijer R and Smith DC (1982) Corrosion of orthodontic bracket bases. *Am J Orthod* 81, 43.

Maijer R and Smith DC (1990) Time saving with self-ligating brackets. *J Clin Orthod* 24, 29–31.

McNamara JA Jr and Bagramian RA (1999) Prospective survey of percutaneous injuries in orthodontic assistants. *Am J Orthod* 115, 72–76.

Miguel JAM, Almeida MA and Chevitarese O (1995) Clinical comparison between a glass ionomer cement and a composite for direct bonding of orthodontic brackets. *Am J Orthod Dentofacial Orthop* 107, 484–487.

Miller JR, Mancl L, Arbuckle G, Baldwin J and Phillips RW (1996) A three-year clinical trial using a glass ionomer cement for the bonding of orthodontic brackets. *Angle Orthod* 66, 309–312.

Miura F, Nakagawasa K and Masuhara E (1971) New direct bonding system for plastic brackets. *Am J Orthod* 59, 350.

Möhlhenrich SC, Alexandridis C, Peters F, Kniha K, Modabber A, Danesh G and Fritz U (2020) Three-dimensional evaluation of bracket placement accuracy and excess bonding adhesive depending on indirect bonding technique and bracket geometry: an in-vitro study. *Head Face Med* Aug 3;16(1), 17.

Mollabashi V, Rezaei-Soufi L, Farhadian M and Reza Noorani A (2019) Effect of Erbium, chromium-doped: Yttrium, scandium, gallium, and garnet and erbium: Yttrium-aluminum-garnet laser etching on Enamel demineralization and shear bond strength of orthodontic brackets. *Contemp Clin Dent* Apr-Jun;10(2), 263–268.

Nagani NI, Ahmed I, Tanveer F, Khursheed HM and Farooqui WA (2020) Clinical comparison of bond failure between two types of mandibular canine-canine bonded orthodontic retainers- a randomized clinical trial. *BMC Oral Health* 20, 180–186.

Nawrocka A and Lukomska-Szymanska M (2020) The indirect bonding technique in orthodontics-A narrative literature review. *Materials (Basel)* Feb 22;13(4), 986–994.

Neugebauer S, Jost-Brinkmann PG, Patzold B and Cacciafesta V (2004) Plasma versus halogen light: the effect of different light sources on the shear bond strength of brackets. *J Orofac Orthop* 65(3), 223–236.

Newman GV (1974) Direct and indirect bonding of brackets. *J Clin Orthod* 8, 264–272.

Nishio C, Da Motta AF, Elias CN and Mucha JN (2004) In vitro evaluation of frictional forces between archwires and ceramic brackets. *Am J Orthod* 125(1), 56–64.

Odegaard J and Segner D (1990) The use of visible light-curing composites in bonding ceramic brackets. *Am J Orthod* 97, 188.

Oliveira SR, Rosenbach G, Brunhard IH, Almeida MA and Chevitarese O (2004) A clinical study of glass ionomer cement. *Eur Orthod* 26(2), 185–189.

Pizzoni L, Ravnholt G and Melsen B (1998) Frictional forces related to self-ligating brackets. *Eur J Orthod* 20, 283–291.

Pratten DH, Popli K, Germane N and Gunsolley JC (1990) Frictional resistance of ceramic and stainless steel orthodontic brackets. *Am J Orthod Dentofacial Orthop* 98, 398–403.

Quick AN, Harris AM and Joseph VP (2005) Office reconditioning of stainless steel orthodontic attachments. *Eur J Orthod* 27(3), 231–236.

Rajagopal R, Padmanabhan S and Gnanamani J (2004) A comparison of shear bond strength and debonding characteristics of conventional, moisture-insensitive, and self-etching primers in vitro. *Angle Orthod* 74(2), 264–268.

Read-Ward GE, Jones SP and Davies EH (1997) A comparison of self-ligating and conventional orthodontic bracket systems. *Br J Orthod* 24, 309–317.

Renkema A-M, Renkema A, Bronkhorst E and Katsaros C (2011) Long-term effectiveness of canine-to-canine bonded flexible spiral wire lingual retainers. *Am J Orthod Dentofac Orthop* 139(5), 614–621.

Reynolds IR (1975) A review of direct orthodontic bonding. *Br J Orthod* 2, 171–178.

Rezk-Lega F and Ogaard B (1991) Tensile bond force of glass ionomer cements in direct bonding of orthodontic brackets: an *in vitro* comparative study. *Am J Orthod Dentofacial Orthop* 100, 357–361.

Rueggerberg FA and Lockwood P (1990) Thermal debracketing of orthodontic resins. *Am J Orthod* 98, 56–65.

Sadat-Khonsari R, Moshtaghy A, Schlegel V, Kahl-Nieke B, Moller M and Bauss O (2004) Torque deformation characteristics of plastic brackets: a comparative study. *J Orofac Orthop* 65(1), 26–33.

Salehi P, Najafi HZ and Roeinpeikar SM (2013) Comparison of survival time between two types of orthodontic fixed retainer: a prospective randomized clinical trial. *Prog Orthod* 14(1), 25.

Scott G (1988) Fracture toughness and surface cracks – the key to understanding ceramic brackets. *Angle Orthod* 58, 5–8.

Scribante A, Vallittu PK, Özcan M, Lassila LVJ, Gandini P and Sfondrini MF (2018) Travel beyond clinical uses of fiber reinforced composites (FRCs) in Dentistry: A review of past employments, present applications, and future perspectives. *Biomed Res Int* Oct 22;2018:1498901. eCollection 2018;, . .

Silverman E, Cohen M, Gianelly AA and Dietz VS (1972) A universal direct bonding system for both metal and plastic brackets. *Am J Orthod* 62(3), 236–244.

Sinha PK and Nanda RS (1997) Esthetic orthodontic appliances and bonding concerns for adults. *Dent Clin North Am* 41(1), 89–109.

Smith GA, McInnes-Ledoux P, Ledoux WR, Weinberg R (1988) Orthodontic bonding to porcelain – bond strength and refinishing. *Am J Orthod* 94, 245.

Sperber RL, Watson PA, Rossouw PE and Sectakof PA (1999) Adhesion of bonded orthodontic attachments to dental amalgam: in vitro study. *Am J Orthod* 116(5), 506–513.

Stolzenberg J (1935) The Russell attachment and its improved advantages. *Int J Orthod Dent Child* 21, 837–840.

Swartz ML (1988) Ceramic brackets. *J Clin Orthod* 24, 91–94.

Tahmasbi S, Shiri A and Badiee M (2020) Shear bond strength of orthodontic brackets to porcelain surface using universal adhesive compared to conventional method. *Dent Res J (Isfahan)* Jan 21;17(1), 19–24.

Theodorakopoulou LP, Sadowsky PL, Jacobson A and Lacefield W Jr (2004) Evaluation of the debonding characteristics of 2 ceramic brackets: an in vitro study. *Am J Orthod* 125(3), 329–336.

Thomas RG (1979) Indirect bonding: simplicity in action. *J Clin Orthod* 13, 93.

Thompson RE and Way DC (1981) Enamel loss due to prophylaxis and multiple bonding/debonding of orthodontic attachment. *Am J Orthod* 79, 282.

Thorstenson G and Kusy R (2003) Influence of stainless steel inserts on the resistance to sliding of aesthetic brackets with second-order angulation in the dry and wet states. *Angle Orthod* 73(2), 167–175.

Uysal T, Sari Z and Demir A (2004) Are the flowable composites suitable for orthodontic bracket bonding? *Angle Orthod* 74(5), 697–702.

Verstrynge A, Ghesquiere A and Willems G (2004) Clinical comparison of an adhesive precoated vs. uncoated ceramic brackets system. *Orthod Craniofac Res* 7(1), 15–20.

Viazis AD (1989) Enamel surface abrasion from ceramic orthodontic brackets. *Am J Orthod Dentofacial Orthop* 96, 514–518.

Vicente A, Bravo LA and Romero M (2005) Influence of a nonrinse conditioner on the bond strength of brackets bonded with a resin adhesive system. *Angle Orthod* 75(3), 400–405.

Vorhies AB, Donly KJ, Staley RN and Wefel JS (1998) Enamel demineralization adjacent to orthodontic brackets bonded with hybrid glass ionomer cements: an *in vitro* study. *Am J Orthod Dentofacial Orthop* 114, 668–674.

Wendl B and Droschl H (2004) A comparative in vitro study of the strength of directly bonded brackets using different curing techniques. *Eur J Orthod* 26(5), 535–544.

Wildman AJ, Hice TL, Lang HM, Lee IF and Strauch EC Jr (1972) Round Table: the Edgelok bracket. *J Clin Orthod* 6, 613–623.

Wilson RM and Donley KJ (2001) Demineralization around orthodontic brackets bonded with resin-modified glass ionomer cement and fluoride-releasing resin composite. *Pediatr Dent* 23, 255–259.

Winchester LJ (1991) Bond strengths of five different ceramic brackets: an *in vitro* study. *Eur J Orthod* 13, 293–305.

Wood DP, Jordan RE, Way DC and Galil KA (1986) Bonding to porcelain and gold. *Am J Orthod* 89(3), 194–205.

Yang X, Xue C, He Y, Zhao M, Luo M, Wang P and Bai D (2018) Transversal changes, space closure, and efficiency of conventional and self-ligating appliances: a quantitative systematic review. *J Orofac Orthop* Jan;79(1), 1–10.

Yi GK, Dunn WJ and Taloumis LJ (2003) Shear bond strength comparison between direct and indirect bonded orthodontic brackets. *Am J Orthod* 124(5), 577–581.

Zachrisson BU (1977a) A posttreatment evaluation of direct bonding in orthodontics. *Am J Orthod* 71, 173.

Zachrisson BU (1977b) Clinical experience with direct-bonded orthodontic retainers. *Am J Orthod* 71(4), 440–448.

Zachrisson BU (1985) Bonding in orthodontics. In Graber TM and Swain BF (eds) *Orthodontics: Current Principles and Techniques*, St Louis: Mosby-Year Book.

Zachrisson BU and Artun J (1979) Enamel surface appearance after various debonding techniques. *Am J Orthod* 75, 121.

Zachrisson BU and Brobakken BO (1978) Clinical comparison of direct versus indirect bonding with different bracket types and adhesives. *Am J Orthod* 74, 62.

Zachrisson BU, Buyukyilmaz T and Zachrisson YO (1995) Improving orthodontic bonding to silver amalgam. *Angle Orthod* 65(1), 35–42.

Zachrisson YO, Zachrisson BU and Buyukyilmaz T (1996) Surface preparation for orthodontic bonding to porcelain. *Am J Orthod* 109(4), 420–430.

10

Material-Related Adverse Reactions in Orthodontics

Dorthe Arenholt Bindslev, Gottfried Schmalz

Introduction

Unintended direct or indirect side effects of orthodontic treatment (e.g., root resorption, bone loss, white spot/caries lesions, dental hard tissue wear or cracking in relation to brackets and bands, discolourations, etc.) are well recognised and quite extensively described in the literature. Before the initiation of treatment, the orthodontic patient must be thoroughly informed and should have consented to the risks along with some degree of discomfort (Perry et al. 2021). Thus, since some degree of mechanically induced functional restrictions, discomfort and pain are recognised to be an experience for a major part of orthodontic patients (Zhou et al. 2014), material-related adverse reactions (toxic/allergic) to orthodontic appliances may – unless particularly severe – be misdiagnosed or go undetected.

Fixed appliances

Metals

Hypersensitivity – general epidemiology

A considerable number of metals are currently used in orthodontic appliances. Some provide strength, some contribute to 'elastic' properties, some are added to improve the resistance to corrosion and some may be used for aesthetic reasons. Although it is confirmed that ions of almost all metals present in orthodontic appliances can be released in the oral cavity and eventually further distributed in the body, nickel (Ni) was for many years the metal of prime biocompatibility concern in the orthodontic field. More recently, also cobalt (Co), chromium (Cr) and titanium (Ti) and a few others have gained increasing attention.

Ni is an allergen which can cause immediate or delayed hypersensitivity reactions. Ni has been found to be the most prevalent chemical contact allergen in the general population of the industrialised world (Ahlström et al. 2019; Alinaghi et al. 2019). The exposure can be through skin, mucous membranes, diet, inhalation or implants (Ahlström et al. 2019). The risk of developing Ni hypersensitivity is high in some industries and occupational settings, whereas for the general population, the risk has been attributed to the wide use of Ni-containing alloys, for example, jewellery, coins, tools, household utensils, cell phones, dental alloys and orthopaedic implants. The prevalences of Ni allergy in the European general population are approximately 8–19% in adults and 8–10% in children and adolescents, with a strong female predominance (Ahlström et al. 2019). A recent meta-analysis reported a prevalence of Ni allergy at 11.4% in the general population (Alinaghi et al. 2019). The relative high prevalence of Ni allergy in females has been attributed mainly to the wearing of Ni-containing alloys in fashion and lifestyle products. Regulations of permissible Ni levels in consumer products intended for intimate and prolonged skin contact appear to have reversed the trend, at least among the younger generations (Ahlström et al. 2017).

The prevalence of contact allergy to cobalt is reported to be 2.7% (3.3% among females and 2.1% for males), and for chromium 1.8% (equal for females and males) in the general population (Alinaghi et al. 2019).

The prevalence of Ti hypersensitivity is not established, but case reports and the fact that Ti alloys are increasingly used for medical implants have raised attention to the release of Ti ions from implants and the potential biocompatibility aspects of further distribution in the body (Fage et al. 2016; Comino-Garayoa et al. 2020).

History of atopy is recognised as having a bearing on irritant contact dermatitis. Contrary to previous opinions, recent evidence suggests that patients with atopic dermatitis may also have an increased risk of sensitisation to certain chemicals, especially those in their regular topical regimens as skincare products, and also to metals such as Ni (Borok et al. 2019).

Nickel applications in orthodontics

In orthodontics, Ni is one of the most commonly used metals, being a component of, for example, stainless steel and superelastic and shape-memory wires. Ni is incorporated in the composition of all austenitic stainless-steel alloys to stabilise the austenite phase. In comparison with the 8–12% Ni in stainless-steel formulations, the Ni content in Ni–titanium (Ni–Ti) and copper Ni–Ti (Cu–Ni–Ti) formulations amounts to 55–65%. The metal composition of archwires as well as brackets may vary slightly among brands (Brantley 2001; Eliades et al. 2001).

Release of nickel from dental alloys

Corrosion aspects laboratory studies

Leakage of metal ions from orthodontic appliances into the saliva is preceded by disintegration of the alloy either by corrosion or mechanical abrasion. Microscopy studies of orthodontic fixed appliances have shown that after 1 month intraoral wear, corrosion is present on all intraoral metal appliances (e.g., Houb-Dine et al. 2018; Velasco-Ibanez et al. 2020).

A number of studies have reported on metal ion release from dental alloys under various laboratory conditions (e.g., Kim and Johnson 1999; Khuta et al. 2009; Luft et al. 2009; Senkutvan et al. 2014; Houb-Dine et al. 2018). The clinical relevance of results obtained in vitro has, however, been questioned, and the lack of similarity with the clinical situation when using non-agitated, non-replenished artificial storage media has been emphasised (Eliades et al. 2002). Laboratory studies clearly demonstrate that physical factors such as surface structure, pH and the oxygen state at the material surface markedly influence the corrosiveness of dental alloys (Khuta et al. 2009; Luft et al. 2009; Martin-Camean et al. 2015). It is thus clear that the presence of passivating oxide films on the surface decreases the corrosion rate, while abrasion, polishing, low pH and high chloride content in the surrounding liquid contribute to the loss of these passivating films and subsequently increase the corrosiveness. Further, inhomogeneous soldered surfaces are more prone to corrosion; in particular, connecting points between different alloys are highly susceptible to corrosion (Eliades et al. 2002). In general, the corrosiveness of a dental alloy depends on several physical and environmental factors and is not directly proportional to, for example, the Ni content.

Due to the methodological limitations of laboratory corrosion models, in vitro results cannot be extrapolated directly to the clinical situation. From studies of retrieved orthodontic appliances, it is, however, evident that corrosion takes place during oral services (Figure 10.1) (see in the following text). Further, discolouration of the underlying bonding material and tooth surface during orthodontic treatment has been linked to corrosion in the crevices of the bracket bases (Maijer and Smith 1982; Eliades et al. 2001).

In general, most of the in vivo studies that have evaluated the release of metal ions from orthodontic appliances in biological fluids have concluded that the levels of released metal ions are well within the levels of average normal daily dietary intake (Martin-Camean et al. 2015).

In vitro studies have documented the cytotoxicity of Ni ions, which, for example, inhibit the proliferation of commonly used cell lines, however, in doses which are far beyond the concentration levels estimated to be released in vivo (for review, see Martin-Camean et al. 2015). On the other hand, Ni ions in clinically relevant doses influence the release of inflammation mediators from human oral

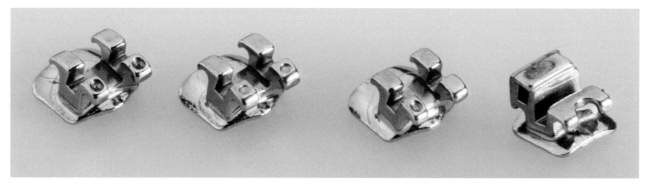

Fig. 10.1 Recycled brackets. Colour discrepancies indicate metallurgic changes compared with as-received brackets.

epithelial cells (Schmalz et al. 1997), activate monocytes and endothelial cells and suppress or promote the expression of intercellular adhesion molecules in endothelial cells (Noda et al. 2002; Wataha et al. 2002). The clinical significance of these observations is so far not clear (Martin-Camean et al. 2015).

Mini-implants for temporary extradental anchorage devices (TADs) have gained much attention in recent years and an increasing number of products with different compositions are available. The majority are made of Ti-6Al-4V alloy (titanium with small amounts of aluminium and vanadium to improve strength and fatigue resistance), and also stainless steel and unalloyed 'pure' titanium devices are available. The biocompatibility of TADs is influenced by a number of factors, such as the composition, the corrosivity, the surface characteristics and the time length of service in the individual patient. Biocompatibility studies on TADs are so far limited (e.g., Chen et al. 2019). In a rabbit model, low amounts of Ti, Al and V were detected in kidneys, liver and lungs after insertion of Ti-6Al-4V TADs (de Morais et al. 2009). The levels found were considered to be significantly below the levels observed with average dietary intake through food and drink and far from reaching toxic concentrations. Szuhanek et al. (2020) recently showed in two different in vitro tests that TADs may have different biocompatibility profiles depending on the composition. The study suggested that unalloyed pure titanium implants should be considered for Ni-sensitive patients rather than Ti alloys and stainless-steel brands.

Contradictory results from genotoxicity tests have been reported on an array of components of orthodontic appliances. Concern raised on the background of these assays has so far not been confirmed by more long-term biocompatibility studies (for review, see Martin-Camean et al. 2015).

Nickel in body fluid samples from orthodontic patients

Saliva

While the corrosion potential of orthodontic alloys has been studied quite intensively in vitro, less information exists on corrosion of orthodontic appliances in the oral cavity environment during orthodontic treatment. Corrosion products

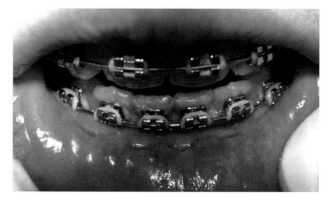

Fig. 10.2 Significant labial impression of a fixed appliance indicating intimate contact between the oral mucosa and the appliance.

may be taken up directly through the oral mucosa, which in orthodontic patients often presents a compromised barrier due to mechanical irritation (Figure 10.2) from intraoral appliances, or through the lining of the gastrointestinal tract.

The study of metal ion levels in saliva is complicated by the continuous release pattern of saliva. It is well known that factors such as temperature, quantity and quality of saliva, plaque, physical and chemical properties of food and liquids and oral health conditions may influence the results. Further, physiological variables, such as time of the day, general health conditions, diet and salivary flow rate, have significant impact. It is therefore generally recognised that large inter- and intra-individual variations are seen when analysing saliva samples for metal content. Despite the methodological limitations, a number of papers have reported on metal ion levels in saliva samples from orthodontic patients (Martin-Camean et al. 2015; Imani et al. 2019). Some studies have found that initial slightly elevated saliva levels of metal ions gradually decline during orthodontic treatment (e.g., Agaoglu et al. 2001; Petoumenou et al. 2009), while others have reported increasing levels of metal ions during the first months of treatment followed by fluctuating raised levels until some months after removal of appliance (Martin-Camean et al. 2015; Velasco-Ibanez et al. 2020). It has been hypothesised that a passivation layer might be formed on the metal surfaces in the oral environment, thereby decreasing the release of metal ions. Disturbance of the passivation layer may cause increased release of ions (Imani et al. 2019).

In general reports on this issue have confirmed the large inter- and intra-individual variations in the concentrations of metal ions in saliva sample studies. The limitations of saliva sampling and processing have been emphasised, and so far no definitive conclusions can be drawn regarding quantification of the range of metal ion release from orthodontic appliances in vivo, which, however, seems to be within that of daily intake through water and food (Eliades et al. 2003a; Martin-Camean et al. 2015).

Blood/serum/urine

Concern has repeatedly been raised that metal ions from intraoral alloys may be released to the saliva and once swallowed may accumulate in blood and organs. A few studies have attempted to elucidate whether metal ions from orthodontic appliances can be retrieved in blood or serum samples drawn from orthodontic patients. The results are conflicting. Some older studies could not find measurable amounts of Ni in blood samples taken before and after orthodontic treatment with full-mouth fixed appliances (e.g., Bishara et al. 1993), while more recent studies have found a statistically significant increase in the amount of Ni, Cr, Ti and zinc during orthodontic treatment (Agaoglu et al. 2001; Quadras et al. 2019; Velasco-Ibanez et al. 2020). The elevated metal ion levels reported are far below known toxic levels. Possible implications on the immune system are discussed, for example, Ni-induced T-lymphocyte production of cytokines may stimulate tissue proliferation and favour gingival hyperplasia (Pazzini et al. 2016).

A few studies found elevated urine Ni and Ti levels related to the fluctuations in the metal ion levels in saliva samples during orthodontic treatment (Menezes et al. 2007; Velasco-Ibanez et al. 2020). The biological significance of these findings is not known and more studies seem warranted.

Influencing clinical factors

Movement of archwires and friction between brackets, wires and ligatures may lead to corrosion-enhanced release of metal ions from fixed orthodontic appliances (Sifakakis & Eliades 2017).

Toothbrushing has been shown to increase elemental release from dental alloys, particularly from base-metal alloys and when toothpaste is used (Wataha et al. 2003). Although these studies did not include orthodontic alloys, it is of interest to the orthodontic field that brushing with toothpaste caused an almost universal increase of metal ions release, particularly from Ni-based alloys. The laboratory data cannot be directly extrapolated to the clinical situation. It has, however, been suggested that the use of low-abrasive toothpastes might be advisable when Ni-based alloys are

used. It has been hypothesised that the high Ni release from the Ni-based alloys might at least partially be due to the loss of protective surface oxides during brushing. Recent reviews have concluded that high fluoride concentrations, long exposures to fluoride ions and an acidic pH decrease the passivation layer and thereby the corrosion resistance also of Ni-free titanium alloys (Houb-Dine et al. 2018).

Recycling

Thermo-recycling of brackets may increase the release of metal ions substantially (Huang et al. 2004; Sfondrini et al. 2010). The higher ion release from recycled brackets has been attributed to the heating of the brackets, which is necessary to remove the bonding material. It has been hypothesised that the solder, porosity of the alloys and grain size of alloy constituents might have caused the differences observed between brands. Differences between wing and base materials and between brands have been reported (Eliades et al. 2003b). Ni loss initiated by corrosion and subsequent recycling may extend more than 5–10 μm below the surface (Eliades et al. 2002).

Nickel hypersensitivity – epidemiology in relation to orthodontics

Reviews concluded that studies on the epidemiology of Ni hypersensitivity among dental patients are sparse (e.g., Gölz et al. 2015; Ahlström et al. 2019). The existing literature however indicates that orthodontic treatment is not significantly associated with an increased risk of Ni hypersensitivity (Gölz et al. 2015). The frequency of diagnosed allergic reactions during orthodontic treatment is low, ranging between 0.03% and 0.3% (Schuster et al. 2004a; Volkman et al. 2007).

A German questionnaire survey of 68 orthodontic offices estimated the prevalence of perceived allergic reactions to be 1:430 (Schuster et al. 2004a). The majority of the reported reactions were extraoral (labial fissures, perioral inflammation and eczema on the face and extremities) and most often related to the use of a headgear. The relative few intraoral reactions comprised erythema, swelling and gingivitis. The perceived allergic reactions led to discontinuation of the orthodontic treatment in only 0.03% of the cases (1:3150). In 0.07% of the cases, the treatment plan and the appliances remained unchanged despite the observed reactions. In 0.13% (1:810) cases, the orthodontic appliances were replaced with those composed of Ni-free or low-Ni materials. In a later, similar American study, a prevalence of perceived Ni-related adverse reactions of 0.03% was reported (Volkman et al. 2007).

Clinical aspects of hypersensitivity reactions to metals in dental alloys

Nickel is capable of evoking both IgE-mediated (immediate type) and cell-mediated (delayed) contact allergic reactions. Particularly in the industrial setting, volatilisation of metals presents a respiratory occupational risk of type I hypersensitivity (e.g., urticaria, asthma, rhinoconjunctivitis, gastrointestinal involvement and anaphylaxis). In contrast to dust

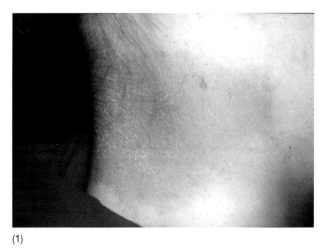

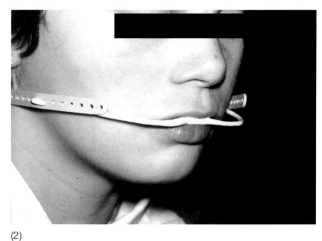

(1)   (2)

Fig. 10.3 Contact dermatitis adjacent to the stainless steel part of a headgear. (Courtesy of Professor A Hensten, University of Tromsø, Norway).

generated in, for example, mining and construction, highly dispersible and respirable aerosols may be formed during processes such as smelting and heating (Hostýnek 2002). The delayed-type hypersensitivity reaction generally presents as dermatitis, eczema and occasionally stomatitis. Dermatitis and urticaria, the primary manifestations of Ni hypersensitivity, are observed in the area of contact as well as at distant sites (secondary eruptions).

Quite a number of allergic reactions related to orthodontic alloys have been described in the literature and demonstrate the diversity of reactions Ni exposure may evoke in sensitised individuals.

Intraoral reactions

Intraoral verified allergic reactions to orthodontic alloys described in case reports have ranged from almost negligible, such as a slight erythema (e.g., Kolokitha and Chatzistavrou 2009), to large erythematous macular lesions or ulcerations (e.g., Veien et al. 1994; Counts et al. 2002) and subjective symptoms ranging from mild to very painful burning sensations compromising normal oral functions (Noble et al. 2008). It has been emphasised that symptoms of Ni hypersensitivity may in rare cases present as hygiene-resistant severe gingivitis (Counts et al. 2002; Pazzini et al. 2009, 2010, 2016). Recent reports suggest that rather than being an allergic reaction gingival hyperplasia may in sensitive individuals be triggered by cytokines released due to a local irritative reaction induced by, for example, Ni (Pazzini et al. 2016). In summary, reports on verified intraoral adverse reactions to Ni or other metals are very rare.

Extraoral reactions

Case reports on hypersensitivity reactions to intraoral Ni-containing orthodontic appliances reveal that in the vast majority of cases the lesions described were extraoral and not accompanied by any intraoral signs or symptoms of discomfort (e.g., Jacobsen and Hensten-Pettersen 2003; Kerusuo and Dahl 2007; Feilzer et al. 2008; Kolokitha and Chatzistavrou 2009). A number of reports have described skin lesions in direct contact with or adjacent to metal parts of headgears (Figure 10.3). Soreness, blisters and ulceration of the contacting skin areas were often seen (e.g., Jacobsen and Hensten-Pettersen 1989, 2003). Further eczematous lesions have, however, been noted in remote locations, for example, face, fingers, eyelids, arms, trunk and feet.

A considerable number of cases with onset or flaring of eczematous skin lesions in relation to insertion, change or activation of intraoral fixed orthodontic appliances have been reported. Very few of these were accompanied by intraoral complaints. Angular cheilitis and fissures of the lips or more severe perioral and facial eczema have frequently been described in relation to Ni-hypersensitive orthodontic patients (e.g., Feilzer et al. 2008; Ehrnrooth and Kerosuo

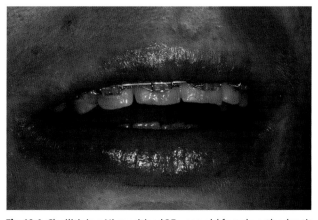

Fig. 10.4 Cheilitis in a Ni-sensitised 25-year-old female orthodontic patient with no intraoral symptoms. She tolerated the fixed orthodontic appliances without any skin reactions, except when Cu–Ni–Ti archwires were inserted.

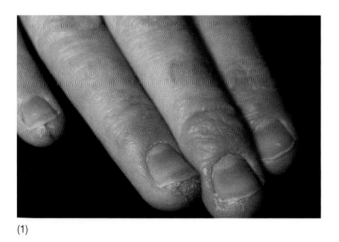 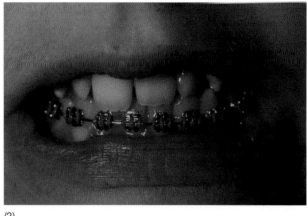

(1)   (2)

Fig. 10.5 Vesicular hand dermatitis following insertion of a fixed orthodontic appliance in a 15-year-old girl with no intraoral symptoms. Positive skin test on chromate. (Courtesy of Dr N Veien, Aalborg, Denmark.)

2009; Kolokitha and Chatzistavrou 2009; Silverberg et al. 2020) (Figure 10.4). More remote eczema lesions, for example, periorbitally, eyelids, ears, scalp, fingers, chest, back, arms and feet, have also been described (e.g., Veien et al. 1994; Bishara 1995; Ehrnrooth and Kerosuo 2009; Silverberg et al. 2020) (Figure 10.5). In a number of cases, it has been reported how the lesions flared up, for example, healed lesions being aggravated when the orthodontic appliance was manipulated (activating archwires or inserting new wires) (Jensen et al. 2003). A number of papers have reported that lesions aggravated when Ni–Ti wires were worn and improved when stainless-steel wires or titanium molybdenum (TMA) alloy wires were used as an alternative to Ni–Ti wires (e.g., Counts et al. 2002; Mancuso and Berdondini 2002; Schultz et al. 2004). Some striking remote reactions, probably secondary eruptions of previous lesions, have also been reported, for example, on the feet and trunk, in the absence of intraoral symptoms (Trombelli et al. 1992; Kerosuo and Kanerva 1997).

On the basis of the available case reports, it can be summarised that hypersensitivity reactions to intraoral orthodontic devices are relatively rare, and when they do occur, in the majority they manifest as extraoral eczematous lesions frequently in locations remote to the oral cavity. Unless particularly severe, such reactions may be misdiagnosed or may go undetected.

Hypersensitivity reactions to chromium, cobalt and titanium in dental alloys

Allergic contact dermatitis caused by chromate salts was first reported in 1925 and is still common. Hexavalent chromium compounds are considered the strongest sensitisers among the Cr ions. On the other hand, it is generally accepted that Cr itself does not act as a hapten, and is accordingly non-sensitising. It is important to emphasise this difference compared with, for example, Ni. Theoretically, sweat or plasma can transform metallic Cr into allergenic chromate

salts. Saliva may have a similar effect on intraoral devices containing Cr (Kanerva and Aitio 1997). It is often not clear whether chromates or other metals and metal salts have caused the allergic reactions elicited by dental alloys. Rare case reports describe patients with generalised eczematoid dermatitis following installation of dentures with metal framework (Pantuzo et al. 2007). Skin tests were strongly positive to Ni and Cr and the dermatitis subsided after discontinuing use of the denture. In most instances in which an allergic reaction is attributed to a metallic chrome object, Ni is the actual sensitiser. A rare case of dermatitis in an orthodontic patient who was allergic to chromate, and negative on patch testing to Ni, has also been described (Veien et al. 1994) (Figure 10.6). The dermatitis appeared shortly after installation of a stainless-steel orthodontic appliance and cleared when the appliance was removed. Rare cases of systemic contact dermatitis from chromate in dental cast crowns have also been reported (Guimaraens et al. 1994).

Hypersensitivity reactions to Co in dental materials are very rare (Vamnes et al. 2004; Mittermüller et al. 2018). Cobalt hypersensitivity may appear together with Ni and/or Cr allergy, but may also be solitary (Duarte et al. 2018). The prevalence of contact allergy to Co in the general population is around 2.5% (Alinaghi et al. 2019; Duarte et al. 2018).

As mentioned in the earlier text, the prevalence of Ti hypersensitivity has not been established and is presently regarded very rare. Standardisation of reliable test regimes for Ti-hypersensitivity is lacking (Fage et al. 2016; Comino-Garayoa et al. 2020). Ti ions are released in the presence of biological fluids and tissue under certain circumstances, in which context dental implants have raised concern due to the communication to the oral cavity environment (e.g., Fage et al. 2016; Comino-Garayoa et al. 2020). A recent study on a group of orthodontic patients described self-reported symptoms to perceived Ti allergy (Zigante et al. 2020). No common pattern of symptoms could be found. The current literature suggests that with the rapidly growing demand for

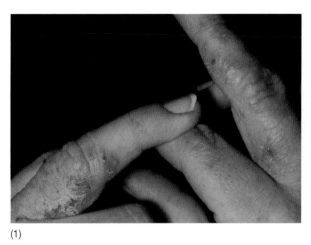
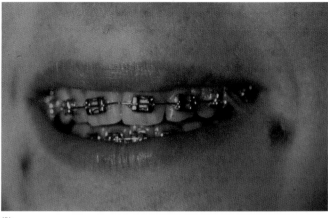

(1)   (2)

Fig. 10.6 Vesicular hand dermatitis which developed some months after insertion of a fixed orthodontic appliance in a 13-year-old girl with no intraoral symptoms. The oral challenge test on Ni was positive. (Courtesy of Dr N Veien, Aalborg, Denmark.)

insertion of medical implants, more knowledge is needed to elucidate the possible importance of hypersensitivity reactions to Ti, impurities in 'pure' Ti and to Ti alloys (e.g., Fage et al. 2016; Comino-Garayoa et al. 2020).

The possible role of oral exposure (orthodontic devices) in preventing sensitisation to nickel

There seems to be increasing evidence that long-term oral exposure to low levels of Ni substantially reduces the prevalence of hypersensitivity on later challenge. Van der Burg et al. (1986) at the first, in a prospective study of hairdressers and nurses, showed that individuals who in childhood had worn some kind of intraoral Ni-containing appliance had a markedly lower incidence of Ni allergy than those who had not had orthodontic treatment. A number of later studies have followed cohorts of adolescents from the onset of orthodontic treatment and confirmed that early oral exposure to Ni-releasing appliances may induce a state of tolerance to Ni (e.g., Todd and Burrows 1989; van Hoogstraten et al. 1991, 1992; Kerosuo et al. 1996; Lindsten and Kurol 1997; Mortz et al. 2002). Reviews have recently concluded that there is a significantly lower risk of developing Ni hypersensitivity when orthodontic treatment preceded piercing than when orthodontic treatment occurred after piercing (Gölz et al. 2015). The American Academy of Paediatrics in a recent policy statement recommended that 'If orthodontic metal braces are anticipated, families should consider delaying ear piercing until after dental work is completed' (Silverberg et al. 2020).

Summary and recommendations, including nickel-free alternatives

According to the available literature, there is no evidence for a risk of primary sensitisation through exposure to intraoral dental alloys, including orthodontic appliances (Kolokitha

et al. 2008; Gölz et al. 2015). Furthermore, patients with diagnostic tests verifying presence of Ni allergy do not necessarily experience adverse intraoral reactions on exposure to Ni-containing dental alloys (Jensen et al. 2003).

Although the vast majority of orthodontic patients – including those with a positive skin patch test to Ni – tolerate the wearing of conventional orthodontic appliances without material-related adverse reactions, there may – as described in the earlier text – be some hypersensitive Ni-allergic patients in whom appliances with high content of Ni (e.g., Cu–Ni–Ti wires) should be avoided. A number of these patients may tolerate stainless-steel appliances. In a few cases, it may, however, be necessary to completely avoid Ni-containing alloys. Alternative products that are Ni-free or have a very low Ni content are available. Different types of coatings reduce the release of metal ions and the adhesion of bacteria by reducing the friction and corrosion. Ni-free wires of TMA or pure titanium, or gold-plated wires, as well as plastic-/resin-coated Ni–Ti archwires with less corrosion potential may be considered. Brackets are available in different ceramic forms, as well as polycarbonate, titanium or even gold plated. It seems justified to recommend that thermo-recycled brackets should not be used in patients with a known allergy to Ni or other metals that may be present in the bracket alloy.

Headgears without extraoral metal components are available; they have plastic studs or plastic-coated metallic studs. The successful use of cast titanium framework for rapid palatal expansion devices and activators for Ni-sensitive patients has been described as case stories (e.g., Maspero et al. 2018).

Increasing efforts are presently focused on improving coating techniques as well as modifying the archwire composition in order to reduce the release of metal ions, reduce friction and minimise bacterial adhesion (Bacela et al. 2020).

Bonding and cementation materials

Optimal material selection and application require an understanding of the chemical differences between and the physical limitations of today's orthodontic bonding and cementation materials. Such materials comprise today a number of material categories, for example, cements (zinc phosphate, polycarboxylate, glass ionomer cements (GICs), etc.), resins, resin-modified glass ionomers and polyacid-modified composite resins. Unfortunately, the information on material composition required by legal regulations (e.g., safety data sheets) is so far limited (Michelsen et al. 2003; van Landuyt et al. 2011), and recent research has documented that numerous non-declared substances of potential harmful nature may be released from, for example, resin-based dental materials (Arenholt-Bindslev et al. 2009; Pelourde et al. 2018). The new EU Medical Devices Regulation (European Commission 2017) coming into force in 2021 may somewhat improve the situation. It specifies that the overall qualitative composition of such materials and quantitative information on the main constituent or constituents responsible for achieving the principal intended action must be provided. Especially, CMR (carcinogenic, mutagenic and reprotoxic) components and endocrine-disrupting substances down to 0.1% must be declared. ISO 4049-Polymer-based Restorative Materials (ISO 2019) require the declaration of components present in the material of ≥1% by mass (irrespective of hazard potential) and any CMR ingredient of ≥0.1% by mass.

Composition, degradation/release

Zinc phosphate cement

This is the reaction product of zinc oxide and a phosphoric acid solution. Some brands further contain around 10% fluoride in the form of stannous fluoride. Apart from the acidity of the phosphoric acid solution, the hazardous potential of these materials is limited, and when used according to the manufacturer's instructions, practically no material-related adverse reactions are relevant according to the literature.

Polycarboxylate cement

This is the reaction product of zinc oxide and a polycarboxylic acid solution. Fluoride salts may be added for anticariogenic purposes. There are no reports on material-related side effects when used according to the instruction manual.

Glass ionomer cements

These consist of calcium fluoroaluminosilicate glass particles, which when mixed with polyacrylic acid undergo an acid–base reaction to form polycarboxylate salts that comprise the cement matrix. No reports of side effects of conventional GICs are available in the literature when used as band cementation material.

Resin-modified GICs and polyacid-modified composite resins (compomers)

Both material categories contain a cement and a resin component, of which mainly the resin part is of interest with regard to biocompatibility. Resin-modified GICs contain ion-releasing glass particles, water-soluble polyacrylic acids and hydrophilic monomers such as hydroxyethyl methacrylate (HEMA) and specific catalysts which allow for light-curing. Compomers were developed in an attempt to combine the fluoride release of GICs with the mechanical properties of composite resins. These materials are composed of ion-releasing glass particles and a polymerisable organic matrix. In addition to conventional monomers, the organic matrix of compomers may contain bi-functional monomers which can react with methacrylates by radical polymerisation and by acid–base reaction to bring about release of ions from glass in the presence of water. Biological effects of these materials are mainly related to the resin phase (see in the following text).

Adhesive resins

These consist of a mixture of monomers, mainly methacrylates (e.g., bisphenol-A-glycidyl dimethacrylate (Bis-GMA), urethane dimethacrylate (UDMA), triethylene glycol dimethacrylate (TEGDMA), / ethylene glycol dimethacrylate (EGDMA) or HEMA), that vary from brand to brand. Based on the polymerisation-initiation mechanism, adhesive resins can be grouped as chemically activated (two-paste), light-cured or dual-cured (chemically activated and light-cured). Additives normally amount to 1–2% of the adhesive resins and the chemical substances added vary according to brand and the type of polymerisation process they initiate and modulate. Filler particles are usually added. These resins are generally applied after etching the enamel with, for example, a 38% phosphoric acid gel. Self-etch resins are less commonly used for bonding brackets, due to the reduced bond strength to enamel. Furthermore, light-curing units (LCUs) are needed for resin polymerisation and presently mainly LED LCUs with a radiant exitance (mW/cm^2) normally between 1000 and 2000 mW/cm^2 are used emitting mainly blue light (between 400 and 500 nm).

Local and systemic toxicity of resin-/polymer-based materials (resin-modified GICs, compomers and adhesive resins)

Common to all resin-/polymer-containing dental materials is incomplete conversion during polymerisation of the resin part, especially when used under metallic brackets. A significant amount of constituents remain unbound in the cured material. Conversion rates within the range of 35–77% have been reported (Fujioka-Kobayashi et al. 2019). Several studies have documented that numerous substances with known harmful potential (e.g., cytotoxic, allergenic, mutagenic and hormone-like effects) can be eluted from resin-based dental materials (van Landuyt et al. 2011). Further, unwanted degradation products, for example, formaldehyde, may over several weeks be released into the oral cavity in clinically relevant concentrations (Oysaed et al. 1988; Ruyter 1995; van Landuyt et al. 2011) and also from certain polymer-based bracket products (polyoxymethylene) (Kusy and Whitley 2005).

A number of studies have specifically documented the cytotoxic and local irritative potential of orthodontic adhesive resins (Huang et al. 2008; Jagdish et al. 2009; Taubmann et al. 2020). The irradiation procedure used for polymerisation of light-curing bonding materials significantly influences the amount of substances leaching from the cured material, and it has been suggested that insufficient available light intensity results in a lower conversion rate and a subsequent increased leaching of unbound substances (Purushothaman et al. 2015). The highest amount of residual monomers was eluted from the chemically cured adhesives. Mixing the base and catalyst pastes has been shown to increase the bulk porosity, which may contribute to increased oxygen inhibition of polymerisation and increased potential for monomer leaching (Eliades et al. 1995; Eliades and Eliades 2001). Also, the longer setting time of chemically cured adhesives may result in increased oxygen inhibition, thus contributing to elevated amounts of monomer elution (Eliades et al. 1995).

Recently, the hazards for patients and dental personnel from intraorally generated nanoparticles, for example, when removing resinous materials have been addressed (van Landuyt et al. 2012). However, the use of copious water spray and high-volume suctions when intraorally grinding resinous materials reduces the risk significantly (Schmalz et al. 2017). Today, the commonly used face masks further reduce the health risks for the dental personnel.

The clinical implications of the harmful potential of the currently available resin-based dental materials are yet to be clarified. So far, it has been documented that due to the variability in composition, the biocompatibility profile of products may vary. Since, however, the biologically relevant constituents (e.g., Bis-GMA, UDMA, TEGDMA or HEMA) and a number of general processes are common for a vast number of materials, including the orthodontic bonding materials, general biocompatibility aspects are shared by the majority of the resin-based products. In vitro studies have shown that shortly after polymerisation the components of resin-based materials may be released in concentrations sufficiently high to cause local irritative mucosa reactions (van Landuyt et al. 2011) (Figure 10.7). Such reactions may be assumed to be short-lasting, as the elution for most leachables declines over time. Since, however, very few case reports are available on this topic, irritative reactions – from a theoretical point of view – seem to be underreported, which may be explained by the low severity but also differential diagnostic aspects. So far,

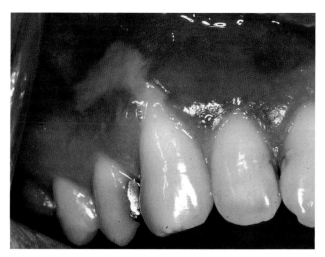

Fig. 10.7 Local irritative mucosa reaction adjacent to 13, which had received a gingival composite restoration 24 hours earlier.

few studies have estimated the amount of substances released following bonding of a full-mouth orthodontic appliance and the results are not directly applicable to the clinical situation (Eliades et al. 1995; Kloukos et al. 2015). Although a single intraorally exposed surface of bonding material is relatively low, the total amount of material and primers inserted in the patient during the bonding procedure for a full-mouth orthodontic appliance is considerably higher than that used for a single or few dental fillings. Further, the resinous component of orthodontic bonding materials is considerably higher than that of dental restoratives, which contain up to 60–80% by weight inorganic filler particles to improve mechanical properties. It can be concluded that at present the total amount of leachable substances to which an orthodontic patient is exposed to during and after bonding of a full-mouth fixed appliance is unknown.

As has been delineated in the earlier text, phosphoric acid gel is generally used for enamel etching before resin application. These preparations may cause eye damage and they are skin-corrosive (Figure 10.8). Therefore, inadvertent spilling of the phosphoric acid gel may lead to skin, eye or soft-tissue damage, and thus these substances should be handled carefully, especially when removing the gel by using cotton wool followed by water spray and high-volume suction. The patient should wear protective glasses and a bib. Also, care should always be taken not to pass any instruments or materials over the patient's face (Evans et al. 2014; Steele et al. 2014).

LCUs may cause intraoral soft-tissue burns after incorrect application (Spranley et al. 2012). Also, eye damage ('blue-light hazard') – mainly for dental personnel – has been addressed (Fluent et al. 2019). The use of protective shields is highly emphasised.

Bisphenol A (BPA), which is a widely used chemical in industry, has been shown to be released e.g. from Bis-GMA-based composite resin filling and bonding such materials

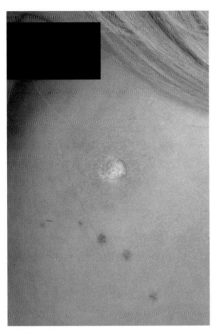

Fig. 10.8 Chemical burn on the left cheek of a 13-year old girl one day following an untended spill of a drop of acid etch gel while bonding orthodontic brackets. As soon as the patient noticed the pain caused by the spill the skin area was rinsed thoroughly with running water for several minutes. The next day the skin lesion was evident, now surrounded by erythema. After a healing period the girl was left with a small scar.

used in restorative dentistry and also from orthodontic bonding materials in both in vitro and in vivo experiments (review by Halimi et al. 2016). The amounts of released BPA were dependent upon the quality of polymerisation, and are generally very low. If properly cured, released BPA quantities were well below the temporary tolerable daily intake (TDI) as set by the European Food Safety Authority (EFSA 2015) of 4 µg/kg bw (body weight) and not detectable after a few days anymore. In a more recent study from 2018, BPA release from orthodontic bonding materials was slightly elevated directly after curing, but not statistically significantly different from the control (Becher et al. 2018). While BPA is not used as an ingredient in materials for bonding, it is needed in the manufacturing process of the respective monomers and thus may be present as impurity. BPA is classified by the WHO (2009) as endocrine disruptor and exhibits a weak estrogenic activity. In animal studies, adverse health effects have been associated with BPA, such as effects on hormonal activity, asthma, diabetes, obesity, behavioural changes, cancer, infertility and genital malformations. However, clinical evidence is inconsistent (Becher et al. 2018). In some studies, mineralisation defects in enamel were observed in male rats after orally administering 5 µg/kg bw BPA (Jedeon et al. 2013, 2014). However, BPA metabolism in rats is different from humans, and the Scientific Committee on Emerging and Newly Identified Health Risks (SCENIHR) (European Commission

2015) concluded that long-term oral exposure to BPA via dental materials is below the temporary TDI of 4 µg/kg bw/ day, thus posing a negligible risk for human health. However, this topic is still under discussion, because for hormone-like substances even at very low concentrations, specific biologic effects are claimed due to their specific interaction with respective cell receptors, which may result in a so-called biphasic dose–response relationship (Mandrup et al. 2016). Furthermore, the EFSA limit value of 4 µg/kg bw is named 'temporarily' due to these unsolved problems (Becher et al. 2018) and therefore the discussion is still ongoing. Very recently (2022) EFSA has proposed to reduce the 2015 limit value for BPA by a factor of 100 000. This may require a new risk assessment also for respective dental resin materials. Still, BPA release from orthodontic bonding materials is very low and only transitory.

Hypersensitivity reactions to resin-based materials

Several reports of the increasing prevalence of allergic reactions because of occupational exposure have clearly emphasised the sensitisation potential of resin-based dental materials (Schmalz and Arenholt-Bindslev 2009; Sananez et al. 2020) (Figures 10.9 and 10.10).

HEMA, TEGDMA, Bis-GMA and UDMA are common allergens (Bishop and Roberts 2020). In the non-dental field (e.g., 'nail industry workers'), HEMA was found to be a common occupational allergen. A 14-year retrospective study of dental technicians also showed HEMA (beside other acrylates) being the predominant allergen (Heratizadeh et al. 2018). In Finland, dentists have been

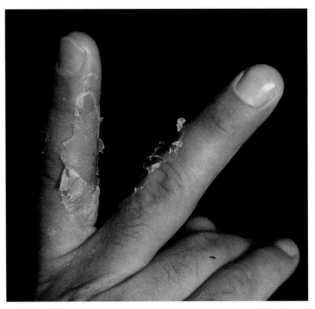

Fig. 10.9 Occupational allergic contact dermatitis caused by dental methacrylates in a 40-year-old male dentist.

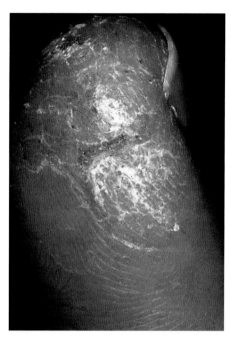

Fig. 10.10 Occupational allergic contact dermatitis caused by dental methacrylates in a 56-year-old male dentist.

reported to be the profession at highest risk of developing occupational allergic contact dermatitis, and dental nurses have the fourth greatest risk (Kanerva et al. 1999). Methacrylate constituents of dental resin-based materials present the most frequently observed causative factor among dentists (Kanerva et al. 1999). In Sweden, 174 persons from the dental profession were referred to an occupational dermatology department in the period 1995–1998 because of hand eczema (Wrangsjo et al. 2001). Twenty-two per cent of the group had positive patch-test reactions to (meth)acrylates (Wrangsjo et al. 2001). Subsequent papers have reported an increasing incidence of occupational asthma and rhinoconjunctivitis caused by dental acrylics, and increasing attention is being paid to the issue (Bishop and Roberts 2020). Also students, who have reported itchy, red skin lesions underneath the area where they placed uncured adhesive resin on a nitrile-gloved hand, were patch-tested positive to HEMA (Sananez et al. 2020).

Few investigations have focused specifically on occupational problems in the orthodontic field (Jacobsen and Hensten-Pettersen 1989, 2003; Kerosuo et al. 2000). Kerosuo et al. (2000) conducted a questionnaire survey on occupational problems among members of the Finnish Orthodontic Society, of whom 72% responded. Forty-two per cent of the respondents reported hand dermatoses (e.g., redness, itching, chapping, etc.). Occupation-related respiratory problems were reported by 28% of the orthodontists. Cough, a blocked or runny nose, bronchitis and difficulties in breathing were the most common complaints. Sixty-three per cent of the individuals with respiratory symptoms attributed the reaction to dry air in

the clinic, whereas 17% assumed the handling of a specific dental material to be the causative factor. Dental materials were considered to cause symptoms by 21.5% of the total group of general practitioners and orthodontists. Methacrylates and latex gloves were the two most commonly reported causes for symptoms. The adverse effects of acrylics were attributed both to the monomer during the handling process of the material and to the acrylic dust generated during grinding of acrylic appliances. In one case, merely being present in the room where dental composites or acrylics had been handled induced a respiratory reaction (Kerosuo et al. 2000).

In another survey (Jacobsen and Hensten-Pettersen 2003) of occupational problems in 121 Norwegian orthodontists who took part in the previous survey (Jacobsen and Hensten-Pettersen 1989), the number of dermatoses had decreased significantly from 40.1% to 17.4%. The decrease was assumed to be caused by the increased awareness of protective measures. Eight per cent of the subjects with dermatoses attributed their symptoms to the handling of composites and acrylics. Five orthodontists reported respiratory/ systemic and eye reactions related to chemical factors. Two of these reactions were caused by the dust generated while grinding acrylic work.

Further, one case report described severe skin problems in a 48-year-old female orthodontic assistant (Hamann et al. 2003). For 10 years she had redness, itching and pustules on both hands, as well as cracked and fissured fingertips. While on disability leave she had experienced complete healing of the skin on her hands. She also tested positive for sensitisation to three methacrylates commonly used in orthodontic bonding materials. By following careful protective working routines such as adopting non-touch routines in relation to bonding materials, she was later able to continue her work as an orthodontic assistant.

So far, there have been relatively few reports on allergic reactions to dental resins in dental patients (Arenholt-Bindslev et al. 2009). An extensive study investigating 500 patients (Mittermüller et al. 2018), who claimed adverse reactions from dental materials, included 416 patients with patch-test results for verification of suspected allergies. Two hundred and thirty four patients had a positive test to one or more compounds of the European standard series including substances relevant to dentistry. However, only 70 patients showed a clinically relevant positive patch-test reaction with clinical symptoms and the positively tested material/component intraorally present. Metals (e.g., Ni, palladium, Co, etc.) were found to be the main allergens followed at much lower frequencies by acrylates such as EGDMA, methyl methacrylate (MMA) or TEGDMA (Mittermüller et al. 2018).

Verified allergic reactions have been observed as intraoral lesions red/white/lichenoid; edema, for example, of lips; facial exanthema; urticaria; asthma-like symptoms and very seldom anaphylactic reactions (Goncalves et al. 2006;

Arenholt-Bindslev et al. 2009; Mittermüller et al. 2018). Very few of the available case reports were related to reactions to orthodontic materials (Hutchinson 1994; Barber et al. 2018). The general society is facing an increasing and widespread exposure to acrylics identical or structurally related to those applied in dentistry, and cross-reactivity has been reported between a great number of methacrylates and acrylates, including those used in dentistry (Kanerva 2001). These facts seem to present a risk that an increasing number of allergic reactions to methacrylates and acrylates can be expected in the future. At present an increasing number of sensitisations and allergic reactions to (meth)acrylates have been presented in relation to non-dental handling of acrylates, for example, in printing industry, and in relation to artificial nail-sculpturing procedures (Arenholt-Bindslev et al. 2009; Bishop and Roberts 2020).

Recommendations

Many orthodontic bonding materials have been rapidly introduced and withdrawn from the market in the past few decades. The orthodontist should be sceptical and request sufficient documentation to be able to select and handle the materials optimally. Due to the well-documented sensitisation potential of constituents of resin-based bonding materials, these materials should be handled with utmost care and any skin contact should be avoided ('no-touch technique'). Disposable (latex and nitrile) gloves offer none or a very limited barrier (Munksgaard 1992; Baumann et al. 2000; Bishop and Roberts 2020; Sananez et al. 2020). Exposure to grinding dusts and aerosols should also be avoided by using sufficient water spray and high-volume suction (Schmalz et al. 2017).

Allergic reactions may be evoked by very low concentrations of released substances from adhesive resins, and so far the information provided by the manufacturer on material composition was regarded to be not sufficient (Bishop and Roberts 2020). The recently extended requirements for manufacturers to declare materials composition are an improvement (see in the earlier text); however, it is yet unclear to which extent allergic reaction can now better be prevented (Bishop and Roberts 2020). Patients' allergic reactions to resin-based dental materials fortunately seem to be rare, but do occur, and may manifest as a wide range of symptoms. In cases of a suspected allergic reaction, the patient should be investigated by a specialist.

Removable appliances

Acrylic base plates and activators

Mucosal reactions are not rare in relation to acrylic appliances (Wishney 2017) and symptoms such as erythema, ulcerations, lichenoid reactions, papules and cheilitis have been described (Vilaplana and Romaguera 2000). It may, however, be a challenge to find out the direct cause of the reaction, which can be

mechanical, microbial, irritative/toxic or allergic (Figure 10.11). Polymethylmethacrylate (PMMA) materials for removable appliances are cured from MMA by activation with heat or by chemical activation using, for example, dimethyl-*p*-toluidine/benzoyl peroxide. Microwave-activated PMMA polymerisation is also used. The composition of light-polymerised denture base resins may vary between products. They are mainly based on the family of dimethacrylates also found in, for example, dental composites, adhesives and orthodontic bonding materials (see in the earlier text). The conversion of MMA to PMMA is not complete and the cured material thus consists of the remaining part of polymer beads from the original powder embedded in an interstitial matrix of newly formed polymer. These materials also include additives such as plasticisers, inhibitors, catalysts and fillers.

Leaching of organic compounds as well as chemical additives and degradation products has been demonstrated from heat-, light- and cold-cured (chemically activated) dental PMMA, for example, MMA, formaldehyde, methacrylic acid, benzoic acid, di-butylphthalate, biphenyl, phenyl benzoate (PB) and phenyl salicylate (PS) (Lygre et al. 1994, 1995; Kopperud et al. 2011). The residual monomer content of PMMA has been determined in a number of studies, which concluded that the degree of polymerisation caused by chemical or light activation is not as high as that produced by heat activation. Subsequently less residual monomer is found in heat-cured PMMA than in chemically or light-cured PMMA, and more MMA is released from chemically or light-cured PMMA than by heat-cured materials (Lygre et al. 1994, 1995).

The polymer to monomer ratio has also been shown to influence the leakage from the cured material; a higher proportion of monomer in the initial mixture results in significantly higher levels of residual monomer as compared with those prepared with a lower monomer ratio (Lamb et al. 1983; Kedjarune et al. 1999).

Baker et al. (1988) found MMA in the saliva of orthodontic patients for up to 1 week after insertion of cold-cured appliances, with a fourfold higher concentration in the salivary film on the fitting surface of the appliance compared with whole saliva. No MMA was detected in blood or urine. This was confirmed in a later study showing that

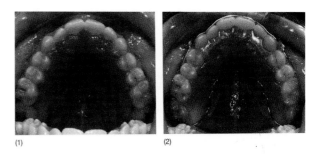

(1)   (2)

Fig. 10.11 Erythematous reaction on the palatal mucosa contacting a removable orthodontic appliance. The reaction was irritative, but mimicked an allergic reaction.

methylmethacrylate from PMMA is released into saliva mainly during the first day after incorporation and then it significantly decreases (Singh et al. 2013). Lygre et al. (1994) found organic compounds and traces of phenyl benzoate (an irritative/toxic agent; probably a degradation product from the initiator benzoyl peroxide) and phenyl salicylate (a known allergen; usually added to plastic as a light absorber) in saliva samples from patients wearing orthodontic cold-cured methacrylate appliances processed by the powdering technique. In 35% of the patients, mucosal reactions were seen beneath the appliances. The study concluded that the powdering technique for processing of cold-cured orthodontic resins seems to give significantly higher quantities of leaching compounds than a pre-mix technique. Also, the residual MMA content was found higher in specimens which were prepared with doughing method compared to the spray-on method (Iça et al. 2014).

According to the release pattern, auto-polymerised resins were more cytotoxic than heat-polymerised materials (Goiato et al. 2015). Therefore, it has been suggested that auto-polymerised PMMA should be heat-treated to decrease cytotoxic effects (Jorge et al. 2003). In line with the variation in product composition, several studies have shown that these materials have different levels of cytotoxicity according to brand (Barron et al. 1993; Schuster et al. 1995) and that the leakage of cytotoxic substances may have prolonged toxic effects on cells (Lindsten and Kurol 1997). Residual monomer, resulting from incomplete conversion of monomers into polymers, and chemical additives released from PMMAs have the potential to cause irritation, inflammation and allergic reactions in the oral mucosa (Lind 1988; Arenholt-Bindslev et al. 2009; Geurtsen 2009; Pituru 2020).

An in vivo study showed that monomers from an Andresen activator may lead to DNA damages in the buccal mucosa epithelial cells (Faccioni et al. 2019). However, the clinical relevance was challenged (Souza et al. 2019) and these effects may no longer be detected after removing the appliances as was shown for metallic appliances (Martin-Camean et al. 2015), and thus more studies are necessary for confirmation.

According to their composition and leakage potential, it can be assumed that light-polymerised denture base materials present an adverse risk profile similar to composite resin filling and bonding materials. So far, no reports on adverse patients' reactions related to orthodontic treatment using these materials have appeared.

Recommendations

Several studies on leachables from PMMAs have suggested that the amount of leachables released is highest during the first 24 hours (Kopperud et al. 2011; Iça et al. 2014), and therefore it is recommended that for minimising release of potentially irritative/allergenic substances, particularly cold-cured/light-polymerised appliances should be immersed for at least 24 hours in water before insertion.

Soft retainers and trainers

Soft orthodontic removable appliances are used for different applications, for example, positioners, retainers and so-called 'trainers'. The popularity of this type of appliance may vary considerably among practitioners. It has been reported that in Finland (around four million inhabitants) approximately 20,000 children use a soft trainer (European Commission 2002). Soft appliances can be made of a variety of materials, for example, polyvinyl chloride (PVC), polyurethane, silicone, ethylencopolymer, etc. PVC-based soft devices contain plasticisers/softeners, of which the most widely used is diethylhexylphthalate (DEHP). During the past decade, increasing concern has emerged about a number of plasticisers, particularly DEHP and other phthalates because of the evidence of their hormone-like characteristics (estrogen-like). Phthalates are found in most PVC products, including soft-squeeze children toys. In a number of countries, DEHP of more than 0.1% is no longer allowed in children's products intended for mouthing, such as teethers, pacifiers and toys for small children (European Commission 2018). Additional to the use as plasticisers in PVC products, phthalates are widely used in, for example, cosmetics, but have also been forbidden (European Commission 2009). Estrogen-like substances such as phthalates or BPA (see in the earlier text) are suspected to play a role in the increasing adverse reproductive health outcomes observed in a number of industrialised countries (European Commission 2016). Reproductive and developmental toxicity of phthalates has been documented in a number of experimental animal models, and wildlife observations support these results. The general public is exposed to estrogen-like substances including phthalates from a vast number of sources, including medical sources. A number of national and international authorities have reviewed the aspects of human exposure to phthalates, particularly DEHP, from medical devices, and extensive reports have been issued (European Commission 2016). The reports reviewed the available knowledge in relation to a great number of medical applications, most importantly intravenous storage bags, infusion sets and all kinds of catheters and tubes, and also dental applications in the form of soft orthodontic appliances (European Commission 2016). It was generally concluded that children, both prenatally and postnatally, are at greater risk of developing adverse effects of DEHP and that the limited but suggestive human exposure data indicate that there may be a dose-dependent association between exposure to these substances and adverse effects on male reproductive tract development (European Commission 2016). DEHP was also suspected to be responsible for precocious puberty of females (Wen et al. 2015). In the new Medical Devices Regulation (European Commission 2017), which is in force since May 2021, the use of phthalates of more than 0.1% must be justified (European Commission 2019) and declared in the labelling information.

The content of phthalates in soft orthodontic PVC-based retainers is not known so far, but might have, according to unpublished data, amounted to 30–40%. In relation to the dental application of DEHP releasing devices, the European Union report further states that autocuring or light-curing methylmethacrylate used in orthodontics may contain 6–8% phthalates (European Commission 2002). Since alternatives are available, reservations were expressed as to the use of DEHP-releasing products in children for orthodontic appliances, which may be worn several hours per day in close mucosal contact and released DEHP being readily absorbed in the gastrointestinal tract. The review concluded that although there are no reports concerning any adverse effects in humans following exposure to DEHP PVC, even in neonates or other groups of relatively high exposure, the use of these products should be considered very carefully and only accepted if the balance between benefits and risk can be justified (European Commission 2002). There are so far no papers reporting on the detailed contents of orthodontic soft removable appliances.

It had been reported that temporary denture soft-lining materials may contain up to around 50% phthalates, which readily leach from the material within a short period (30 days). For two of the materials, the average amount of leached phthalates within the first day exceeded the proposed TDI by about 11 and 32 times, respectively, for an average adult person (Munksgaard 2004). Calculations based on 30-day release data showed a daily leached average amount of plasticisers, which for one material amounted to 6.6 times the TDI. Further, it has been documented that dibutyl phthalate is released from denture base material and can be retrieved in small amounts in saliva collected from patients wearing new dentures (Lygre et al. 1993). The data from denture-release studies cannot be extrapolated to the orthodontic situation, since the products do not have identical compositions. So far, none of the published studies on the release of substances from orthodontic methacrylate-based devices have focused on the release of DEHP.

In contrast with denture base materials and denture liners, soft orthodontic appliances are mostly used in children who are more susceptible to adverse effects of hormone-like substances than elderly patients. Based on the available literature, it can be concluded that this orthodontic issue needs further elucidation.

Also, bisphenol A (see in the earlier text) has been shown to be released in vitro from a series of orthodontic materials used, for example, for retainers. After vigorous mechanical treatment and thermocycling, quantifiable amounts of leached BPA were observed from one thermoformed orthodontic retainer material within the first 3 days of artificial saliva immersion (Kotyk and Wiltshire 2014), later no BPA was detectable. Other tested materials for retainers did not release any BPA. Quantities of leached BPA were below the temporary TDI of 4 µg/kg bw (European Food Safety Authority 2015). In a clinical study, BPA was released into saliva from removable Hawley retainers (containing polypropylene/ethylene copolymer); the released amount decreased over a week (Raghavan et al. 2017). Other

heat- and chemical-cured materials (containing methacrylates) released less BPA, especially when heat-cured. The authors report that the amount of BPA leached is extremely low compared with temporary tolerable daily intake of 4 µg/kg bw. Cell-culture studies on estrogenic properties of a clear thermoplastic polyurethane retainer displayed no estrogenic activity in vitro (Al Naqbi et al. 2018). As was delineated in the earlier text, BPA release is product-specific. The amount released is low and after a couple of days not detectable anymore.

Recommendations

In cases where the use of soft orthodontic appliances is relevant, orthodontists should request adequate information from the supplier to be able to evaluate the material composition carefully, which is in line with the new EU legislation (European Commission 2017). Since appropriate alternatives are available, a product documenting no release of hormone-like substances is preferred. Based on evidence from release studies on similar but not identical materials, it is recommended to let the soft appliances soak in water for at least 24 hours before being inserted in the patient (Figure 10.12).

Aligners

The use of so-called aligners for tooth correction has increased significantly during recent years. As for other treatment modalities in orthodontics (e.g., see in the earlier text), thermoplastic materials are also used for aligners. They are composed of polyurethane and together with other

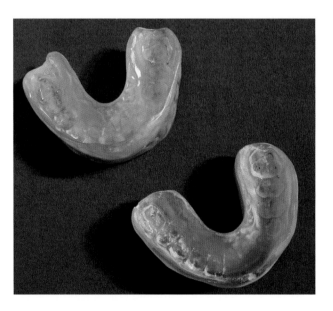

Fig. 10.12 Soft retainers/positioners that had been used for 1 and 1.5 years, respectively. The colour changes and changes in material softness indicate altered material characteristics, which may partially be due to leakage of unbound substances from the material and water uptake.

elastomer (Gracco et al. 2009) or polypropylene, polycarbonate, thermoplastic polyurethanes and ethylene-vinyl acetate. In one in vitro study (Schuster et al. 2004b), aged samples of polyurethane-based material (Invisalign®) did not release traceable monomers or by-products after immersion in an ethanol–water solvent. Accordingly, no release of BPA from the same material was found in a later study (Kotyk and Wiltshire 2014). No evidence of cytotoxicity on human gingival fibroblasts and no estrogenic activity in vitro were found for Invisalign® appliances (Eliades et al. 2009). This was confirmed in 2018 with a similar material used as retainer (Al Naqbi et al. 2018).

Miscellaneous materials

Elastic bands and chains

Latex rubber bands and chains are commonly used in orthodontics. The power-chain types will typically serve for a longer (visit to visit) period than the rubber-band types, which are placed by the patient and may be replaced with new ones more than once per day. The prevalence of natural rubber latex sensitisation in the general population varies internationally, but is generally reported to be in the range of 1–2% (Nguyen and Kohli 2020). During the last decades, hypersensitivity to ingredients of latex products has been considered an increasing health problem internationally with special concern focused on problems in relation to the health sector, most importantly as occupational exposure, and also due to serious patient reactions (Nguyen and Kohli 2020). Initiatives have been taken to minimise general exposure to natural rubber proteins as well as chemicals used in the manufacturing of latex products (De Jong et al. 2002).

Together with the methacrylates, natural rubber latex and latex manufacturing chemicals have been reported to be the most prevalent causes of allergic contact dermatitis among dental personnel (Munksgaard et al. 1996; Kanerva et al. 1999; Wrangsjö et al. 2012). Some concern has been expressed as to the widespread use of latex elastomers in orthodontics. While a number of studies have addressed the physical and mechanical properties of orthodontic elastomers, only a few papers have focused on biocompatibility aspects. In two consecutive Norwegian questionnaire surveys among orthodontists, prevalence of patient reactions to latex, including rubber elastics, was around 3:10,000, which seemed to have increased slightly between the two surveys (Jacobsen and Hensten-Pettersen 2003).

A few studies investigated the biocompatibility of latex and non-latex orthodontic elastics. In general, latex elastics were found to be more irritative than non-latex (e.g., Martinez-Colomer et al. 2016) and exhibit a more porous surface structure under identical experimental conditions.

Adverse reactions to natural rubber latex are well known in relation to exposure to, for example, latex gloves and medical catheters. Despite the widespread use of latex elastics in orthodontics, only very few reports exist on clinical side effects of latex in this context. Allergic reactions to orthodontic rubber elastics were most frequently described as soreness, burning or itching of the buccal or labial mucosa with or without objective findings which might present as erythema and/or swelling (Hain et al. 2007).

Recommendations

Although reactions to rubber elastics among orthodontic patients seem to be rare, the orthodontist has to be aware of this potential source of difficulty. Non-latex alternatives are available to use in patients with a verified latex allergy or those who are strongly suspected of having such an allergy. Improvement in the physical and mechanical properties has, however, been recommended before more widespread replacement of the traditional latex elastics can occur (Hain et al. 2007).

Concluding remarks

The orthodontic patient may be exposed to a wide variety of potentially hazardous substances. On the basis of the limited amount of literature on this topic, the prevalence of material-related adverse reactions among orthodontic patients is in the range of 1:300–400. As mentioned in the opening section of this chapter, discomfort – mechanical irritation, pain and the challenge of maintaining oral hygiene– is part of daily life for orthodontic patients, and thus has to be tolerated and accepted by them and the orthodontists. With this background, material-related adverse reactions may be overlooked and therefore not diagnosed.

For the benefit of the patient, the orthodontist should be aware of possible material-related side effects and take actions to prevent, alleviate or at least partially reduce those where possible, for example, by modifying the appliance into a more tolerable version. In particular, orthodontists should be aware that hypersensitivity reactions to Ni may present in locations remote to the oral cavity. In some areas, in particular concerning aspects of leachable substances from soft removable appliances, more research is clearly needed.

Furthermore, as was outlined in this chapter, the orthodontist and the assisting team should be aware that they are a risk group concerning possible adverse effects derived from the materials they use. They have frequent contact with such materials and – for setting products – are potentially exposed to the more reactive material components. Especially, for resinous materials, standard gloves do not provide sufficient protection against direct skin contact and therefore a no-touch technique should be exercised whenever possible.

In the light of the rapid introduction of new materials and formulations within the orthodontic field together with growing public awareness of biocompatibility aspects, it is strongly recommended that the orthodontists evaluate critically the material properties and biocompatibility aspects of a product before choosing to use it.

References

Agaoglu G, Arun T, Izgi B and Yarat A (2001) Ni and chromium levels in the saliva and serum of patients with fixed orthodontic appliances. *Angle Orthod* 71, 375–379.

Ahlström MG, Thyssen JP, Menne T and Johansen JD (2017) Prevalence of Ni allergy in Europe following the EU Ni Directive – a review. *Contact Dermatitis* 77, 193–200.

Ahlström MG, Thyssen JP, Wennervaldt M, Menne T and Johansen JD (2019) Ni allergy and allergic contact dermatitis: a clinical review of immunology, epidemiology, exposure, and treatment. *Contact Dermatitis* 81, 227–241.

Al Naqbi SR, Pratsinis H, Kletsas D, Eliades T and Athanasiou AE (2018) In vitro assessment of cytotoxicity and estrogenicity of Vivera® retainers. *J Contemp Dent Pract* 19, 1163–1168.

Alinaghi F, Bennike NH, Egeberg A, Thyssen JP and Johansen JD (2019) Prevalence of contact allergy in the general population: a systematic review and meta-analysis. *Contact Dermatitis* 80, 77–85.

Arenholt-Bindslev D, Jolanki R and Kanerva L (2009) Diagnosis of side effects of dental materials, with special emphasis on delayed and immediate allergic reactions. In Schmalz G and Arenholt-Bindslev D (eds) *Biocompatibility of Dental Materials*, pp. 335–366. Heidelberg: Springer.

Bacela J, Labowska MB, Detyna J, Ziety A and Michalak I (2020) Functional coatings for orthodontic arch wires – a review. *Materials* 13, 3257–3283.

Baker S, Brooks SC and Walker DM (1988) The release of residual monomeric methyl methacrylate from acrylic appliances in the human mouth: an assay for monomer in saliva. *J Dent Res* 67, 1295–1299.

Barber SK and Dhaliwal HK (2018) Allergy to acrylate in composite in an orthodontic patient: a case report. *J Orthod* 45, 203–209.

Barron DJ, Schuster GS, Caughman GB and Lefebvre CA (1993) Biocompatibility of visible light-polymerized denture base resins. *Int J Prosthodont* 6, 495–501.

Baumann MA, Rath B, Fischer JH and Iffland R (2000) The permeability of dental procedure and examination gloves by an alcohol based disinfectant. *Dent Mater* 16, 139–144.

Becher R, Wellendorf H, Sakhi AK, Samuelsen JT, Thomsen C, Bølling AK and Kopperud HM (2018) Presence and leaching of bisphenol a (BPA) from dental materials. *Acta Biomater Odontol Scand* 27, 56–62.

Bishara SE (1995) Oral lesions caused by an orthodontic retainer: a case report. *Am J Orthod Dentofacial Orthop* 108, 115–117.

Bishara SE, Barrett RD and Selim MI (1993) Biodegradation of orthodontic appliances. Part II. Changes in the blood level of Ni. *Am J Orthod Dentofacial Orthop* 103, 115–119.

Bishop S and Roberts H (2020) Methacrylate perspective in current dental practice. *J Esthet Restor Dent* 32, 673–680.

Borok J, Matiz C, Goldenberg A and Jacob SE (2019) Contact dermatitis in atopic dermatitis children – past, present, and future. *Clin Rev Allergy Immunol* 56, 86–98.

Brantley WA (2001) Orthodontic wires. In Brantley WA and Eliades T (eds) *Orthodontic Materials*, pp. 77–103. Stuttgart: Thieme Verlag.

Chen Z, Patwari M and Liu D (2019) Cytotoxicity of orthodontic temporary anchorage devices on human periodontal ligament fibroblasts in vitro. *Clin Exp Dent Res* 5, 648–654.

Comino-Garayoa R, Brinkmann JC, Peláez J, López-Suárez C, Martínez-González JM and Suáre MJ (2020) Allergies to Titanium dental implants: what do we really know about them? A scoping review. *Biology*, 9, 404; doi:10.3390/biology9110404

Counts AL, Miller MA, Khakhria ML and Strange S (2002) Ni allergy associated with a transpalatal arch appliance. *J Orofac Orthop* 63, 509–515.

De Jong WH, Geertsma RE and Tinkler JJ (2002) Medical devices manufactured from latex: European regulatory initiatives. *Methods* 27, 93–98.

De Morais LS, Serra GG, Palermo EFA, Andrade LR, Küller CA, Meyers MA and Elias CN (2009) Systemic levels of metallic ions released from orthodontic mini-implants. *Am J Orthodont Denntofac Orthoped* 135, 522–529.

Duarte I, Korkes KL, Hafner MFS, Mendonca RF and Lazzarini L (2018) Ni, chromium and cobalt: the relevant allergens in allergic contact dermatitis. Comparative study between two periods: 1995–2002 and 2003–2015. *An Bras Dermatol* 93, 59–62.

Ehrnrooth M and Kerosuo H (2009) Face and neck dermatitis from a stainless steel orthodontic appliance. *Angle Orthod* 79, 1194–1196.

Eliades T and Eliades G (2001) Orthodontic adhesive resins. In Brantley WA and Eliades T (eds) *Orthodontic Materials. Scientific and Clinical Aspects*, pp. 201–219, Stuttgart: Thieme Verlag.

Eliades T, Eliades G and Brantley WA (2001) Orthodontic brackets. In Brantley WA and Eliades T (eds) *Orthodontic Materials. Scientific and Clinical Aspects*, pp. 144–172. Stuttgart: Thieme Verlag.

Eliades T, Eliades G, Brantley WA and Johnston WM (1995) Residual monomer leaching from chemically cured and visible light- cured orthodontic adhesives. *Am J Orthod Dentofacial Orthop* 108, 316–321.

Eliades T, Pratsinis H, Athanasiou AE, Eliades G and Kletsas D (2009) Cytotoxicity and estrogenicity of Invisalign appliances. *Am J Orthod Dentofacial Orthop* 136, 100–103.

Eliades T, Trapalis C, Eliades G and Katsavrias E (2003a) Salivary metal levels of orthodontic patients: a novel methodological and analytical approach. *Eur J Orthod* 25, 103–106.

Eliades T, Zinelis S, Eliades G and Athanasiou AE (2003b) Characterization of as-received, retrieved, and recycled stainless steel brackets. *J Orofac Orthop* 64, 80–87.

Eliades T, Zinelis S, Eliades G and Athanasiou AE (2002) Ni content of as-received, retrieved, and recycled stainless steel brackets. *Am J Orthod Dentofacial Orthop* 122, 217–220.

European Commission (2002) Health and Costumer Protection Directorate- General. Opinion on medical devices containing DEHP plasticised PVC; Neonates and other groups possibly at risk from DEHP toxicity. Adopted by the Scientific Committee on Medicinal Products and Medical Devices on 26 September 2002, pp. 1–34.

European Commission (2009) Regulation (EC) No 1223/2009 of 30 November 2009 on Cosmetic Products. Official Journal of the European Union 22.12.2009 L 342/59.

European Commission (2015) Scientific Committee on Emerging and Newly-Identified Health Risks (SCENIHR) Opinion on the safety of the use of bisphenol A in medical devices. https://ec.europa.eu/health/scientific_committees/emerging/docs/scenihr_o_040.pdf

European Commission (2016) Scientific Committee on Emerging and Newly-Identified Health Risks (SCENIHR): the safety of medical devices containing DEHP plasticized PVC or other plasticizers on neonates and other groups possibly at risk (2015 update). https://op.europa.eu/en/publication-detail/-/publication/9c14b179-d3ae-11e5-a4b5-01aa75ed71a1/language-en

European Commission (2017) Regulation (EU) 2017/745 of 5 April 2017 on Medical Device Regulation. Official Journal of the European Union, 5.5.2017, L 117/1.

European Commission (2018) Regulation 2018/2005 of 17 December 2018 as regards bis(2-ethylhexyl) phthalate (DEHP), dibutyl phthalate (DBP), benzyl butyl phthalate (BBP) and diisobutyl phthalate (DIBP). https://eur-lex.europa.eu/legal-content/EN/TXT/?uri=CELEX%3A32018R2005

European Commission (2019) Scientific Committee on Health, Environmental and Emerging Risks (SCHEER) Guidelines on the benefit-risk assessment of the presence of phthalates in certain medical devices covering phthalates which are carcinogenic, mutagenic, toxic to reproduction (CMR) or have endocrine-disrupting (ED) properties. http://ec.europa.eu/health/scientific_committees/experts/declarations/scheer_wg_en

European Food Safety Authority (EFSA) (2015) Scientific Opinion on the risks to public health related to the presence of bisphenol A (BPA) in foodstuffs. *EFSA Journal* 13 (1) 3978. www.efsa.europa.eu/efsajournal

Evans R and Johnston D (2014) Facial burns: reducing risks. *Br Dent J* 217, 162

Faccioni P, De Santis D, Sinigaglia S, Pancera P, Faccioni F and Nocini PF (2019) Short-term "in vivo" study on cellular DNA damage induced by acrylic Andresen activator in oral mucosa cells. *Orthod Craniofac Res* 22, 208–212.

Fage SW, Muris J, Jakobsen SS and Thyssen JP (2016) Titanium: a review on exposure, release, penetration, allergy, epidemiology, and clinical reactivity. *Contact Dermatitis* 74, 323–345.

Feilzer A, Laeijendecker R, Kleverlaan CJ, van Schendel P and Muris J (2008) Facial eczema because of orthodontic fixed retainer wires. *Contact Dermatitis* 59, 118–120.

Fluent MT, Ferracane JL, Mace JG, Shah AR and Price RB (2019) Shedding light on a potential hazard: dental light-curing units. *J Am Dent Assoc* 150, 1051–1058.

Fujioka-Kobayashi M, Miron RJ, Lussi A, Gruber R, Ilie N, Price RB and Schmalz G (2019) Effect of the degree of conversion of resin-based composites on cytotoxicity, cell attachment, and gene expression. *Dent Mater* 35, 1173–1193.

Geurtsen W (2009) Polymethylmethacrylate resins. In Schmalz G and Arenholt-Bindslev D (eds) *Biocompatibility of Dental Materials*, pp. 255–292. Heidelberg: Springer.

Goiato MC, Freitas E, dos Santos D, de Medeiros R and Sonego M (2015) Acrylic resin cytotoxicity for denture base–literature review. *Adv Clin Exp Med* 24, 679–686.

Gölz L, Papageorgiou SN and Jäger A (2015) Ni hypersensitivity and orthodontic treatment: a systematic review and meta-analysis. *Contact Dermatitis* 73, 1–14.

Goncalves TS, Morganti MA, Campos LC, Rizzatto SM and Menezes LM (2006) Allergy to auto-polymerized acrylic resin in an orthodontic patient. *Am J Orthod Dentofacial Orthop* 129, 431–435.

Gracco A, Mazzoli A, Favoni O, Conti C, Ferraris P, Tosi G, et al (2009) Short-term chemical and physical changes in Invisalign appliances. *Aust Orthod J* 25, 34e40.

Guimaraens D, Gonzalez MA and Conde-Salazar L (1994) Systemic contact dermatitis from dental crowns. *Contact Dermatitis* 30, 124–125.

Hain MA, Longman LP, Field EA and Harrison JE (2007) Natural rubber latex allergy: implications for the orthodontist. *J Orthod* 34, 6–11.

Halimi A, Benyahia H, Bahije L, Adli H, Azeroual MF and Zaoui F (2016) A systematic study of the release of bisphenol A by orthodontic materials and its biological effects. *Int Orthod* 14, 399–417.

Hamann CP, Rodgers PA and Sullivan K (2003) Allergic contact dermatitis in dental professionals: effective diagnosis and treatment. *J Am Dent Assoc* 134, 185–194.

Heratizadeh A, Werfel T, Schubert S and Geier J (2018) IVDK Contact sensitization in dental technicians with occupational contact dermatitis. Data of the Information Network of Departments of Dermatology (IVDK) 2001–2015. *Contact Dermatitis* 78, 266–273.

Hostýnek JJ, Reagan KE and Maibach HI (2002) Ni allergic hyper- sensitivity: prevalence and incidenc by country, gender, age and occupation. In Hostýnek JJ and Maibach HI (eds) *Ni and the Skin. Absorption, Immunology, Epidemiology, and Metallurgy*, pp. 39–82. Boca Raton, FL: CRC Press.

Houb-Dine A, Bahije L and Zaoui F (2018) Fluoride induced corrosion affecting Titanium brackets: a systematic review. *Int Orthod* 16, 603–612.

Huang TH, Ding SJ, Min Y and Kao CT (2004) Metal ion release from new and recycled stainless steel brackets. *Eur J Orthod* 26, 171–177.

Huang TH, Liao PH, Li HY, Ding SJ, Yen M and Kao CT (2008) Orthodontic adhesives induce human gingival fibroblast toxicity and inflammation. *Angle Orthod* 78, 510–516.

Hutchinson I (1994) Hypersensitivity to an orthodontic bonding agent. A case report. *Br J Orthod* 21, 331–333.

Içẚ RB, Öztürk F, Ates B, Malkoc MA and Ü K (2014) Level of residual monomer released from orthodontic acrylic materials. *Angle Orthod* 84, 862–867.

Imani MM, Mozzafarri HR, Ramezani M and Saghedi M (2019) Effect of fixed orthodontic treatment on salivary Ni and chromium levels: a systematic review and meta-analysis of observational studies. *Dent J* 7, 21–36.

ISO 4049:2019 Dentistry – polymer-based restorative materials. International Organizations for Standardization: Chemin de Blandonnet 8, 1214 Vernier, Genève, Switzerland, 2014.

Jacobsen N and Hensten-Pettersen A (1989) Occupational health problems and adverse patient reactions in orthodontics. *Eur J Orthod* 11, 254–264.

Jacobsen N and Hensten-Pettersen A (2003) Changes in occupational health problems and adverse patient reactions in orthodontics from 1987 to 2000. *Eur J Orthod* 25, 591–598.

Jagdish N, Padmanabhan S, Chitharanjan AB, Revathi J, Palani G, Sambasivam M, Sheriff M and Saravanamurali K (2009) Cytotoxicity and degree of conversion of orthodontic adhesives. *Angle Orthod* 79, 1133–1138.

Jedeon K, De la Dure-Molla M, Brookes SJ, Loiodice S, Marciano C, Kirkham J, Canivenc-Lavier MC, Boudalia S, Bergès R, Harada H, Berdal A and Babajko S (2013) Enamel defects reflect perinatal exposure to bisphenol A. *Am J Pathol* 183, 108–118.

Jedeon K, Loiodice S, Marciano C, Vinel A, Canivenc Lavier MC, Berdal A and Babajko S (2014) Estrogen and bisphenol A affect male rat enamel formation and promote ameloblast proliferation. *Endocrinology* 155, 3365–3375.

Jensen CS, Menne T, Lisby S, Kristiansen J and Veien NK (2003) Experimental systemic contact dermatitis from Ni: a dose-response study. *Contact Dermatitis* 49, 124–132.

Jorge JH, Giampaolo ET, Machado AL and Vergani CE (2003) Cytotoxicity of denture base acrylic resins: a literature review. *J Prosthet Dent* 90, 190–193.

Kanerva L (2001) Cross-reactions of multifunctional methacrylates and acrylates. *Acta Odontol Scand* 59, 320–329.

Kanerva L and Aitio A (1997) Dermatotoxicological aspects of metallic chromium. *Eur J Dermatol* 7, 79–84.

Kanerva L, Lahtinen A, Toikkanen J, Forss H, Estlander T, Susitaival P and Jolanki R (1999) Increase in occupational skin diseases of dental personnel. *Contact Dermatitis* 40, 104–108.

Kedjarune U, Charoenworaluk N and Koontongkaew S (1999) Release of methyl methacrylate from heat-cured and autopolymerized resins: cytotoxicity testing related to residual monomer. *Aust Dent J* 44, 25–30.

Kerosuo E, Kerosuo H and Kanerva L (2000) Self-reported health complaints among general dental practitioners, orthodontists, and office employees. *Acta Odontol Scand* 58, 207–212.

Kerosuo H and Kanerva L (1997) Systemic contact dermatitis caused by Ni in a stainless steel orthodontic appliance. *Contact Dermatitis* 36, 112–113.

Kerosuo H, Kullaa A, Kerosuo E, Kanerva L and Hensten-Pettersen A (1996) Ni allergy in adolescents in relation to orthodontic treatment and piercing of ears. *Am J Orthod Dentofacial Orthop* 109, 148–154.

Kerusuo HM and Dahl JE (2007) Adverse patient reactions during orthodontic treatment with fixed appliances. *Am J Orthod Dentofacial Orthop* 132, 789–795.

Khuta M, Pavlin D, Slaj M, Varga S, Lapter-Varga M and Slaj M (2009) Type of archwire and level of acidity: effects on the release of metal ions from orthodontic appliances. *Angle Orthod* 79, 102–110.

Kim H and Johnson JW (1999) Corrosion of stainless steel, Ni-titanium, coated Ni-titanium, and titanium orthodontic wires. *Angle Orthod* 69, 39–44.

Kloukos D, Sifakakis I, Voutsa D, Doulis I, Eliades G, Katsaros C and Eliades T (2015) BPA qualtitative and quantitative assessment associated with orthodontic bonding in vivo. *Dent Mater* 31, 887–894.

Kolokitha OE and Chatzistavrou E (2009) A severe reaction to Ni-containing orthodontic appliances. *Angle Orthod* 79, 186–192.

Kolokitha OE, Kaldamanos EG and Papadopouos MA (2008) Prevalence of Ni hypersensitivity in orthodontic patients: a meta-analysis. *Am J Orthod Dentofacial Orthop* 134, 722.e1–722.e12.

Kopperud HM, Kleven IS and Wellendorf H (2011) Identification and quantification of leachable substances from polymer-based orthodontic base-plate materials. *Eur J Orthod* 33, 26–31.

Kotyk MW and Wiltshire WA (2014) An investigation into bisphenol-A leaching from orthodontic materials. *Angle Orthod* 84, 516–520.

Kusy RP and Whitley JQ (2005) Degradation of plastic polyoxymethylene brackets and the subsequent release of toxic formaldehyde. *Am J Orthod Dentofacial Orthop* 127, 420–407.

Lamb DJ, Ellis B and Priestley D (1983) The effects of process variables on levels of residual monomer in autopolymerizing dental acrylic resin. *J Dent* 11, 80–88.

Lind PO (1988) Oral lichenoid reactions related to composite restorations. Preliminary report. *Acta Odontol Scand* 46, 63–65.

Lindsten R and Kurol J (1997) Orthodontic appliances in relation to Ni hypersensitivity. A review. *J Orofac Orthop* 58, 100–108.

Luft S, Keilig L, Jäger A and Bourauel C (2009) In-vitro evaluation of the corrosion behavior of orthodontic brackets. *Orthod Craniofac Res* 12, 43–51.

Lygre H, Klepp KN, Solheim E and Gjerdet NR (1994) Leaching of additives and degradation products from cold-cured orthodontic resins. *Acta Odontol Scand* 52, 150–156.

Lygre H, Solheim E and Gjerdet NR (1995) Leaching from denture base materials in vitro. *Acta Odontol Scand* 53, 75–80.

Lygre H, Solheim E, Gjerdet NR and Berg E (1993) Leaching of organic additives from dentures in vivo. *Acta Odontol Scand* 51, 45–51.

Maijer R and Smith DC (1982) Corrosion of orthodontic bracket bases. *Am J Orthod* 81, 43–48.

Mancuso G and Berdonini RM (2002) Eyelid dermatitis and conjunctivitis as sole manifestations of allergy to Ni in an orthodontic appliance. *Contact Dermatitis* 46, 245.

Mandrup K, Boberg J, Isling LK, Christiansen S and Hass U (2016) Low-dose effects of bisphenol A on mammary gland development in rats. *Andrology* 4, 673–683.

Martin-Camean A, Jos A, Mellado-Garcia P, Iglesias-Linares A, Solano E and Camean A (2015) In vitro and in vivo evidence of the cytotoxic and genotoxic effects of metal ions released by orthodontic appliances: a review. *Environment Toxocol Pharmacol* 40, 86–113.

Martinez-Colomer S, Gaton-Hernandez P, Romano FL, De Rossi A, Fukada SY, Nelson-Filho P, Consolaro A, Silva RAB and Silva LAB (2016) Latex and nonlatex orthodontic elastics: in vitro and in vovo evaluations of tissue compatibility and surface structure. *Angle Orthodont* 46, 278–284.

Maspero C, Galbiati G, Giannini L, Guenza G, Esposito L and Farronato G (2018) Titanium TSME appliance for patients allergic to Ni. *Eur J Paediatr Dent* 19, 67–69.

Menezes LM, Quintao CA and Blognese AM (2007) Urinary excretion levels of Ni in orthodontic patients. *Am J Orthod Dentofacial Orthop* 131, 635–638.

Michelsen VB, Lygre H, Skalevik R, Tveit AB and Sollnehn E (2003) Identification of organic eluates from four polymer-based dental filling materials. *Eur J Oral Sci* 111, 263–271.

Mittermüller P, Hiller KA, Schmalz G and Buchalla W (2018) Five hundred patients reporting on adverse effects from dental materiale: frequencies, complaints, symptoms, allergies. *Dent Mater* 34, 1756–1768.

Mortz C, Lauritsen J, Bindslev-Jensen C and Andersen K (2002), Ni sensitization in adolescents and association with ear piercing, use og dental braces and hand eczema *Acta Derm Venerol* 82, 359–364.

Munksgaard EC (1992) Permeability of protective gloves to (di)methacrylates in resinous dental materials. *Scand J Dent Res* 100, 189–192.

Munksgaard EC (2004) Leaching of plasticizers from temporary denture soft lining materials. *Eur J Oral Sci* 112, 101–104.

Munksgaard EC, Hansen EK, Engen T and Holm U (1996) Self-reported occupational dermatological reactions among Danish dentists. *Eur J Oral Sci* 104, 396–402.

Nguyen K and Kohli A Latex Allergy (2020) [Updated 2020 Nov 21]. In: StatPearls [Internet]. Treasure Island (FL): StatPearls Publishing https://www.ncbi.nlm.nih.gov/books/NBK545164/.s3

Noble J, Ahing SI, Karaiskos E and Wiltshire WA (2008) Ni allergy and orthodontics, a review and report of two cases. *Br Dent J* 204, 207–300.

Noda M, Wataha JC, Lockwood PE, Volkmann KR, Kaga M and Sano H (2002) Low-dose, long-term exposures of dental material components alter human monocyte metabolism. *J Biomed Mater Res* 62, 237–243.

Oysaed H, Ruyter IE and Sjovik KI (1988) Release of formaldehyde from dental composites. *J Dent Res* 67, 1289–1294.

Pantuzo MC, Zenobio EG, de Andrade MH and Zenobio MA (2007) Hypersensitivity to conventional and to Ni-free orthodontic brackets *Braz Oral Res* 21, 298–302.

Pazzini CA, Junior FO, Marques LS, Pereira CV and Pereira LJ (2009) Prevalence of Ni allergy and longitudinal evaluation of periodontal abnormalities in orthodontic allergic patients. *Angle Orthod* 79, 922–927.

Pazzini CA, Pereira LJ, Marques LS, Generoso R and Oliveira G (2010) Allergy to Ni in orthodontic patients: clinical and histopathologic evaluation. *Gen Dent* 5, 58–61.

Pazzini CA, Pereira LJ, Peconick AP, Marques LS and Paiva SM (2016) Ni allergy: blood and periodontal evaluation after orthodontic treatment. *Acta Odontol Latinoam* 29, 42–48.

Pelourde C, Bationo R, Boileau MJ, Colat-Parros J and Jordana F(2018) Monomer release from orthodontic retentions: an in vitro study. *Am J Orthod Dentofacial Orthop* 153, 248–254

Perry J, Popat H, Johnson I, Farnell D and Morgan MZ (2021) Professional consensus on orthodontic risks: what orthodontists should tell their patients. *Am J Orthod Dentofacial Orthop* 159, 41–52.

Petoumenou E, Arndt M, Keilig L, Reimann S, Hoederath H, Eliades T, Jäger A and Bourauel C (2009) Ni concentration in the saliva of patients with Ni-titanium orthodontic appliances. *Am J Orthod Dentofacial Orthop* 135, 59–65.

Pituru SM, Greabu M, Totan A, Imre M, Pantea M, Spinu T, Tancu AMC, Popoviciu NO, Stanescu A and Ionescu E (2020) A review on the biocompatibility of PMMA-based dental materials for interim prosthetic restorations with a glimpse into their modern manufacturing techniques. *Materials (Basel)* 13, 2894.

Purushothaman D, Kailasam V and Chitharanjan A (2015) Bisphenol A release from orthodontic adhesives and its correlation with the degree of conversion. *Am J Orthod Dentofacial Orthop* 147, 29–36.

Quadras DD, Nayak USK, Kuman NS, Priyadarshini HR, Gowda S and Fernandes B (2019) In vivo study on the release of Ni, chromium, and zinc in saliva and serum from patients treated with fixed orthodontic appliances *Dent Res J* 16, 209–215.

Raghavan AS, Pottipalli Sathyanarayana H, Kailasam V and Padmanabhan S (2017) Comparative evaluation of salivary bisphenol A levels in patients wearing vacuum-formed and Hawley retainers: an in-vivo study. *Am J Orthod Dentofacial Orthop* 151, 471–476.

Ruyter IE (1995) Physical and chemical aspects related to substances released from polymer materials in an aqueous environment. *Adv Dent Res* 9, 344–347.

Sananez A, Sanchez A, Davis L, Vento Y and Rueggeberg F(2020) Allergic reaction from dental bonding material through nitrile gloves: clinical case study and glove permeability testing. *J Esthet Restor Dent* 32, 371–379.

Schmalz G and Arenholt-Bindslev D (eds) (2009) *Biocompatibility of Dental Materials*. Heidelberg: Springer.

Schmalz G, Arenholt-Bindslev D, Hiller KA and Schweikl H (1997) Epithelium-fibroblast co-culture for assessing mucosal irritancy of metals used in dentistry. *Eur J Oral Sci* 105, 86–91.

Schmalz G, Hickel R, van Landuyt KL and Reichl FX (2017) Nanoparticles in dentistry. *Dent Mater* 33, 1298–1314.

Schultz JC, Connelly E, Glesne L and Warshaw EM (2004) Cutaneous and oral eruption from oral exposure to Ni in dental braces. *Dermatitis* 15, 154–157.

Schuster G, Reichle R, Bauer RR and Schopf PM (2004a) Allergies induced by orthodontic alloys: incidence and impact on treatment. Results of a survey in private orthodontic offices in the Federal State of Hesse, Germany. *J Orofac Orthop* 65, 48–59.

Schuster GS, Lefebvre CA, Dirksen TR, Knoernschild KL and Caughman GB (1995) Relationships between denture base resin cytotoxicity and cell lipid metabolism. *Int J Prosthodont* 8, 580–586.

Schuster S, Eliades G, Zinelis S, Eliades T and Bradley TG (2004b) Structural conformation and leaching from in vitro aged and retrieved Invisalign appliances. *Am J Orthod Dentofacial Orthop* 126, 725–728.

Senkutvan RS, Jacob S, Charles A, Vadgaonkar V, Jatol-Tekade S and Gangurde P (2014) Evaluation of Ni ion release from various orthodontic arch wires: an in vitro study. *J Int Soc Prev Community Dent* 4, 12–16. *Am J Contact Dermat* 10, 18–30.

Sfondrini MF, Cacciafesta V, Maffia E, Scribante A, Alberti G, Biesuz R and Klersy C (2010) Ni release from new conventional stainless stee, recycled, and Ni-free orthodontic brackets: an in vitro study. *Am J Orthod Dentofacial Orthop* 137, 809–815.

Sifakakis I and Eliades T (2017) Adverse reactions to orthodontic materials. *Austr Dent J* 62, 20–28.

Silverberg NB, Pelletier JL, Jacob SE and Schneider LC (2020) Nickel allergic contact dermatitis: identification, treatment, and prevention *Pediatrics* 145, e20200628.

Singh RD, Gautam R, Siddhartha R, Singh BP, Chand P, Sharma VP and Jurel SK (2013) High performance liquid chromatographic determination of residual monomer released from heat-cured acrylic resin. An in vivo study. *J Prosthodont* 22, 358–361.

Souza ACF, Galvani MG, de Souza DV, Vasconcelos JRC and Ribeiro DA (2019) Is orthodontic therapy able to induce genetic damage on oral cells? *Orthod Craniofac Res* 22, 222–223.

Spranley TJ, Winkler M, Dagate J, Oncale D and Strother E (2012) Curing light burns. *Gen Dent* 60, e210–4.

Steele JE, Parker K, Atkins JL and Gill DS (2014) Facial burns: acid drops. *Br Dent J* 217, 56.

Szuhanek CA, Watz CG, Avram S, Moaca E-A, Mihali CV, Popa A, Campan AA, Nicolov M and Dehelean CA (2020) *Materials* 13, 5690. doi:10.3390

Taubmann A, Willershausen I, Walter C, Al-Maawi S, Kaina B and Gölz L (2020) Genotoxic and cytotoxic potential of methacrylate-based orthodontic adhesives. *Clin Oral Investig* doi:10.1007/s00784-020-03569-x

Todd DJ and Burrows D (1989) Ni allergy in relationship to previous oral and cutaneous Ni contact. *Ulster Med J* 58, 168–171.

Trombelli L, Virgili A, Corazza M and Lucci R (1992) Systemic contact dermatitis from an orthodontic appliance. *Contact Dermatitis* 27, 259–260.

Vamnes JS, Lygre GB, Grönningsæter AG and Gjerdet NR (2004) Four years of clinical experience with an adverse reaction unit for dental biomaterials. *Community Dent* 32, 150–157.

van der Burg CK, Bruynzeel DP, Vreeburg KJ, von Blomberg BM and Scheper RJ (1986) Hand eczema in hairdressers and nurses: a prospective study. I. Evaluation of atopy and Ni hypersensitivity at the start of apprenticeship. *Contact Dermatitis* 14, 275–279.

van Hoogstraten I, Andersen KE, von Blomberg BM, Boden D, Bruynzeel DP, Burrows D, Camarasa JG, Dooms-Goossens A, Kraal G and Lahti A

(1991) Reduced frequency of Ni allergy upon oral Ni contact at an early age. *Clin Exp Immunol* 85, 441–445.

van Hoogstraten I, Boden D, von Blomberg ME, Kraal G and Scheper RJ (1992) Persistent immune tolerance to Ni and chromium by oral administration prior to cutaneous sensitization. *J Invest Dermatol* 99, 608–616.

Van Landuyt KL, Nawrot T, Geebelen B, De Munck J, Snauwaert J, Yoshihara K, Scheers H, Godderis L, Hoet P and Van Meerbeek B (2011) How much do resin-based dental materials release? A meta-analytical approach. *Dent Mater* 27, 723–747.

Van Landuyt KL, Yoshihara K, Geebelen B, Peumans M, Godderis L, Hoet P and Van Meerbeek B (2012) Should we be concerned about composite (nano-)dust? *Dent Mater* 28, 1162–1170.

Veien NK, Borchorst E, Hattel T and Laurberg G (1994) Stomatitis or systemically-induced contact dermatitis from metal wire in orthodontic materials. *Contact Dermatitis* 30, 210–213.

Velasco-Ibanez R, Lara-Carillo E, Morales-Luckie RA, Romero-Guzman ET, Toral-Rizo VH, Ramires-Cardona M, Garcia-Hernandez V and Medina-Solis CE (2020) Evaluation of the release of Ni and titanium under orthodontic treatment. *Sci Rep* 10, 22280.

Vilaplana J and Romaguera C (2000) Contact dermatitis and adverse oral mucous membrane reactions related to the use of dental prostheses. *Contact Dermatitis* 43, 183–185.

Volkman KK, Inda MJ, Reichl PG and Zacharisen MC (2007) Adverse reactions to orthodontic appliances in Ni-allergic patients. *Allergy Asthma Proc* 28, 480–483.

Wataha JC, Lockwood PE, Mettenburg D and Bouillaguet S (2003) Toothbrushing causes elemental release from dental casting alloys over extended intervals. *J Biomed Mater Res B Appl Biomater* 65, 180–185.

Wataha JC, Lockwood PE, Schedle A, Noda M and Bouillaguet S (2002) Ag, Cu, Hg and Ni ions alter the metabolism of human monocytes during extended low-dose exposures. *J Oral Rehabil* 29, 133–139.

Wen Y, Liu SD, Lei X, Ling YS, Luo Y and Liu Q (2015) Association of PAEs with precocious puberty in children: a systematic review and meta-analysis. *Int J Environ Res Public Health* 12, 15254–15268.

Wishney M (2017) Potential risks of orthodontic therapy: a critical review and conceptual framework. *Aust Dent J* 62(Suppl 1), 86–96.

World Health Organization (WHO) (2009) Food and agriculture organization of the united nations, toxicological and health aspects of bisphenol A. http://www.who.int/foodsafety/publications/bisphenol-a/en

Wrangsjö K, Boman A, Lidén C and Meding B (2012) Primary prevention of latex allergy in healthcare-spectrum of strategies including the European glove standardization. *Contact Dermatitis* 66, 165–171.

Wrangsjo K, Swartling C and Meding B (2001) Occupational dermatitis in dental personnel: contact dermatitis with special reference to (meth) acrylates in 174 patients. *Contact Dermatitis* 45, 158–163.

Zhou Y, Wang Y, Wang XY, Volière G and Hu RD (2014) The impact of orthodontic treatment on the quality of life, a systematic review. *Oral Health* 14, 66–73.

Zigante M, Mlinaric MR, Kastelan M, Perkovic V, Zrinski MT and Spalj S (2020) Symptoms of titanium and Ni allergic sensitization in orthodontic treatment. *Progr Orthod* 21. doi:10.1186/s40510-020-00318-4

11

Patients with Periodontal Problems

Birte Melsen

Prevalence of periodontal disease

Periodontal problems contribute to the development of malocclusion in a substantial number of adult orthodontic patients. Indeed, as is commonly seen in the Western world, the risk of gingival recessions, attachment loss and probing depth > 4 mm increases significantly with age (Hugoson et al. 1995; Albandar 2002a, 2002b) (Figure 11.1). Both general and local factors have been described as influencing the development of periodontal disease (Table 11.1).

The periodontal condition is crucial when considering orthodontic treatment in older adults. This is not the case in adolescent or young adults where the correlation between gingivitis and periodontitis is only weak. Shei et al. (1959) found that with increasing age, oral hygiene had a significantly greater impact on the marginal bone level (Figure 11.2). This was confirmed by a study in which students below 25 years of age and teachers above 40 years were compared following a 21-day period of oral hygiene abstention. The older group not only accumulated more plaque but also developed gingivitis more rapidly than the young individuals (Figure 11.3) (Holm-Pedersen et al. 1975).

Malocclusion and periodontal disease

A malocclusion has no direct influence on periodontal breakdown (Geiger et al. 1972, Shaw et al. 1980). However, it has been indicated that untreated occlusal discrepancies are associated with more rapid progression of periodontal disease and that occlusal treatment reduces the progression (Harrel and Nunn 2001; Reichwage and Rydesky 2002). Several studies propose that certain malocclusion traits can be considered risk factors due to the strong correlation between them and aspects of periodontal disease, for example, pocketing and crowding (el-Mangoury et al. 1987; Staufer and Landmesser 2004), bone level and crowding (Jensen and Solow 1989) and bone loss and tooth rotation (Peretz and Machtei 1996). The relationship between periodontal disease and crowding is most likely indirect, since several studies have demonstrated that plaque accumulation is more pronounced in crowded areas (Ingervall et al. 1977; Buckley 1981). In addition, Chung et al. (2000) demonstrated an increased number of periopathogenic species such as spirochaetes, motile rods, *Fusobacterium* species, *Capnocytophaga* species, *Campylobacter rectus* and

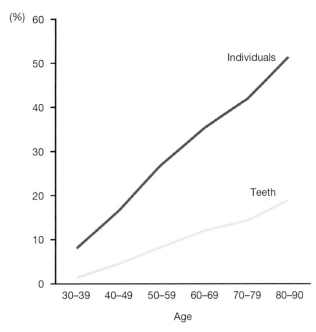

Fig. 11.1 Increase in the loss of periodontal support in relation to age. (Redrawn from Albandar (2002b), with permission.)

Table 11.1 Factors influencing the development of periodontal disease.

General factors	Local factors
Gender	Oral hygiene
Genetic factors	Untreated dental caries
Social status	Dental restorations
General health	Microbiological factors
Host-immune factors	Crowding
Smoking	Occlusion

Peptostreptococcus micros in crowded compared to non-crowded areas. Diedrich (2000) also points to the relevance of crowding, not only with respect to plaque retention but also with respect to the altered topography of the gingiva and the alveolar bone. To limit the effect of crowding on the periodontium, Helm and Petersen (1989) stated that the special topography of the crowded areas calls for special professional efforts of hygiene education and therapy.

The relationship between crowding and periodontitis does work both ways, as the migration of anterior teeth occurs more frequently in the presence of periodontal disease, leading to more crowding in the lower arch, which then makes it more difficult to maintain a healthy periodontium (Towfighi et al. 1997). The only malocclusion in which there is a direct correlation between malocclusion and attachment loss is a deep-bite impinging either lingually to the upper incisors or/and labially to the lower incisors (Sanavi et al. 1998) (Figure 11.4). Another way in which

occlusion leads to periodontal disease may be via the distribution of occlusal forces. It has also been demonstrated repeatedly (Ericsson and Lindhe 1982, 1984; Svanberg et al. 1995) that although jiggling forces from occlusal trauma do not in themselves produce loss of connective tissue attachment if the periodontium is healthy, jiggling will, in the presence of periodontitis, accelerate the loss of attachment (Burgett 1995).

The indirect effect of traumatic occlusion may be explained by the fact that it frequently results in the loosening of the teeth, which has been shown to be a risk factor, as the prevalence of specific periodontopathogens increases and thereby leads to a more rapid breakdown of the attachment (Grant et al. 1995; Melsen et al. 1998). Increased mobility is conversely also seen in relation to orthodontic treatment whereby the treatment in itself constitutes a risk factor if the periodontal health is not completely under control.

Orthodontics and periodontal disease

Adult orthodontics and periodontal disease have been the focus of increasing attention over the past 25 years. Miethke and Melsen (1993) searched the literature, from between 1984 and 1993, using the keywords adult orthodontics and periodontal disease and found 104 papers. Thirty-one were case reports, 24 longitudinal studies and 9 cross-sectional studies. A similar search done with the same keywords between 1994 and 2003 disclosed 261 papers (Table 11.2).

Most patients ask for orthodontic treatment in anticipation that it will improve both the aesthetics and overall prognosis of the dentition. However, patients should be informed that orthodontic treatment in itself cannot be considered protective in relation to further development of periodontitis.

The influence of orthodontic treatment on the periodontium has been described as both beneficial and detrimental. Zachrisson and collaborators showed that orthodontics can contribute to the development of the loss of attachment especially in relation to space closure following extraction (Sjolien and Zachrisson 1973; Zachrisson and Alnaes 1973). The beneficial impact of the treatment result on the oral hygiene might, on the other hand, explain that when the same authors performed a longitudinal study on 38 children (Alstad and Zachrisson 1979), they found that the treated patients seemed to maintain even better hygiene following treatment than the control group.

However, the detrimental effect of orthodontic treatment in the absence of an adequate oral hygiene programme has been shown both in papers describing iatrogenic damages and in animal experiments. It has been invariably found that moving a tooth into an infected infrabony defect will

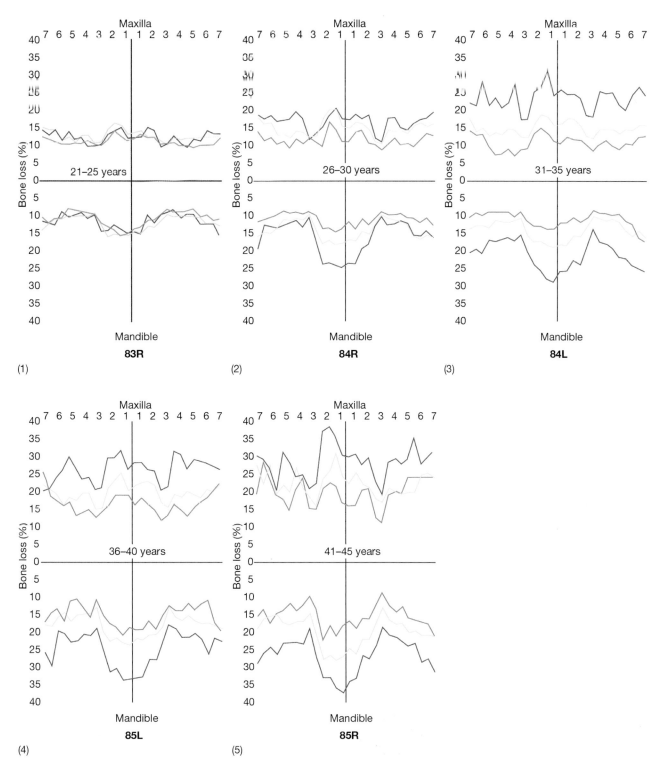

Fig. 11.2 (1)–(5) Relationship between oral hygiene and marginal bone level at different ages. It is obvious that the relation between oral hygiene and marginal bone level becomes more significant with increasing age. (Redrawn from Shei O, Waerhaug J, Lovdal A and Arnulf A (1959) Alveolar bone loss as related to oral hygiene and age. J Periodontol 26, 7–16.)

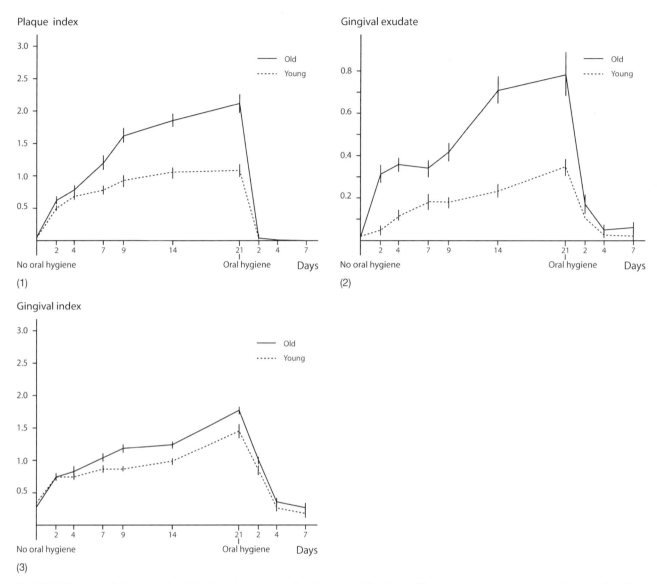

Fig. 11.3 Influence of absence of oral hygiene in young and older adults. The figure illustrates the consequences of abstention from oral hygiene for 3 weeks. Both (1) plaque accumulation and (2) inflammation manifested as gingival exudate and (3) gingival index were greater in the older than in the young probands. (Redrawn from Holm Pedersen P, Agerbaek N and Theilade E (1975) Experimental gingivitis in young and elderly individuals. J Clin Periodontol 2, 14–24, with permission.)

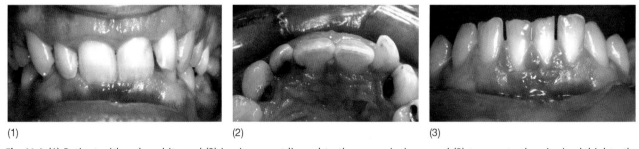

Fig. 11.4 (1) Patient with a deep bite and (2) impingement lingual to the upper incisors, and (3) trauma to the gingiva labial to the lower incisors.

Table 11.2 Papers with the keywords adult orthodontics and periodontal disease.

	1984–1993	1994–2002	2010–2020
Total number	104	261	670
Case report	31	116	197
Clinical trial	33	24	156
Technique described	20	85	197
Review	19	28	92

enhance the destruction of connective tissue attachment (Ericsson and Thilander 1978; Wennström et al. 1993). The experiments were carried out on dogs with experimentally induced periodontal disease. The periodontium of adult patients with periodontal disease can be expected to react even less favourably, since their resistance can be anticipated to be less than that of the dogs in which the disease was provoked.

Iatrogenic damage in orthodontics seems to be age-dependent, rendering the orthodontic treatment of older adults even more risky. When the periodontal status of young adults who had received orthodontic treatment at least 10 years earlier was compared with that of adults with untreated malocclusions, no differences were found in any of the periodontal variables including plaque inflammation, bleeding on probing pockets' depth, recessions, loss of attachment and crestal bone level (Polson et al. 1988). Conversely, Lupi et al. (1996) studied 88 adult patients who had had orthodontic treatment and found that the percentage of patients with loss of alveolar height exceeding 2 mm from the cementoenamel junction to the alveolar crest increased during treatment from 19% to 37%. However, in this study, there was no information about the hygiene of the individuals. The importance of good oral hygiene was stressed both by Eliasson et al. (1982) and Boyd et al. (1989), who both found that when periodontal health was maintained during treatment, orthodontics had no iatrogenic effects and might even be beneficial.

Vanarsdall (1995), on the other hand, addressed oral hygiene from a more pragmatic aspect, stating that not all patients can be expected to comply with the recommended maintenance schedule. He still recommended to compromise treatment that may reduce the chances of a reinfection following adequate periodontal treatment.

The recent trend towards non-extraction treatments with self-ligation brackets was introduced with a lot of promises regarding expansion. However, the 'bone price' in terms of marginal bone was high. When assessing the level of marginal bone on the upper premolars on CBCT images, it was found that 80% of the patients had lost more than 20% marginal bone when treated with Damon, while the average loss in the In-Ovation group was 14% (Cattaneo et al. 2011).

Indications for orthodontic treatment in periodontally involved patients

Before starting treatment, several questions could be posed:

- What are the characteristics of patients with periodontal disease seeking orthodontic treatment?
- Who can realistically benefit from orthodontic treatment?

Patients' concern for their teeth is more closely related to the perceived need for treatment rather than to the objective need judged by the orthodontist (Tervonen and Knuuttila 1988; Lundegren et al. 2004). The patient will seek treatment when he or she no longer finds their dentition acceptable. Most patients with periodontal breakdown have experienced migration of teeth in relation to the development of their periodontal disease (Figure 11.5). It is, however, important to determine whether the periodontal disease along with the development of the malocclusion is a slowly developing process or whether the patients can relate the migration of the teeth to any specific change in the local (extractions) or general environment (changes in bone metabolism).

Tooth migrations leading to unacceptable malocclusions are closely related to change in the marginal bone level. This can be caused by periodontitis (Hugoson et al. 1998; Albandar and Rams 2002), and can also be an adverse effect of a toothbrushing habit (Pattison 1983; Smukler and Landsberg 1984; Spieler 1996; Litonjua et al. 2003). With changes in the marginal bone level, the centre of resistance is displaced apically, whereby occlusal forces on the incisors will lead to tipping and extrusion, as the horizontal forces acting on the oblique alveolar wall will lead to shearing. Thereby, a vicious circle commences, consisting of further migration and shearing forces (Figure 11.6).

The most common symptoms of malocclusion in patients with periodontal disease are deepening of the bite, increased overjet and development of spacing between the upper incisors and lower incisor crowding. In the incisor region, general flaring is typically seen, but extrusion of single teeth with local periodontal disease may occur (Diedrich 1999). This is often seen in relation to the upper lateral incisors and has been attributed to the particular anatomy of these teeth. A fissure on the lingual aspect of these teeth as a result of an

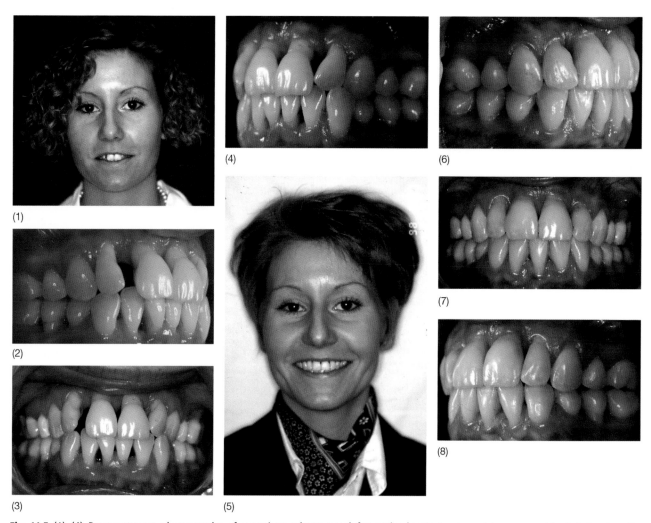

Fig. 11.5 (1)–(4) Pre-treatment photographs of a patient whose need for orthodontic treatment became evident following the periodontal surgery that had led to opening of spaces and 'black' spaces between the incisors. She now felt that she was pressing the tongue against the spaces when speaking and that she was starting to lisp. (5)–(8) Following orthodontic treatment with intrusion and retraction of the upper incisors. Note the shortening of the clinical crowns.

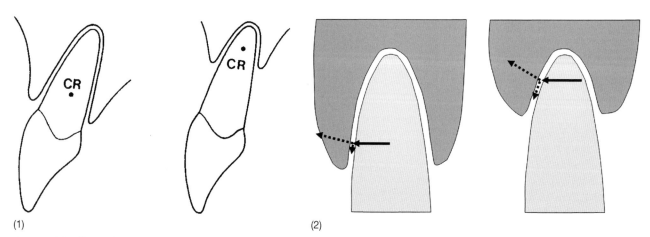

Fig. 11.6 (1) Effect of marginal bone loss on the location of the centre of resistance (CR). (2) When the tooth is submitted to a horizontal force, this is converted to a shearing force in the periodontal ligament leading to relative extrusion. The more oblique the surface, the more is the shearing force leading to extrusion.

invagination, sometimes referred to as dens in dente, allows for the development of inflammation leading to localised bone loss due to the increased intra-periodontal pressure, which secondarily can lead to extrusion of the involved teeth (Chen et al 1990, Ploud and Molven 1998) (Figure 11.7). When flaring starts to occur, it may influence the balance between the internal and the external muscle matrices. Once the lower lip is positioned behind the upper incisors during swallowing and/or speech or para-function, it can lead to rapid deterioration of the dentition or aggravation of the malocclusion. Increase in overjet may also occur as a result of collapse due to loss of posterior teeth (Figure 11.8). For most patients, impaired aesthetics is the reason for seeking treatment.

So, can all patients with periodontal disease and malocclusions benefit from orthodontic treatment? Before planning orthodontic treatment in patients with periodontal disease, it should be ascertained that the patient will be willing to go through the necessary periodontal preparation and is able to maintain a healthy but, in their case, reduced periodontium. Even so, it should be borne in mind that patients with a history of earlier periodontal disease are high-risk patients (Loe and Morrison 1986). Patients who have developed a secondary malocclusion or in whom there is aggravation of an existing malocclusion in relation to periodontal breakdown cannot be treated to a satisfactory result by periodontal and prosthodontic treatment without involving orthodontics. Loading of the spontaneously

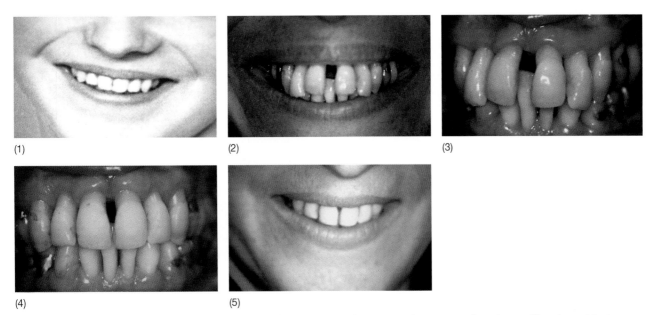

Fig. 11.7 (1) Personal photograph taken when the patient was around 20 years of age. Note that the maxillary lateral incisors are shorter than the central incisors. (2) and (3) Twenty-six years later, the lateral incisors appear longer than the central incisors. These teeth have extruded due to periodontal disease. The periodontium is healthy following periodontal surgery, but the occlusion is not satisfactory. (4) and (5) Following orthodontic treatment, a nice smile was re-established.

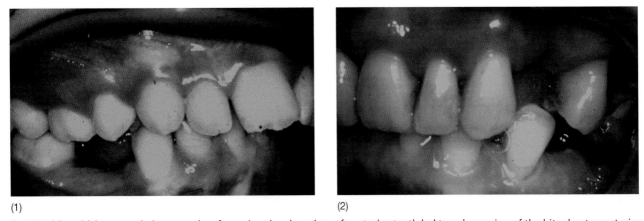

Fig. 11.8 (1) and (2) Intraoral photographs of a patient in whom loss of posterior teeth led to a deepening of the bite due to posterior tipping of the lower anterior teeth.

migrated teeth during normal function will often be detrimental and migration will continue in spite of a healthy periodontium. Solving the problem by prosthetic rehabilitation alone is rarely advisable, as the patient's aesthetic needs can seldom be fulfilled. The majority of patients will therefore benefit from orthodontic treatment that re-establishes a functional equilibrium, if possible, or creates an occlusion that allows for satisfactory prosthodontic rehabilitation.

Malocclusions in adult patients that may be considered as indications for orthodontic treatment are:

- *Intra-arch problems*, anomalies that interfere with maintenance of optimal oral hygiene or necessary replacement of missing teeth.
- *Inter-arch problems*, deviations in occlusion that do not allow normal function.
- *Functional deviations*, malocclusions related to forced bites.

In many patients, the problems fit into more than one category:

- *Intra-arch problems* include: adverse gingival topography, poor crown-to-root ratio, uneven bone level, osseous defects, diastema (flaring), excessive root proximity, crowding, tipping and rotation, poor distribution of the existing teeth.
- *Inter-arch problems* comprise: sagittally (increased overjet or inversion); vertically (both deep bite and open bite); transversely (crossbite and scissor bite).
- *Signs of malfunction* that may contribute to aggravation of a malocclusion include flared incisors with lip catch and posterior and lateral forced bites reflected in abnormal wear of teeth.

The treatment goal for orthodontic treatment in such patients is to establish an occlusion that allows optimisation of the necessary oral rehabilitation and maintenance. In addition, the treatment should aim for an aesthetically satisfactory result, thus taking the patient's chief complaint into consideration.

The tooth movements required in periodontally involved patients include sagittal and transverse movements to relieve crowding, uprighting of teeth tilted into extraction spaces and intrusion, often combined with retraction or protraction and closure of diastema. When attempting to move teeth horizontally, it should be appreciated that the bone loss results in an apical displacement of the centre of resistance and that the moment-to-force ratio therefore has to be adjusted to the individual situation (Figure 11.6). In addition, it is important to remember that in order to avoid shearing, the applied forces have to comprise an intrusive component.

Treatment of patients with flared and extruded upper incisors

Correction of flared anterior teeth in patients with horizontal bone loss as a result of combined proclination and extrusion of these teeth involves a combination of retraction and intrusion. Mere retroclination of the flared teeth would lead to a deepening of the bite. Melsen et al. (1989) studied the effect of intrusion on the periodontium in the patients with horizontal bone loss in 30 consecutive patients (5 men and 25 women, aged 22–26 years) with deep bite and need for intrusion. In 24 patients, the malocclusion had developed or worsened in relation to progressive periodontal disease, and in six patients, deepening of the bite had occurred following extraction of posterior teeth.

Before orthodontic treatment, all patients received conservative periodontal treatment including scaling and root planing and oral hygiene instruction. In addition, a modified Widman flap operation was necessary in 15 patients to reduce the pockets to the acceptable 3–4 mm or less (Figure 11.9). An unavoidable and undesirable side effect of surgery was that the clinical crowns became longer. As the dentition had severely deteriorated, the patients were (partly as a joke) asked: 'Do you want your incisors longer or no longer?' All patients accepted orthodontic

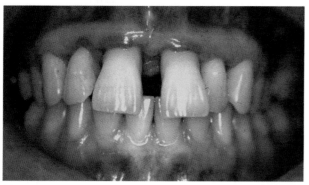
(1)

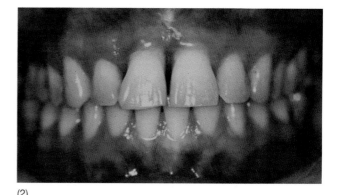
(2)

Fig. 11.9 A patient requesting treatment for flared upper incisors. (1) The pre-treatment photograph was taken after periodontal preparation leading to elongation of the clinical crowns. (2) The post-treatment photograph demonstrates the shortening of the clinical crowns as a result of intrusion of the extruded teeth.

treatment. One week after surgery, active intrusion started using a segmented appliance approach. The anchorage unit comprised two rigid buccal segments including the available molars and premolars. These segments were connected across the palate with one or two 0.036-inch stainless-steel transpalatal arches. A stiff stainless-steel full-size segment consolidated the anterior teeth that had to be intruded and maybe retracted (Figure 11.10). The active appliance consisted of a titanium–molybdenum alloy (TMA) base arch or two cantilevers delivering an intrusive force of 5–20 g per tooth depending on the periodontal support. The point of force application and the configuration of the wire were chosen based on the estimated centre of resistance, so that the desired combination of intrusion and proclination or retroclination could be generated (Dalstra and Melsen 1999). The appliance design is discussed in Chapter 7.

During the treatment, which lasted between 6 and 8 months, the patients received continuous periodontal follow-up, including instruction for home care and regular check-ups with the periodontologist. The changes occurring as a result of the treatment were evaluated on intraoral photographs, head films, periapical radiographs of the upper incisors and study casts, all taken at the start and end of the treatment. The alveolar bone level was evaluated on the periapical radiographs with the aid of a special film holder that ensured the reproducibility of the intraoral radiographs (Figure 11.11). The periapical radiographs demonstrated a coronal displacement of the marginal bone level. Based on drawings of the superimposed intraoral radiographs, the changes occurring over treatment were calculated.

The mean increase in the area of the osseous alveolus of 7% varied from a gain of 22% to a loss of 15% (Table 11.3). Nineteen of the 30 patients demonstrated improvement in alveolar support; five exhibited no change, while five patients had lost bone, in two of these patients, this could be attributed to inadequate maintenance of oral hygiene and one patient had pronounced tongue pressure counteracting the retraction, for which reason the treatment resulted in a loosening of the incisors during retraction.

The movement of the incisors was evaluated on the head films in relation to a coordinate system comprising of the hard palate as the X-axis and the perpendicular to the reference point pterygomaxillary as the Y-axis (Figure 11.12). As all the

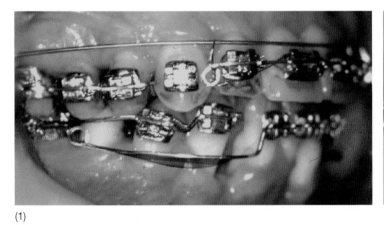 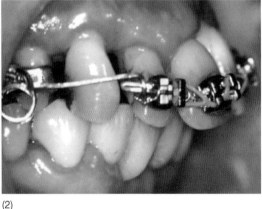

(1)   (2)

Fig. 11.10 Appliance used for intrusion. (1) A base arch made of 0.018-inch titanium–molybdenum alloy (TMA). This was used when maximum intrusion and little retraction were required. (2) Three-piece mechanics used for combined retraction and intrusion.

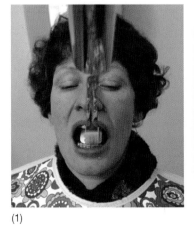 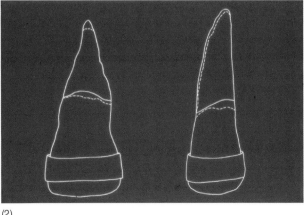

(1)   (2)

Fig. 11.11 (1) Special film holder allowing identical exposure of the individual tooth. (2) Tracing of the periapical radiographs indicating the marginal bone level before and after the intrusion. Slight apical resorption could also be verified in most cases.

Table 11.3 Change in bone support area of alveolus (%).

Mean	Minimum	Maximum
6.76	−1.5	+22

Table 11.4 True intrusion (mm).

	Minimum	Maximum
Apex	−2	5
Centre of resistance	−0	4
Incision	−2	6

Table 11.5 Reduction in crown length (mm).

Mean	Minimum	Maximum
−1.08	+2.1	−3.8

28 out of 30 had reduction.

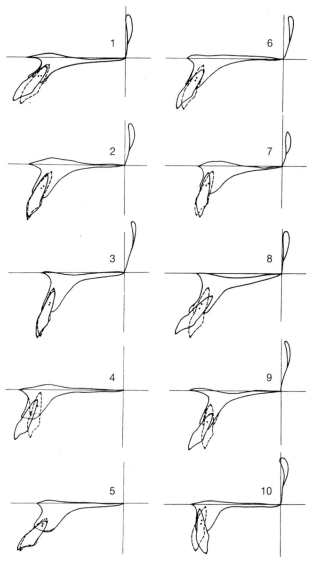

Fig. 11.12 (1)–(10) Tracings demonstrating the movement of the upper incisors during treatment in 10/30 patients.

patients were adults, these reference points were stable. A template of the central incisor was made for each patient and the best possible estimate of the centre of resistance, 40% from the marginal bone level was indicated on the templates. The templates were placed according to the best fit on the pre- and post-treatment head films. The vertical movement of the apex varied between 2 mm extrusion and 5 mm intrusion. Extrusion of the apex was seen when retroclined incisors were proclined in combination with intrusion of the crown (Table 11.4). The maximum intrusion of the apex occurred when proclined teeth were retroclined in combination with the intrusion. The intrusion of the centre of resistance varied between 0 and 4 mm, while the displacement of the incisal edge was between 2 mm extrusion and 6 mm intrusion.

In addition to the change in overbite, an average reduction of 1.08 mm in the height of the clinical crown was noted on the study casts (Table 11.5). Twenty-eight patients exhibited a shortening of the clinical crown, whereas further retraction of the gingiva and the marginal bone was observed in two patients. This was related to absence of a healthy periodontium. The results of this prospective clinical study led to the conclusion that in the case of bite deepening resulting from extrusion and horizontal bone loss, orthodontic intrusion results in an improvement of the marginal bone level. As no increase in probing depth could be verified, this was interpreted as either gain of attachment or a long epithelial attachment (Figure 11.13).

Post-treatment periapical radiographs demonstrated a cone-shaped vertical defect surrounding the intruded teeth. This defect disappeared after some months and the density of the surrounding alveolar bone increased (Figure 11.14). The latter was attributed to the improved loading situation

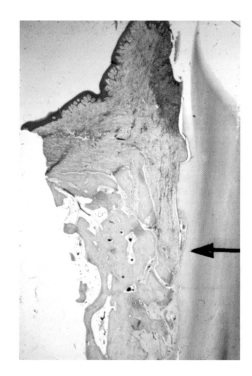

Fig. 11.13 Long epithelial attachment.

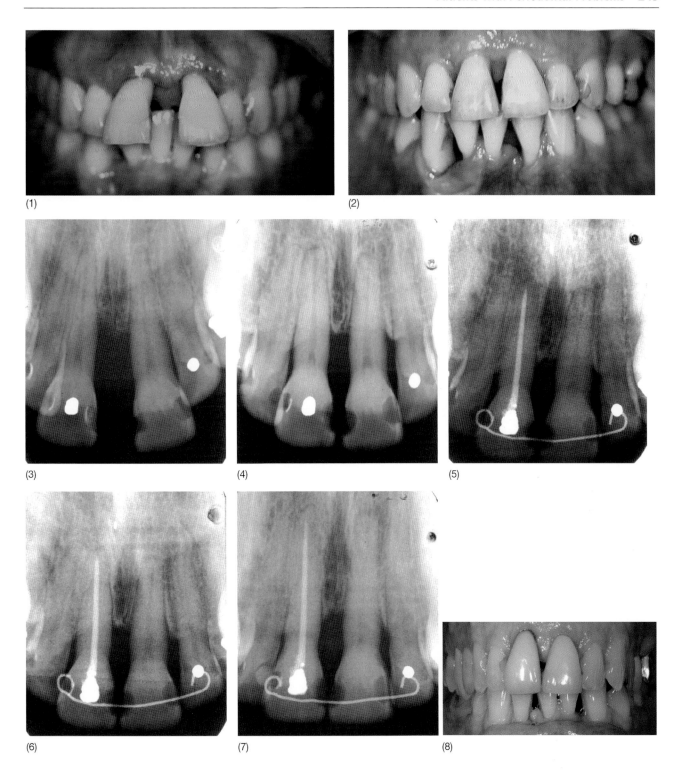

Fig. 11.14 (1) Intraoral photograph after periodontal treatment with exposure of cementum. (2) Following treatment, no cementum is visible and no pockets could be measured. (3)–(7) Radiographs taken in: (3) 1977, (4) 1979, (5) 1985, (6) 1995 and (7) 2000. There were no measurable pockets following treatment and the bone density was increased. (8) Clinical image 40 years following treatment. A porcelain veneer was placed on the endodontically treated incisor. The patient lost 2 lower molars and as the tooth 'pyjama' was removed when the veneer was done, an eruption of two upper molars took place. The result of the intrusion was however maintained, but a treatment of the lateral segments is necessary to maintain the dentition.

achieved with the treatment. Sixteen patients were reviewed after more than 30 years. No significant reduction of the bone level had occurred and the bone density had been maintained during the intervening period (Figures 11.15 and 11.16).

The results of the above-mentioned study contradict those of previous studies carried out on dogs. Those studies failed to show that true intrusion into bone could be done. However, the mechanics used in the dogs differed significantly from those used in the above-mentioned

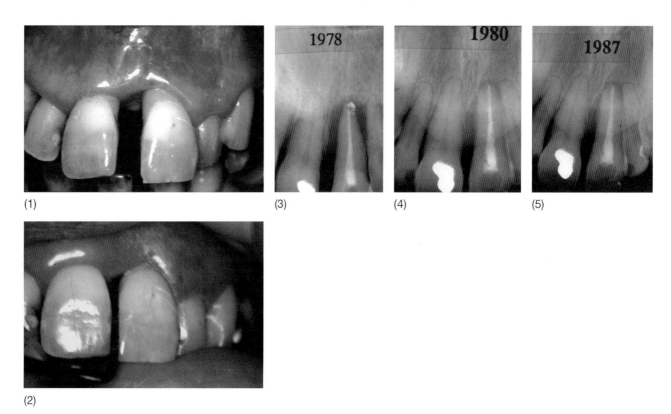

Fig. 11.15 Patient treated with intrusion. (1) Before treatment. (2) Following treatment. The clinical crown height was reduced and no pockets were found. (3)–(5) Periapical radiographs revealed that the connecting marginal and apical defects healed following the combined endodontic, periodontic and orthodontic intrusion.

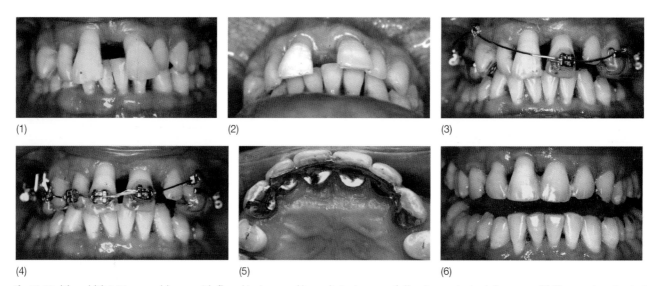

Fig. 11.16 (1) and (2) A 36-year-old man with flared incisors and long clinical crowns following periodontal surgery. (3) The most protruded and extruded tooth was retracted and intruded first. (4) Then, the three flared incisors were retracted and intruded to the level of 22. (5) The treatment result was maintained with a cast splint connecting the incisors to the canines and fabricated such that there was group contact to the anterior teeth at articulation. (6) Post-treatment situation. (7) Tracing demonstrating the tooth movements during treatment. (8) and (9) Five years post treatment. (10) and (11) Ten years post treatment. (12) 25 years following treatment.

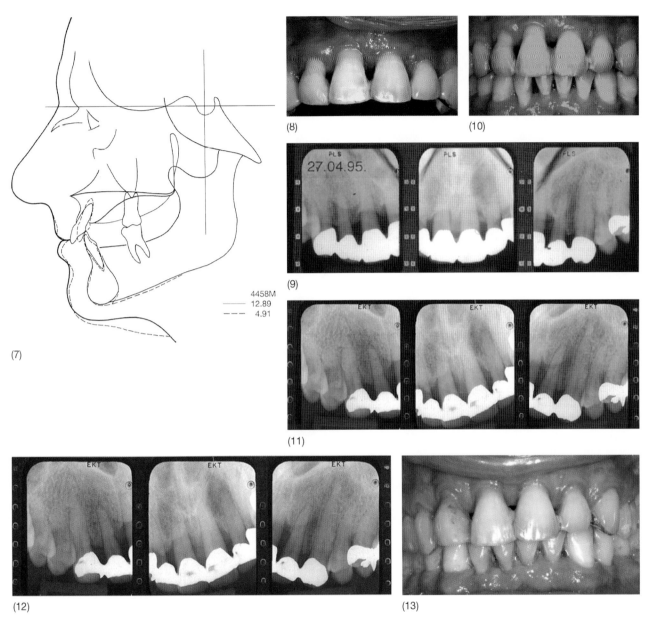

(7)

(8)

(10)

(9)

(11)

(12)

(13)

Fig. 11.16 (*Continued*)

human study. Several authors (Ericsson et al. 1977, 1978; Ericsson and Thilander 1978; Polson et al. 1984) have warned against intrusion, as it may displace supragingival plaque and calculus into a subgingival position. The patients included in the study by Melsen et al. (1989) were controlled with respect to plaque, calculus and any sign of active periodontal disease and had no increased probing depth apart from one patient with a vertical defect. In addition, the force level applied was significantly lower than that advocated in the literature (Burstone 1977; Ricketts 1980) and delivered continuously without jiggling, as is often the case when intrusion arches are combined with extraoral traction or when intermaxillary elastics are used.

Tissue reaction to intrusion of teeth with horizontal bone loss

In spite of the clinically beneficial effect of intrusion on periodontal status shown in the above-mentioned study and later corroborated by Diedrich (1996c) and Corrente et al. (2003), it is still not clear whether intrusion leads to attachment gain or to an establishment of a long epithelial attachment. This question was addressed in several animal experiments. The tipping of teeth in dogs (Ericsson and Thilander 1978; Polson et al. 1984), however, could not be compared with intrusion carried as apical translation. In the case of tipping, the periodontal ligament is compressed on the intrusive side and the stress concentrated at the marginal

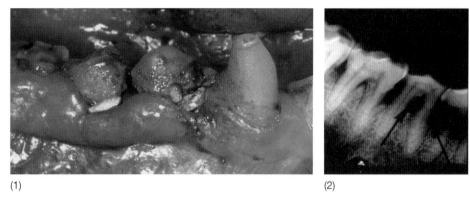

(1) (2)

Fig. 11.17 (1) Clinical image of the generation of attachment loss by the placement of elastic surrounding the collum of the molars and premolars in rhesus macaque monkeys. (2) Periapical radiograph illustrating the attachment loss.

bone level. This is not the case with true intrusion, where the line of action of the force passes close to the centre of resistance of the tooth to be intruded.

A study was therefore designed with the purpose of evaluating the tissue reaction to intrusion of premolars and incisors in rhesus macaque monkeys (Melsen et al. 1988). All 12 adult *Macaca fascicularis* monkeys included in the study showed signs of general gingivitis, and intraoral radiographs demonstrated a normal marginal bone level. Periodontal breakdown was generated by placing cotton threads and orthodontic elastics around the upper incisors and the upper and lower premolars. After 3–4 months, 4–5 mm pockets were found on probing and confirmed on intraoral radiographs (Figure 11.17). The pathologically deepened pockets were then treated by reverse bevel surgery (Caton and Nyman 1980), the root surfaces were thoroughly scaled and the pocket epithelium and granulation tissue carefully removed from the bony margin without contouring the edges. During the surgical procedure, a reference notch was prepared with a small round bur on the mesial and the distal surfaces of all the experimental teeth just coronal to the margin of the alveolar bone at the most apical part of the epithelial junction (Figure 11.18). This notch served as the reference for measurement on the histological sections. The flap was repositioned apically in order to eliminate the pockets. Following surgery, toothbrushing with 0.2% chlorhexidine digluconate solution was performed on one side three times a week. One week after surgery, the sutures were removed and an orthodontic appliance was inserted in all four quadrants. Three molars in each segment were consolidated with a cast metal splint, onto which double rectangular tubes were soldered buccally and lingually at the level of the second molars. The appliance used for intrusion of the premolars was a U-shaped segment of 0.018-inch TMA®, inserted into the tubes of the molar segment and resting on the occlusal surfaces. The incisors were bonded with small brackets, consolidated with a segment of 0.021 × 0.021-inch stainless steel and intruded

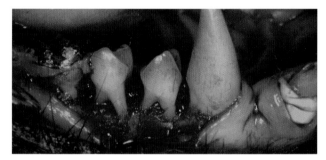

Fig. 11.18 Clinical view of the flap surgery illustrating the marginal bone loss following the breakdown of the attachment. A notch was made with a round bur above the bone margin.

with a base arch made of TMA. The force level was approximately 10 cN per tooth. In two monkeys, only one of the incisors or one of the premolars was intruded, the others serving as controls.

The period of intrusion was 3 weeks or 3–4 months prior to termination. The monkeys were euthanised by perfusion with 10% buffered formalin and the jaws were excised and prepared for parasagittal serial sectioning. On the histological sections, the distances from the most apical aspect of the notch to the gingival margin, the epithelial junction and the bone level were measured. The influence of time, hygiene and intrusion on the measured parameters was evaluated with a three-way analysis of variance.

After 3 weeks, a slight reduction in clinical crown height was noted and significant inflammation was seen on the non-hygiene side where the intrusion appliance had been placed. This was not the case in relation to the control teeth without appliance. On histological examination, no change was observed in the level of the attachment of the control teeth where no intrusion and oral hygiene had been performed (Figure 11.19). Conversely, in the teeth that had been subjected to intrusion and hygiene, the notch was always below the level of the marginal bone (Figure 11.20).

After an observation period of 3–4 months, the control teeth that had been subjected to surgical treatment only followed by neither hygiene regimen nor orthodontic treatment showed the same results as 3 weeks after surgery; that is, no change in attachment level was observed. On the non-hygiene side, the clinical crowns of the teeth subjected to intrusion were shortened. The gingiva surrounding the intruded teeth on the non-hygiene side was swollen, inflamed and bled on probing, and the alveolar bone level appeared significantly lower than that of the non-intruded neighbouring tooth (Figure 11.21). On the hygiene side, the clinical crowns were likewise shortened, but the gingiva was adapted closely to the teeth and no pathological pockets were noted (Figure 11.22). Histologically, the position of the notch on both the mesial and the distal aspects of the roots was below the bone level, clearly indicating that mainly apical translation into bone had taken place.

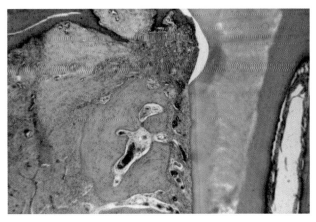

Fig. 11.19 Histological section of the marginal bone following weeks of intrusion. The notch is still above the bone level and the marginal bone is being resorbed.

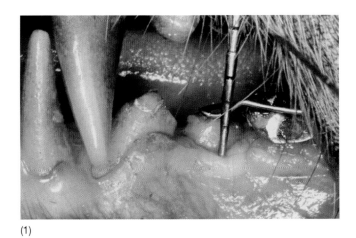

(1)

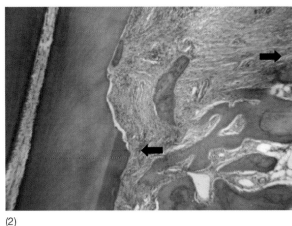

(2)

Fig. 11.20 (1) Intrusion of one premolar over three weeks with maintenance of hygiene. The appliance consisted of a 0.018-inch TMA wire extending from the molar region and resting on the occlusal surface. (2) The histological section shows that the notch is below the bone level. A bony island can be identified and resorption is occurring of the notch area, probably as part of a repair process.

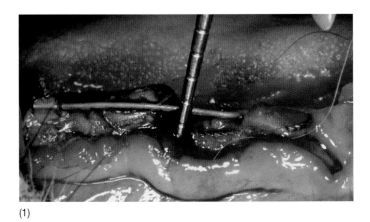

(1)

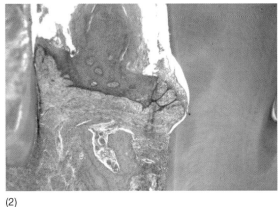

(2)

Fig. 11.21 (1) Clinical photograph of the side without oral hygiene after 3 months of intrusion. Two premolars were intruded simultaneously with a 0.018-inch TMA wire resting on the occlusal surface. The gingiva was heavily inflamed and bleeding on probing. (2) The corresponding histological section shows that the notch of the intruded tooth had reached the level of the apex of the adjacent tooth. Note the active resorption of the marginal bone.

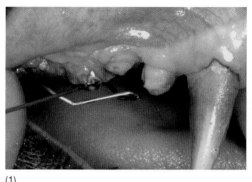
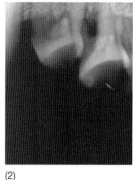
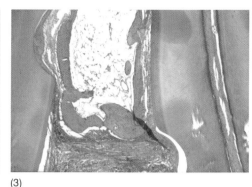

(1)   (2)   (3)

Fig. 11.22 (1) Clinical image of intrusion on the side on which oral hygiene was provided. One lower premolar was intruded for 6 months with a 0.018-inch TMA wire resting on the occlusal surface. The gingiva was healthy and no pockets could be probed. (2) Periapical radiograph of the premolar that has been intruded for 3 months. (3) Histological section where the different levels of the notches illustrate the amount of intrusion achieved. Note that the attachment level of the intruded tooth has regained its normal level. On the adjacent tooth that has not been intruded, cellular cementum is extending into the notch, but the level of attachment of the two teeth is significantly different.

The histomorphometric analysis demonstrated that when intrusion was done under a strict periodontal regimen, the teeth were indeed intruded into bone without reduction in the height of the alveolar process and without inflammation (Figure 11.23). The reference notch was situated on an average 1.5 mm apical to the epithelial junction and 1.3 mm apical to the bone level. The notch area was lined with a layer of cellular cementum and continued from the notch in a coronal direction. The epithelial junction was re-established to its original level, very close to the marginal bone level, slightly above in some cases and slightly below in others. Collagen fibres stretched from bone into the periodontal ligament in an apical direction. The bone surface bordering the periodontal ligament was lined with formative cells apart from the apical area in which the ligament appeared to be compressed. In the case in which only one of the neighbouring premolars was intruded, there was a distinct difference in the level of connective-tissue attachment of the intruded and the non-intruded teeth. In the latter, the periodontal treatment had resulted in new cementum formation covering the apical half of the notch, thus corroborating the findings of Caton et al. (1980) (Figure 11.22). No active root resorption could be detected, but apically some of the resorption lacunae had undergone repair (Figure 11.24).

The three-way analysis of variance clearly demonstrated that both hygiene and intrusion were factors of major significance for the explanation of the results. It was also obvious that a significant interaction existed between intrusion and hygiene. The results of the measurements are summarised in Tables 11.6 and 11.7.

The conclusion from several repeated studies was that given a healthy periodontium and absence of increased probing depth, a new attachment could be generated in relation to teeth with horizontal bone loss, provided the movement was carried out as an apically directed intrusion with low, constant forces.

Treatment of patients with vertical bone defects

The treatment of patients with vertical pockets has been the subject of many studies, which found that the movement of a tooth into a vertical defect does not result in attachment gain even in cases with significant improvement of the gingival level, and the risk for attachment loss should not be overlooked when moving teeth associated with pathological pockets. Depending on the type of the desired tooth movement, the treatment approach will be different.

In cases in which intrusion will be part of the movement, the probing depth has to be reduced before orthodontic treatment. This is usually done by apical displacement of the gingival margin, but may be difficult in the presence of vertical defects. In these cases, guided tissue regeneration (GTR) and/or the application of growth factors before orthodontic treatment is the approach followed (Figures 11.25 and 11.26). Both GTR with membranes and regenerative therapy with Emdogain® have been successfully used in cases with two or three wall pockets, and when combined with orthodontic intrusion, the benefit is even greater (Kraal et al. 1980; Diedrich 1996a, 1996b; Diedrich et al. 2003).

In cases where rehabilitation of the periodontally involved tooth is planned, an alternative strategy would be to extrude the tooth with the vertical defect. This would also be the case when the marginal gingival level is more apical than that of the other teeth. The influence of levelling generally has a beneficial effect on the bone level. The specific effect of extrusion has been studied both clinically (Ingber 1974, 1989; Mantzikos and Shamus 1997, 1999; Roth et al. 2004) and experimentally (van Venrooy and Yukna 1985), and there is general agreement that orthodontic extrusion is a recommendable way of building up the alveolar process. This can be done before prosthetic rehabilitation including implant insertion (Figure 11.27).

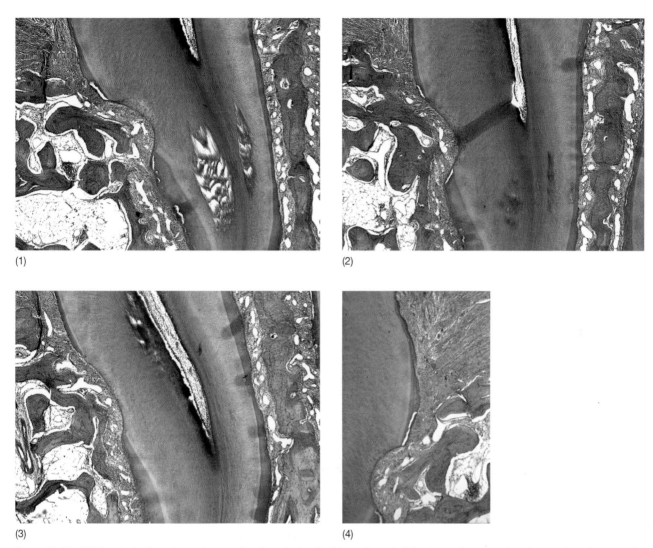

Fig. 11.23 (1)–(4) Histological sections of a sample of teeth that had been intruded for 3 months. Note that the notch is always under the marginal bone level and the attachment level is above the marginal bone.

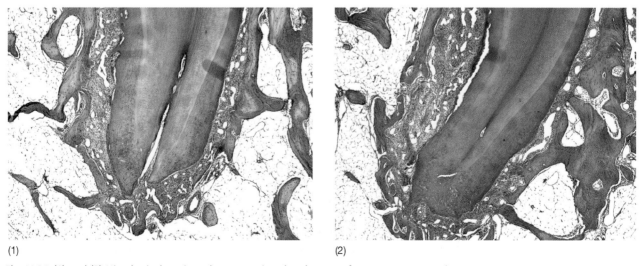

Fig. 11.24 (1) and (2) Histological sections demonstrating the absence of severe root resorption.

Table 11.6 Changes in attachment level as a result of intrusion. AM-EJ: apical limit of the notch to cementoenamel junction.

Orthodontic treatment	Periodontal treatment	Variable	N	Mean	SD
Without intrusion	Without hygiene	AM-EJ	6	−0.1	0.67
	With hygiene	AM-EJ	8	0.3	0.32
With intrusion	Without hygiene	AM-EJ	10	0.9	0.75
	With hygiene	AM-EJ	24	1.5	0.76

Table 11.7 Changes in attachment level as a result of intrusion. AM-BL: apical limit of the notch to bone level.

Orthodontic treatment	Periodontal treatment	Variable	N	Mean	SD
Without intrusion	Without hygiene	AM-BL	6	0.1	0.50
	With hygiene	AM-BL	8	0.4	0.31
With intrusion	Without hygiene	AM-BL	10	0.3	0.28
	With hygiene	AM-BL	24	1.5	0.29

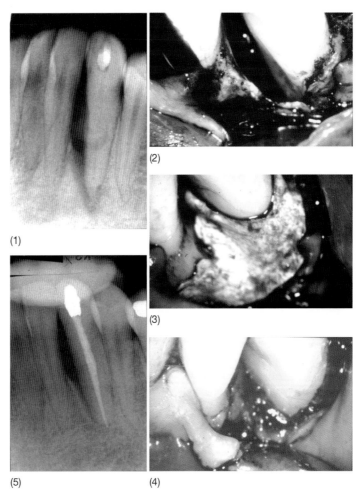

Fig. 11.25 (1) and (2) Lower canine with a vertical defect. (3) Following mechanical debridement, a GORE-TEX® membrane was applied and the gingiva repositioned. (4) When the membrane was removed 6 months later, the vertical defect had filled in and a more coronal attachment level had been established. (5) Periapical radiograph following treatment. (Courtesy of Kirsten Warrer.)

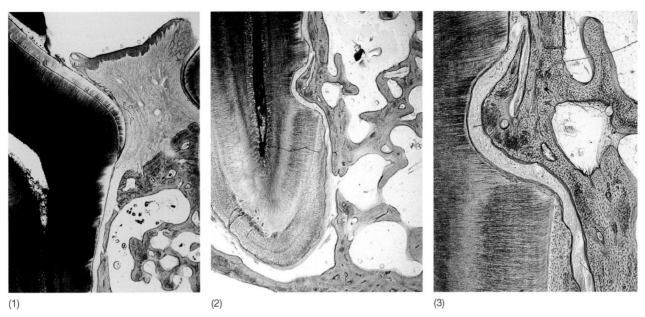

(1)   (2)   (3)

Fig. 11.26 Histological section of a periodontally affected tooth that was orthodontically intruded following mechanical/chemical debridement and regenerative therapy (Emdogain®). (1) Marginal bone level, and (2) the area where a notch had been made during surgery before intrusion, corresponding to the deepest point of instrumentation. (3) Larger magnification of the notch area. (From Diedrich P, Fritz U, Kinzinger G and Angelakis J (2003) Movement of periodontally affected teeth after guided tissue regeneration (GTR) – an experimental pilot study in animals. J Orofac Orthop 64, 214–227. Reproduced with kind permission of Springer Science + Business Media.)

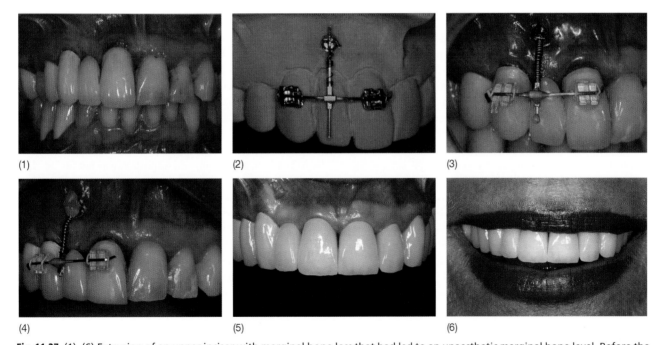

(1)   (2)   (3)

(4)   (5)   (6)

Fig. 11.27 (1)–(6) Extrusion of an upper incisor with marginal bone loss that had led to an unaesthetic marginal bone level. Before the porcelain crown was redone, the incisor was extruded 'with' bone to regenerate the marginal bone level. A mini-implant was used for anchorage. (From Roth A, Yildirim M and Diedrich P (2004) Forced eruption with microscrew anchorage for preprosthetic levelling of the gingival margin. Case report. J Orofac Orthop 65, 513–519. Reproduced with kind permission of Springer Science + Business Media.)

Frequently, vertical defects are related to tipped teeth and the effect of the uprighting on the attachment has been described as beneficial (Kraal et al. 1980). Brown (cited in Cohen (1984)) performed histological studies of human molars and demonstrated new attachment and new bone formation in relation to the uprighting of the tipped teeth, and Geraci et al. (1990) also demonstrated new attachment following the displacement of teeth into infrabony defects in monkeys. In both these studies, periodontal treatment was carried out before orthodontics and the periodontium maintained during treatment.

Polson et al. (1984), however, found no change in attachment level when tipping teeth into infrabony defects. The detrimental effect of moving teeth into vertical defects was demonstrated by Wennström et al. (1993), who investigated the influence of orthodontic tooth movement on artificially created vertical defects in beagle dogs. They found that tooth movement into inflamed infrabony pockets resulted in an increased rate of destruction of the periodontium. The health of the periodontium seems to be the determining factor when performing tooth movement involving intrusion.

What are the periodontal limits for orthodontic tooth movement?

Sagittal movement

A crucial question in relation to the majority of orthodontic patients is whether to extract or to expand. This question is especially important in relation to adult patients, as extraction will frequently lead to undesirable side effects on the soft-tissue profile. Protrusion of the lower incisors is an alternative to extraction in the lower arch in cases of crowding and to extraction in the upper arch in cases of increased overjet. Protraction of the lower incisors is desirable in cases in which it will have a beneficial effect on the soft-tissue profile through smoothing of the mentolabial sulcus. The decision regarding the optimal position of the lower incisors is still a matter of debate. Diedrich (1996c) concluded that provided the specific anatomy was taken into consideration, the gingival health and the force system were carefully monitored, and teeth could be moved with their surrounding periodontium. This explains why several authors have found no association between proclination and gingival recession (Artun and Krogstad 1987; Wennström et al. 1987; Ruf et al. 1998; Artun and Grobety 2001), while other authors consider proclination of lower incisors a risk (Dorfman 1978; Hollender et al. 1980; Steiner et al. 1981; Genco 1996; Djeu et al. 2002; Joss-Vassalli et al. 2010; Renkema et al. 2015).

The question regarding sagittal expansion as a possible risk factor for the creation of dehiscences in relation to the lower incisors was finally addressed in a case–control study carried out on 150 consecutive patients aged 33.7 ± 9.5 years. They all had their lower incisors displaced significantly labially. The patients were matched by age and sex with a control group waiting for similar treatment (Allais and Melsen 2003). The arch length was increased during treatment on an average by 3.4 mm (Figure 11.28).

The intraoral slide recordings revealed a difference in the numbers of individuals with gingival recession in the case and control groups, but there was no significant difference in the mean recession value. To investigate changes in prevalence and severity of gingival recession at the lower incisors occurring during proclination of incisors in the 150 above-mentioned patients, gingival recession, width of keratinised gingival biotype, inflammation and visual plaque were recorded on standard intraoral slides taken before and after treatment. The amount of labial movement was assessed on cast measurements as the difference between the pre- and post-treatment positions (Melsen and Allais 2005).

No significant increase in mean gingival recession was observed during treatment. The mean recession value at the beginning of treatment was 0.20 mm and at the end of treatment 0.34 mm. The difference of 0.14 mm was below the error of the measurement and of no clinical relevance (Baumrind and Frantz 1971). The prevalence of gingival recession >1.0 mm increased from 21% before to 35% after treatment ($p < 0.05$), but only 2.8% acquired recessions >2 mm and 5% of the pre-existing gingival recession improved.

When an attempt was made to identify skeletal, dentoalveolar, occlusal and soft tissue parameters that could be useful predictors for the dehiscences by a logistic regression analysis, only the presence of baseline recession ($p <$ gingival biotype ($p < 0.01$), gingival inflammation ($p < 0.003$)) and none of the orthodontically related variables were significantly associated with the development of recession.

When Lindtoft (2015) made a recall, she managed to find that in 100 out of the 150 patients, the development of periodontal loss was due to the mean increase in gingival recession that was 0.44 mm with a range of 0.26–0.70 mm. The predictors were: older age (>45), traumatic occlusion and presence of a bonded retainer and a thin biotype. The oral hygiene which most likely was important was not included, as all the patients who turned up had maintained their oral hygiene regimen. Also, the error in registration of inflammation was so high that the results had only low validity.

Considering the results of the above-mentioned reviews, it seems most likely that the attitude towards anterior movement of lower incisor is based on dogmas regarding incisor inclination and findings of studies in which neither the force systems nor the maintenance of the periodontal health during treatment was taken into account. Differences in the force systems applied may result in tooth movement with or through bone (Melsen 1999), thereby contributing to the explanation for the detrimental findings found by some authors. When displacing lower incisors anteriorly, it is important that it is not done with a tipping which will lead to a bending of the marginal bone and a local necrosis. If, on the other hand, the displacement is initiated with a root movement, a formation is occurring at the labial aspect of the alveolar process. This was the case for most of the patients in the Aarhus study (Figure 11.28(1),(2)). Intraoral images of a patient with increased overbite and anterior crowing are shown in Figure 11.28(3),(4). The upper incisors were proclined and intruded to solve the increased overbite and the crowding. In the lower arch, the lower incisors were protruded in order to obtain a normal overjet and generate space for the replacement of the second premolars with implants. The heights of the lower incisors were not increased (Figure 11.28(5),(6)). The status of the gingival level was not changed after 20 years.

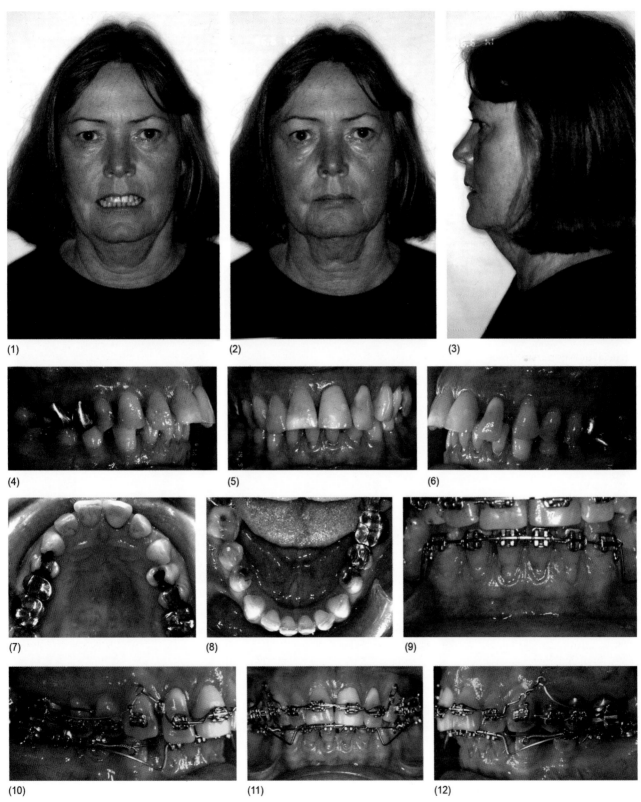

(1) (2) (3)

(4) (5) (6)

(7) (8) (9)

(10) (11) (12)

Fig. 11.28 (*Continued*)

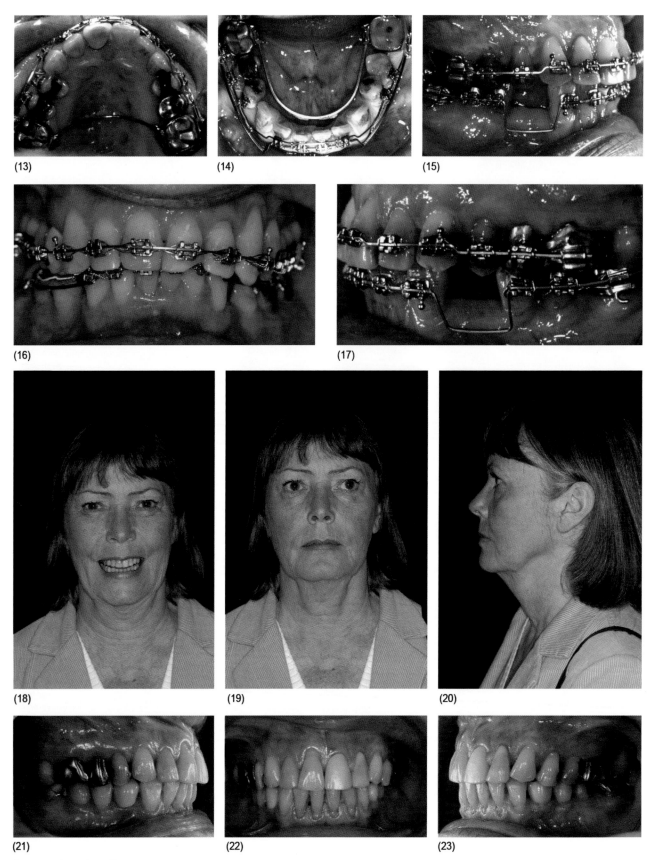

(13) (14) (15)

(16) (17)

(18) (19) (20)

(21) (22) (23)

Fig. 11.28 (*Continued*)

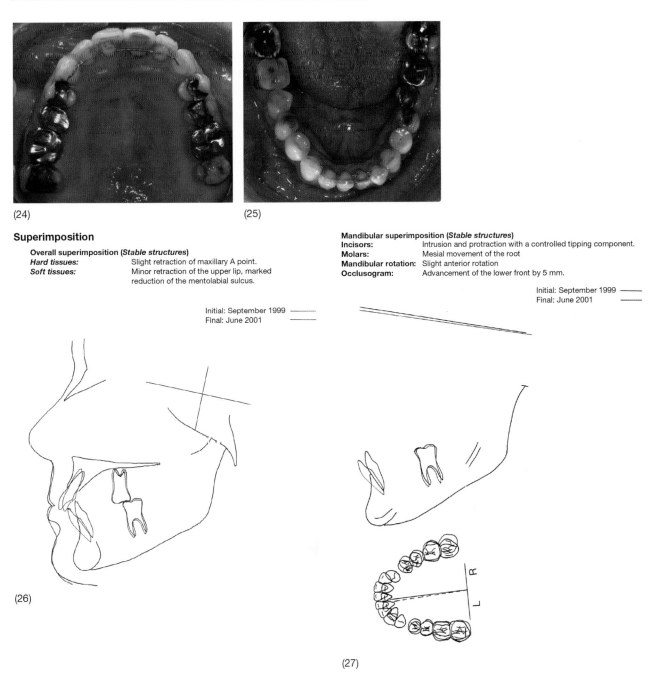

Superimposition

Overall superimposition (*Stable structures*)
Hard tissues: Slight retraction of maxillary A point.
Soft tissues: Minor retraction of the upper lip, marked
                         reduction of the mentolabial sulcus.

Mandibular superimposition (*Stable structures*)
Incisors: Intrusion and protraction with a controlled tipping component.
Molars: Mesial movement of the root
Mandibular rotation: Slight anterior rotation
Occlusogram: Advancement of the lower front by 5 mm.

Initial: September 1999 ————
Final: June 2001   ————

Initial: September 1999 ————
Final: June 2001   ————

(24)   (25)   (26)   (27)

Fig. 11.28 (1)–(8) A 56-year-old woman with increased overjet partly caused by retroclination of the lower anterior teeth following extraction of the lower first molars when she was still a child. Due to her age, surgery was not an option, and extraction of the upper premolars and retraction of the upper anterior segment were considered inappropriate due to profile considerations. It was therefore decided to protract the lower anterior teeth to create space for an implant distal to the canines. (9) The marginal gingiva at the start of treatment. (10)–(14) Sagittal expansion was done with a torque arch combined with a bypass arch. (15)–(17) Root uprighting was done with a vertical step down in the TMA continuous arch. (18)–(25) Status at the end of treatment. The treatment was finished by insertion of implants in the first premolar region. The patient then had 'three premolars' on each side. The protrusion of the lower anterior segment involved controlled tipping, without loss of attachment or creation of any dehiscences. (26) and (27) Tracing demonstrating the tooth movements during treatment.

Transverse movement

Transverse expansion is also considered a periodontal risk according to the hypothesis put forward by Wennström et al. (1987, 1993) 'that teeth could not be moved out of the dentoalveolar envelope'. This opinion was shared with Vanarsdall and Secchi (2005), who warned against transverse expansion in adult patients after demonstrating an increase in dehiscence following transverse maxillary expansion in adult patients. Riedel and Brandt (1976) also advised against transverse expansion as a treatment subject to high risk of relapse. However, it does seem as if the type of expansion is important. Handelman and colleagues (Riedel and Brandt 1976; Handelman 1997; Handelman et al. 2000) found no significant differences between the pre- and post-treatment crown height in a group of adult patients treated with a tooth- and tissue-borne palatal expander and nor did Bassarelli et al. (2005). Recent studies on expansion with broad arches and self-ligating brackets indicate that bone loss is a common side effect (Cattaneo et al. 2011).

Surgically assisted expansion has been recommended as a solution to transverse problems in adult patients. Carmen et al. (2000) found less periodontal damage following surgically assisted expansion compared with following orthodontic expansion, and this was later confirmed by Garib (2006). On the other hand, Cureton and Cuenin (1999) described periodontal damage to the incisors following surgically assisted expansion. The risk related to expansion is thus yet a matter of controversy. The answer to the question on the limit therefore seems to be dependent on the local environment and the type of tooth movement. The recommendation of widening is completely without scientific background and will frequently lead to loss of marginal bone (Cattaneo et al. 2011)

Sequence of treatment in periodontally involved patients

The periodontium has to be healthy before and maintained in a healthy state during and after the treatment. No orthodontic treatment should be started if the periodontal condition is not under control.

Any orthodontic treatment should therefore always be initiated by motivation and instruction followed by scaling and removal of factors such as overhanging fillings interfering with a good oral hygiene. Other pathologies interfering with oral health, such as caries and/or periapical lesions, should be taken care of before proceeding to active orthodontic treatment (Box 11.1). It is important that the patient feels co-responsibility for the treatment and for the maintenance of the result. The resources required in terms of time and money should be made clear to the patient before starting treatment. Only when the patient is well informed and has accepted the conditions, the detailed planning can be worked up involving the establishment of the plan for interdisciplinary collaboration with other colleagues.

Spontaneous tooth migrations that have led to development of a secondary malocclusion are never horizontal movements but combined horizontal and extrusive displacements. The required force system will therefore generally include an intrusive component when replacing the flared or migrated teeth. As this tooth movement includes the risk of displacing supragingival plaque and calculus subgingivally, a perfect periodontal health is crucial in order to avoid iatrogenic damage (Ericsson and Thilander 1978).

It is imperative that no pockets of >3 mm probing depth are present around the tooth to be moved orthodontically. State-of-the-art periodontal therapy recommends a conservative approach even in the case of deep pockets. This is acceptable as long as no tooth movements are to take place (Badersten et al. 1985a, 1985b, 1985c, 1987a, 1987b). However, as the tissue reaction responsible for tooth movement resembles inflammation, it is crucial that the periodontium is also healthy on a tissue level. Waerhaug (1952) performed thorough scaling of teeth before extraction and found that in cases with pockets between 3 mm and 5 mm only 60% of the teeth were satisfactorily scaled, and the results were even worse if the probing depth was above 5 mm (Table 11.8). If the teeth therefore have to be periodontally healthy, an open scaling and root planning is required. In the case of a horizontal bone loss, a Widman modified flap surgery is the preferred surgery, as the advantage of this surgery offers the possibility of obtaining a close adaptation of the soft tissues to the root surfaces with a minimum of trauma to the tissue exposed and a minimum of exposure of the roots.

Having reduced the pockets, the orthodontic treatment can be initiated. Once the appliances are inserted, the patient should be given additional instructions in personal oral hygiene, taking the appliance into consideration. In addition, it should be ensured that the appliance does not in any way compromise the maintenance of a healthy periodontal status. Following the orthodontic treatment, additional periodontal treatment including eventual mucogingival surgery may be required (Figure 11.28).

The final question naturally concerns stability. In adult patients, post-treatment stability cannot be predicted.

Box 11.1 The essential procedures

- Oral prophylaxis
- Restorative therapy
- Endodontics
- Extractions
- Temporary restorations

Table 11.8 Rate of success or failure as a result of subgingival plaque control and as influenced by pocket depth[a].

	Pocket depth 3 mm		Pocket depth 3–5 mm		Pocket depth >5 mm		Total	
	No.	%	No.	%	No.	%	No.	%
Success	52	83	36	39	6	11	94	44
Failure	11	17	56	61	51	89	118	56
Total	63	100	92	100	57	100	212	100

[a] Evaluations made on 212 surfaces of 53 teeth.

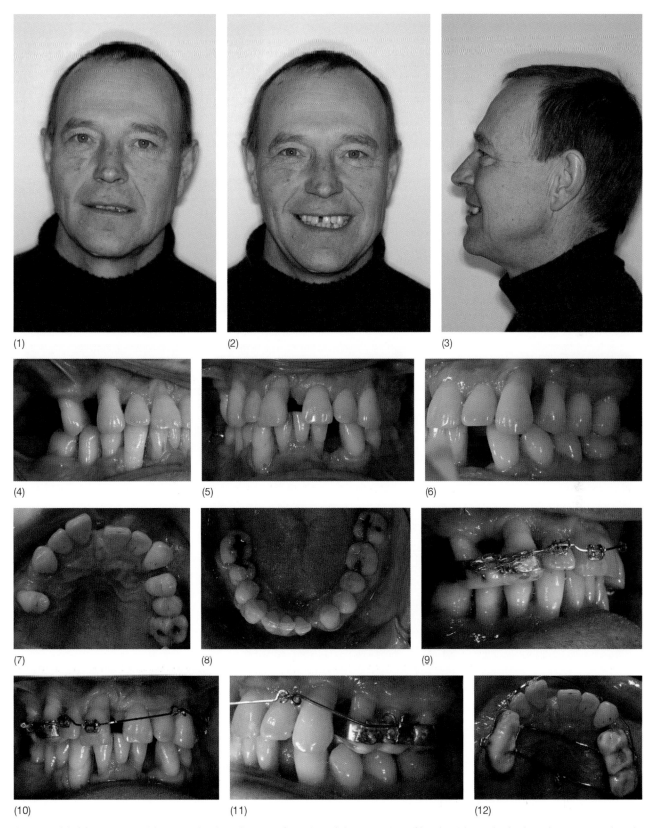

(1)

(2)

(3)

(4)

(5)

(6)

(7)

(8)

(9)

(10)

(11)

(12)

Fig. 11.29 (1)–(8) A 55-year-old man with a long history of continued deterioration of his dentition, who had not been aware that the process could be avoided. A 'new' dentist made him aware of the treatment possibilities. When he was referred to the orthodontist, he had already had periodontal surgery. (9)–(12) The most deviated tooth in the upper arch was intruded and displaced towards the midline with a cantilever. A double transpalatal arch and reinforcement of the occlusion were used as anchorage. (13)–(17) Following movement of 11, the other incisors were included in the appliance. In the lower arch, the lack of buccal bone in relation to 43 was preventing midline correction. (18) At the end of the orthodontic treatment, a connective tissue graft was applied on the labial aspect of 11. (19)–(26) Post-treatment status. A cast upper retainer was bonded to the upper anterior segment and a bonded bridge served as retainer in the lower arch. (27) and (28) Pre- and post-treatment periapical status. Note the improvement in the marginal bone level.

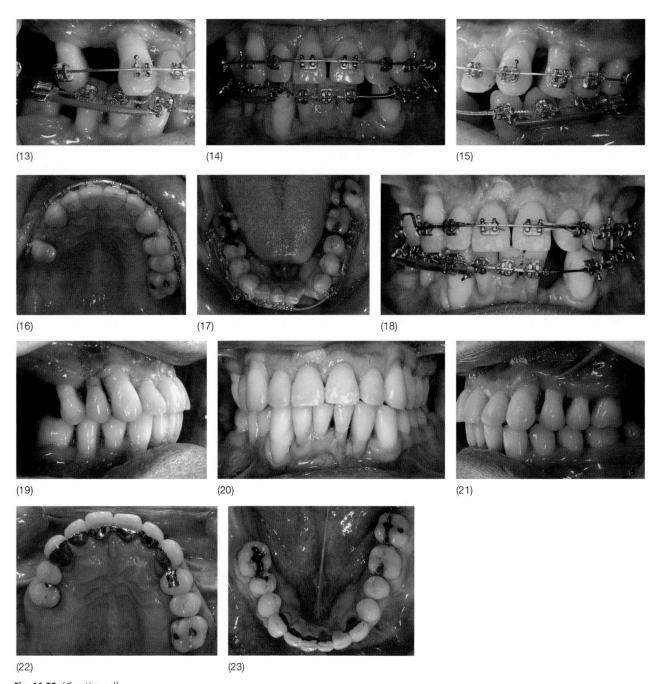

(13)　　　　　(14)　　　　　(15)

(16)　　　　　(17)　　　　　(18)

(19)　　　　　(20)　　　　　(21)

(22)　　　　　(23)

Fig. 11.29 (*Continued*)

Frequently, these treatments will be compromise treatments, and as a rule, these patients need lifelong maintenance and retention either with fixed or removable retention devices. Long-term follow-up, however, demonstrates that treatment results can be preserved provided the periodontal health and mechanical retention are maintained. The treatment sequence is discussed in detail in Chapters 12 and 13.

Conclusion regarding influence of orthodontic treatment on periodontal status

Both clinical studies and animal experiments have demonstrated that a combination of periodontal therapy and orthodontics not only prevents further deterioration but also improves the periodontal status. An example of a patient with severe deterioration of the dentition is shown in Figure 11.29.

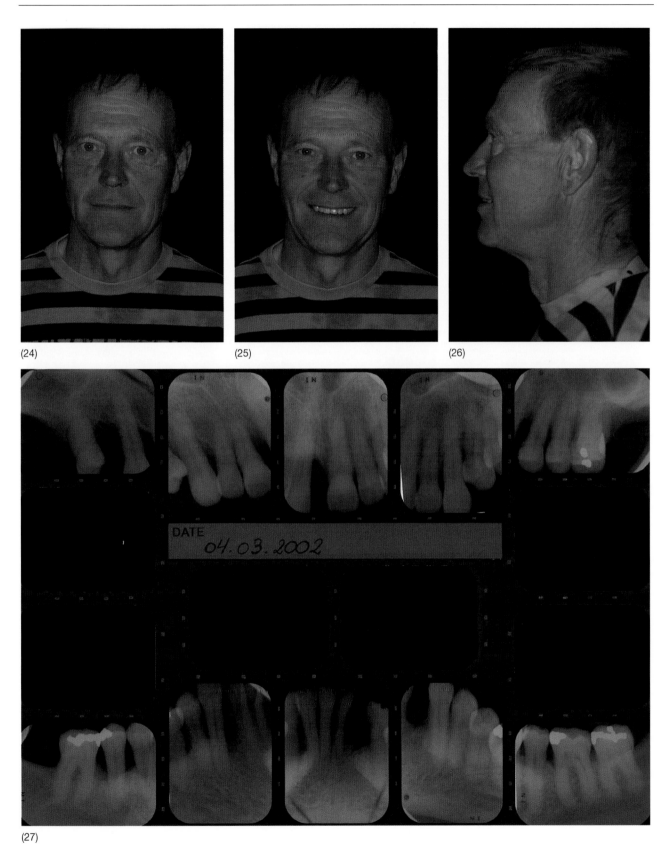

(24)   (25)   (26)

DATE 04.03.2002

(27)

Fig. 11.29 (*Continued*)

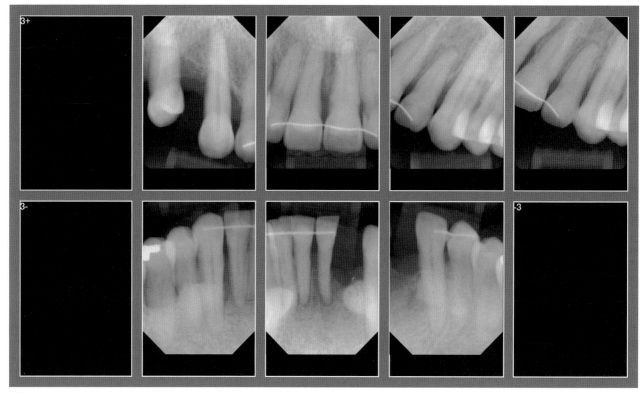

(28)

Fig. 11.29 (*Continued*)

References

Albandar JM (2002a) Global risk factors and risk indicators for periodontal diseases. *Periodontol 2000* **29**, 177–206.

Albandar JM (2002b) Periodontal diseases in North America. *Periodontol 2000* **29**, 31–69.

Albandar JM and Rams TE (2002) Risk factors for periodontitis in children and young persons. *Periodontol 2000* **29**, 207–222.

Allais D and Melsen B (2003) Does labial movement of lower incisors influence the level of the gingival margin? A case-control study of adult orthodontic patients. *Eur J Orthod* **25**, 343–352.

Alstad S and Zachrisson BU (1979) Longitudinal study of periodontal condition associated with orthodontic treatment in adolescents. *Am J Orthod* **76**, 277–286.

Artun J and Grobety D (2001) Periodontal status of mandibular incisors after pronounced orthodontic advancement during adolescence: a follow-up evaluation. *Am J Orthod Dentofacial Orthop* **119**, 2–10.

Artun J and Krogstad O (1987) Periodontal status of mandibular incisors following excessive proclination. A study in adults with surgically treated mandibular prognathism. *Am J Orthod Dentofacial Orthop* **91**, 225–232.

Badersten A, Nilveus R and Egelberg J (1985a) Effect of non-surgical periodontal therapy (IV). Operator variability. *J Clin Periodontol* **12**, 190–200.

Badersten A, Nilveus R and Egelberg J (1985b) Effect of non-surgical periodontal therapy. VI. Localization of sites with probing attachment loss. *J Clin Periodontol* **12**, 351–359.

Badersten A, Nilveus R and Egelberg J (1985c) Effect of nonsurgical periodontal therapy. VII. Bleeding, suppuration and probing depth in sites with probing attachment loss. *J Clin Periodontol* **12**, 432–440.

Badersten A, Nilveus R and Egelberg J (1987a) Effect of nonsurgical periodontal therapy (VIII). Probing attachment changes related to clinical characteristics. *J Clin Periodontol* **14**, 425–432.

Badersten A, Niveus R and Egelberg J (1987b) 4-year observations of basic periodontal therapy. *J Clin Periodontol* **14**, 438–444.

Bassarelli T, Dalstra M and Melsen B (2005) Changes in clinical crown height as a result of transverse expansion of the maxilla in adults. *Eur J Orthod* **27**, 121–128.

Baumrind S and Frantz RC (1971) The reliability of head film measurements. 1. Landmark identification. *Am J Orthod* **60**, 111–127.

Boyd RL, Leggott PJ, Quinn RS, Eakle WS and Chambers D (1989) Periodontal implications of orthodontic treatment in adults with reduced or normal periodontal tissues versus those of adolescents. *Am J Orthod Dentofacial Orthop* **96**, 191–198.

Buckley LA (1981) The relationships between malocclusion, gingival inflammation, plaque and calculus. *J Periodontol* **52**, 35–40.

Burgett FG (1995) Trauma from occlusion. Periodontal concerns. *Dent Clin North Am* **39**, 301–311.

Burstone CR (1977) Deep overbite correction by intrusion. *Am J Orthod* **72**, 1–22.

Carmen M, Marcella P, Giuseppe C and Roberto A (2000) Periodontal evaluation in patients undergoing maxillary expansion. *J Craniofac Surg* **11**, 491–494.

Caton J and Nyman S (1980) Histometric evaluation of periodontal surgery. I. The modified Widman flap procedure. *J Clin Periodontol* **7**, 212–223.

Caton J, Nyman S and Zander H (1980) Histometric evaluation of periodontal surgery. II. Connective tissue attachment levels after four regenerative procedures. *J Clin Periodontol* **7**, 224–231.

Cattaneo P, Treccani M, Carlsson K, Thorgeirsson T, Myrda A, Cevidanes L and Melsen B (2011) Transversal maxillary dento-alveolar changes in patients treated with active and passive self-ligating brackets: a randomized clinical trial using CBCT-scans and digital models. *Orthod Craniofac Res* **14**(4), 222–233. doi:10.1111/j.1601-6343.2011.01527.x

Chen RJ, Yang JF and Chao TC (1990) Invaginated tooth associated with periodontal abscess. *Oral Surg Oral Med Oral Pathol* **69**, 659.

Chung CH, Vanarsdall RL, Cavalcanti EA, Baldinger JS and Lai CH (2000) Comparison of microbial composition in the subgingival plaque of adult crowded versus non-crowded dental regions. *Int J Adult Orthod Orthog Surg* **15**, 321–330.

Cohen DW (1984) Areas of common concern to orthodontics and periodontics. In McNamara JA and Ribbens KA (eds) *Malocclusion and the Periodontium*, pp. 67–76. Ann Arbor, MI: University of Michigan.

Corrente G, Abundo R, Re S, Cardaropoli D and Cardaropoli G (2003) Orthodontic movement into infrabony defects in patients with advanced periodontal disease: a clinical and radiological study. *J Periodontol* **74**, 1104–1109.

Cureton SL and Cuenin M (1999) Surgically assisted rapid palatal expansion: orthodontic preparation for clinical success. *Am J Orthod Dentofacial Orthop* **116**, 46–59.

Dalstra M and Melsen B (1999) Force systems developed by six different cantilever configurations. *Clin Orthod Res* **2**, 3–9.

Diedrich P (1996a) Preprosthetic orthodontics. *J Orofac Orthop* **57**, 102–116.

Diedrich PR (1996b) Guided tissue regeneration associated with orthodontic therapy. *Semin Orthod* **2**, 39–45.

Diedrich PR (1996c) Orthodontic procedures improving periodontal prognosis. *Dent Clin North Am* **40**, 875–887.

Diedrich P (1999) The eleventh hour or where are our orthodontic limits? Case report. *J Orofac Orthop* **60**, 60–65.

Diedrich P (2000) Periodontal relevance of anterior crowding. *J Orofac Orthop* **61**, 69–79.

Diedrich P, Fritz U, Kinzinger G and Angelakis J (2003) Movement of periodontally affected teeth after guided tissue regeneration (GTR) – an experimental pilot study in animals. *J Orofac Orthop* **64**, 214–227.

Djeu G, Hayes C and Zawaideh S (2002) Correlation between mandibular central incisor proclination and gingival recession during fixed appliance therapy. *Angle Orthod* **72**, 238–245.

Dorfman HS (1978) Mucogingival changes resulting from mandibular incisor tooth movement. *Am J Orthod* **74**, 286–297.

Eliasson LA, Hugoson A, Kurol J and Siwe H (1982) The effects of orthodontic treatment on periodontal tissues in patients with reduced periodontal support. *Eur J Orthod* **4**, 1–9.

el-Mangoury NH, Gaafar SM and Mostafa YA (1987) Mandibular anterior crowding and periodontal disease. *Angle Orthod* **57**, 33–38.

Ericsson I and Lindhe J (1982) Effect of longstanding jiggling on experimental marginal periodontitis in the beagle dog. *J Clin Periodontol* **9**, 497–503.

Ericsson I and Lindhe J (1984) Lack of significance of increased tooth mobility in experimental periodontitis. *J Periodontol* **55**, 447–452.

Ericsson I and Thilander B (1978) Orthodontic forces and recurrence of periodontal disease. An experimental study in the dog. *Am J Orthod* **74**, 41–50.

Ericsson I, Thilander B and Lindhe J (1978) Periodontal conditions after orthodontic tooth movements in the dog. *Angle Orthod* **48**, 210–218.

Ericsson I, Thilander B, Lindhe J and Okamoto H (1977) The effect of orthodontic tilting movements on the periodontal tissues of infected and non-infected dentitions in dogs. *J Clin Periodontol* **4**, 278–293.

Fristad I and Molven O (1998) Root resorption and apical breakdown during orthodontic treatment of a maxillary lateral incisor with dens invaginatus. *Endodont Dent Traumatol* **14**, 241–244.

Garib DG, Henriques JF, Janson G, de Freitas MR and Fernandes AY (2006) Periodontal effects of rapid maxillary expansion with tooth-tissue-borne and tooth-borne expanders: a computed tomography evaluation. *Am J Orthod Dentofacial Orthop* **129**(6), 749–758.

Geiger AM, Wasserman BH, Thompson RH Jr and Turgeon LR (1972) Relationship of occlusion and periodontal disease. V. Relation of classification of occlusion to periodontal status and gingival inflammation. *J Periodontol* **43**, 554–560.

Genco RJ (1996) Current view of risk factors for periodontal diseases. *J Periodontol* **67**, 1041–1049.

Geraci TF, Nevins M, Crossetti HW, Drizen K and Ruben MP (1990) Reattachment of the periodontium after tooth movement into an osseous defect in a monkey. 1. *Int J Periodont Restorative Dent* **10**, 184–197.

Grant DA, Grant DA, Flynn MJ and Slots J (1995) Periodontal microbiota of mobile and non-mobile teeth. *J Periodontol* **66**, 386–390.

Handelman CS (1997) Nonsurgical rapid maxillary alveolar expansion in adults: a clinical evaluation. *Angle Orthod* **67**, 291–305.

Handelman CS, Wang L, BeGole EA and Haas AJ (2000) Nonsurgical rapid maxillary expansion in adults: report on 47 cases using the Haas expander. *Angle Orthod* **70**, 129–144.

Harrel SK and Nunn ME (2001) The effect of occlusal discrepancies on periodontitis. II. Relationship of occlusal treatment to the progression of periodontal disease. *J Periodontol* **72**, 495–505.

Helm S and Petersen PE (1989) Causal relation between malocclusion and periodontal health. *Acta Odontol Scand* **47**, 223–228.

Hollender L, Ronnerman A and Thilander B (1980) Root resorption, marginal bone support and clinical crown length in orthodontically treated patients. *Eur J Orthod* **2**, 197–205.

Holm-Pedersen P, Agerbaek N and Theilade E (1975) Experimental gingivitis in young and elderly individuals. *J Clin Periodontol* **2**, 14–24.

Hugoson A, Koch G, Bergendal T, Hallonsten AL, Slotte C, Thorstensson B and Thorstensson H (1995) Oral health of individuals aged 3–80 years in Jonkoping, Sweden in 1973, 1983, and 1993. II. Review of clinical and radiographic findings. *Swed Dent J* **19**, 243–260.

Hugoson A, Norderyd O, Slotte C and Thorstensson H (1998) Oral hygiene and gingivitis in a Swedish adult population 1973, 1983 and 1993. *J Clin Periodontol* **25**, 807–812.

Ingber JS (1974) Forced eruption. I. A method of treating isolated one and two wall infrabony osseous defects-rationale and case report. *J Periodontol* **45**, 199–206.

Ingber JS (1989) Forced eruption: alteration of soft tissue cosmetic deformities. *Int J Periodontics Restorative Dent* **9**, 416–425.

Ingervall B, Jacobsson U and Nyman S (1977) A clinical study of the relationship between crowding of teeth, plaque and gingival condition. *J Clin Periodontol* **4**, 214–222.

Jensen BL and Solow B (1989) Alveolar bone loss and crowding in adult periodontal patients. *Commun Dent Oral Epidemiol* **17**, 47–51.

Joss-Vassalli I, Grebenstein C, Topouzelis N, Sculea C and Katsaros C (2010) Orthodontic therapy and gingival recession: a systematic review. *Orthod Craniofac Res* **13**(3), 127–141.

Kraal JH, Digiancinto JJ, Dail RA, Lemmerman K and Peden JW (1980) Periodontal conditions in patients after molar uprighting. *J Prosthet Dent* **43**, 156–162.

Lindtoft H (2015) Post treatment changes in the clinical crown height and periodontal health occurring following an orthodontic treatment involving proclination of lower incisors A prospective clinical study in adult orthodontic patients. Master thesis Aarhus University Denmark.

Litonjua LA, Andreana S, Bush PJ and Cohen RE (2003) Toothbrushing and gingival recession. *Int Dent J* **53**, 67–72.

Loe H and Morrison E (1986) Periodontal health and disease in young people: screening for priority care. *Int Dent J* **36**, 162–167.

Lundegren N, Axtelius B, Hakansson J and Akerman S (2004) Dental treatment need among 20 to 25-year-old Swedes: discrepancy between subjective and objective need. *Acta Odontol Scand* **62**, 91–96.

Lupi JE, Handelman CS and Sadowsky C (1996) Prevalence and severity of apical root resorption and alveolar bone loss in orthodontically treated adults. *Am J Orthod Dentofacial Orthop* **109**, 28–37.

Mantzikos T and Shamus I (1997) Forced eruption and implant site development: soft tissue response. *Am J Orthod Dentofacial Orthop* **112**, 596–606.

Mantzikos T and Shamus I (1999) Forced eruption and implant site development: an osteophysiologic response. *Am J Orthod Dentofacial Orthop* **115**, 583–591.

Melsen B (1999) Biological reaction of alveolar bone to orthodontic tooth movement. *Angle Orthod* **69**, 151–158.

Melsen B, Agerbaek N, Eriksen J and Terp S (1988) New attachment through periodontal treatment and orthodontic intrusion. *Am J Orthod* **94**, 104–116.

Melsen B, Agerbaek N and Markenstam G (1989) Intrusion of incisors in adult patients with marginal bone loss. *Am J Orthod Dentofacial Orthop* **96**, 232–241.

Melsen B and Allais D (2005) Factors of importance for the development of dehiscences during labial movement of mandibular incisors: a retrospective study of adult orthodontic patients. *Am J Orthod Dentofacial Orthop* **127**, 552–561.

Melsen B, Petersen JK and Costa A (1998) Zygoma ligatures: an alternative form of maxillary anchorage. *J Clin Orthod* **32**, 154–158.

Miethke RR and Melsen B (1993) Adult orthodontics and periodontal diseases – a 9 year review of the literature from 1984–1993. *Praktisher Kieferorthopadie* **7**, 249–262.

Pattison GL (1983) Self-inflicted gingival injuries: literature review and case report. *J Periodontol* **54**, 299–304.

Peretz B and Machtei EE (1996) Tooth rotation and alveolar bone loss. *Quintessence Int* **27**, 465–468.

Polson A, Caton J, Polson AP, Nyman S, Novak J and Reed B (1984) Periodontal response after tooth movement into intrabony defects. *J Periodontol* **55**, 197–202.

Polson AM, Subtelny JD, Meitner SW, Polson AP, Sommers EW, Iker HP and Reed BE (1988) Long-term periodontal status after orthodontic treatment. *Am J Orthod Dentova Facial Orthop* **93**, 51–58.

Reichwage DP and Rydesky S (2002) The loss of anterior guidance as an etiological factor in periodontal pocketing. *Dent Today* **1**(10), 86–89.

Renkema AM, Navratilova Z, Mazuro K, Katzaros C and Fudalej PS (2015) Gingival labial recessions and post-treatment proclination of mandibular incisors *Eur J. Orthod* Oct;**37**(5), 508–513.

Ricketts RM (1980) *Bioprogressive Therapy*. Denver, CO: Rocky Mountain Orthodontics.

Riedel RA and Brandt S (1976) Dr. Richard A. Riedel on retention and relapse. *J Clin Orthod* **10**, 454–472.

Roth A, Yildirim M and Diedrich P (2004) Forced eruption with microscrew anchorage for preprosthetic leveling of the gingival margin. Case report. *J Orofac Orthop* **65**, 513–519.

Ruf S, Hansen K and Pancherz H (1998) Does orthodontic proclination of lower incisors in children and adolescents cause gingival recession? *Am J Orthod Dentofacial Orthop* **114**, 100–106.

Sanavi F, Weisgold AS and Rose LF (1998) Biologic width and its relation to periodontal biotypes. *J Esthet Dent* **10**, 157–163.

Shaw WC, Addy M and Ray C (1980) Dental and social effects of malocclusion and effectiveness of orthodontic treatment: a review. *Commun Dent Oral Epidemiol* **8**, 36–45.

Shei O, Waerhaug J, Lovdal A and Arnulf A (1959) A alveolar bone loss as related to oral hygeine and age. *J Periodontol* **26**, 7–16.

Sjolien T and Zachrisson BU (1973) Periodontal bone support and tooth length in orthodontically treated and untreated persons. *Am J Orthod* **64**, 28–37.

Smukler H and Landsberg J (1984) The toothbrush and gingival traumatic injury. *J Periodontol* **55**, 713–719.

Spieler EL (1996) Preventing toothbrush abrasion and the efficacy of the Alert toothbrush: a review and patient study. *Compend Contin Educ Dent* **17**, 478–5.

Staufer K and Landmesser H (2004) Effects of crowding in the lower anterior segment–a risk evaluation depending upon the degree of crowding. *Journal of Orofacial Orthopedics* **65**, 13–25.

Steiner GG, Pearson JK and Ainamo J (1981) Changes of the marginal periodontium as a result of labial tooth movement in monkeys. *J Periodontol* **52**, 314–320.

Svanberg GK, King GJ and Gibbs CH (1995) Occlusal considerations in periodontology. *Periodontology* 2000 **9**, 106–117.

Tervonen T and Knuuttila M (1988) Awareness of dental disorders and discrepancy between "objective" and "subjective" dental treatment needs. *Community Dentistry and Oral Epidemiology* **16**, 345–348.

Towfighi PP, Brunsvold MA, Storey AT, Arnold RM, Willman DE and McMahan CA (1997) Pathologic migration of anterior teeth in patients with moderate to severe periodontitis. *Journal of Periodontology* **68**, 967–972.

van Venrooy, Jr. and Yukna RA (1985) Orthodontic extrusion of single-rooted teeth affected with advanced periodontal disease. *American Journal of Orthodontics* **87**, 67–74.

Vanarsdall RL and Secchi A (2005) Periodontal-Orthodontic Interrelatioship. In *Orthodontics: Current principles and techniques,fourth edition* Graber T.M,V.R.L.V.K.W.L., ed. pp. 901–936, Elsevier.

Vanarsdall RL (1995) Orthodontics and periodontal therapy. *Periodontology* 2000 **9**, 132–149.

Waerhaug J (1952) The gingival pocket; anatomy, pathology, deepening and elimination. *Odontologisk Tidskrift* **60**, 1–186.

Wennstrom JL (1990) The significance of the width and thickness of the gingiva in orthodontic treatment. *Dtsch. Zahnarztl. Z.* **45**, 136–141.

Wennstrom JL, Lindhe J, Sinclair F and Thilander B (1987b) Some periodontal tissue reactions to orthodontic tooth movement in monkeys. *J Clin. Periodontol* **14**, 121–129.

Wennstrom JL, Lindhe J, Sinclair F and Thilander B (1987a) Some periodontal tissue reactions to orthodontic tooth movement in monkeys. *Journal of Clinical Periodontology* **14**, 121–129.

Wennstrom JL, Stokland BL, Nyman S and Thilander B (1993) Periodontal tissue response to orthodontic movement of teeth with infrabony pockets. *American Journal of Orthodontics and Dentofacial Orthopedics* **103**, 313–319.

Zachrisson BU (1976) Cause and prevention of injuries to teeth and supporting structures during orthodontic treatment. *American Journal of Orthodontics* **69**, 285–300.

Zachrisson BU (2003) Poor crown-root ratio - increased mobility and thooth survival. *World Journal of Orthodontics* **4**, 359–365.

Zachrisson BU and Alnaes L (1973) Periodontal condition in orthodontically treated and untreated individuals. I. Loss of attachment, gingival pocket depth and clinical crown height. *The Angle Orthodontist* **43**, 402–411.

12

A Systematic Approach to the Orthodontic Treatment of Periodontally Involved Anterior Teeth

Jaume Janer

Single tooth gingival recession

This section focuses on isolated labial gingival recession in relation to the anterior teeth, either present or likely to occur, in patients who are going to receive orthodontic treatment. It does not cover the hard toothbrushing-related recession, which is primarily seen in canines, or multiple tooth recession affecting individual patients with thin-type gingiva.

Etiology and prevalence

A tooth has gingival recession when its gingival margin is located apical to the cementoenamel junction (CEJ). There is scant information about the prevalence of solitary gingival recession in children and adults. After examining the lower incisor region in 15-year-old children, Stoner and Mazdyasna (1980) reported a prevalence of 17% for pseudo-gingival recession, that is, a longer clinical crown without root exposure, and 1% for gingival recession. Ainamo et al. (1986), in a sample of 7-, 12- and 17-year-old children, found the prevalence of gingival recession to be 5%, 39% and 74%, respectively. Evaluating the periodontal status among American children older than 13 years, Brown et al. (1996) found that gingival recession and loss of attachment increased with age, although the extent or number of affected sites with advanced conditions was not large in any age group; these findings were in agreement with Gorman (1967), Löe et al. (1992) and Khocht et al. (1993). Gingival recession is present in populations with both good and poor dental hygiene, although in the former it affects the buccal surfaces more (Löe et al. 1992). The teeth most frequently affected by isolated gingival recession are the lower central incisors, followed, but to a much smaller extent, by the upper and lower canines.

It has been suggested but not proved that gingival recession follows alveolar bone dehiscence. Bone dehiscence is a common finding when examining human dry skulls (Elliot and Bowers 1963; Rupprecht et al. 2001) and is positively correlated with thin alveolar bone. One should bear in mind that before computed topography was introduced, there were no reliable indirect means (conventional radiographs) for measuring the thickness of the alveolar bone of the teeth. During the surgical treatment of 113 teeth with gingival recession, Löst (1984) found that the average distance between the lowest point of recession and alveolar dehiscence was 2.8 mm, with considerable individual variation. With computed tomography, it has been demonstrated that the thickness of both the labial and lingual plates of the alveolar bone of the lower incisors

Adult Orthodontics, Second Edition. Edited by Birte Melsen and Cesare Luzi.
© 2022 John Wiley & Sons Ltd. Published 2022 by John Wiley & Sons Ltd.
Companion Website: http://www.wiley.com/go/melsen-adult-orthodontics

decreases when these teeth are orthodontically retracted, developing in some instances bony dehiscences that do not cause gingival recession (Sarikaya et al. 2002). This study only lasted 3 months, so the formation of new alveolar bone afterwards cannot be ruled out. Nonetheless, it showed that dehiscence does not always lead to gingival recession.

Various factors have been implicated in the development of gingival recession: plaque-induced inflammation, malalignment of teeth, toothbrushing, orthodontic movement, high muscle/frenal attachment, caries and subgingival restorations, and a combination of these factors (Snyder 1982; Khocht et al. 1993). With regard to single tooth recession, especially in labially displaced lower central incisors or in canines blocked out of the arch, the insufficient amount of hard and/or soft tissue covering the labial side of these teeth seems to be the major factor in the presence or the potential for developing gingival recession with or without orthodontics.

Amount of keratinised gingiva

A number of studies aimed to determine the minimal amount of keratinised gingiva necessary to prevent gingival recession. There is a general agreement that teeth with minimal or no keratinised gingiva will not necessarily be associated with gingival recession (Bowers 1963; Lang and Löe 1972; Kennedy et al. 1985; Wennström et al. 1987; Freedman et al. 1992, 1999). In healthy periodontal patients with no gingival recession who underwent orthodontic treatment, Coatoam et al. (1981) reported that teeth with less than 2 mm of keratinised gingiva were capable of tolerating the treatment.

In children, gingival recession around the lower central incisors may improve when gingival inflammation is reduced (Powell and McEniery 1982) and self-correction of labially displaced incisors has occurred (Andlin-Sobocki et al. 1991; Andlin-Sobocki and Persson 1994). The more prominent a lower incisor is in the arch, the less keratinised gingiva it will have (Bowers 1963; Rose and App 1973), and when a labially proclined incisor is moved lingually, the width of its keratinised gingiva increases (Dorfman 1978; Nygan et al. 1991). The thickness of the labial marginal soft tissue appears to be more relevant than the width when considering its resistance to the proclination of the teeth, especially in the presence of plaque-induced inflammation of the gingiva (Steiner et al. 1981; Wennström et al. 1993).

Gingival recession and proclination of lower incisors

In contemporary orthodontics, crowding of the lower incisors is largely resolved through the expansion of the dental arch and the proclination of the incisors, and more seldom by extraction of one central incisor or two lower premolars.

Various studies have been performed in humans and animals to ascertain the influence of tooth position on gingival recession. It has been demonstrated that orthodontic proclination of the lower incisors in youngsters and adults does not cause gingival recession (Ruf et al. 1998; Artun and

Grobety 2001; Djeu et al. 2002; Allais and Melsen 2003), but there are no data on long-term effects. Artun and Krogstad (1987), in a study of surgically treated patients with Class III malocclusions, reported a mild increase in the clinical crown height following proclination, greater than 10°, of the lower incisors. When reviewing animal studies, one should keep in mind that:

- The experiments were carried out in healthy animals, mainly monkeys and dogs.
- Maxillary instead of the mandibular incisors were used in some instances (Karring et al. 1982; Wennström et al. 1987).
- Mechanotherapy and appliance design varied among the studies and differed from those used in regular human orthodontics.

a. In sum, proclination of the lower incisors in animals may result in:
   i. Minimal increase of crown length.
   ii. Bone dehiscence.
   iii. No loss of connective tissue attachment or only in a few teeth when the measurements were done on histological sections analysed in the microscope, or when the assessment was done clinically following an elevation of a mucoperiosteal flap.

b. Moreover, if the tooth was moved back to the original position, the bone loss – dehiscence – was reverted, possibly owing to a healthy supracrestal soft tissue with the capacity to form bone after its resorption caused by traumatic forces (Batenhorst et al. 1974; Steiner et al. 1981; Engelking and Zachrisson 1982; Karring et al. 1982; Nyman et al. 1982; Wennström et al. 1987).

Based on the studies cited in the earlier text, it is likely that when lower incisors with a thin band of keratinised gingiva are proclined to resolve severe crowding, bone dehiscence, a thinning of the gingiva and an apical shift of the gingival margin may occur. This, in turn, may serve as a *locus minoris resistentiae* to the development of gingival recession if bacterial plaque is present (Steiner et al. 1981; Wennstrom 1996).

Clinical guidelines

When deciding to increase the band of keratinised gingiva around a tooth, it makes sense to distinguish between (1) lower and upper anterior teeth, (2) adults and children, (3) orthodontic and non-orthodontic patients as well as (4) presence of, or potential for, gingival recession. In the presence of a minimal band of keratinised gingiva, if no orthodontic treatment is implemented, surgically increasing the width of the band of gingiva to improve the periodontal health is not indicated, regardless of age (Hangorsky and Bissada 1980; Wennstrom and Lindhe 1983; Persson and Lennartsson 1986). However, when adults with gingival recession affecting the upper anterior teeth and with a high smile line request treatment for aesthetic reasons, surgical correction of the recession is indicated.

Periodontal plastic surgery for root covering or gingival augmentation is effective in reducing gingival recession, but the proportion of partial and complete root coverage shows marked variability both between and within surgical techniques (Roccuzzo et al. 2002). In orthodontic patients with or the risk of gingival recession, free, epithelialised or connective, rather than pedicle, grafts are recommended, as the resulting gain in gingival thickness is larger. According to the few articles published on the subject, the type of gingival attachment that develops on the grafted site is, to a limited extent, the connective tissue type in the most apical and lateral parts of the recession and the epithelial type on the major portion of the covered root (Wennstrom and Pini Prato 2003). Free epithelialised gingival grafts should be reserved for the lower anterior teeth, where the colour match is not an issue, while the connective tissue type can be used in both arches. Coronal migration of the gingival margin of the graft, known as creeping effect, is sometimes observed during the maturation period in young patients who have received the free epithelialised graft long before the initiation of the orthodontic treatment.

It is worth emphasising that with the use of superelastic archwires and self-ligating low-friction brackets, teeth can be moved orthodontically with truly light forces which are much more gentle on the periodontal support. This, in turn, may allow expansion and proclination of teeth without causing bone resorption (Handelman 1996), but with bone remodelling. Although there is no scientific evidence to support this claim, clinical experience indicates that larger dental movements can be implemented without risking the periodontal tissues.

In adults, the most commonly affected teeth are the upper and lower canines which are partially or completely blocked out of the dental arch, and crowded and labially positioned lower central incisors. In adults with recession, a gingival graft is most times placed before the orthodontic treatment is initiated (Figures 12.1 and 12.2).

When aligning a blocked-out lower central incisor with an appropriate band of keratinised gingiva by marked proclination of the tooth, a gingival graft may or may not be indicated to prevent thinning out of the gingiva and thereafter gingival recession during or long after the orthodontic treatment (Figures 12.3 and 12.4).

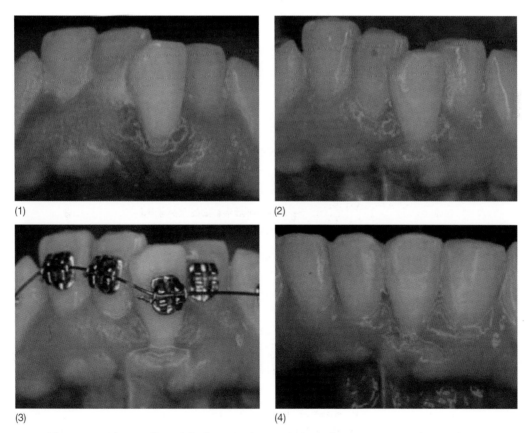

(1)   (2)

(3)   (4)

Fig. 12.1 A 36-year-old woman with crowding of the lower incisors and gingival recession on tooth 31. A free epithelialised gingival graft was placed before non-extraction orthodontic treatment. (1)–(4) Tooth 31 before treatment after the gingival graft and during and after the orthodontic treatment. (5) and (6) Occlusal view before and after the treatment. (7) and (8) Frontal view before and after the treatment.

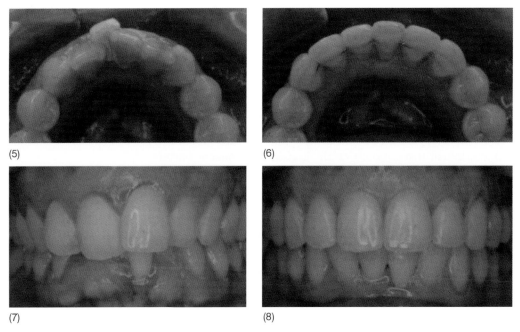

(5) (6)

(7) (8)

Fig. 12.1 (*Continued*)

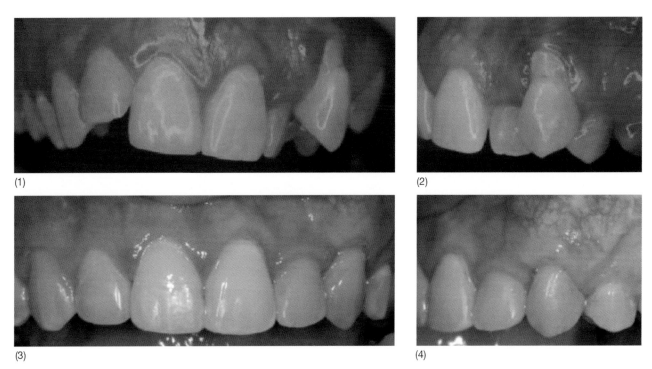

(1) (2)

(3) (4)

Fig. 12.2 A 37-year-old woman with a very narrow maxillary arch showing a blocked out maxillary left canine with severe gingival recession. Tooth 23 received a free subepithelial connective tissue graft before the orthodontic treatment. Before and after the interdisciplinary treatment: (1)–(4) upper front teeth, (5) and (6) frontal view, (7) and (8) occlusal view and (9) and (10) smile.

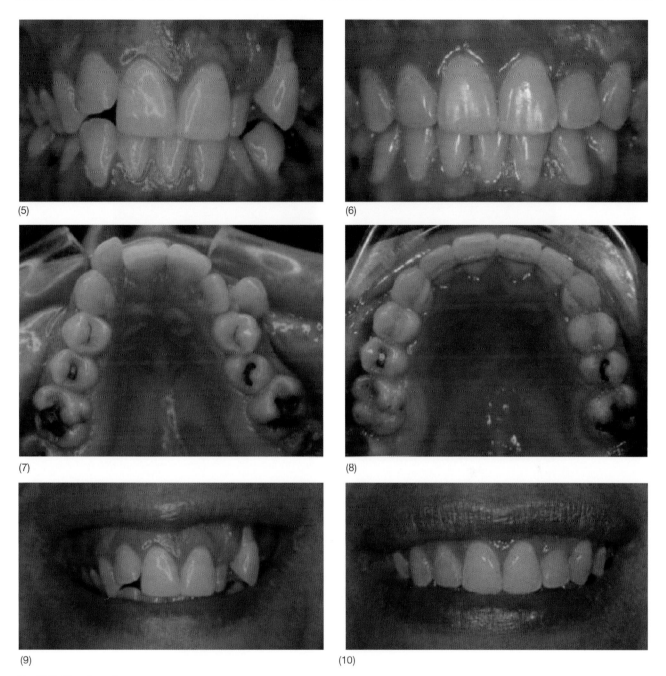

(5)

(6)

(7)

(8)

(9)

(10)

Fig. 12.2 (*Continued*)

Progressive spacing of incisors

Etiology, prevalence and differential diagnosis

In the periodontal literature, progressive spacing of the incisors (PSI) is known as pathological tooth migration and defined as a change in tooth position resulting from disruption of the forces that maintain teeth in a normal position with reference to the skull (Chasens 1979).

PSI is the most evident sign of the pathological change in the position of the teeth, in opposition to the 'physiological' dental crowding that usually occurs with ageing; the affected teeth are the incisors, especially the upper ones; and spacing,

at least initially, is progressive. However, some forms of spacing should not be termed as PSI, although they increase with time. These are:

- Dentitions which have always had spacing, for example, due to Bolton discrepancies, some dental Class III malocclusions, alteration of the function or form of the tongue (very seldom).
- Dentitions with missing anterior teeth where neighbouring teeth may have migrated into the edentulous space created by extraction or agenesis.
- Dentitions with gingival hyperplasia.

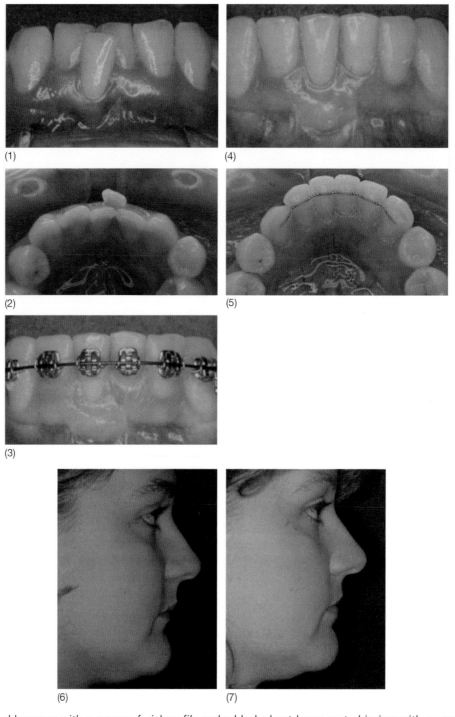

Fig. 12.3 A 22-year-old woman with a concave facial profile and a blocked-out lower central incisor with an appropriate band of keratinised gingiva. The incisor received a free epithelialised gingival graft before non-extraction orthodontic treatment to increase the thickness of the gingival margin and thus prevent the risk of gingival recession after dental alignment. (1) and (2) Before, (3) during and (4) and (5) after the orthodontic treatment. (6)–(9) Facial profile and cephalometric radiograph before and after the orthodontic treatment.

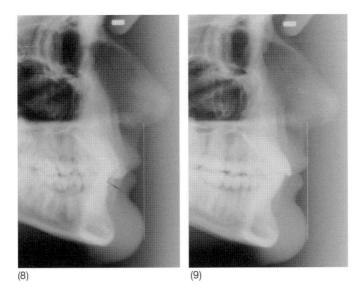

(8)   (9)

Fig. 12.3 (*Continued*)

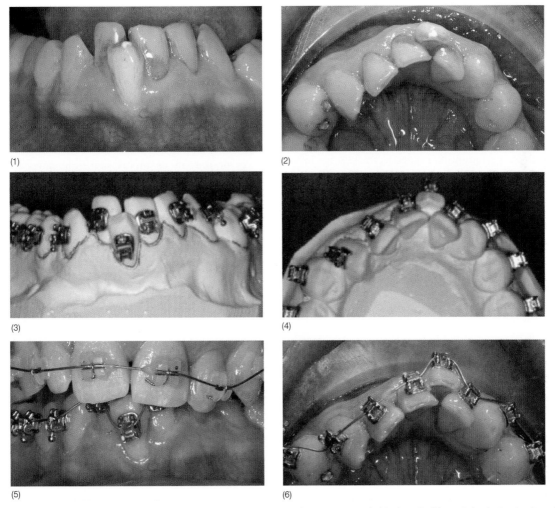

(1)   (2)

(3)   (4)

(5)   (6)

Fig. 12.4 A 42-year-old patient with crowding of the lower incisors and a narrow and thin band of keratinised gingiva in relation to 41. It was decided to check the soft-tissue response to orthodontic treatment with expansion of the dental arch and proclination of the incisors. Non-extraction treatment, using low-friction self-ligating brackets and superelastic archwires, was initiated; no augmentation of the gingival band was needed. (1) and (2) Before treatment, (3) and (4) patient's casts with bonded bracket, (5) and (6) at bonding appointment, (7) and (8) 5 months into otreatment, (9) after three-dimensional tooth remodelling of the lower anterior teeth and (10) after the orthodontic treatment.

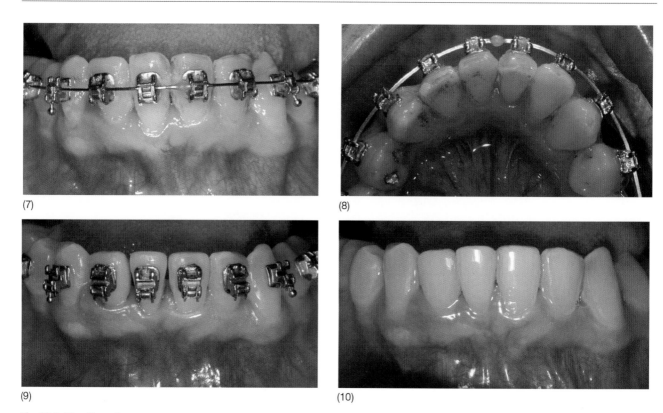

(7)

(8)

(9)

(10)

Fig. 12.4 (*Continued*)

The causes of PSI have not yet been established, but we know from Towfighi et al. (1997) and Martínez-Canut et al. (1997) that the prevalence of PSI in patients with moderate and severe periodontitis ranges from 30% to 56%, respectively. Moreover, the loss of more than three posterior teeth raises the odds of developing PSI (Martínez-Canut et al. 1997). It is likely that the periodontal bone loss could by itself explain the developing of PSI. Based on the *equilibrium theory* of tooth position, the periodontium together with the cheeks and lips counteracts the pressure exerted by the tongue at rest (Proffit 1978). When bone loss occurs, the centre of resistance of the teeth changes and the tongue pressure on the incisors results in tooth migration leading to spacing.

The minor spacing in the anterior teeth that sometimes occurs in the acute periodontal phases and that partially or completely reverses after conventional or surgical periodontal treatment may be considered as an initial stage of PSI (Hirschfeld 1933; Manor et al. 1984; Brunsvold et al. 1997; Gaumet et al. 1999; Singh and Deshpande 2002). The evolution of bone loss with or without presence of deep overbite and/or tooth loss will determine whether the condition will progress to true PSI.

In summary, the term PSI should be restricted to those individuals with chronic periodontitis who, in any given time of their lives, develop spacing between the anterior teeth as a result of their proclination, with or without the presence of mutilated dentitions and/or deep overbites (Figure 12.5).

Management

It should be emphasised that in patients with established PSI, periodontal treatment only will not close the interdental spaces or prevent its progression. Therefore, a combined interdisciplinary periodontal and orthodontic approach along with restorative prosthetic treatment if tooth loss is present is the appropriate way of managing these patients. The clinician should not underestimate the devastating effect that PSI has on the patient's smile. Patients often seek a solution for their unsatisfactory smiles on their own and are therefore highly motivated to undergo interdisciplinary treatment which would include orthodontics (Figure 12.6).

Closing spaces between anterior upper teeth with orthodontics is easy and predictable, provided there is enough overjet between the upper and the lower incisors to retract the former. In the presence of a reduced vertical dimension with a deep overbite, the treatment of PSI is more challenging. In the patients, opening the bite will be the first treatment objective, which in turn will create an overjet into which the fanned-out upper incisors can be retracted. There are various possibilities for opening the bite including: the use of a modified Hawley's bite plane (see Box 12.1) with an anterior bite plane; uprighting the inclined posterior teeth and placement of temporary prosthesis before the orthodontic treatment is initiated in patients with posterior mutilated dentitions. Three patients with PSI, deep bite of dental origin and insufficient overjet are presented in the following text showing different ways of opening the bite. For the figures illustrating these cases, please visit the book's companion website at www.wiley.com/go/melsen.

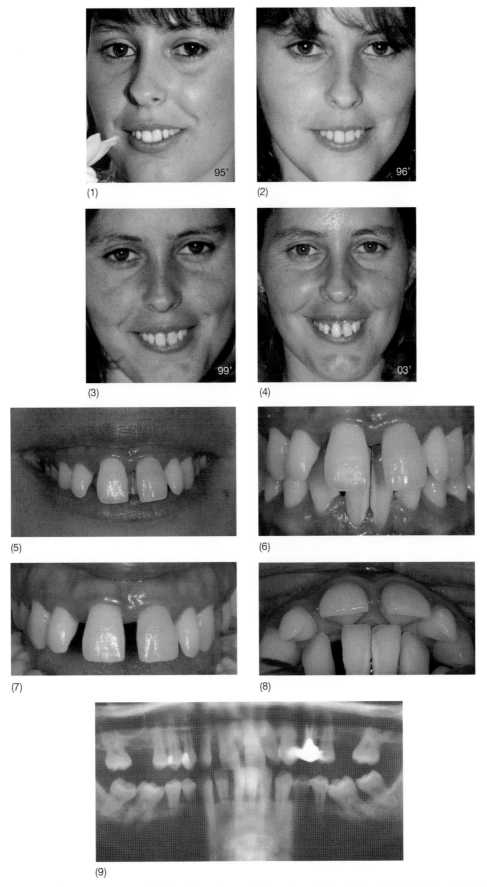

Fig. 12.5 (1)–(4) Evolution of PSI in a 35-year-old female patient with chronic periodontitis and (5)–(9) clinical situation at the initial orthodontic records.

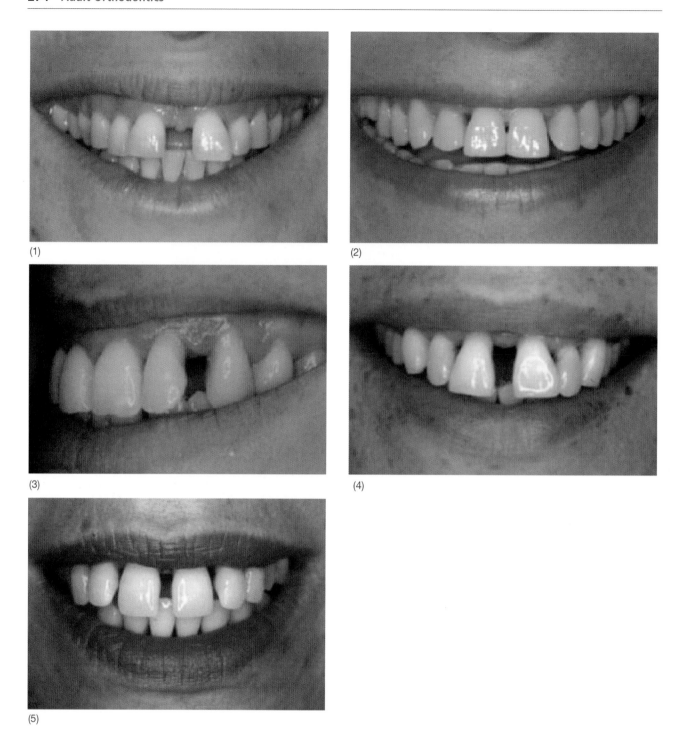

(1)

(2)

(3)

(4)

(5)

Fig. 12.6 (1)–(5) Handicapped smiles of patients with PSI and chronic periodontitis.

Box 12.1   Modified Hawley's bite plane

- **Description**: A removable acrylic palatal plate supported by Adams' clasp or similar on the molars, with or without a labial bow, which carries an anterior bite plane immediately behind the upper incisors and canines onto which the lower anterior teeth, incisors and canines have contact leaving at the same time the posterior teeth slightly out of contact. In order to avoid an overloading, the lower incisors should contact the bite plane.
- **Effect**: It temporarily opens the dental bite via passive eruption of the posterior lower teeth left out of contact which, in turn, as the mandible rotates clockwise, will develop or increase the overjet. The overjet so created will permit the closing of the spaced upper incisors without interference from the lower anterior teeth (Figure 12.7).

- **Usage**: In the active part of the orthodontic treatment, Hawley's bite plane is worn 24 hours per day except during the meals. In chronic periodontal patients, the bite opening required for the treatment of PSI is usually achieved in 3–4 months. The standard sequence consists of: (1) bite opening with Hawley's bite plane, (2) bonding of the fixed appliances in the lower arch while maintaining Hawley's bite plane until the lower teeth are aligned, (3) ceasing wear of Hawley's bite plane with bonding of the fixed appliances in the upper arch to close the spaces and (4) at end of orthodontic treatment, placement of fixed lingual retainers in both arches and a new Hawley's bite plane for night use.

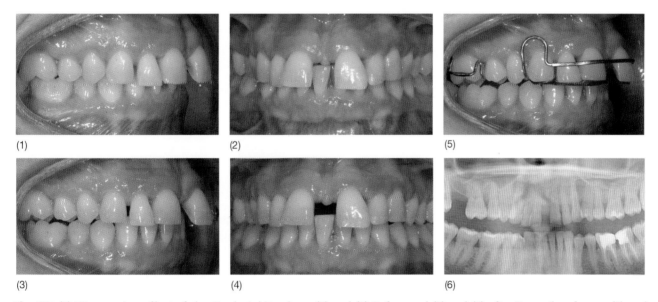

(1)   (2)   (5)

(3)   (4)   (6)

Fig. 12.7 (5) Bite opening effect of the Hawley's bite plane. (1) and (2) Before and (3) and (4) after 3 months of wear. (3) and (4) Appliance just removed at the time of photograph. (6) Initial panoramic radiograph showing periodontal bone loss.

Case reports

Case 1

A 47-year-old woman was referred by her general dentist for chronic periodontitis, PSI, impacted upper canines and mutilated dentition (see Box 12.2 for details). Bite opening was achieved with a combination of (1) prosthetic design, (2) proclination of the incisors and (3) reduction of the crown-to-root ratio. For the photographs for this case, visit www.wiley.com/go/melsen.

- Prosthetic design: The bite opening was mainly achieved by increasing the height of the clinical crowns of the posterior teeth. Since full-arch prosthetic rehabilitation of the upper arch to replace both canines and stabilise the anterior segment was planned for the patient, the

logical interdisciplinary treatment sequence was altered. Before the start of the orthodontic treatment, the patient received two vertically over-elongated provisional prosthesis in the posterior segments to establish a working vertical dimension to which the position of the upper and lower incisors was orthodontically adjusted.

- Proclination of the incisors: The overjet produced by the opening of the bite was utilised to procline the lower incisors, creating a new incisal relationship compatible with the new occlusal vertical dimension that had been established.
- Decreasing the crown-to-root ratio of the incisors: The clinical crowns especially of the upper incisors were reduced just before the start of the orthodontic treatment.

Box 12.2 Patient 1: diagnosis, treatment plan and sequence

Diagnosis: Brachyfacial (3)[a] · PSI (3) · Missing teeth 17, 27, 36, 37, 47 · Upper canines impacted in the palate · Angle Class I dental and skeletal · Retroclined upper and lower incisors (3) · Dental and skeletal deep bite (3/2)
Posterior bite collapse · Chronic periodontitis (3) · Primary and secondary occlusal trauma

Treatment plan: orthodontics, periodontics and prosthetics
- Objectives: pleasing smile + closing the interdental spaces of the anterior segment + opening the bite + coordination of the dental arches to allow the aesthetic prosthetic rehabilitation of the dentition
- Appliances: multibracket + elastics + modified provisional prosthesis
- Retention: indefinitely, with a fixed lingual arch in the lower anterior segment
- Possible limitations: degree of overbite and periodontal bone loss extension. Retention

[a] (1) mild, (2) moderate, (3) severe.
[b] Tooth 26 was extracted due to an endodontic accident.

- The upper incisors were orthodontically tested during a short period of time before any irreversible treatment was implemented
- Financial limitations: only certain aspects of dental treatment could be carried out

Sequence:
- Periodontal treatment and monitoring periodontal status throughout the orthodontic phase
- Orthodontics – start
- Implants: tooth 36
- Dental extractions: teeth 13 and 23, upper canines, and tooth 26[b]
- Modified provisional prosthesis in the upper posterior segments, markedly increasing the dental vertical dimension
- Orthodontics – end + retention
- Provisional prosthesis: from tooth 16 to 25
- Final prosthesis: Tooth-borne from tooth 16 to 25, in one piece; implant-borne for teeth 36 and 26

Case 2

A 40-year-old woman was referred by her periodontist for chronic periodontitis and PSI. It is worth noting how the periodontal bone loss, in an almost intact dentition, could lead to PSI by itself. The overjet necessary to retract the spaced upper incisors was created with the bite-opening effect of a modified removable Hawley bite plane (Box 12.1). For the photographs for this case, visit www.wiley.com/ go/ melsen.

Case 3

A 37-year-old man was referred by his general dentist for chronic periodontitis, PSI, deep overbite and mutilated dentition (see Box 12.3 for details).

A Hawley's bite plane was used to open the bite and create an overjet (see Case 2).

Management of periodontally involved teeth

Chronic periodontitis is defined by the American Academy of Periodontology (2000) as inflammation of the gingiva extending into the adjacent attachment apparatus. The disease is characterised by loss of clinical attachment due to destruction of the periodontal ligament and loss of the adjacent supporting bone.

When performing comprehensive treatment of periodontally involved anterior teeth, aesthetic results are almost as important as the eradication of periodontal disease and the achievement of adequate tooth alignment. If the patient's smile is to be improved, it is necessary to: prevent any unnecessary further loss of soft tissue; safely

Box 12.3 Patient 2: diagnosis, treatment plan and sequence

Diagnosis: Brachyfacial (2)[a] · PSI (2) · Crowding lower incisors (1) · Angle Class I dental and skeletal · Dental and skeletal deep bite (1/2) · Posterior bite collapse · Chronic periodontitis (2) · Primary and secondary occlusal trauma

Treatment plan: periodontics and orthodontics
- Objectives: pleasing smile + closing the interdental spaces of the anterior segment + aligning the lower incisors
- Appliances: multibracket + elastics + modified Hawley's bite plane
- Retention: indefinitely, by a fixed lingual arch in the upper and lower anterior segments + a new modified Hawley's bite plane, night time
- Possible limitations: retention

Sequence:
- Periodontal treatment and monitoring periodontal status throughout the orthodontic phase
- Orthodontics – start
- Orthodontics – end + retention

[a] (1) mild, (2) moderate, (3) severe.

perform the orthodontic treatment; modify, when required, tooth anatomy to make the teeth resemble their original form and size as much as possible and position the incisors to mask the negative effects that the soft tissue and bone loss have had on the patient's smile over time.

In spite of the fact that patients with reduced periodontal support will be closely monitored before, during and after orthodontic treatment by their periodontist or general dentist, it is imperative that orthodontists involved in combined ortho–perio treatments are knowledgeable with

Box 12.4   Patient 3: diagnosis, treatment plan and sequence

Diagnosis: Brachyfacial (3) · Lower smile line · PSI (3) · Missing teeth 17, 27, 36, 37, 47 · Hopeless tooth 21 · Angle Class I dental and skeletal · Retroinclined upper and lower incisors (1) · Dental and skeletal deep bite (2/2) · Posterior bite collapse · Chronic periodontitis (3) · Primary and secondary occlusal trauma · Heavy smoker 1.5 packs/day

Treatment plan: orthodontics, periodontics and prosthesis
- Objectives: pleasing smile + closing the interdental spaces of the anterior segment + creating the appropriate space for the missing anterior upper teeth + opening the bite + coordination of the dental arches to allow the aesthetic prosthetic rehabilitation of the upper dentition
- Appliances: HBP + multibrackets + elastics
- Retention: indefinitely, by a fixed lingual arch in the lower anterior segment and a HBP at night time
- Possible limitations: bruxism · Smoking · Aesthetic management of tooth 21 · Retention

Sequence:
- Non-surgical periodontal treatment: leaving tooth 21 for aesthetic reasons
- Orthodontics – start: HBP
- Surgical periodontal treatment: upper posterior segments
- Fixed lower appliances
- Stop HBP + fixed upper appliances
- Remove lower fixed appliances + placement of a lower fixed 3–3 lingual arch
- Orthodontics – end: remove upper fixed appliances + deliver a HPB at night time
- Prosthesis I: upper provisional prosthesis from tooth 16 to tooth 26 in one piece, with extraction of tooth 21
- Prosthesis II: final prosthesis

(1) mild, (2) moderate, (3) severe

regard to periodontics, so that they can assess both the effect of the periodontal therapy and evaluate the impact that the orthodontic tooth movement has on the periodontal support of the affected teeth during follow-up.

When the orthodontist, the periodontist or the general dentist is considering an interdisciplinary treatment for a patient with reduced periodontal support, it is worth deliberating the following:

- Is it realistic to expect a zero bacterial plaque level in patients undergoing orthodontic treatment? Probably, not.
- How well do periodontally involved teeth resist orthodontics? In a plaque-controlled dentition, most teeth with bone loss do satisfactorily with well-controlled force systems (Ericsson et al. 1978; Eliasson et al. 1982; Polson et al. 1984; Artun and Urbye 1988; Boyd et al. 1989; Nelson and Ärtun 1997; Re et al. 2000) (Figures 12.8 and 12.9).
- Are periodontal patients with crowded or spaced incisors and with traumatised anterior teeth better off when left untreated? Most times, not.

Preliminary considerations

Posterior teeth available for orthodontic therapy

From the orthodontic standpoint, posterior teeth are required for anchorage and control of the vertical dimension. If there are already several missing posterior teeth and/or the remaining ones have a poor prognosis, altering the standard interdisciplinary treatment sequence should be considered. The teeth with poor prognosis should be extracted and implants with provisional prostheses are placed before the orthodontic treatment is initiated.

Anterior tooth/teeth requiring extraction or an extraction site already present

This poses a double-fold challenge: first, an aesthetic problem because it dramatically worsens the patient's smile, and, second, it complicates the orthodontic mechanotherapy. A Maryland prosthesis only supported by one of the teeth next to the edentulous space could be chosen if a tooth is extracted just before the orthodontic treatment starts. If, on the other hand, a tooth fails during the treatment, for example, periodontal abscess, it may be used as a pontic without its root. Whenever possible, extraction of anterior teeth should be postponed until after the orthodontic treatment has finished.

The occlusion

The worst scenario is by far a Class III incisor relationship with either an edge-to-edge or an anterior crossbite. Camouflage through proclination of the upper incisors with reduced bone support is hardly ever an option (Figure 12.10).

Trauma from occlusion

This had been defined as 'an injury to the attachment apparatus as a result of excessive occlusal force' by the American Academy of Periodontology. In dentitions with markedly reduced periodontal support, minimising trauma may be beneficial. Although results of animal studies on the effect of trauma from occlusion superimposed on plaque-associated periodontitis may not be extrapolated to humans, under certain circumstances, tooth mobility may increase the destruction of the periodontal support, that is, loss of connective tissue and apical migration of the dentogingival epithelium (Lindhe and Svanberg 1974; Ericsson and Lindhe 1982).

The bone level

The minimum amount of bone support necessary for teeth to withstand orthodontic forces in a plaque-controlled environment has not yet been established. Reduced bone support by itself is not a contraindication to orthodontic therapy. The prognosis for severely periodontally affected teeth is assessed before the interdisciplinary treatment is

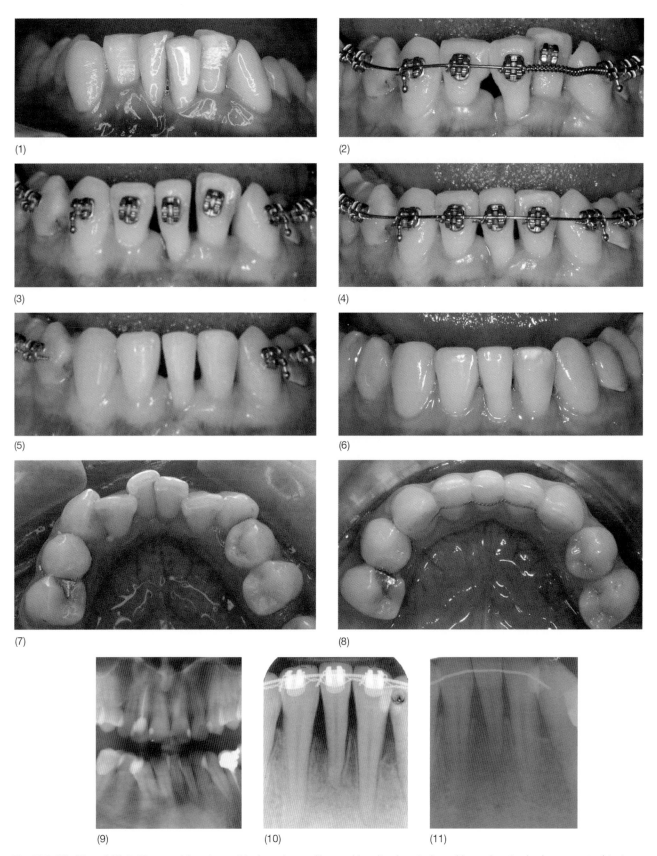

Fig. 12.8 (1), (7) and (9) A 32-year-old patient with dental crowding and localised periodontal bone loss in the lower central incisors. (3) and (4) The right central incisor was extracted due to poor prognosis. (2)–(6) and (8) The treatment plan consisted of dental alignment and closure of the extraction space. (10) and (11) The lower left central incisor with reduced periodontal support withstood satisfactorily well the orthodontic treatment that included extrusion and extensive tooth remodelling.

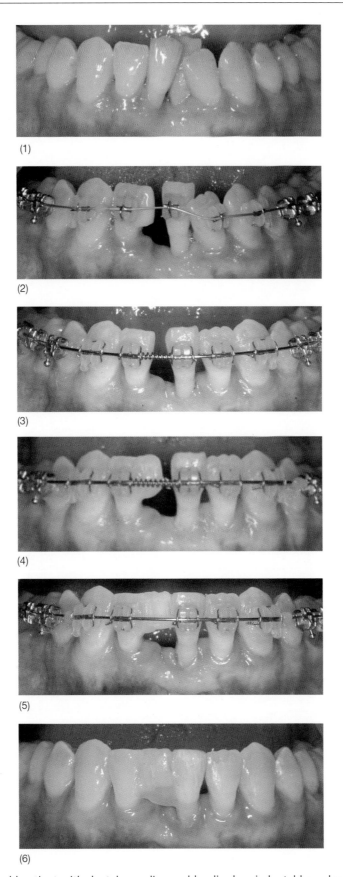

(1)

(2)

(3)

(4)

(5)

(6)

Fig. 12.9 (1) and (7) A 53-year-old patient with dental crowding and localised periodontal bone loss in the lower central incisors. (2)–(6) The hopeless right central incisor was extracted. The treatment plan consisted of: dental alignment, arch width correction and opening appropriate space for the replacement of tooth 41. (8) and (9) Note the response of the lower left central incisor to the extensive orthodontic tooth movement.

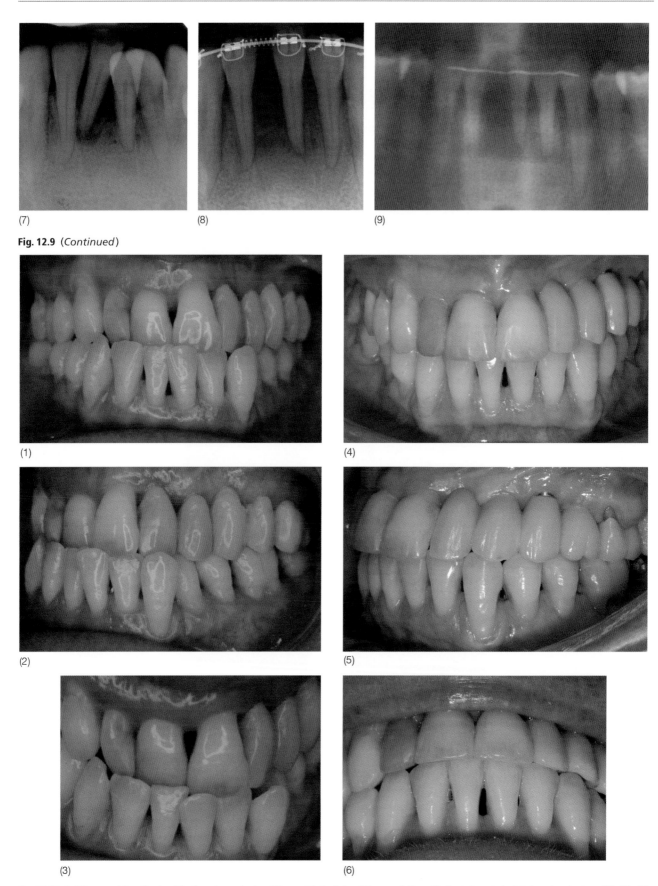

(7)   (8)   (9)

Fig. 12.9 (*Continued*)

(1)

(2)

(3)

(4)

(5)

(6)

Fig. 12.10 A 45-year-old patient with chronic periodontitis, mutilated dentition and Class III dental and skeletal malocclusion. (1)–(3), (7) and (10) Initial condition. (4)–(6), (9) and (11) Final result of the interdisciplinary treatment. Cephalograms: (7) and (9) before and after treatment and (8) before orthognathic surgery. Treatment performed: elimination of dental compensation followed by surgical maxillary advancement. In these types of malocclusion, proclination of the upper incisors to eliminate the anterior crossbite is hardly ever an option.

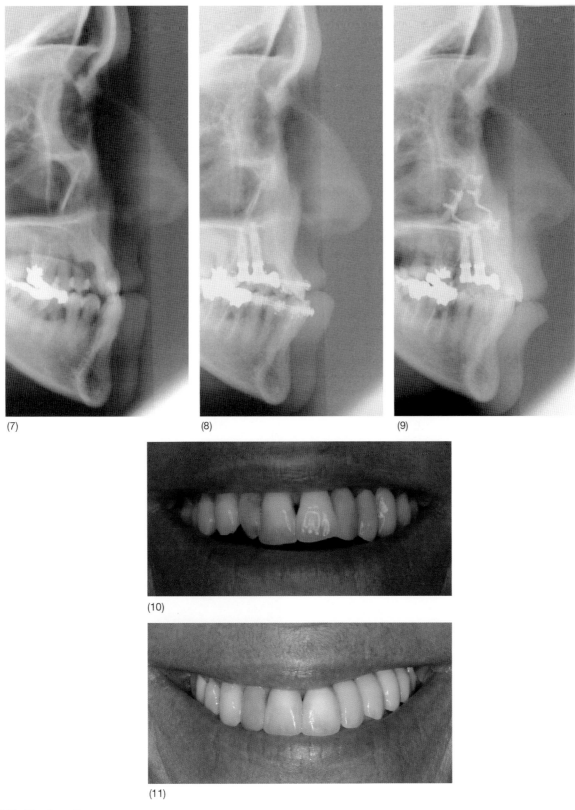

(7)

(8)

(9)

(10)

(11)

Fig. 12.10 (*Continued*)

initiated, based on the amount of bone loss, the aesthetic relevance of the affected teeth, the possibility of the tooth being used as a bridge abutment or placement of implants next to it, the presence of furcation involvement, the patient's financial status, etc. Alternative treatment plans for teeth with uncertain prognosis should be considered before comprehensive treatment begins.

Aesthetic considerations

Orthodontic appliances

Labially bonded appliances are mostly used. Although ceramic brackets are brittle and more delicate to manipulate than stainless-steel appliances, for exclusively aesthetic reasons, they are often used on upper anterior teeth and to a lesser degree in the lower anterior teeth. In order to give the orthodontic labial appliance a low profile, the following steps can be taken:

- Excess composite around the brackets should be avoided; remove the excess with a dental probe or scaler before it sets or with a handpiece and high-speed bur if it has set. If it is not removed, it will soon discolour and the ceramic brackets will appear yellowish.
- Plain arches without hooks or loops should be used where possible.
- Instead of common-tied ligatures from canine to canine for space maintenance, composite stops distal to each canine are recommended.
- Any stain or accumulation of calcified plaque should be eliminated at every orthodontic appointment.

The most significant aesthetic limitation when treating upper incisors with reduced periodontal support is the frequent absence of the gingival papilla. The greater the amount of bone loss and gingival recession, the lesser the capacity to reduce the open embrasures or black triangles already present, or those which may develop, or enlarge, as malaligned teeth are being orthodontically aligned. This issue should be fully explained to the patients before the beginning of the treatment.

Appropriateness, type or extent of the anterior periodontal surgery

The appropriateness, type or extent of the periodontal surgery in the upper anterior segment is of utmost importance. In patients with bone loss and pocket formation after unsuccessful conservative periodontal therapy, it is highly advisable to perform conservative periodontal surgery to minimise any increase in the tooth clinical crown height, root exposure and the development of, or increase in size of already present, black triangles.

The gingival contour

When teeth with healthy periodontal tissues are orthodontically moved in a vertical fashion, the gingival contour

accompanies the incisors and the length of the clinical crown remains unchanged (Figure 12.11). Orthodontic establishment of the gingival contour of upper anterior teeth with bone loss with either recession or pocket formation on the other hand is unpredictable (Figures 12.12 and 12.13).

Tooth anatomy

- Orthodontists usually encounter adult patients with unevenly abraded teeth due to their malpositioning of teeth and with different degrees of gingival recession, resulting in dissimilar clinical crown lengths of the incisors. In these cases, the orthodontist can often camouflage the discrepancies in tooth anatomy with tooth reshaping in the three planes of space during the orthodontic treatment. In patients with very long clinical crowns due to bone loss and gingival recession, improving the crown-to-root ratio through tooth reshaping will not only have a positive impact on the aesthetics of the patient's smile but also on the mechanical functioning of the anterior segment.

Intrusion versus extrusion

When healthy periodontal teeth are orthodontically intruded, their clinical crown length may shorten. So far, it has not been reported if dental intrusion affects their relationship to the periodontal structures in humans, including the possible gain in connective tissue attachment, as this can only be ascertained by histological means, which is not

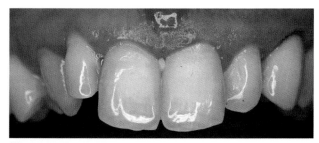

(1)

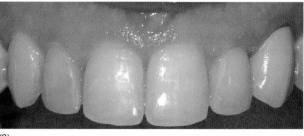

(2)

Fig. 12.11 (1) and (2) In a dentition with healthy periodontium, the gingival contour is readily restored with orthodontics. The effect is not so predictable in crowned teeth (the left canine). Note that the gingival contour has been maintained on the right lateral incisor after its extrusion prior to restorative treatment.

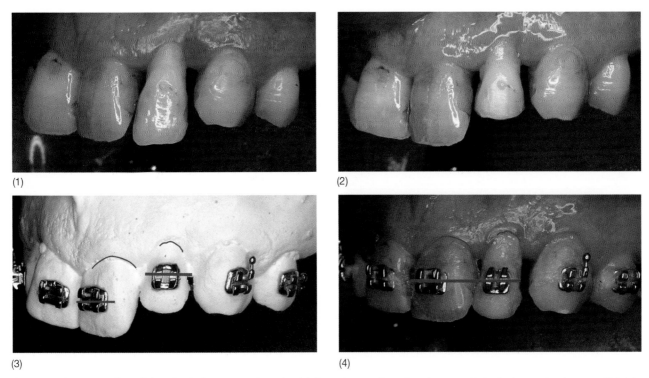

Fig. 12.12 The restoration of the gingival contour of teeth with bone loss and varying degrees of gingival recession is unpredictable. (3) Bracket placement intended to restore the gingival margin of tooth 22, and (4) the orthodontic result after levelling of the bracket slots. (1) Before treatment and (2) after initial reduction of tooth 22.

feasible for obvious reasons. In a monkey study on orthodontic intrusion, Murakami et al. (1989) found that the gingiva moved only approximately 60% as far as the crowns did and the clinical crowns shortened and gingival sulcus deepened, both approximately 40% as much as the tooth intrusion. Unfortunately, the data from the study were taken right after the intrusion, so it could not rule out if the changes were permanent or temporary. Moreover, the overgrowth of the gingiva reported in the study is rarely seen during the orthodontic treatment of either adults or children. It is worth mentioning that in all experimental teeth, the junctional epithelium ended at the CEJ and no apical migration was observed.

In another research study performed in monkeys in which teeth with reduced periodontal support were intruded, Melsen et al. (1988) reported a gain in connective tissue attachment ranging from 0.7 to 2.3 mm. In all teeth, the CEJ was below the marginal bone level. When orthodontic intrusion was performed in patients with bone loss and deep overbite, it was found that the amount of alveolar support as assessed with intraoral radiographs increased in 19 of the 30 patients studied. It was thought that infrabony pockets had developed during intrusion even though they could not be measured, being too narrow for the periodontal probe. It could not be concluded that a gain in connective tissue attachment had been obtained. Rather, it was proposed that the junctional epithelium was extended

below the marginal bone level. A reduction of the clinical crown length by 0.5–1 mm, with large variability, was also reported (Melsen et al. 1989).

Cardaropoli et al. (2001) intruded 10 maxillary central incisors with bone loss and infrabony defects, which were also spaced and extruded. After the orthodontic treatment, they reported reduced probing pocket depth and improved clinical crown length and amount of bone seen on intraoral radiographs. Vanarsdall (1985) recommended levelling the crestal bone between the adjacent CEJs of teeth with reduced periodontal support. Teeth with greater bone loss are extruded in relation to their neighbours and their clinical crowns reduced with a high-speed handpiece. However, if there is horizontal bone loss, orthodontic movement should involve intrusion or extrusion as necessary.

Whether elongated upper incisors are intruded, extruded or a combination of the two is used will depend on the individual patient's needs. If only one incisor with minor gingival recession is extruded, which is an uncommon situation, intrusion is recommended regardless of the attachment gain it may lead to. A more common scenario consists of a combination of homologous incisors with long clinical crowns of different lengths and amount of gingival recession combined with an uneven marginal gingival contour. In this condition, some teeth will be intruded and some extruded, and thereafter reduced in length, in relation to their neighbours (Figure 12.13). As mentioned in the

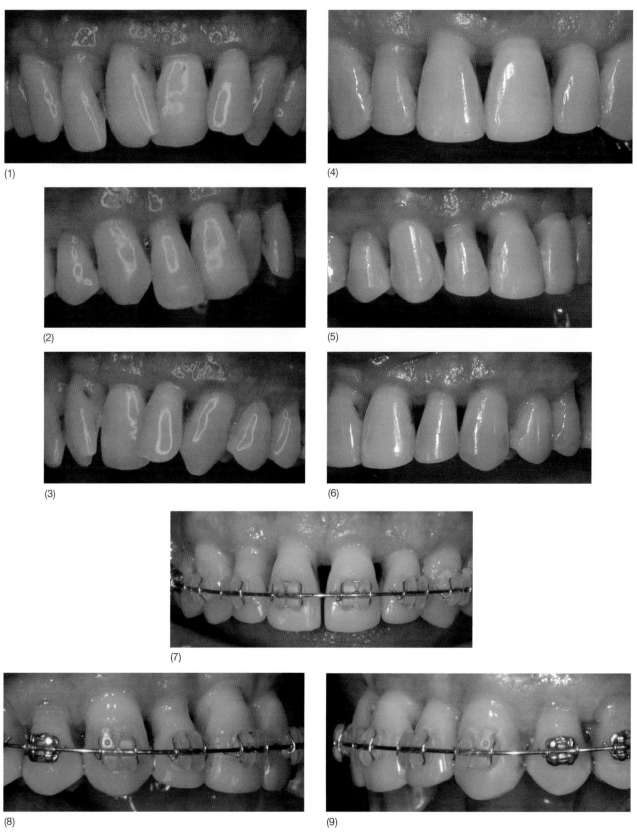

Fig. 12.13 (1)–(3) A 54-year-old patient with chronic periodontitis, gingival recession and crowding of the anterior teeth. (7)–(9) Six to eight months into orthodontic treatment, bracket placement and tooth position were re-evaluated and three-dimensional tooth reshaping was carried out to (a) reduce the open embrasures, (b) enhance the smile line and (c) improve the crown-to-tooth ratio. (4)–(6), (10) and (11) One year after the orthodontic treatment.

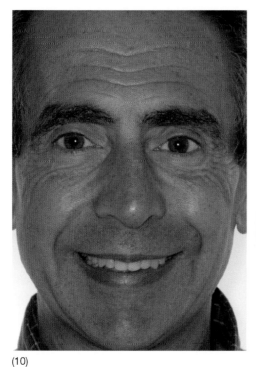

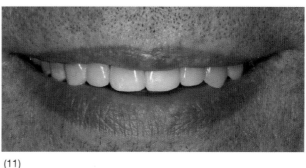

(10)

(11)

Fig. 12.13 (*Continued*)

earlier text, in dentitions with reduced periodontal support, the levelling of the periodontal contour is not predictable. Bearing in mind that the reduction in clinical crown length obtained in human studies amounted at the most to 1 mm, intruding incisors with long clinical crowns and exposed roots will not improve the aesthetics, as the anterior teeth will continue to appear too long. Moreover, if the incisors are prosthetically restored after the orthodontic treatment, extrusion rather than intrusion seems more appropriate. The alveolar bone remodelling frequently observed on radiographs after the orthodontic treatment should be interpreted with care. It is possible that volume of bone remains stable, but its morphology changes. If so, it would explain both the improvement of the clinical probing depth and the reduction of the infrabony defects.

Clinical examination

The orthodontist must perform the basic periodontal clinical examination to determine the actual periodontal status regardless of whether a patient has already received periodontal therapy. The following basic information about the periodontal and dental condition of the anterior teeth should be collected by the orthodontist before orthodontic treatment is started:

- Oral hygiene status.
- Presence of bleeding on probing.

- Amount of bone loss: most times a high-quality panoramic radiograph should suffice to assess the bone levels in relation to the anterior teeth, but if severe crowding is present, complementary periapical radiographs are recommended.
- Clinical probing pocket depth: especially relevant in patients with bone loss and gingival pockets with proportionally less gingival recession.
- Gingival recession and the presence or absence of interdental gingiva.
- Tooth position: whether crowded or spaced, and if the latter, stable or progressive.
- Tooth anatomy: square versus triangular tooth shape, amount of root exposure, presence and extension of dental abrasion, thickness of the incisal edges and the crown-to-root length ratio.
- Tooth mobility and presence of dental fremitus (tooth vibration or mobility upon closing) of the upper incisors.

Management

Chronic periodontitis is the most frequent type of periodontitis present in patients receiving an interdisciplinary dental treatment for their anterior teeth. The amount of bone loss and the outcome of the periodontal treatment determine the severity of the condition and the prognosis of the case.

Before orthodontic treatment

Patients with mild to moderate periodontitis without significant occlusal trauma or deep periodontal pockets should be educated regarding oral hygiene in the following ways:

- There is no evidence that interdental cleaning should be recommended to the whole population as a means of preventing gingivitis and periodontitis. However, in patients with periodontitis, meticulous cleaning of the interdental surfaces is of utmost importance, since plaque deposition in these areas, which appears early and is more prevalent, will cause further loss of supporting bone and gingiva (Echeverría et al. 2003). Moreover, the interproximal areas are the most frequently affected by periodontitis (Warren and Charter 1996). Interproximal plaque removal is performed with dental floss, as toothbrushing is relatively ineffective in these areas. Flossing is carried out with a special dental floss (Superfloss®, Oral-B®) supplied with three components: a stiff-end threader to bypass the orthodontic arch between neighbouring teeth, a spongy floss to clean the interdental surfaces and regular dental floss. Patients are instructed to floss once a day, after dinner, before toothbrushing and informed about the detrimental effect that bleeding when flossing will have on the remaining interdental bone support and gingiva.
- Electric toothbrushes are preferred rather than manual toothbrushes even though the literature shows contradictory results (Boyd and Rose 1994; Heintze et al. 1996; Heasman et al. 1998; Thienpont et al. 2001). As patients will have to dedicate extra time to clean the interdental spaces, facilitating this with the use of an electrical toothbrush seems reasonable, and more so when the length of the orthodontic treatment exceeds the average 2 months period employed in studies on electric toothbrush efficacy. The estimated brushing duration for the anterior segments, upper or lower, should probably be well over 90 seconds and mainly spent on the buccal tooth surfaces (Van der Weijden et al. 1993).
- Interdental toothbrushes are recommended to remove the plaque around and between the brackets, but not for interdental cleaning under the contact point, to prevent traumatising the remaining interdental gingiva.
- Non-surgical periodontal treatment – scaling and root planing: although the benefit of smoothing the root surfaces by removing the exposed root cementum may not influence the healing process following periodontal treatment – hygiene level, bleeding index, probing depth and clinical attachment gain (Rosenberg and Ash 1974; Nyman et al. 1988; Oberholzer and Rateinschack

1996) – keeping the exposed roots of the anterior teeth smooth, especially in the interproximal surfaces, will reduce the accumulation of plaque that patients undergoing orthodontic treatment tend to have due to the retentive plaque effect of the orthodontic fixed appliances, in spite of the dentine hypersensitivity that may occur initially.

Patients with moderate to severe periodontitis

- Patient education: when gingival recession is extensive and the dental papillae are missing, interproximal toothbrushes rather than dental floss are more effective and easy to use in cleaning the exposed interdental surfaces.
- Non-surgical periodontal treatment: Badersten et al. (1984) evaluated the effect of non-surgical periodontal therapy in patients with severe chronic periodontitis and reported a marked reduction in bleeding scores and probing pocket depths even in the deepest pockets, up to 12 mm. This proves the efficacy of scaling and root planing. After a successful phase of scaling and root planing, an extended junctional epithelium will most times develop, helping the gingiva to adhere to the cementum. Although it is not the most resistant scenario against a reactivation of the periodontitis, it seems an acceptable compromise when waged against longer unaesthetic anterior teeth as a result of surgically eliminating the deep gingival pockets.
- Some studies have reported on the negative influence of tooth mobility on the outcome of periodontal treatment (Fleszar et al. 1980; Pihlstrom et al. 1986; Burgett et al. 1992). If occlusal trauma and tooth mobility are present, especially in the upper anterior sextant, a modified Hawley's appliance with an anterior bite plane is recommended to temporarily disclude the teeth.
- When open flap debridements are performed in sites with infrabony defects where scaling and root planing have not eliminated periodontal inflammation and bleeding on probing persists, any further unnecessary loss of gingiva, apart from that inherent to the surgery itself, should be prevented, as it leads to an irreversible unaesthetic effect on the patient's smile. The latter also applies to the lower anterior segment in patients with very low smile lines. Therefore, surgical elimination of periodontal pockets may not always be an option, even though pocking probing depths equal to or greater than 6 mm involve a higher risk for further attachment loss than shallower pockets (Caffey and Egelbert 1995).

Procedures for periodontal regeneration, for example, guided tissue regeneration (GTR), in combination with use of grafting materials and enamel matrix proteins are ways to improve the periodontal status of affected anterior teeth undergoing periodontal surgery (Cortellini and Tonetti 2000).

- Patients will be ready to start the orthodontic treatment when:
  - The plaque levels are satisfactory.
  - Periodontal status is healthy.
  - Motivation is high.

During orthodontic treatment

- The total orthodontic treatment time for periodontally involved adult patients should be under 16 months.
- An interim panoramic radiograph should be taken approximately 6 months into treatment to make a general assessment of bone levels. The radiograph is also used to evaluate the tooth position–bracket placement relationship.
- Professional oral hygiene procedures should be performed every 4–6 months. The gingiva should be probed and any plaque that is present should be removed at every orthodontic appointment for the appliance adjustment, especially between the lower incisors, and to a lesser degree between the upper anterior teeth.

General considerations

- Consider use of light forces.
- Bracket placement:
  When placing the brackets, gingival margin, smile line, root parallelism and crown height should be taken into account.
  - Indirect bonding allows the operator to place the brackets much more accurately than directly in the patient's mouth, as the anatomy and position of the teeth on the dental casts can be evaluated from every possible angle without any interference.
- Tooth reshaping: sometimes it is beneficial to perform gross modification of the tooth anatomy before the orthodontic treatment is initiated. In that case, it is advantageous to outline the reshaping required on the patient's cast and then carrying it out on the actual teeth. Interproximal reshaping is not carried out at this time (Figure 12.14).During orthodontics: revaluate approximately 6–8 months into treatment, with an interim panoramic radiograph and before stainless-steel or beta-titanium rectangular arches (TMA© Ormco) are placed. Special attention should be paid to the tooth contact points and to the management of open embrasures and black triangles, particularly

between the upper central incisors. First, the length of the teeth and the thickness of the incisal edges are modified. Then, the contact points are opened to allow elimination or reduction of the black triangles, while avoiding narrowing the incisors or approximating their roots too much. The created interdental spaces are readily closed with orthodontics. Slight mesial tipping of the roots of the central incisors may be necessary to reduce the interdental space further, so that the interdental gingiva fills the space in cases where additional reduction in the width of the crowns is not recommended (Figure 12.15).

After orthodontic treatment

It is widely accepted that patients with bone loss should be monitored for life by their periodontist or general dentist (Lindhe et al. 1983; Badersten et al. 1984; Becker et al. 1984; Lindhe and Nyman 1984).

Retention

- Retention after adult orthodontics, whether or not associated with reduced periodontal support, is for life. The only means that have proved reliable at maintaining the position of the anterior teeth, canine to canine, invariable over long periods of time, is bonded lingual arches.
- The fixed lingual arches and the composite used for bonding should be kept away from the lingual gingival papilla and should not interfere with the interdental spaces below the contact points so that the patient can floss that area. At the appointment when the retainers are bonded, patients should be informed about the purpose of the retainers and how important they are for maintaining the tooth positions achieved. They should be instructed on the use of Superfloss and to check regularly with a mouth mirror that the composite pads are bonded on every tooth.
- Unfortunately, sometimes, the maintenance of the fixed lingual arches is overlooked. It is advisable that, after an initial period of 6 months following the ending of the orthodontic treatment (which usually includes three appointments), the patient should be seen regularly every 12–16 months by the orthodontist.
- Lingual arches have an added beneficial splinting effect on incisors with reduced periodontal support despite the lack of literature supporting this aspect. Tooth mobility is markedly reduced when teeth are splinted with a bonded lingual arch.
- In deep bite cases with PSI, a modified Hawley's bite plane is recommended at night time.

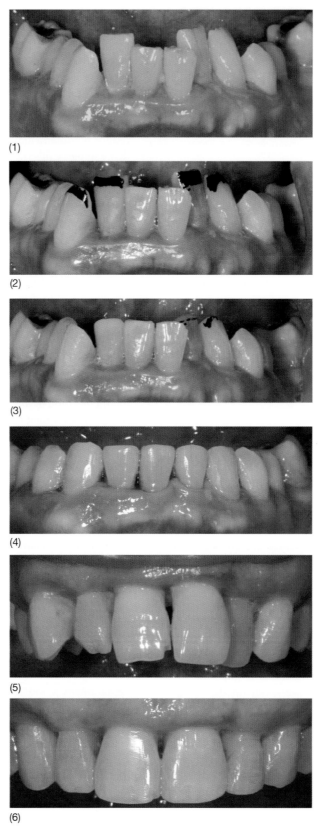

Fig. 12.14 A 55-year-old patient with chronic periodontitis and malocclusion with dental crowding who received orthodontic treatment with extraction of 31. (1)–(3) Before the initiation of the orthodontic treatment, a marked modification of the height of the lower front teeth was performed, and (4)–(10) later on into the treatment, both the upper and the lower front teeth were remodelled again, this time, three dimensionally. (11) and (12) The treatment not only resulted in much better occlusion but also a significantly aesthetic change in the patient's smile due to a great extent to the aggressive tooth remodelling carried out.

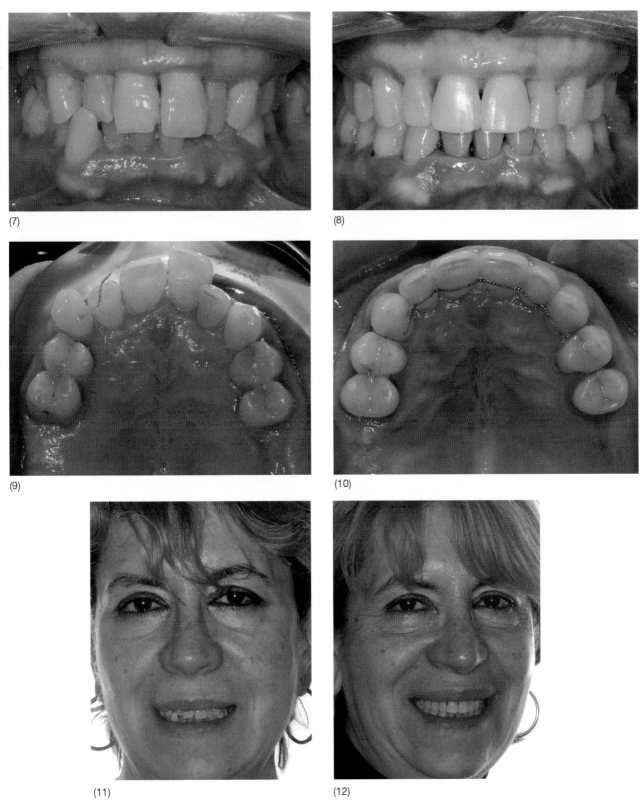

Fig. 12.14 (*Continued*)

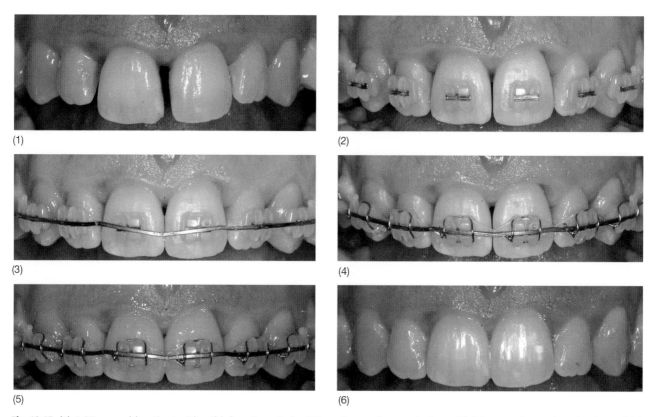

Fig. 12.15 (1) A 35-year-old patient with mild chronic periodontitis and spaced upper incisors. (2) After gentle tooth reshaping, which included the interdental areas between the central incisors, an open embrasure remained. (3) and (4) Second-order bends were placed in a 0.019 × 0.025-inch titanium molybdenum (TMA) archwire to tip mesially the roots of the central incisors. (5) Four weeks later, the embrasure was closed. (6) Final result.

References

Ainamo J, Polohemio L, Nordblad A and Murtomaa H (1986) Gingival recession in schoolchildren at 7, 12 and 17 years of age in Espoo, Finland. *Commun Dent Oral Apidemiol* 14, 283–286.

Allais D and Melsen B (2003) Does labial movement of lower incisors influence the lebel of the gingival margin? A case-control study of adult orthodontic patients. *Eur J Orthod* 25, 343–352.

Andlin-Sobocki A, Marcusson A and Persson M (1991) 3-year observations on gingival recession in mandibular incisors in children. *J Clin Periodontol* 18(3), 155–159.

Andlin-Sobocki A and Persson M (1994) The association between spontaneous reversal of gingival recession in the mandibular incisors and dentofacial changes in children. A 3-year longitudinal study. *Eur J Orthod* 16(3), 229–239.

Artun J and Grobety D (2001) Periodontal status of mandibular incisors after pronounce orthodontic advancement during adolescence: a follow-up evaluation. *Am J Orthod Dentofacial Orthop* 119, 2–10.

Artun J and Krogstad O (1987) Periodontal status of mandibular incisors following excessive proclination. A study in adults with surgically treated mandibular prognathism. *Am J Orthod Dentofacial Orhop* 91(3), 225–232.

Artun J and Urbye K (1988) The effect of orthodontic treatment on periodontal bone support in patients with advanced loss of marginal periodontium. 93, 143–148.

Badersten A, Nilvéus R and Egelbert J (1984) Effect of non-surgical periodontal therapy. II. Severely advanced periodontitis. *J Clin Periodont* 11, 63–76.

Batenhorst KF, Bowers GM and Williams JE (1974) Tissue changes resulting from facial tipping and extrusion of incisors in monkeys. *J Periodontol* 45, 660–668.

Becker W, Becker BE and Berg LE (1984) Periodontal treatment without maintenance. A retrospective study in 44 patients. *J Periodontol* 55, 505–509.

Bowers G (1963) A study of the width of attached gingiva. *J Periodontol* 34, 201–209.

Boyd RL, Leggott PJ, Quinn RS, Eakle WS and Chambers D (1989) Periodontal implications of orthodontic treatment in adults with reduced or normal periodontal tissues versus those of adolescents. *Am J Orthod Dentofacial Orthop* 96, 191–199.

Boyd RL and Rose MR (1994) Effect of rotatory electric toothbrush versus manual toothbrush on decalcification during orthodontic treatment. *Am J Orthod Dentofacial Orthop* 105, 450–456.

Brown LJ, Brunelle JA and Kingman A (1996) Periodontal status in the United States, 1988–1991: prevalence, extent, and demographic variation. *J Dent Res* 75(Spec Iss), 672–683.

Brunsvold MA, Zammit KW and Dongari AI (1997) Spontaneaous correction of pathologic tooth migration following periodontal therapy. *Int J Periodont Restorative Dent* 17, 183–189.

Burgett F, Ramfjord S, Nissle R, Morrison E, Chabernau T and Cafesse R (1992) A randomized trial of occlusal adjustment in the treatment of periodontitis patients. *J Clin Periodont* 19, 381–387.

Caffey N and Egelbert J (1995) Clinical indications of probing attachment loss following initial periodontal treatment in advanced periodontitis patients. *J Clin Periodont* 22(9), 690–696.

Cardaropoli D, Re S, Corrente G and Abundo R (2001) Intrusion of migrated incisors with infrabony defects in adult periodontal patients. *Am J Orthod Dentofacial Orthop* 120, 671–675.

Chasens AI (1979) Peridontal disease, pathologic tooth migration, and adult orthodontics. *N Y State Dent J* 49, 40–43.

Coatoam G, Behrents R and Bissada N (1981) The width of keratinized gingiva during orthodontic treatment: its significance and impact on periodontal status. *J Periodontol* 52, 307–313.

Cortellini P and Tonetti MS (2000) Focus on intrabony defects: guided tissue regeneration (GTR). *Periodontol 2000* 22, 104–132.

Djeu G, Hayes C and Zawaideh S (2002) Correlation between mandibular central incisor proclination and gingival recession during fixed appliance therapy. *Angle Orthod* 72, 238–245.

Dorfman H (1978) Mucogingival changes resulting from mandibular tooth movement. *Am J Orthod* 74, 286–297.

Echeverría JJ, Sanz M and Rylander H (2003) Mechanical supragingival plaque control. In Lindhe J, Karting T and Lang N (eds) *Clinical Periodontology and Implant Dentistry*, 4th edn, p. 454. Oxford: Blackwell Publishing.

Eliasson LA, Hugoson A, Kurol J and Siwe H (1982) The effects of orthodontic treatment on periodontal tissues in patients with reduced periodontal support. *Eur J Orthod* 4, 1–9.

Engelking G and Zachrisson BU (1982) Effects of incisor repositioning on monkey periodontium after expansion through the cortical plate. *Am J Orthod* 82, 23–32.

Ericsson I and Lindhe J (1982) Effect of longstanding jiggling on the experimental marginal periodontitis in the beagle dog. *J Clin Periodontol* 9, 497–503.

Ericsson I, Thilander B and Lindhe J (1978) Periodontal condition after orthodontic tooth movement in the dog. *Angle Orthod* 48, 210–218.

Fleszar TJ, Knowels JW, Morrison EC, Burgett FG, Nissle RR and Ramfjord SP (1980) Tooth mobility and periodontal therapy. *J Clin Periodont* 7, 495–505.

Freedman AL, Green K, Salkin LM, Stain MD and Mellado JR (1999) An 18-year longitudinal study of untreated mucogingival defects *J Periodontol* 70, 1174–1176.

Freedman AL, Salkin LM, Stein MD and Green K (1992) A 10-year longitudinal study of untreated mucogingival defects. *J Periodontol* 63, 71–72.

Gaumet PE, Brunsvold MI and McMahan CA (1999) Spontaneous repositioning of pathologically migrated teeth. *J Periodontol* 70(10), 1177–1184.

Gorman WJ (1967) Prevalence and etiology of gingival recession. *J Periodontol* 38, 316–322.

Handelman CS (1996) The anterior alveolus: its importance in limiting orthodontic treatment and its influence on the occurrence of iatrogenic sequelae. *Angle Orthod* 66(2), 95–110.

Hangorsky U and Bissada NF (1980) Clinical assessment of free gingival graft effectiveness on the maintenance of periodontal health. *J Periodontol* 51, 274–278.

Heasman P, Wilson Z, Macgregor I and Kelly P (1998) Comparative study of electric and manual toothbrushes compare with manual technique in orthodontic patients. *Am J Orthod Dentofacial Orthop* 114, 45–49.

Heintze SD, Jost-Brinkmann P and Laudus J (1996) Effectiveness of three different types of electrical toothbrushes compare with manual technique in orthodontic patients. *Am J Orthod Dentofacial Orthop* 110, 630–638.

Hirschfeld I (1933) The dynamic relationship between pathologically migrated teeth and inflammatory tissue in periodontal pockets: a clinical study. *J Periodontol* 4, 35–47.

Karring T, Nyman S, Thilander B and Magnusson I (1982) Bone regeneration in orthodontically produced alveolar bone dehiscences. *J Periodont Res* 17, 309–315.

Kennedy JE, Bird WC, Palcanis KG and Dorfman HS (1985) A longitudinal evaluation of varying width of attached gingiva. *J Clin Periodontol* 12, 667–675.

Khocht A, Simon G, Person P and Denepitiya JL (1993) Gingival recession in relation to history of hard toothbrush use. *J Periodontol* 64, 900–905.

Lang NP and Löe H (1972) Relationship between the width of KG and gingival health. *J Periodontol* 43, 623.

Lindhe I and Svanberg G (1974) Influences of trauma from occlusion on progression of experimental periodontitis in the Beagle dog. *J Clin Periodont* 1, 3–14.

Lindhe J, Haffajee AD and Socransky SS (1983) Progression of periodontal disease in adult subjects in the absence of periodontal therapy. *J Clin Periodontol* 10, 433–442.

Lindhe J and Nyman S (1984) Long-term maintenance of patients treated for advanced periodontal disease. *J Clin Periodontol* 11, 504–514.

Löe H, Anerud A, Boysen H and Morrison E (1992) The natural history of periodontal disease in man: prevalence, severity, and extent of gingival recession. *J Periodontol* 63, 489–495.

Löst C (1984) Depth of alveolar bone dehiscences in relation to gingival recessions. *J Clin Periodontol* 11, 583 589.

Manor A, Kaffe I and Littner MM (1984) 'Spontaneous' repositioning of migrated teeth following periodontal surgery. *J Clin Periodontol* 11, 540–545.

Martinez-Canut P, Carrasquer A, Magan R and Lorca A (1997) A study on factors associated with pathologic tooth migration. *J Clin Periodontol* 24, 492–497.

Melsen B, Agerbaek N, Eriksen J and Terp S (1988) New attachment through periodontal treatment and orthodontic intrusion. *Am J Orthod Dentofacial Orthop* 94, 104–116.

Melsen B, Agerbaek N and Markenstam G (1989) Intrusion of incisors in adult patients with marginal bone loss. *Am J Orthod Dentofacial Orthop* 96, 232–241.

Murakami T, Yokota S and Takahama Y (1989) Periodontal changes after experimentally induced intrusion of the upper incisors in Macaca fuscata monkeys. *Am J Orthod Dentofacial Orthop* 95, 115–126.

Nelson PA and Ärtun J (1997) Alveolar bone loss of maxillary anterior teeth in adult orthodontic patients. *Am J Orthod Dentofacial Orthop* 111, 328–334.

Nygan PW, Burch JG and Wei SH (1991) Grafted and ungrafted labial gingival recession in pediatric orthodontic patients: effect of retraction and inflammation. *Quintessence Int* 22(2), 103–111.

Nyman S, Karring T and Bergenholtz G (1982) Bone regeneration in alveolar bone dehiscences produced by jiggling forces. *J Periodont Res* 17, 316–322.

Nyman S, Westfelt E, Sarhed G, Ericsons I and Karring T (1988) The role of 'disease' root cementum in healing following treatment of periodontal disease. A clinical study. *J Clin Periodont* 15, 464–468.

Oberholzer R and Rateinschack KH (1996) Root planing or root smoothing. *J Clin Periodont* 3, 326–330.

Persson M and Lennartsson B (1986) Improvement potential of isolated gingival recession in children. *Swed Dent J* 10, 45–51.

Pihlstrom BL, Anderson KA, Aeppli D and Schaffer EM (1986) Association between sings of trauma from occlusion and periodontitis. *J Periodontol* 57, 1–6.

Polson A, Caton J, Polson AP, Nyman S, Novak J and Reed B (1984) Periodontal response after tooth movement into infrabony defects. *J Periodontol* 55, 197–202.

Powell RN and McEniery TM (1982) A longitudinal study of isolated gingival recession in the mandibular central incisor region of children age 6–8 years. *J Clin Periodontol* 9, 357–364.

Proffit WR (1978) Equilibrium theory revisited: factors influencing pocition of the teeth. *Angle Orthod* 48, 75–186.

Re S, Corrente G, Abundo R and Cardaropoli D (2000) Orthodontic treatment in periodontally compromised patients: 12-year report. *Int J Periodont Restorative Dent* 20, 31–39.

Roccuzzo M, Bunino M, Needleman I and Sanz M (2002) Periodontal plastic surgery for treatment of localized gingival recessions: a systematic review. *J Clin Periodontol* 29, 178.

Rose ST and App GR (1973) A clinical study of the development of the attached gingiva along the facial aspect of the maxillary and mandibular anterior teeth in deciduous, transitional and permanent dentitions. *J Periodontol* 44, 131.

Rosenberg RM and Ash NN Jr (1974) The effect of root roughness on plaque accumulation and gingival inflammation. *J Periodontol* 7, 457–462.

Ruf S, Hansen K and Pancherz H (1998) Does orthodontic proclination of lower incisors in children and adolescents cause gingival recession? *Am J Orthod Dentofacial Orthop* 114, 100–106.

Rupprecht RD, Horning GM, Nicoll BK and Cohen ME (2001) Prevalence of dehiscences and fenestrations in modern American skulls. *J Periodontol* 72(6), 722–729.

Sarikaya S, Haydar B, Ciger S and Ariyurek M (2002) Changes in the alveolar bone thickness due to retraction of anterior teeth. *Am J Orthod Dentofacial Orthop* 122, 15–26.

Singh J and Deshpande RH (2002) Pathologic migration – spontaneous correction following periodontal therapy: a case report. *Quintessence Int* 33(1), 65–68.

Snyder MB (1982) Gingival recession: a review of causative factors and treatment. Part I. Diagnostic and treatment considerations. *Comp Cont Educ Dent* 3, 195–200.

Steiner GG, Pearson JK and Ainamo J (1981) Changes of the marginal periodontium as a result of labial tooth movements in monkeys. *J Periodontol* 52, 314–320.

Stoner J and Mazdyasna S (1980) Gingival recession in the lower incisor region of 15-year-old subjects. *J Periodontol* 51, 74–76.

The American Academy of Periodontology (2000) Parameter on chronic periodontitis with slight to moderate loss of periodontal support. *J Periodontol* 71, 353–355.

Thienpont V, Dermart LR and Van Maele G (2001) Comparative study of 2 electric and 2 manual toothbrushes in patients with fixed orthodontic appliances. *Am J Orthod Dentofacial Orthop* 120, 353–360.

Towfighi PP, Brunsvold MA, Story AT, Arnold RM, Willman DE and McMahan CA (1997) Pathologic migration of anterior teeth in patients with moderate to severe periodontitis. *J Periodontol* 68, 967–972.

Van der Weijden GA, Timmerman MF, Nijboer A and Van der Velden U (1993) A comparative study of electrical toothbrushes and the effectiveness of plaque removal in relation to toothbrushing duration. *J Clin Periodont* 20, 476–481.

Vanarsdall RL (1985) Periodontal orthodontic relationships. In Graber TM and Vanarsdall RL (eds) *Orthodontics. Current Principles and Techniques*, 2nd edn, pp. 123–124. St Louis, MO: Mosby.

Warren PR and Charter BV (1996) An overview of established interdental cleaning methods. *J Clin Dent* 7, 65–69.

Wennstrom J and Lindhe J (1983) Role of attached gingiva for maintenance of periodontal health. Healing following excisional and grafting procedures in dogs. *J Clin Periodontol* 10, 206–221.

Wennström J, Lindhe J, Sinclair F and Thilander B (1987) Some periodontal tissue reactions to orthodontic tooth movement in monkeys. *J Clin Periodontol* 14, 121–129.

Wennstrom JL (1996) Mucogingival considerations in orthodontic treatment. *Semin Orthod* 2, 46–54.

Wennström JL, Lindskog-Stokland B, Nyman S and Thilander B (1993) Periodontal tissue response to orthodontic movement of teeth with infrabony pockets. *Am J Orthod Dentofacial Orthop* 103, 313–319.

Wennstrom JL and Pini Prato GP (2003) Mucogingival therapyperiodontal plastic surgery. In Lindhe J, Karring T and Lang N (eds) *Clinical Periodontology and Implant Dentistry*, 4th edn, p. 616. Oxford: Blackwell Publishing.

13

Interdisciplinary Collaboration between Orthodontics and Periodontics

Francesco Milano, Laura Guerra Milano

Introduction

When treating adult patients, the periodontist's awareness of the benefits of orthodontics is as important as the orthodontist's ability to recognise which of his or her patients requires a referral, a periodontic diagnosis and possible periodontal therapy. It is necessary to identify the periodontal problems that must be kept under control throughout the orthodontic treatment phase. Each orthodontic patient with a healthy periodontium must undergo periodic professional hygiene-maintenance sessions. Hence, interdisciplinary collaboration is necessary to achieve an optimal functional and aesthetic therapeutic result.

Advances within periodontal therapy have greatly broadened the horizons of orthodontic treatment, and, similarly, the latter has improved the prospects of the results achievable solely with periodontics. This chapter provides an overview of the fundamental principles necessary for the understanding of the periodontist's role in interdisciplinary treatment, followed by some examples illustrating the range of possible combined treatments in which interdisciplinary work resulted in a more efficient and/or aesthetically satisfying therapeutic outcome.

It is obvious, however, that often there is no choice; the collaboration may prove to be indispensable in cases in which overlooking this is associated with the risk, if not the

Adult Orthodontics, Second Edition. Edited by Birte Melsen and Cesare Luzi.
© 2022 John Wiley & Sons Ltd. Published 2022 by John Wiley & Sons Ltd.
Companion Website: http://www.wiley.com/go/melsen-adult-orthodontics

certainty, of further compromising previously reduced periodontal support of some teeth. When considering a combined treatment plan, it is important to standardise the procedures that allow for correct planning, independent of whether the patient has first been seen by the orthodontist or by the periodontist (Melsen and Milano 1993a, 1993b). At the appointment when the treatment decision is to be made, it is essential that all the team members are involved and the patient too, within the teamwork approach. This could be an ideal moment to explain to the patient the necessity of supportive periodontal treatment before, during and after orthodontic therapy.

Periodontal diagnosis

Periodontitis is defined as a multifactorial disease that is initiated by microbial dental plaque accumulation, but whose progression and form are influenced by specific interactions between genetic susceptibility and environmental factors (Tonetti 1998; Kinane 1999). The periodontal status of each individual undergoing an orthodontic check-up or therapeutic visit must be evaluated and kept under control.

History taking and clinical and radiographic examination

History taking

During the periodontal visit, data regarding general medical condition, dental and periodontal data must be collected in order to correctly establish the periodontal diagnosis and determine any subsequent therapy required. In addition, a subjective analysis of the patient is performed compiling a 'problem list' and evaluating his/her capacity for compliance.

A comprehensive collection of data may reveal the presence of risk indicators with either a high or a low predictive value. The predictive value of some risk factors such as diabetes, smoking and the presence of certain types of bacteria found in dental plaque – *Porphyromonas gingivalis*, *Tannerella forsythia* (*Bacteroides forsythus*) and *Actinobacillus actinomycetemcomitans* – is supported by evidence. Other variables, such as age, race, environment, stress, nutrition, genetic predisposition, systemic disease and immunodepression, are considered to be probable risk factors (Offenbacher 1996; Zambon 1996; Tonetti 1998; Kinane 1999; McGuire and Nunn 1999; Taylor 2001; Meisel et al. 2002; Ezzo and Cutler 2003; Nunn 2003).

Clinical examination

The clinical examination evaluates:

- Number, status and position of present teeth.
- Level of oral hygiene, plaque index and bleeding score.
- Probing depth and furcation probing.
- Presence of hypertrophy and/or gingival recession.
- Presence and degree of tooth mobility and migration.

A probe is inserted in the gingival sulcus of each tooth with approximately 20–25 g of pressure. In absence of inflammation, the application of this pressure should not result in the probe penetrating the connective tissue (Polson et al. 1980; Caton et al. 1981; Sild et al. 1987a, 1987b). Probing thus demonstrates the loss of clinical attachment and furcation involvement, and is a measure of periodontal pocket depth and gingival recession.

Deep pockets increase the risk of the progression of periodontitis (Armitage 1996). The bleeding score, if repeatedly positive during periodic probing, has a high predictive value for the risk of further attachment loss. If, on the contrary, it is repeatedly negative, it is a valid confirmation of stable periodontal health. The absence of supragingival plaque is highly indicative of stable periodontal health (Armitage 1996).

Physiological tooth mobility is about 0.2 mm (more or less 50%). Tooth mobility is expressed using the following mobility index:

0 = normal mobility.
1 = horizontal mobility up to 1 mm.
2 = horizontal mobility > 1 mm.
3 = horizontal and vertical mobility.

Tooth mobility and migration can be provoked by occlusal trauma, presence of edentulous spaces, unbalanced intraoral forces (such as altered tongue and/or lip pressure) and/or significant loss of supporting periodontal tissue. All information collected must be transferred to the periodontal clinical chart (Figure 13.1).

Radiographic examination

A complete periapical radiographic examination using the Rinn centring device is usually undertaken to evaluate the level of alveolar bone and the presence of root resorption. This examination also indicates the space occupied by the periodontal ligament, the lamina dura, the periapical region and the excessive proximity of roots.

The radiographic examination should always be correlated with the clinical examination, which in itself is insufficient for a diagnosis, given its low sensitivity and the lack of correlation between the measurement of the level of clinical attachment and the radiographic height of the bone. This leads to an underestimation of the severity of the periodontal defects (Hammerle et al. 1990; Akesson et al. 1992).

Screening for periodontal disease

Even if it may not seem relevant to describe probing techniques at this point, it is useful to remind the orthodontist of the screening test suggested by the American Academy of Periodontology (AAP) and the American Dental Association (ADA) (Anon 1993, 1996). The PSR logo (Periodontal Screening and Recording) is a registered mark of the American Dental Association. This simple, fast test can be

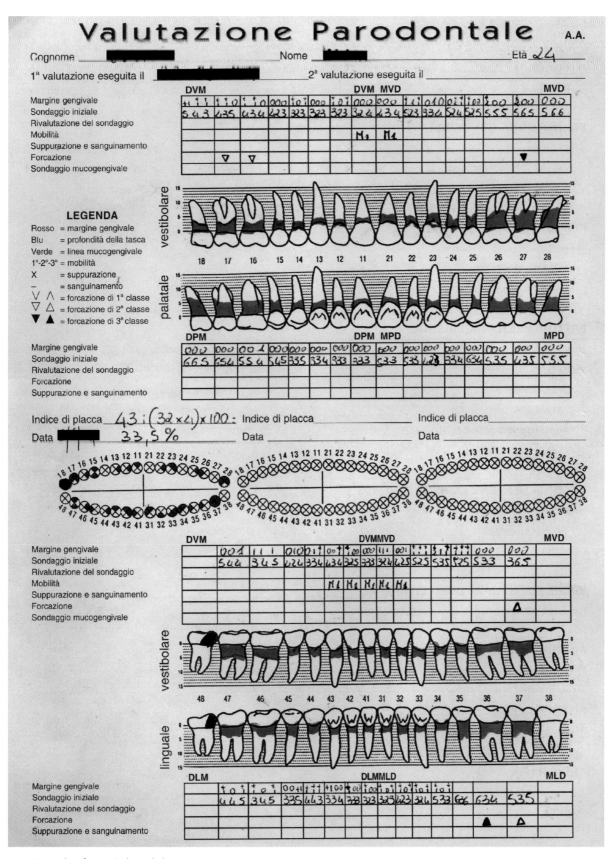

Fig. 13.1 Example of a periodontal chart.

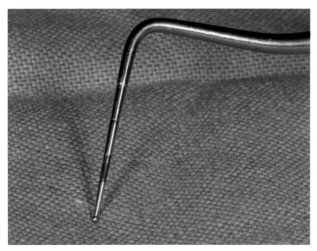

Fig. 13.2 PSR probe: the coloured portion of the probe facilitates immediate reading.

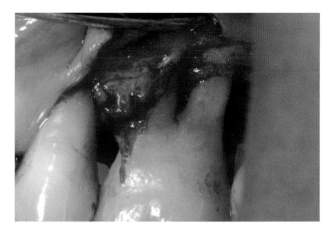

Fig. 13.3 The mesial and distal buccal roots of 26 are slightly divergent, creating a situation that is anatomically favourable for rapid destruction of the deep bone once periodontitis sets in.

Table 13.1 The six dental arch segments for periodontal recording.

1.8–1.4	1.3–2.3	2.4–2.8
4.8–4.4	4.3–3.3	3.4–3.8

implemented routinely in order to immediately differentiate subjects who are periodontally healthy from those who are not, and to periodically monitor their periodontal condition throughout the orthodontic treatment phase.

PSR is a simplified method of recording information collected during probing using a special probe (Figure 13.2) with coloured areas ranging from 3.5 to 5.5 mm. The mouth is divided in six segments as shown in Table 13.1. Only the highest measurement of severity is recorded in each sextant utilising a series of codes:

- 0: the coloured portion of the probe is completely visible.
- 1: the coloured portion of the probe is completely visible, but detects bleeding upon probing.
- 2: the coloured portion of the probe is completely visible, but it detects the presence of calculus and/or restoration overhang, either with or without bleeding.
- 3: the coloured portion of the probe is only partially visible at the maximum probing point of the sextant, indicating the presence of a pocket between 3.5 and 5.5 mm in depth.
- 4: the coloured portion of the probe disappears completely at the maximum probing point of the sextant, indicating the presence of a pocket > 5 mm in depth.

An asterisk (*) is placed next to the code for each sextant, when there is:

- Furcation involvement.
- Dental hypermobility.

- Mucogingival pathologies.
- Recessions > 3.5 mm.

Patients in whom Code 0 is recorded for all areas should commence with a, or continue their previous, prevention programme. Patients with areas in which codes between 1 and 2 without asterisks (*) are recorded should proceed with a prevention programme including oral hygiene instruction, and removal of subgingival and supragingival plaque, calculus deposits and restorations with marginal overhang. Patients presenting areas with codes between 3 and 4 or areas with asterisks (*) require a more detailed periodontal examination, including a comprehensive periodontal chart recording and a complete evaluation of the periapical status. In more complex cases, laboratory investigations should be requested: microbiological and/or haematological, or investigations useful for identifying genetic susceptibility to periodontitis (Cortellini et al. 1999).

Local factors predisposing to periodontal therapy

Local factors, relating to either the anatomy and morphology of teeth or dental restorations which are considered as predisposing to periodontal disease, are as follows:

- Factors relating to tooth anatomy and morphology:
  - Proximity of the roots, particularly between upper molars.
  - Close proximity between the cementoenamel junction (CEJ) and the roof of the furcation area.
  - Ectopic enamel at the furcation.
  - Ridges of dentine covered with a thin layer of cement at the level of the furcation.
  - Reduced divergence of the roots (Figure 13.3).
  - Lingual grooves in the anterior teeth (Figure 13.4).
  - Severe crowding (Figure 13.5).

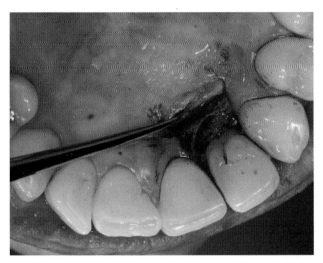

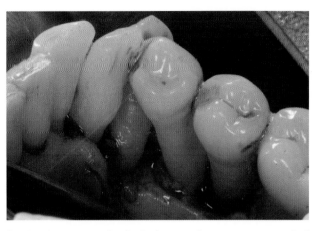

Fig. 13.4 A palatal sulcus that extends beyond the cementoenamel junction favours the accumulation of plaque and the formation of defects of the deep bone. The presence of a bone defect is evident once a flap is raised.

Fig. 13.5 Severe crowding in the lower arch creates an anatomical environment that is favourable for plaque accumulation and makes maintenance of hygiene more difficult and laborious. A raised flap showing severe loss of deep bone in a patient who neglected practising dental hygiene at home and professionally.

- Factors relating to dental restorations:
  - Overhanging fillings.
  - Porous restorative materials capable of holding greater amounts of plaque.
  - Incongruous prosthetic restorations (Figure 13.6).

Timing of ortho–perio treatment

While establishing the treatment plan, it is important to define the treatment to be performed by the periodontist *prior to* starting orthodontic treatment as well as *during* and *after* orthodontic treatment. This should be done both to be able to perform tooth movement in a healthy environment and to optimise the function of the existing periodontal support and to enhance the final aesthetic result (Mathews and Kokich 1997).

Procedures performed prior to orthodontic treatment

- Oral hygiene motivation.
- Prophylaxis or therapy to control inflammation.
- Surgery to eliminate deep pockets.
- Augmentation of attached gingiva.
- Frenulectomy (frenectomy) and frenulotomy (frenotomy).
- Elimination of gingival clefts.

Procedures performed during orthodontic treatment

- Prophylaxis to control inflammation.
- Surgical exposure of impacted teeth according to periodontal concepts.
- Fibrotomy and curettage during forced eruption.

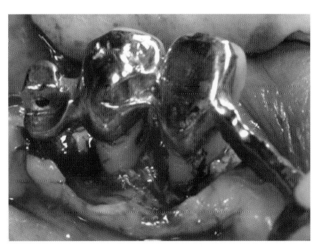

Fig. 13.6 The thick and irregular edges of the prosthetic crowns constitute an obstacle for oral hygiene maintenance and facilitate the accumulation of plaque and formation of calculus.

Procedures performed during and/or post orthodontic treatment

- Prophylaxis to control inflammation.
- Clinical crown lengthening.
- Gingivoplasty.
- Root coverage.

Procedures performed post orthodontic treatment

- Supportive therapy.

The above-mentioned outline is only indicative, as all decisions depend on the individual diagnosis and tailoring the timing of treatment to each patient's unique situation to achieve both the functional and aesthetic therapeutic goals. When labial orthodontic movement is planned, if needed, a periodontal surgical procedure to increase the thickness of the attached gingiva prior to initiating orthodontic treatment can serve to optimise the final result. The same holds true for cases where tooth migrations have resulted in spaces opening and loss of the papilla and eventually a reduction or total lack of attached gingiva. In these cases, surgery is performed before orthodontic closure of the spaces. If only the orthodontic closure or only surgical procedures are performed, the aesthetic and/or functional result will be compromised (Figures 13.7–13.9).

In patients treated with guided tissue regeneration (GTR), simultaneous or almost simultaneous orthodontic treatment may lead to an accentuation of the results (Figure 13.10).

Periodontal therapy

Preventive therapy

This includes oral hygiene education and prophylaxis for inflammation control. Orthodontic treatment in adult patients should only be initiated in the presence of a healthy periodontium. Based on the premise that the most important aetiological agent of periodontitis is plaque, one must consider that the orthodontic appliance increases the risk of plaque accumulation and the difficulty of performing daily oral hygiene at home. Changes in the quality of the microflora in periodontal sites around orthodontic bands have been described in literature (Diamanti-Kipioti et al. 1987; Huser et al. 1990; Turkkahraman et al. 2005). Therefore, in order to avoid complications during orthodontic treatment, it is important to:

- Give detailed oral hygiene instructions. Toothbrushing can be made more effective through the use of an electric toothbrush with a circular head (Sicilia et al. 2002; Heanue et al. 2003), supplemented with rinsing with chlorhexidine to control gingivitis (Sicilia et al. 2002; Heanue et al. 2003; Sekino et al. 2003). At this time, it is opportune to proceed with general oral health behaviour education including motivation and a recommendation to stop or reduce cigarette smoking, avoid or reduce parafunctions and/or residual 'bad hygiene habits'.
- To have quarterly recall visits (Boyd and Baumrind 1992) for professional oral-hygiene sessions to control plaque and supragingival and subgingival calculus.
- To arrange recall visits with the periodontist to register probing depth, the plaque index and bleeding score, tooth mobility and gingival recession.

Non-surgical mechanical therapy

Non-surgical mechanical therapy, scaling and root planing, is performed using manual, sonic or ultrasonic instruments to remove plaque, calculus, necrotic cement and bacteria until the root surface is clean, smooth and hard. This serves to obtain and maintain a healthy periodontal state with reduced bleeding and probing depth. After this primary therapy, the patient is re-evaluated and the need for possible surgical therapy is assessed (Heitz-Mayfield et al. 2002) (Figure 13.11).

Local and systemic antimicrobial therapy

Antimicrobic therapy, administered systemically or applied locally as a support for mechanical therapy, may be prescribed by the periodontist based on the specific diagnosis formulated (Herrera et al. 2002; Haffajee et al. 2003; Hallmon and Rees 2003; Hanes and Purvis 2003).

Surgical therapy

Surgical elimination or reduction of deep pockets

If the periodontal status is controlled, orthodontic tooth movement in adults can be performed even in the case of advanced loss of marginal periodontium (Artun and Urbye 1988; Zachrisson 1997). Before initiating orthodontic treatment, it is necessary to perform periodontal surgical therapy on teeth that, at the completion of preventive therapy and root planing, have deep residual pockets (>4–5 mm) with persistent clinical signs of disease.

The specific goal is to eliminate pockets and to obtain a shallow sulcus in order to facilitate plaque control. According to Armitage (1996), when the pocket depth is 5 mm or more, there is a high risk of relapse. The surgical procedures for pocket reduction require access flaps as the modified Widman flap, while the techniques for pocket elimination include gingivectomy and the apically positioned flap, with or without osseous resective surgery. When performing a gingivectomy, a gingivoplasty is also performed (Goldman 1951), aiming to eliminate suprabony pockets to facilitate access for root planing and to establish a gingival architecture that is favourable for maintenance.

Access flaps consist of lifting of a flap that preserves marginal gingival tissues and gives access to root-planing instruments and removal of the granulation tissue. In this way, healthy tissue is adapted to the root surface and sutured. The modified Widman flap (Ramfjord and Nissle 1974) consists of a vestibular and palatal incision of approximately 1 mm from the gingival margin, which is highly scalloped in such a way that the maximum amount possible of interdental gingiva is included interproximally in the flap. This ensures adequate coverage of interproximal bone while suturing. Having eliminated the collar of gingival tissue from around the alveolar bone, the surgeon proceeds with root planing and curettage of the bone defects. Finally, the flaps are positioned on the alveolar bone and sutured (Figure 13.12). The apically positioned flap (Friedman 1962) is a mucoperiosteal internal bevelled flap, positioned at the level of the bone crest. This permits pocket elimination and keratinised tissue preservation and allows proceeding with bone surgery, osseous resective surgery and/or osteoplasty.

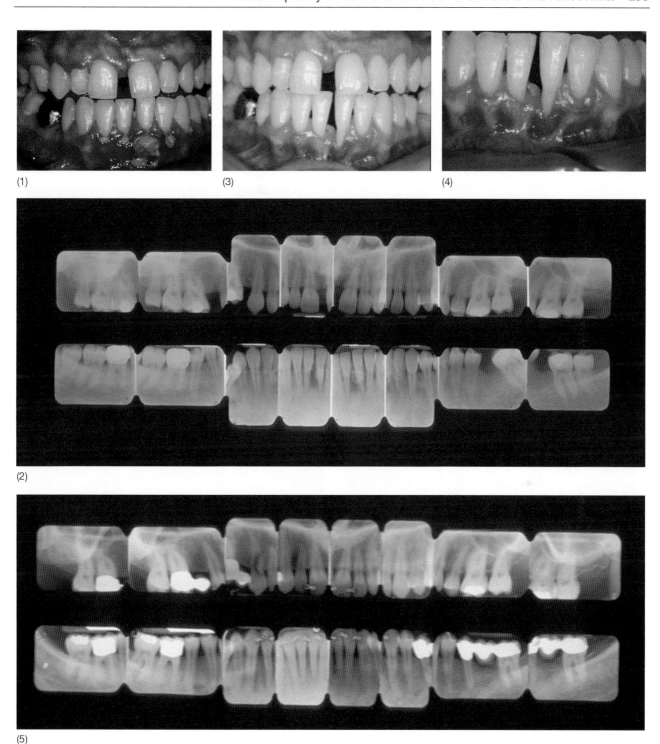

Fig. 13.7 (1) and (2) A 22-year-old woman with a midline diastema, treated in 1982. The patient had extremely poor oral hygiene with plaque and calculus, especially in relation to the lower incisors. Three upper premolars were missing and the space on the right side was partially closed. The patient stated that the midline diastema was increasing in size. (3) and (4) Motivation, scaling and root planing have led to a distinct improvement in the oral hygiene. There is gingival recession in relation to the lower incisors with loss of attachment and interdental alveolar bone, and reduction of the interdental papilla height. (5) and (6) With orthodontic treatment, space was opened for one tooth in the upper right premolar region with closure of the medial diastema. After prosthetic rehabilitation, the upper and the lower incisors were splinted. The gingival recession on 31 and 41 with loss of interdental periodontal tissue was still present, as was the lack of attached gingiva and the presence of a frenulum. (7) and (8) An autogenous free soft-tissue graft was placed in order to eliminate the frenulum and to increase the thickness and the quantity of the attached gingiva. (9) Now the case is finished. (10) At 10-year follow–up, the overall status is still maintained. (11) The clinical situation 22 years later.

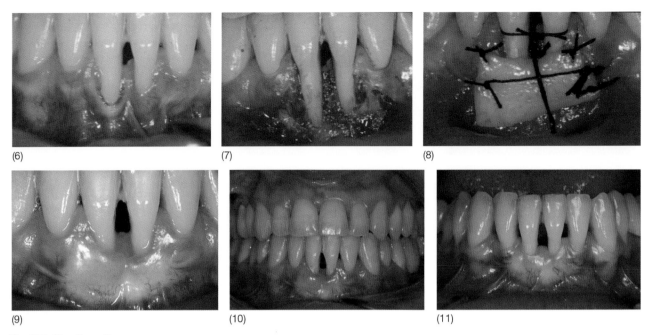

(6)　(7)　(8)

(9)　(10)　(11)

Fig. 13.7 (*Continued*)

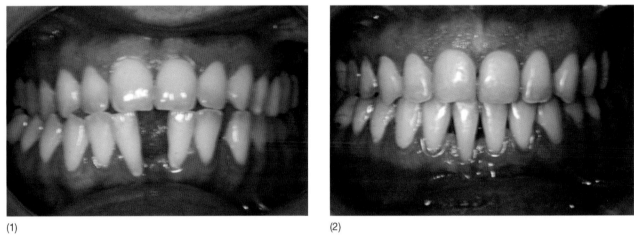

(1)　(2)

Fig. 13.8 (1) A 44-year-old woman treated in 1995 complained of a progressively increasing diastema between the lower incisors with recession and attachment loss at the interproximal surfaces. The diastema made plaque removal more difficult. (2) After being motivated, and after the scaling and root planing, the patient became more attentive regarding hygiene maintenance. At the end of the orthodontic treatment, the occlusion and the aesthetics were restored. Bonded retainers from canine to canine were fitted in both arches. At the end of the treatment, a redistribution of the interdental periodontal tissue was noted, although, due to the thin marginal tissue, root coverage and normal papillary height were not achieved.

Mucogingival and aesthetic surgery

Mucogingival surgery has been given several definitions. In 1957, Friedman described it as surgery 'designed to preserve attached gingiva, to remove frenal or muscle attachment and to increase the depth of the vestibule'. In 1992, the American Academy of Periodontology defined it as surgery consisting of a series of 'plastic surgical procedures designed to correct defects in the morphology, position and/or amount of gingivae surrounding the teeth' (Anon

1992). The most significant factors provoking gingival recession are periodontal disease caused by plaque accumulation and incorrect oral hygiene practices, thin gingiva, prominent root surface, excessively labial/buccal tooth position, short frena and bony dehiscences (Löe et al. 1992a, 1992b). In the light of current knowledge, mucogingival surgery is no longer indicated for augmentation of attached gingiva, but it is indicated for the correction of aesthetic problems mainly if associated with the presence of hypersensitivity often experienced. The

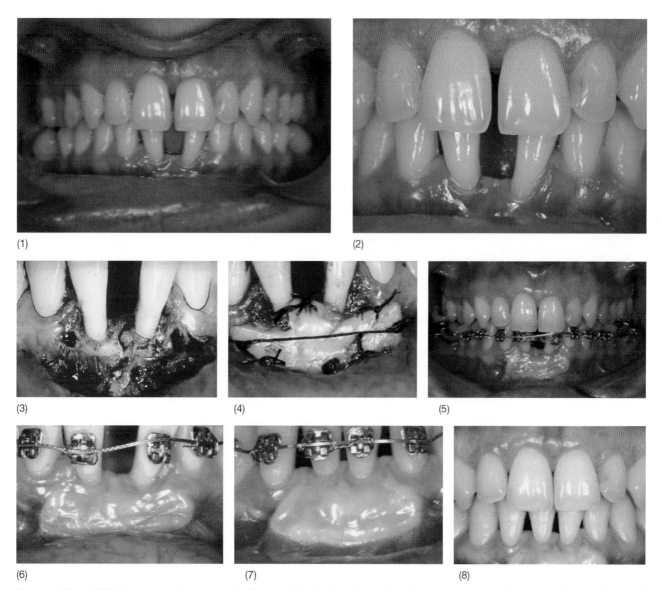

Fig. 13.9 (1) and (2) A 33-year-old woman (1988) complained of an increasing diastema between the lower incisors with speech problems and spraying of saliva through the wide open space. The lower first molars had been extracted a long time ago with mesial migration of second molars. There was total absence of attached gingiva, thin gingival margins and gingival recession with loss of interdental papilla height. (3) and (4) After patient motivation, scaling and root planing, a free gingival graft was placed to increase the thickness of connective tissue before orthodontic treatment to be 'squeezed' during the orthodontic closure of the diastema. In this patient, periodontal surgery alone would be insufficient to obtain root coverage and papilla height. (5) and (6) Orthodontic treatment was performed only in the lower arch, as elimination of the traumatic occlusion between the lower and upper incisors was sufficient to allow spontaneous closure of the upper diastema. (7) At near completion of the orthodontic treatment, complete root coverage was obtained and the papilla filled the interdental space up to the cementoenamel junction, but total recovery of the papilla was not possible due to the triangular shape of the lower incisors. (8) Improvement of the periodontal situation was maintained with a lingual retainer.

following surgical procedures have been among those indicated for coverage of root recessions:

- Laterally positioned pedicle flap (Grupe and Warren 1956).
- Free gingival grafts (Sullivan and Atkins 1968).
- Coronally positioned flap (Allen and Miller 1989).
- Several bilaminar techniques with connective-tissue graft (Langer and Langer 1985; Raetzke 1985).

- GTR techniques (Langer and Langer 1985; Tinti et al. 1992; Prato et al. 1996).

All mucogingival surgical procedures (periodontal plastic surgery) have been proved effective to obtain root coverage with a gain in attachment level (Roccuzzo et al. 2002; Clauser et al. 2003; Pagliaro et al. 2003); even from a systematic review of the literature, it appears that there is a certain advantage in root coverage obtained with the

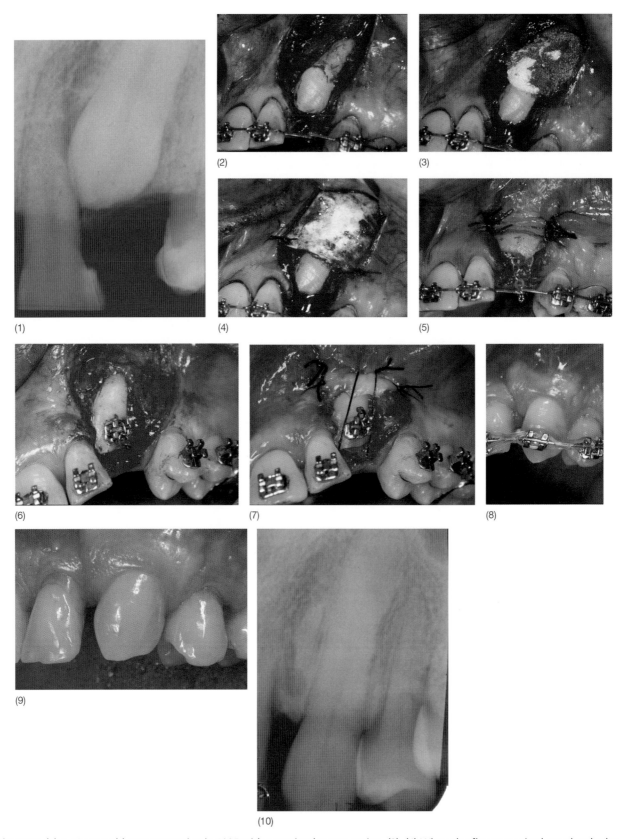

Fig. 13.10 (1) A 42-year-old man presenting in 1995 with a retained upper canine. (2)–(4) When the flap was raised, no alveolar bone was seen on the buccal aspect of the root of the canine. Guided tissue regeneration periodontal therapy was performed, using a resorbable collagen membrane (Paroguide®) and a layer of Biostite® between the root and the membrane. (5) A bracket with a gold chain was bonded to the crown and the flap sutured. (6) At the reopening, it is possible to see the new periodontal tissue. (7) An apically positioned flap was carried out to improve the attached gingiva. (8) The treatment is almost finished. (9) and (10) Clinical and radiographic situation 10 years later (2005).

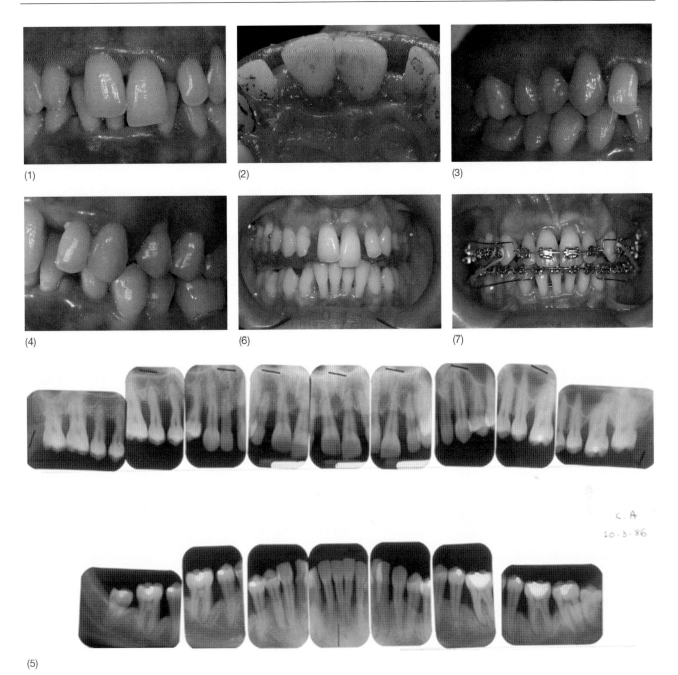

(1)   (2)   (3)

(4)   (6)   (7)

(5)

Fig. 13.11 (1)–(4) In 1986, a 25-year-old woman showed a Class II division 2 malocclusion with deep bite, a deep curve of Spee, a gingival impingement, a periodontal compromised situation and spontaneous migrations. In addition, she had also temporomandibular joint (TMJ) symptoms due to the loss of vertical dimension. (5) The initial full-mouth radiographic examination shows loss of supporting tissues. (6) and (7) After patient motivation, scaling and root planing, oral hygiene and periodontal condition improved. The treatment plan consisted of orthodontic treatment, including intrusion of the upper incisors. (8) At the end of the combined orthodontic and non-surgical periodontal therapy. (9) Radiographs at the end of treatment. Supportive periodontal therapy was strictly followed. (10) and (11) The smile before and after interdisciplinary treatment.

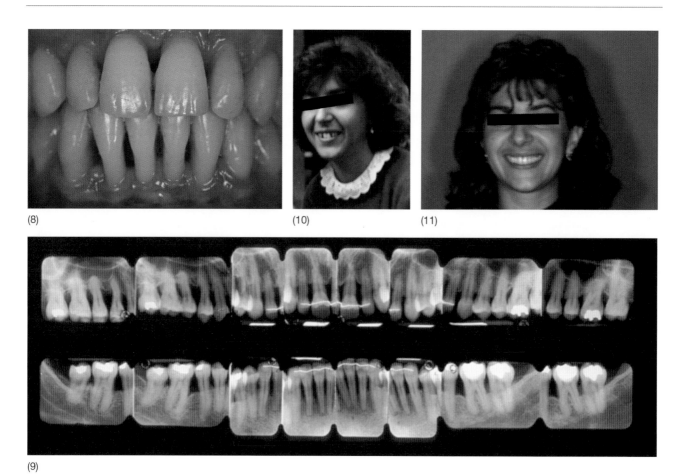

(8)   (10)   (11)

(9)

Fig. 13.11 (*Continued*)

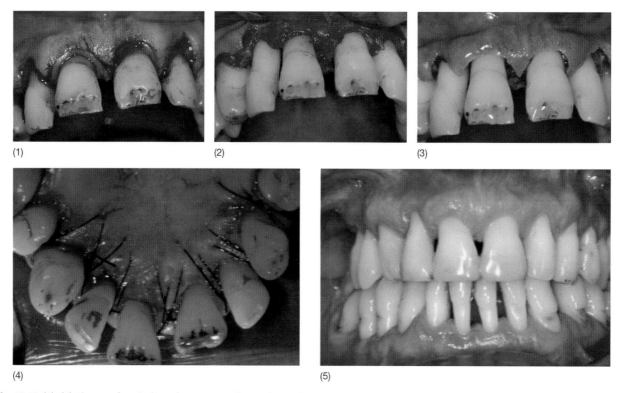

(1)   (2)   (3)

(4)   (5)

Fig. 13.12 (1)–(4) Phases of periodontal surgery performed to reduce probing depth. Exaggerated scalloped incisions, both vestibular and palatal, with maximum preservation of interproximal tissue are evident. Vertical mattress suture. (5) Final view at the conclusion of periodontal and orthodontic treatment.

connective-tissue graft (CTG) procedure compared with that of GTR. The combination of these procedures with orthodontics has long been called for (Boyd 1978; Diedrich 1996). Interrelations between fibrotomy, frenulotomy, frenulectomy, removal of gingival clefts and orthodontics have frequently been mentioned.

Augmentation of attached gingiva and root coverage

The buccolingual position in which teeth erupt influences the quantity of attached gingiva (Maynard and Ochsenbein 1975). In the presence of gingival recession, root coverage treatment can be carried out at the completion of orthodontic treatment. Total resolution of gingival recession will be obtained only when there is no bone or soft-tissue loss at an interdental level (Lindhe et al. 1997). There is no risk of recession associated with orthodontics if the tooth has displaced within the context of its alveolar support, regardless of whether there is adequate or there is not adequate attached gingiva (Wennstrom et al. 1987). However, in the absence of adequate gingival thickness, labial movement that tends to displace the tooth out of its alveolar housing can be the cause of gingival recession (Steiner et al. 1981; Wennstrom et al. 1987; Wennstrom 1994). In this case, the loss of tissue is associated with insufficient gingival thickness and not with the inadequate apical–coronal height. In cases with plaque and incorrect brushing techniques, the thin attached gingiva constitutes a *locus minoris resistentiae*.

Hence, before the initiation of orthodontic treatment that involves labial movement associated with a risk of creating a bone dehiscence, the periodontist must consider whether to proceed with surgery to augment the thickness of the attached gingiva to reduce the risk of recessions (Figures 13.13–13.15). If recessions appear during the course of orthodontic treatment, the patient may lose confidence in the orthodontist. This could also negatively influence the patient's compliance, both of which are fundamental to a successful orthodontic treatment in adults (Figure 13.16).

Miller (1985) classified gingival recession as follows:

- Class I: gingival recession does not extend to the mucogingival junction and there is no loss of bone and soft tissue at the interdental level.
- Class II: marginal tissue recession reaches or extends beyond the mucogingival junction. There is no bone or soft-tissue loss at the interdental level.
- Class III: gingival recession reaches or extends beyond the mucogingival junction. Bone or soft-tissue loss at the interdental level is apical to the CEJ, but coronal to the apical extremity of the recession.
- Class IV: gingival recession extends beyond the mucogingival junction. Interproximal bone loss extends apical to the apical extremity of the recession itself.

In the case of space closure in patients with Miller's Class III or IV gingival recession, it could be useful to increase the thickness of gingival tissue prior to starting the orthodontic

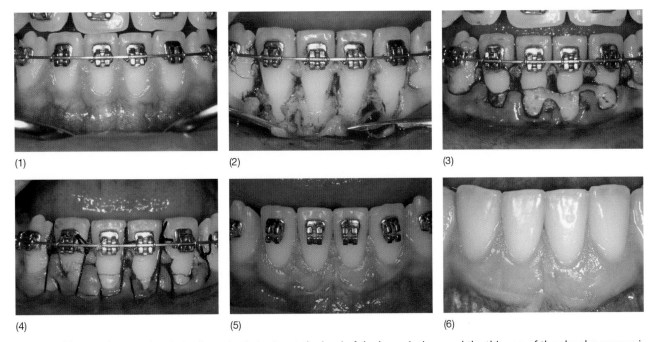

(1) (2) (3)

(4) (5) (6)

Fig. 13.13 (1) Note the complete lack of attached gingiva at the level of the lower incisors and the thinness of the alveolar mucosa in the marginal area. In this case, increasing the thickness of the attached gingiva before labial orthodontic movements is required. (2) A connective-tissue graft with envelope technique graft was performed (Raetzke 1985). Following incision and flap release, note the absence of alveolar bone below the alveolar mucosa margin. (3) and (4) Connective graft harvested from the palate and inserted under the flap. The flap is then sutured. (5) and (6) 5 months and 5 years post surgery.

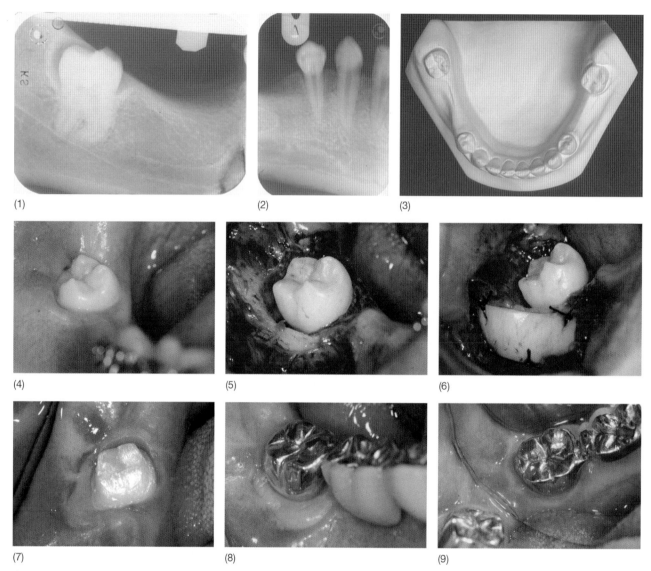

Fig. 13.14 (1) Patient with several missing teeth in the lower arch (in 1984, it was not in common to replace missing teeth with implants). (2) and (3) X-rays showing a partially impacted third molar. As implant surgery was not available, the partially impacted third molar was extruded for use later as a posterior prosthetic abutment. (4)–(6) Following orthodontic extrusion, there was an absolute lack of attached gingiva; therefore, a free epithelial graft was used to increase the depth of the vestibule and obtain an amount of attached gingiva surrounding the tooth. (7) Prosthetic tooth preparation of the molar. An adequate amount of attached gingiva is now present and appropriate hygiene maintenance is now possible. (8) and (9) Buccal and lingual views of the prosthetic bridge.

procedures. With mucogingival surgery alone, little or no gain in root coverage is obtained. In these cases, it is more appropriate to proceed with surgically increasing the thickness of the gingiva before proceeding with orthodontics. In this way, the subsequent orthodontic movement may result in papilla gain and aesthetic and/or functional improvement with the root coverage (Figure 13.17).

Regeneration and reconstruction of the interdental papilla

Due to the reduction of bone support, patients affected by periodontal disease often exhibit migration of teeth leading to opening of spaces in the anterior region, frequently associated with extrusion or labial inclination (Figure 13.9).

This leads to a reduction and/or loss of interdental papilla height.

Nordland and Tarnow (1998) classified loss of papillary height as:

- Normal: the interdental papilla fills the entire interdental space.
- Class I: the tip of the papilla is between the interdental contact point and the most coronal extension of the interproximal CEJ.
- Class II: the tip of the interdental papilla reaches, or is apical to, the interproximal CEJ level, but is coronal to the apical extension of the facial CEJ.
- Class III: the tip of the interdental papilla is at the facial level or apical to the CEJ.

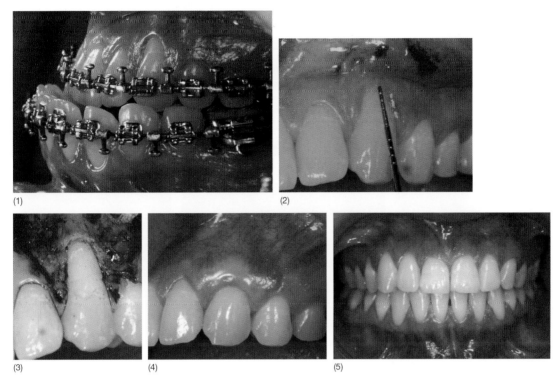

Fig. 13.15 Intraoral lateral view in a patient with skeletal Class III malocclusion. (1) The upper left canine presents Miller's Class I gingival recession. The treatment plan took into consideration the possibilities of a periodontal surgical procedure for root coverage after completion of the orthodontic–surgical treatment. However, that site was monitored monthly to assure that there was no loss of attachment in the area of the papillae, mesial and distal to 23. If such loss had been detected, immediate mucogingival surgical therapy would have been necessary. Due to the orthodontic decompensation in labial direction, the recession is increased, without altering the favourable prognosis for the root coverage procedure. (2) Recession of canine following treatment. (3) and (4) The recession was treated with a bilaminar periodontal flap. Upon healing, total coverage of the recession is achieved, as is predictable, and the integrity of the interproximal attachment was preserved. (5) The case 5 years following treatment.

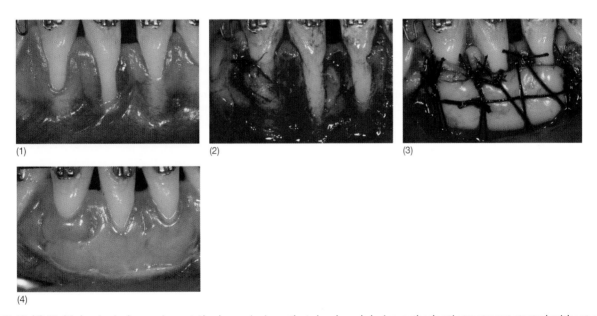

Fig. 13.16 (1) Multiple gingival recessions at the lower incisors that developed during orthodontic treatment started without prior periodontal assessment. The unexpected occurrence of deep recessions during treatment reduced the trust and compliance of the patient. (2) A connective-tissue pedicle graft was performed (Carvalho technique, 1982) because of the shape and quality of the interdental papillae. Prior to placing and suturing the free gingival graft at the recipient site, a multi-papillary pedicle connective-tissue flap was raised and positioned laterally on the recession areas. Suture of the first of three flaps can be seen here. (3) The free gingival graft sutured above the multi-papillary pedicle connective flap. (4) After a few months, considerable attached gingiva was evident with satisfactory results. This patient was treated in 1985.

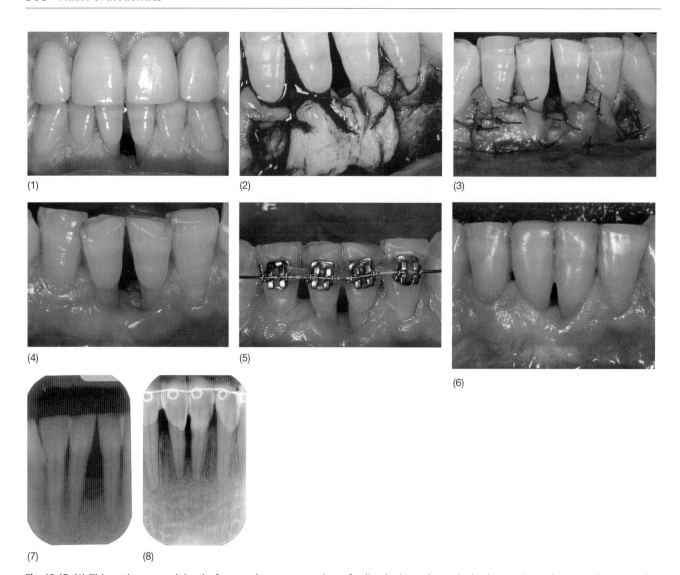

Fig. 13.17 (1) This patient complained of an unpleasant sensation of saliva leaking through the large triangular space between the lower incisors that had developed because of the loss of papilla. The abrasions of the incisal edges masked the divergence of the roots. Combined periodontal and orthodontic therapy was planned. The aim of the periodontal surgery was to increase the thickness of the tissues that would then be compressed by orthodontic approximation of the roots of lower incisors. (2)–(4) The sub-pedicle connective-tissue graft surgical flap (Nelson 1987) led to thickening of the tissue in the interdental zone, but no gain in the papilla. (5) The orthodontist moved the root closer by adjusting the bracket position with respect to the axial inclination. (6) The papilla was improved and the result was maintained by a lingually bonded retainer. (7) and (8) Pre- and post-treatment radiographs demonstrated the root movement.

In 1992, Tarnow et al. confirmed that the presence of the papilla is dependent on the distance between the alveolar crest and the dental contact point; to have a papilla that fills in the space between two adjacent teeth, this distance must be less than or equal to 5 mm. In a total of 288 examined sites in 30 patients, the papilla was present in 56% of the sites with a distance of 6 mm and only in 27% of the sites with a distance greater or equal to 7 mm.

The predictability of papillary regeneration after combined ortho–perio treatment was evaluated by

Cardaropoli et al. (2004) in 28 periodontal patients between 29 and 60 years of age. All patients underwent scaling and root planing prior to initiating orthodontic treatment and all had a low plaque index. After 7–10 days following surgical therapy, consisting of root planing and elimination of granulation tissue from the infrabony defects, orthodontic treatment was commenced. The teeth were realigned and intruded and the spaces were closed. At the end of treatment, the papilla completely filled the interproximal space in 43% of the patients; in 54% of the patients, the papilla was

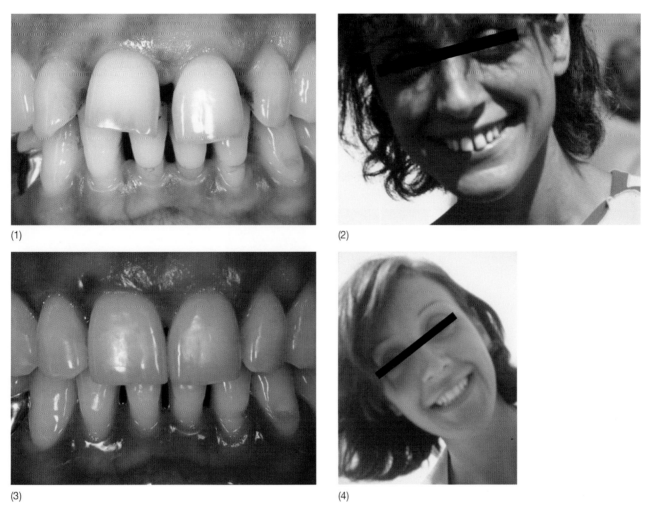

(1) (2) (3) (4)

Fig. 13.18 (1)–(4) Migration and lack of contact between the upper incisors leading to the loss of the interdental papilla and unaesthetic smile in a 37-year-old woman. Non-surgical periodontal treatment and orthodontic space closure were carried out to re-establish the interdental contact points, with the distance between the alveolar crest and each interdental contact point not greater than 5 mm. Thus, complete restoration of all the papillae and the desired aesthetic improvement were achieved. After repositioning, the incisors were retained with intracoronal lingual splinting. In this case, orthodontics replaced a mucogingival and non-surgical therapy.

between the contact point and the CEJ. In only one patient, the papilla height was at the CEJ of the two adjacent teeth. This study confirmed the importance of collaboration between orthodontists and periodontologists in achieving papilla regeneration (Figure 13.18).

Interdental papillae of adequate width, which allows for their inclusion in the flap design, are key to obtaining maximum root coverage (De Sanctis and Zucchelli 1997).

Gingivectomy and clinical crown lengthening

The aesthetic result depends on the contour of the gingival margins, particularly around the upper incisors and canines

(Kokich et al. 1984; Chiche et al. 1994; Kokich 1996). Passive eruption is a physiological process that consists of apical migration of the dentogingival junction over the years. Delayed passive eruption is defined as the condition in which the junctional epithelium is situated at the convexity of the tooth crown, which results in the clinical crown being shorter than the anatomical tooth crown. This occurs either in the presence of gingival hyperplasia or an excessive apico-coronal extension of the alveolar crest (altered passive eruption) (Coslet et al. 1977). This defect can be corrected with gingivectomy or clinical crown lengthening by means of apically repositioned flap surgery and osteoplasty (Bragger et al. 1992).

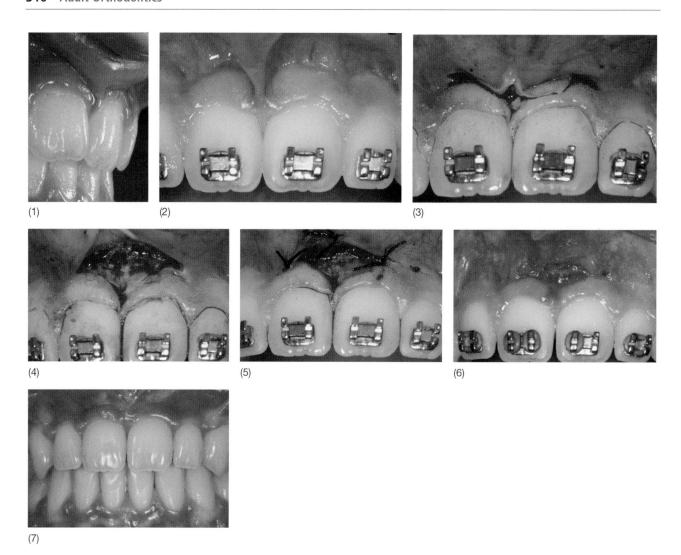

(1)   (2)   (3)

(4)   (5)   (6)

(7)

Fig. 13.19 (1) and (2) A 17-year-old girl presenting a high labial frenulum with a fanned insertion in the upper arch. In such cases, the risk of relapse of the orthodontic closure of the interincisal space is high and surgical removal of the frenulum should be planned before completion of orthodontic treatment. (3)–(5) Surgical phases steps of the frenulectomy procedure. (6) Gingival appearance 15 days post surgery. (7) Stable closure of the median diastema 5 years after combined ortho–perio treatment.

Frenectomy (frenulectomy)

During the eruption of the permanent teeth, the role of the labial frenum in the development of the maxillary median diastema is controversial. Self-correction has been described and therefore only hyperplastic frena with fanned attachments should be removed or repositioned, although it is advisable to wait for spontaneous improvement until the eruption of the first permanent molars (Edwards 1977) (Figure 13.19). If, however, the frenum is present in relation to an interincisal or lateral diastema once the permanent dentition is complete (Figure 13.20), frenectomy is indicated. In addition, frenectomy is indicated in patients presenting a high labial *frenum* with thin gingiva in the mandibular arch (Zachrisson 1997).

Fibrotomy

In 1970 and in 1993, Edwards proposed supracrestal circumferential fibrotomy with the purpose of reducing the risk of relapse after orthodontic rotation, closure of extraction sites and closure of median diastemas. In fact, one of the orthodontic movements at higher risk of relapse is rotation. Retention after this movement must be continued for at least 12 months to allow for remodelling of the supracrestal fibres and periodontal ligament around the teeth (Proffit and Fields 1993). According to Reitan (1969), the ideal time to perform a fibrotomy is at the end of orthodontic treatment, since the greatest risk is present during the first 5 hours post debanding.

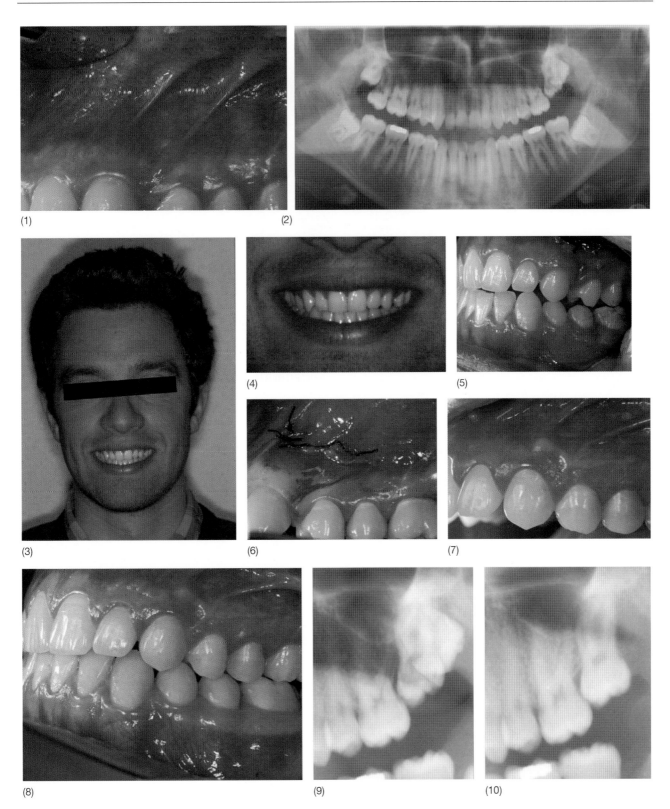

Fig. 13.20 (1) and (2) A 22-year-old man with a lateral diastema between 23 and 24 due to a high buccal frenulum. The radiographs showed that 27 and 28 were impacted. Surgical removal of the frenulum, extraction of 28 and mesialisation of 24, 25 and 26 were planned for allowing eruption and optimal positioning of 27 in the arch. (3) and (4) The frenulum interposed between 23 and 24 is visible and unaesthetic during smiling. (5) and (6) Frenulectomy with apical positioning of the flap. (7) and (8) With time, the diastema closed permanently. (9)–(12) The radiographic sequence showing the impacted 27 and 28, the extraction of impacted 28, the orthodontically positioned 27, which was spontaneously erupted after the extraction of 28, and the mesialisation of 24, 25 and 26 into the area where the frenulum was surgically removed.

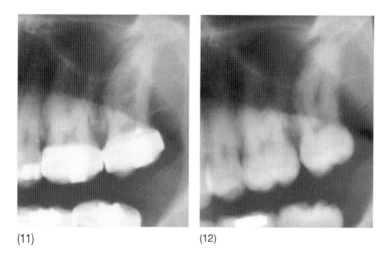

(11)   (12)

Fig. 13.20 *(Continued)*

Another surgical procedure that an orthodontist can request the periodontist to perform is an intrasulcular fibrotomy and curettage during orthodontic forced extrusion. This permits clinical crown lengthening of the tooth by minimising migration of the gingiva, and the attachment of the alveolar bone towards the occlusal surface of the tooth (Kozlovsky et al. 1988). The fibrotomy should be performed every 7–10 days, three or four times, during the entire extrusive phase, to maintain an inflammatory response that prevents the alveolar bone from following the radicular movement (Pontoriero et al. 1987) (Figures 13.21 and 13.22). Six weeks of stabilisation follows, during which a full-thickness periodontal flap can be performed if it is thought to be useful to refine both the gingival and the osseous areas.

Exposure of impacted teeth according to periodontal concepts

According to the classification proposed by Kokich and Mathews in 1993, impacted teeth can be divided into two categories: submucosal and osseous. The aim of orthosurgical treatment is to move the retained tooth to its correct position without causing periodontal damage (Prato et al. 1995). Gingivectomy (Thilander et al. 1973; Archer 1975) and apical flap repositioning are indicated for the exposure of teeth impacted under the alveolar mucosa, the latter being more effective in guaranteeing the correct thickness of the keratinised gingiva surrounding the surface of the erupting tooth (Levin and D'Amico 1974; Vanarsdall and Corn 1977; Shiloah and Kopczyk 1978). The surgical procedure for teeth deeply impacted in the bone consists of raising a full-thickness flap and opening an osseous window that allows access to the dental crown (Thilander et al. 1973; Wisth et al. 1976; Kokich and Mathews 1993). Removal of a significant quantity of osseous tissue facilitates dental eruption, but may lead to loss of support (Kohavi et al. 1984). Thanks to the advances in adhesive techniques, the impacted

tooth, once bonded, can be covered once again with the gingival flap (Figures 13.14 and 13.23).

Regenerative surgical therapy

GTR is based on the principle of guiding the regrowth of various periodontal tissue components during healing after periodontal surgery (Karring et al. 1993). The idea originated in studies carried out by Karring et al. (1980) and Nyman et al. (1982). The technique consists of the application of a subgingival barrier to protect the coagulum. Its function is to impede the apical migration of epithelial cells interposed between the root surface and connective tissue. In this way, the connective tissue of the flap is kept at a distance from the healing sites and the progenitor cells of the periodontal ligament can repopulate the root surface leading to a newly formed periodontium (Gottlow et al. 1984; Caton et al. 1987). Regenerative surgical therapy is used to obtain an increase in the reduced support apparatus and the results are predictable in the correction of angular defects (Murphy and Gunsolley 2003; Tonetti et al. 2004; Cortellini and Tonetti 2005; Needleman et al. 2005). Presently, there are several known regenerative approaches, such as the use of resorbable and non-resorbable membranes, barrier effect, bone grafts and induced periodontal regeneration with enamel matrix derivate (Esposito et al. 2003). Regenerative surgery can be usefully implemented together with orthodontics (Diedrich 1996) (Figure 13.10).

Supportive periodontal treatment

It is of utmost importance to note that supportive periodontal treatment is an active component of periodontal therapy and indispensable for the maintenance of a healthy periodontal state and prevention of recurrence of disease.

Supportive treatment consists of monitoring and of periodic periodontal and hygiene check-ups. The frequency

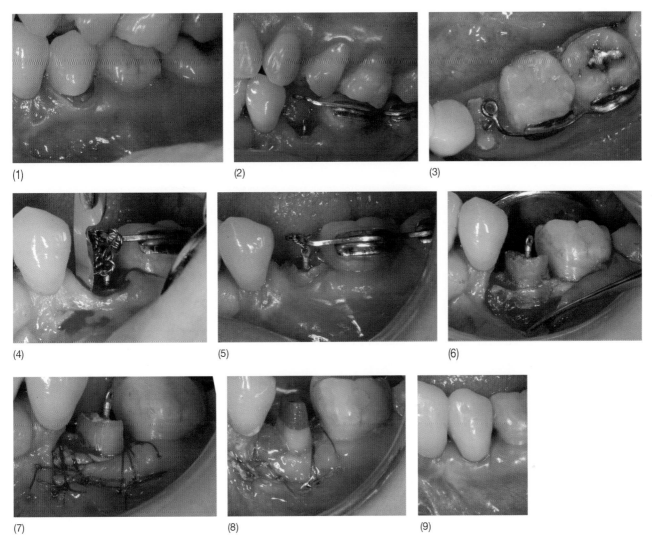

Fig. 13.21 (1) Tooth 35, previously endodontically treated, had a large carious lesion below the prosthetic crown. The root was extruded using rapid extrusion mechanics combined with fibre resection periodically performed during the extrusion phase. (2) and (3) After removal of the crown, a custom-preformed post with an eyelet was inserted into the root. Rigid anchorage was prepared with a stainless-steel 0.022 × 0.028-inch rectangular archwire soldered on orthodontic mesh bases. Buccally, the soldered sectional wire was extended and shaped to allow for the application of the extrusive forces. The patient was able to easily use an interdental toothbrush and floss with a flosser for maintaining oral hygiene between 36 and 37. Fibre resection was carried out periodically. (4) At the completion of extrusion, the achieved root position was retained with a metallic ligature. (5)–(8) At the end of the orthodontic stabilisation, a periodontal flap was performed to improve the relationship of the soft tissue and the root. The open flap shows that the bony level had not followed the extrusion of the root. On the day of suture removal, the prosthetic abutment was constructed. (9) The prosthetic restoration.

of this regimen is established individually for each patient (Wilson 1996a, 1996b).

Ortho–perio and multidisciplinary clinical cases

This section presents typical examples of combined ortho–perio treatment requiring further prosthetic or implant-prosthetic treatment.

In order to emphasise that interdisciplinary procedures have been in use for some time, we have given the dates of treatment. In each case, it is evident that ultimate goal of

interdisciplinary treatment is to re-establish or achieve improved or ideal aesthetics. This objective can be fulfilled with the support of periodontal and/or implant surgical techniques to a more or less significant degree.

Case 1

This 47-year-old patient, treated in 1993, had progressive migration of 22 with extrusion. This caused an unacceptable aesthetic condition for the patient. On probing, a deep pocket was found. The radiographic examination revealed evidence of severe periodontal loss. A combined treatment plan of

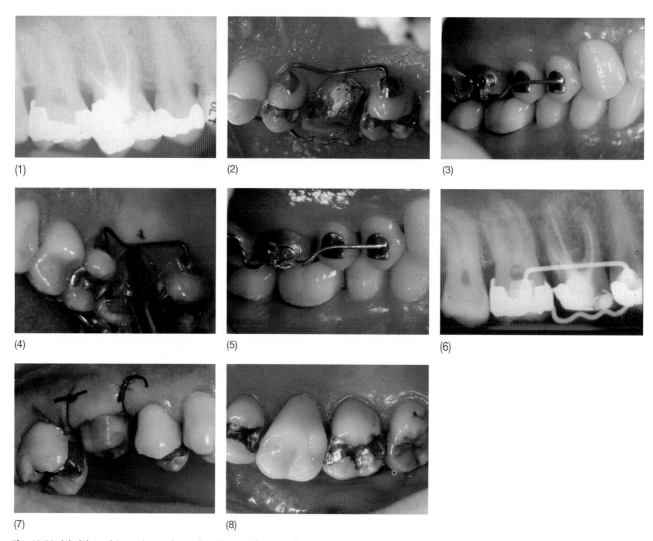

Fig. 13.22 (1)–(3) In this patient, the palatal root of upper first right molar, which had been endodontically treated, had fractured, with the fracture extending beyond the gingival margin. Buccal and palatal sectional wires were bonded to the neighbouring teeth, with a stainless-steel 0.022 × 0.028-inch rectangular archwire adapted for application of elastic forces and soldered onto orthodontic mesh bases. The molar was trimmed occlusally and approximately to eliminate all friction and occlusal contact. (4) To facilitate extrusion through bone, circumferential sulcular fibres resection and curettage were performed and repeated each week for a short period of time. (5) and (6) Clinical and radiographic views following the forced eruption. (7) A gingival flap was performed to refinish the gingival area at the completion of extrusion. (8) A prosthetic crown was prepared for the recovered tooth.

GTR and orthodontic intrusion was proposed as an alternative to tooth extraction (Figure 13.24). On completion, the tooth was intracoronally splinted to the adjacent elements.

In the presence of plaque, intrusion may cause a loss of attachment and formation of angulated bone defects (Ericsson et al. 1977, 1978), but with optimal periodontal control and absence of pathological pockets, orthodontic intrusion can be recommended for treatment of teeth with horizontal bone loss (Melsen et al. 1988, 1989; Melsen and Kragskov 1992). Melsen et al. (1989) demonstrated that orthodontic intrusion resulted in a reduction of the clinical crown length (from 0.3 to 2.3 mm) and an improvement of the bone level. In a subsequent histological study, the authors formulated the hypothesis that the formation of new attachment was due to the increase in the activity of the ligament cells and the movement of the formative cells towards the tooth surface (Melsen and Kragskov 1992). In a clinical study conducted on 10 patients presenting extruded teeth with pocket depth greater than or equal to 6 mm, Corrente et al. (2003) reported that the probing depth was reduced to an average of 4.35 mm following surgical treatment of the pockets and orthodontic intrusion. Radiologically, the horizontal bone defects appeared to have improved by 1.4 mm and vertical defects were filled by 1.35 mm. In the present case of orthodontic intrusion, regenerative techniques were applied (Diedrich 1996).

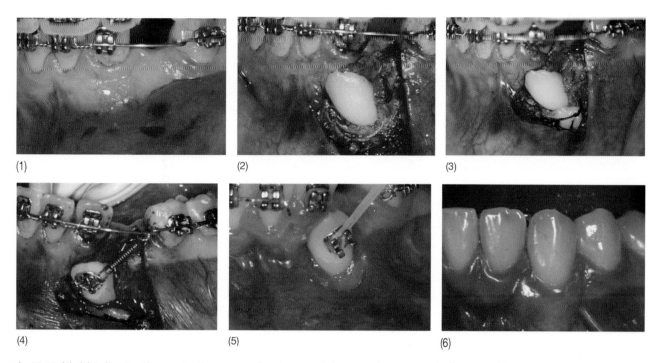

(1)   (2)   (3)

(4)   (5)   (6)

Fig. 13.23 (1)–(3) Following the required space opening the ectopic lower canine was surgically exposed by an apical–lateral positioned flap combined with osteoplasty. The flap was sutured along the long axis of the root. (4) and (5) Orthodontic traction of 33. (6) At the end of the treatment.

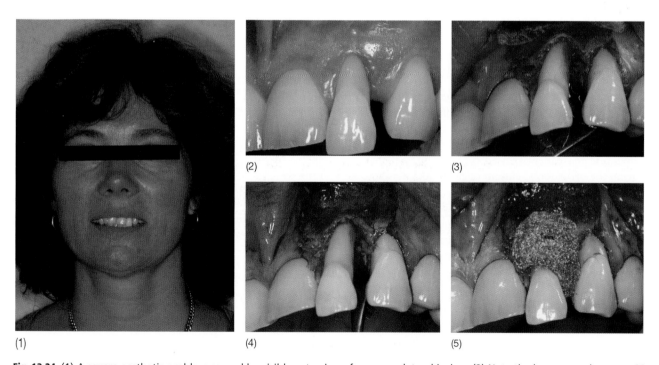

(1)   (2)   (3)

(4)   (5)

Fig. 13.24 (1) A severe aesthetic problem caused by visible extrusion of an upper lateral incisor. (2) Note the large space between 22 and 23. 22 had migrated and extruded due to the severe and advanced loss of periodontal tissue support. (3) and (4) GTR periodontal surgery was done before orthodontic correction. Surgery began with the raising of the flap and debridement with root planing. (5) and (6) The bone defect was filled with Biostite® as support for the resorbable membrane (Paroguide®). (7) The flap was sutured. (8) Partial recovery of supporting bone can be observed. (9) The aesthetics of the smile were restored. (10) 12 years later, the treatment result has been maintained (1994–2006). Views following orthodontic intrusion and space closure. (11) and (12) Pre- and post-treatment radiographs of 22.

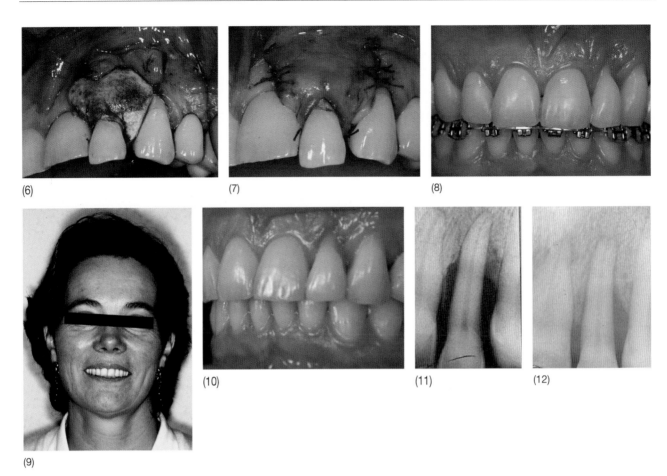

(6)   (7)   (8)

(9)   (10)   (11)   (12)

Fig. 13.24 (*Continued*)

Case 2

This 40-year-old man required ortho–perio prosthetic treatment to replace the left central incisor that had been subject to repeated trauma. While discussing an interdisciplinary approach, perio–ortho prosthetic rehabilitation was agreed on because the patient refused complex implant therapy. During the orthodontic closure of the spaces between the incisors, 21 was extracted, the root cut, the crown pulpal space filled and the tooth opportunely trimmed and used as a replacement. At the time of extraction, for aesthetic purposes, a connective-tissue graft was carried out in the same site. The subsequent prosthetic treatment finally consisted of insertion of a Maryland bridge (Figure 13.25).

Case 3

This 23-year-old woman presented with agenesis of the left lateral upper incisor. A shift of the midline to the left was evident when she smiled. A decision was made to create symmetry in the upper arch by distal displacement on the right side with creation of space for the insertion of an implant in the place of the missing incisor. At the end of the orthodontic phase, the space was maintained with a temporary tooth supported by a palatal orthodontic appliance inserted in the vertical lingual slots welded onto the molar

bands. This type of retainer has several advantages: the temporary tooth presses the gingiva slightly, thereby giving natural aesthetics; it cannot be removed by the patient; it can be removed at the time of implant surgery, giving the periodontist maximum space in the operating field and finally it can be reinserted at the end of surgery.

In order to obtain the best aesthetics in the anterior segment, the ridge defect, slightly visible as a darker concavity, was filled at the time of implant-reopening surgery following a roll-flap procedure (Abrams 1971, 1980). Once healing was achieved, a gold–porcelain crown was fitted on the abutment (Figure 13.26).

Case 4

This 44-year-old woman with chronic periodontitis and severe loss of bone support and gingival recession underwent periodontal rehabilitation prior to orthodontic and prosthetic treatment. All the necessary endodontic treatments were also performed. Given the patient's excellent compliance and good plaque control, orthodontic treatment was then carried out to align the teeth in their correct positions and to recreate functional guidance. At the end of the orthodontic treatment, prior to prosthetic rehabilitation, gingival aesthetics were improved in the area of 11 where

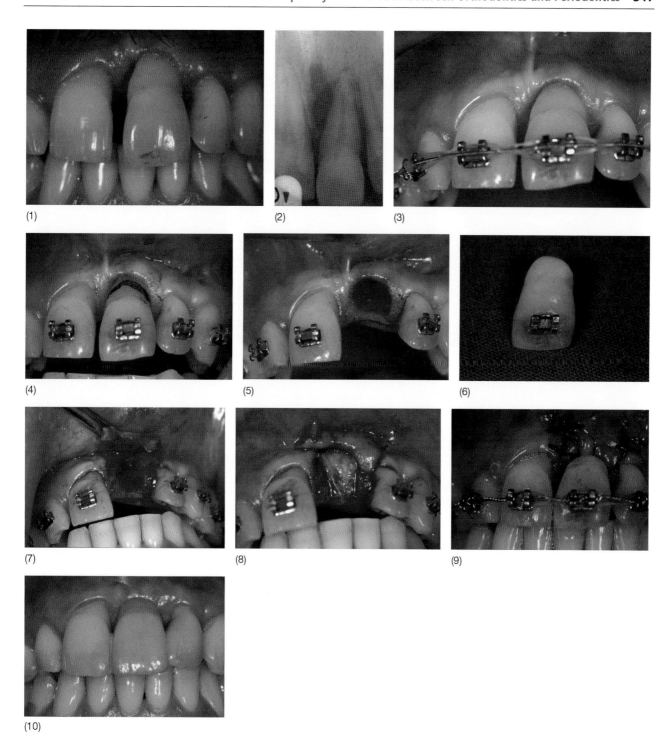

Fig. 13.25 (1) and (2) The left upper central incisor had been subject to several instances of trauma and could not be saved. Financial constraints did not allow for an implant. (3) Prior to proceeding with the extraction, the anterior diastema was partially closed. (4)–(6) The level of the gingival margin of the contralateral tooth was reproduced on the tooth to be extracted. Following extraction, the tooth was appropriately trimmed, reinserted and used as a provisional pontic while the space closure was completed. (7)–(9) A connective-tissue graft was performed at the extraction site to fill the extraction space and was kept under pressure during final space closure. As planned, the natural tooth was used as a temporary pontic. (10) The prosthetic rehabilitation with a Maryland bridge. (Courtesy of Dr G Anderlini.)

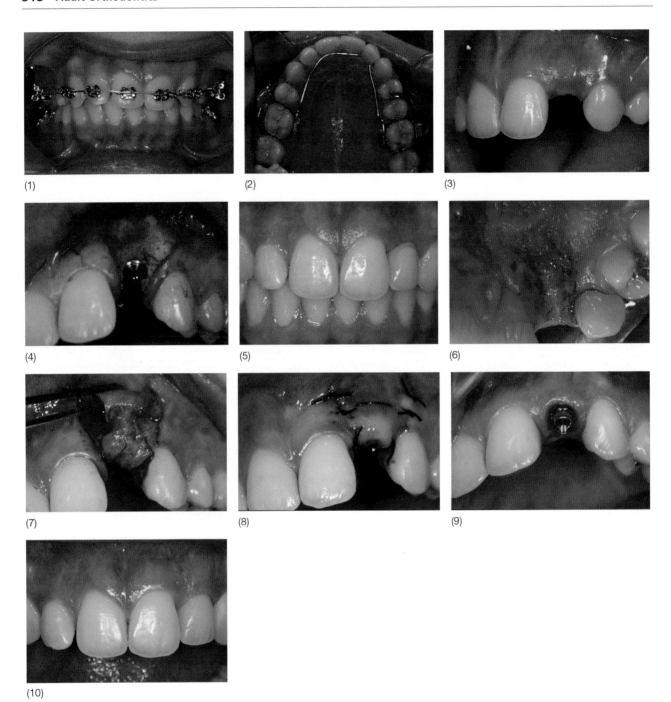

(1) (2) (3)

(4) (5) (6)

(7) (8) (9)

(10)

Fig. 13.26 (1) Patient with agenesis of 22. The goal of the orthodontic treatment was to centre the upper midline with reopening of the space for 22 implant substitution. (2) At the end of the orthodontic treatment, a temporary resin crown was supported by a provisional orthodontic appliance inserted in vertical lingual slots welded on molar bands. (3) The site ready for implant surgery. (4) The implant with cover screw. A ridge Class I defect is evident (Seibert 1983). (5) The presence of a dark concavity due to tissue thinness is evident at the implant site. (6)–(8) To improve aesthetics and function in this area, a roll-flap procedure was performed (Abrams 1980). In this procedure, the epithelium at the palatal level is removed, a pedicle connective-tissue flap is raised and two release incisions are made from the palate to and beyond the mucogingival line in the vestibular site. The palatal connective-tissue flap is folded and sutured under the vestibular epithelial connective-tissue flap. (9) Abutment has been inserted. (10) The dental–gingival complex is now harmonious, resulting in renewal of the correct convexity of the supporting tissues. The gold–ceramic crown has aesthetically integrated with the natural teeth.

the blackish colour of the root of the devitalised tooth showed through the thin gingiva. A combined flap was performed to increase the thickness of the gingiva (Milano 1998) (Figure 13.27).

Conclusion

Interdisciplinary collaboration should be considered an indispensable approach to achieving the best aesthetic and therapeutic results as well as full patient satisfaction. Several surgical and orthodontic techniques exist that can be combined according to the different requests of each clinical case. The diagnostic basis for periodontics has been discussed and various surgical techniques have been demonstrated in this chapter. Presently, the bilaminar techniques offer the greatest possibilities for success, also from a strictly cosmetic and aesthetic perspective. The diagnosis remains fundamental in relation to how timing and the relative procedural sequences will be assessed. Patient compliance remains fundamental to achieve therapeutic success and for long-term maintenance of the obtained results. It can only be reiterated that for long-term maintenance, supportive therapy is of primary importance.

Acknowledgements

The authors would like to thank Heather Dawe for her help in English translation.

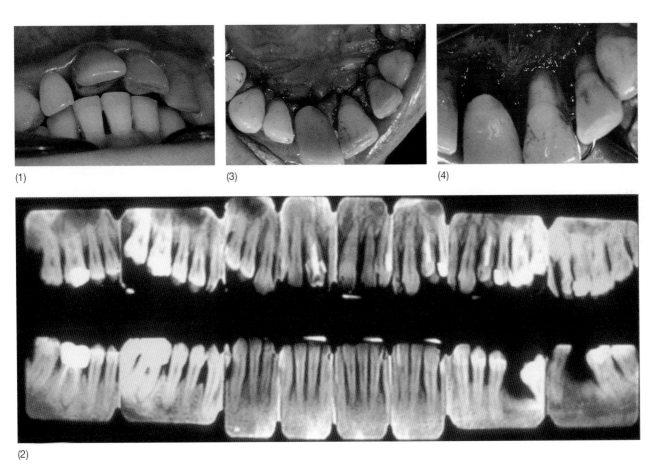

(1) (3) (4)

(2)

Fig. 13.27 (1) The patient had a Class II division 1 malocclusion with visible labial displacement of 21 resulting in unfavourable smile aesthetics. Chronic periodontitis is present with pockets > 5 mm and gingival recession. (2) Full X-ray status demonstrating severe marginal bone loss. (3)–(6) After patient motivation, scaling and root planing, surgical periodontal therapy was performed in all sextants. Some phases of surgery in the anterior zone are shown here. In order to limit post-surgical aesthetic damage, papillary preservation technique was performed (Takei et al. 1985; Kenney et al. 1989). The upper labial frenum was removed. (7) Once healing was stabilised and achieved, orthodontic treatment was performed (courtesy of Professor B Melsen). At completion, an excellent degree of correction was obtained. (8)–(12) A combined flap (Milano 1998) was performed to correct the aesthetic problem of gingival translucency of 11. In fact, the dark colour of the endodontically treated root reflected through the thin gingival tissue. (13) The result obtained at the end of surgery can be judged satisfactory because the thickened gingiva is no longer translucent. (14) The patient's smile before periodontal and orthodontic therapy. (15) The patient's smile after periodontal and orthodontic therapy. (16) The post-treatment full-mouth periapical radiographs show the situation 13 years post treatment.

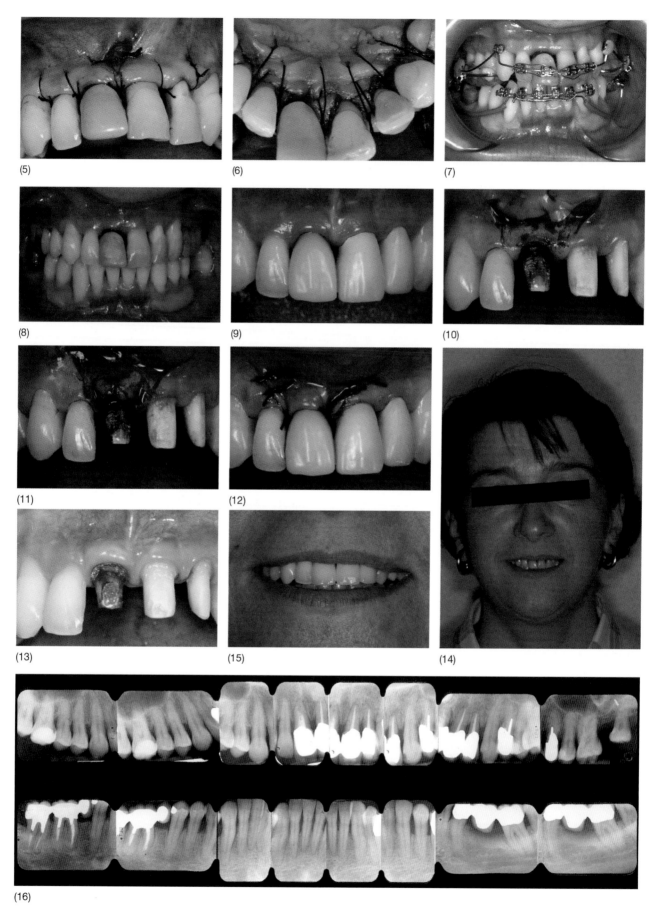

(5)

(6)

(7)

(8)

(9)

(10)

(11)

(12)

(13)

(15)

(14)

(16)

Fig. 13.27 (*Continued*)

References

Abrams L (1971) *Esthetics in Fixed Prosthesis*. Harrisburg: Dental Society.

Abrams L (1980) Augmentation of the deformed residual edentulous ridge for fixed prosthesis. *Compend Contin Educ Gen Dent* 1, 205–213.

Akesson L, Hakansson J and Rohlin M (1992) Comparison of panoramic and intraoral radiography and pocket probing for the measurement of the marginal bone level. *J Clin Periodontol* 19, 326–332.

Allen EP and Miller PD Jr (1989) Coronal positioning of existing gingiva: short term results in the treatment of shallow marginal tissue recession. *J Periodontol* 60, 316–319.

Anon (1992) *Glossary of Terms in Periodontology*. Chicago, IL: The American Academy of Periodontology.

Anon (1993) Periodontal screening and recording an early detection system. *J N J Dent Assoc* 64, 7–9, 11.

Anon (1996) Consensus report. Periodontal diseases: epidemiology and diagnosis. *Ann Periodontol* 1, 216–222.

Archer WH (1975) Oral and maxillofacial surgery. In *Oral and Maxillofacial Surgery*, 5th edn, pp. 338–342. Philadelphia: WB Saunders.

Armitage GC (1996) Periodontal diseases: diagnosis. *Ann Periodontol* 1, 37–215.

Artun J and Urbye KS (1988) The effect of orthodontic treatment on periodontal bone support in patients with advanced loss of marginal periodontium. *Am J Orthod Dentofacial Orthop* 93, 143–148.

Boyd RL (1978) Mucogingival considerations and their relationship to orthodontics. *J Periodontol* 49, 67–76.

Boyd RL and Baumrind S (1992) Periodontal considerations in the use of bonds or bands on molars in adolescents and adults. *Angle Orthod* 62, 117–126.

Bragger U, Lauchenauer D and Lang NP (1992) Surgical lengthening of the clinical crown. *J Clin Periodontol* 19, 58–63.

Cardaropoli D, Re S, Corrente G and Abundo R (2004) Reconstruction of the maxillary midline papilla following a combined orthodontic- periodontic treatment in adult periodontal patients. *J Clin Periodontol* 31, 79–84.

Carvalho JC, Pustiglioni FE and Kon S (1982) Combination of a connective tissue pedicle flap with a free gingival graft to cover localized gingival recession. *Int J Periodontics Restorative Dent* 2(4), 26–33.

Caton J, Greenstein G and Polson AM (1981) Depth of periodontal probe penetration related to clinical and histologic signs of gingival inflammation. *J Periodontol* 52, 626–629.

Caton JG, DeFuria EL, Polson AM and Nyman S (1987) Periodontal regeneration via selective cell repopulation. *J Periodontol* 58, 546–552.

Chiche G, Kokich VG and Caudill R (1994) Diagnosis and treatment planning of esthetic problems. In Pinault A and Chiche G (eds) *Esthetics in Fixed Prosthodontics*, pp. 33–52. Quintessence.

Clauser C, Nieri M, Franceschi D, Pagliaro U and Pini-Prato G (2003) Evidence-based mucogingival therapy. Part 2: ordinary and individual patient data meta-analyses of surgical treatment of recession using complete root coverage as the outcome variable. *J Periodontol* 74, 741–756.

Corrente G, Abundo R, Re S, Cardaropoli D and Cardaropoli G (2003) Orthodontic movement into infrabony defects in patients with advanced periodontal disease: a clinical and radiological study. *Journal of Periodontology* 74, 1104–1109.

Cortellini P, Gagliardi G, Merli M and Tonetti M (1999) *Progetto Diagnosi Parodontale della Società Italiana di Parodontolgia*. Florence, Italy.

Cortellini P and Tonetti MS (2005) Clinical performance of a regenerative strategy for intrabony defects: scientific evidence and clinical experience. *J Periodontol* 76, 341–350.

Coslet JG, Vanarsdall R and Weisgold A (1977) Diagnosis and classification of delayed passive eruption of the dentogingival junction in the adult. *Alpha Omegan* 70, 24–28.

De Sanctis M and Zucchelli GM (eds) (1997) *Atlante di chirurgia estetica mucogengivale*. Bologna, Italy: Edizoni Martina.

Diamanti-Kipioti A, Gusberti FA and Lang NP (1987) Clinical and micro-biological effects of fixed orthodontic appliances. *J Clin Periodontol* 14, 326–333.

Diedrich PR (1996) Guided tissue regeneration associated with orthodontic therapy. *Semin Orthod* 2, 39–45.

Edwards JG (1970) A surgical procedure to eliminate rotational relapse. *Am J Orthod* 57, 35–46.

Edwards JG (1977) The diastema, the frenum, the frenectomy: a clinical study. *Am J Orthod* 71, 489–508.

Edwards JG (1993) Soft-tissue surgery to alleviate orthodontic relapse. *Dent Clin North Am* 37, 205–225.

Ericsson I, Thilander B and Lindhe J (1978) Periodontal conditions after orthodontic tooth movements in the dog. *Angle Orthod* 48, 210–218.

Ericsson I, Thilander B, Lindhe J and Okamoto H (1977) The effect of orthodontic tilting movements on the periodontal tissues of infected and non-infected dentitions in dogs. *J Clin Periodontol* 4, 278–293.

Esposito M, Coulthard P and Worthington HV (2003) Enamel matrix derivative (Emdogain) for periodontal tissue regeneration in intrabony defects. *Cochrane Database Syst Rev* 2, CD003875.

Ezzo PJ and Cutler CW (2003) Microorganisms as risk indicators for periodontal disease. *Periodontol 2000* 32, 24–35.

Friedman N (1962) Mucogingival surgery. The apically repositioned flap. *J Periodontol* 33, 328–340.

Goldman HM (1951) Gingivectomy. *Oral Surg Oral Med Oral Pathol* 4, 1136–1157.

Gottlow J, Nyman S, Karring T and Lindhe J (1984) New attachment formation as the result of controlled tissue regeneration. *J Clin Periodontol* 11, 494–503.

Grupe HE and Warren RF (1956) Repair of gingival defects by a sliding flap operation. *J Periodontol* 27, 92–95.

Haffajee AD, Socransky SS and Gunsolley JC (2003) Systemic anti-infective periodontal therapy. A systematic review. *Ann Periodontol* 8, 115–181.

Hallmon WW and Rees TD (2003) Local anti-infective therapy: mechanical and physical approaches. A systematic review. *Ann Periodontol* 8, 99–114.

Hammerle CH, Ingold HP and Lang NP (1990) Evaluation of clinical and radiographic scoring methods before and after initial periodontal therapy. *J Clin Periodontol* 17, 255–263.

Hanes PJ and Purvis JP (2003) Local anti-infective therapy: pharmacological agents. A systematic review. *Ann Periodontol* 8, 79–98.

Heanue M, Deacon SA, Dery C, Robinson PG, Walmsley AD, Worthington HV and Shaw WC (2003) Manual versus powered toothbrushing for oral health. *Cochrane Library* 1st edn, 002281.

Heitz-Mayfield LJ, Trombelli L, Heitz F, Needleman I and Moles D (2002) A systematic review of the effect of surgical debridement vs non-surgical debridement for the treatment of chronic periodontitis. *J Clin Periodontol* 29(Suppl 3), 92–102.

Herrera D, Sanz M, Jepsen S, Needleman I and Roldan S (2002) A systematic review on the effect of systemic antimicrobials as an adjunct to scaling and root planing in periodontitis patients. *J Clin Periodontol* 29(Suppl 3), 136–159.

Huser MC, Baehni PC and Lang R (1990) Effects of orthodontic bands on microbiologic and clinical parameters. *Am J Orthod Dentofacial Orthop* 97, 213–218.

Karring T, Nyman S, Gottlow J and Laurell L (1993) Development of the biological concept of guided tissue regeneration – animal and human studies. *Periodontol 2000* 1, 26–35.

Karring T, Nyman S and Lindhe J (1980) Healing following implantation of periodontitis affected roots into bone tissue. *J Clin Periodontol* 7, 96–105.

Kenney EB, Carranza FA, Takei HH, Lekovic V, Han TJ and Elbaz JJ (1989) Porous hydroxylapatite. *J Calif Dent Assoc* 17(1), 53–58.

Kinane DF (1999) Periodontitis modified by systemic factors. *Ann Periodontol* 4, 54–64.

Kohavi D, Becker A and Zilberman Y (1984) Surgical exposure, orthodontic movement, and final tooth position as factors in periodontal breakdown of treated palatally impacted canines. *Am J Orthod* 85, 72–77.

Kokich VG (1996) Esthetics: the orthodontic-periodontic restorative connection. *Semin Orthod* 2, 21–30.

Kokich VG and Mathews DP (1993) Surgical and orthodontic management of impacted teeth. *Dent Clin North Am* 37, 181–204.

Kokich VG, Nappen DL and Shapiro PA (1984) Gingival contour and clinical crown length: their effect on the esthetic appearance of maxillary anterior teeth. *Am J Orthod* 86, 89–94.

Kozlovsky A, Tal H and Lieberman M (1988) Forced eruption combined with gingival fiberotomy. A technique for clinical crown lengthening. *J Clin Periodontol* 15, 534–538.

Langer B and Langer L (1985) Subepithelial connective tissue graft technique for root coverage. *J Periodontol* 56, 715–720.

Levin MP and D'Amico RA (1974) Flap design in exposing unerupted teeth. *Am J Orthod* 65, 419–422.

Lindhe J, Karring T and Lang NP (1997) *Clinical Periodontology and Implant Dentistry*. Copenhagen: Munksgaard.

Löe H, Anerud A and Boysen H (1992a) The natural history of periodontal disease in man: prevalence, severity, and extent of gingival recession. *J Periodontol* 63, 489–495.

Löe H, Anerud A and Boysen H (1992b) The natural history of periodontal disease in man: prevalence, severity, and extent of gingival recession. *J Periodontol* 63, 489–495.

Mathews DP and Kokich VG (1997) Managing treatment for the orthodontic patient with periodontal problems. *Semin Orthod* 3, 21–38.

Maynard JG Jr and Ochsenbein C (1975) Mucogingival problems, prevalence and therapy in children. *J Periodontol* 46, 543–552.

McGuire MK and Nunn ME (1999) Prognosis versus actual outcome. IV. The effectiveness of clinical parameters and IL-1 genotype in accurately predicting prognoses and tooth survival. *J Periodontol* 70, 49–56.

Meisel P, Siegemund A, Dombrowa S, Sawaf H, Fanghaenel J and Kocher T (2002) Smoking and polymorphisms of the interleukin-1 gene cluster (IL-1alpha, IL-1beta, and IL-1RN) in patients with periodontal disease. *J Periodontol* 73, 27–32.

Melsen B, Agerbaek N, Eriksen J and Terp S (1988) New attachment through periodontal treatment and orthodontic intrusion. *Am J Orthod Dentofacial Orthop* 94, 104–116.

Melsen B, Agerbaek N and Markenstam G (1989) Intrusion of incisors in adult patients with marginal bone loss. *Am J Orthod Dentofacial Orthop* 96, 232–241.

Melsen B and Kragskov J (1992) Tissue reaction to intrusion of periodontally involved teeth. In Davidovitch Z (ed.) *Biomechanical Mechanism of Tooth Movement and Craniofacial Adaption*, pp. 423–430. Columbus: Ohio State University, College of Dentistry.

Melsen B and Milano F (1993a) Lavoro déquipe: perchè? Il futuro dell'odontoiatria. *Dental Cadmos* 7, 64–69.

Melsen B and Milano F (1993b) Lavoro d'equipe: quale aiuto reciproco? Il futuro dell'odontoiatria. *Dental Cadmos* 8, 104–108.

Milano F (1998) A combined flap for root coverage. *Int J Periodontics Restorative Dent* 18, 544–551.

Miller PD Jr (1985) A classification of marginal tissue recession. *Int J Periodontics Restorative Dent* 5, 8–13.

Murphy KG and Gunsolley JC (2003) Guided tissue regeneration for the treatment of periodontal intrabony and furcation defects. A systematic review. *Ann Periodontol* 8, 266–302.

Needleman I, Tucker R, Giedrys-Leeper E and Worthington H (2005) Guided tissue regeneration for periodontal intrabony defects – a Cochrane Systematic Review. *Periodontol 2000* 37, 106–123.

Nelson SW (1987) The subpedicle connective tissue graft. A bilaminar reconstructive procedure for the coverage of denuded root surfaces. *J Periodontol* 58(2), 95–102.

Nordland WP and Tarnow DP (1998) A classification system for loss of papillary height. *J Periodontol* 69, 1124–1126.

Nunn ME (2003) Understanding the etiology of periodontitis: an overview of periodontal risk factors. *Periodontol 2000* 32, 11–23.

Nyman S, Gottlow J, Karring T and Lindhe J (1982) The regenerative potential of the periodontal ligament. An experimental study in the monkey. *J Clin Periodontol* 9, 257–265.

Offenbacher S (1996) Periodontal diseases: pathogenesis. *Ann Periodontol* 1, 821–878.

Pagliaro U, Nieri M, Franceschi D, Clauser C and Pini-Prato G (2003) Evidence-based mucogingival therapy. Part 1: a critical review of the literature on root coverage procedures. *J Periodontol* 74, 709–740.

Polson AM, Caton JG, Yeaple RN and Zander HA (1980) Histological determination of probe tip penetration into gingival sulcus of humans using an electronic pressure-sensitive probe. *J Clin Periodontol* 7, 479–488.

Pontoriero R, Celenza F Jr, Ricci G and Carnevale G (1987) Rapid extrusion with fiber resection: a combined orthodontic-periodontic treatment modality. *Int J Periodontics Restorative Dent* 7, 30–43.

Prato GP, Clauser C and Cortellini P (1995) Periodontal plastic and mucogingival surgery. *Periodontol 2000* 9, 90–105.

Prato GP, Clauser C, Tonetti MS and Cortellini P (1996) Guided tissue regeneration in gingival recessions. *Periodontol 2000* 11, 49–57.

Proffit WR and Fields HW (1993) *Contemporary Orthodontics*. St. Louis, MO: Mosby.

Raetzke PB (1985) Covering localized areas of root exposure employing the 'envelope' technique. *J Periodontol* 56, 397–402.

Ramfjord SP and Nissle RR (1974) The modified widman flap. *J Periodontol* 45, 601–607.

Reitan K (1969) Principles of retention and avoidance of posttreatment relapse. *Am J Orthod* 55, 776–790.

Roccuzzo M, Bunino M, Needleman I and Sanz M (2002) Periodontal plastic surgery for treatment of localized gingival recessions: a systematic review. *J Clin Periodontol* 29(Suppl 3), 178–194.

Seibert JS (1983) Reconstruction of deformed, partially edentulous ridges, using full thickness onlay grafts. Part II. Prosthetic/periodontal inter-relationships. *Compend Contin Educ Dent* 4(6), 549–562.

Sekino S, Ramberg P, Uzel NG, Socransky S and Lindhe J (2003) Effect of various chlorhexidine regimens on salivary bacteria and de novo plaque formation. *J Clin Periodontol* 30, 919–925.

Shiloah J and Kopczyk RA (1978) Mucogingival considerations in surgical exposure of maxillary impacted canines: report of case. *ASDC J Dent Child* 45, 79–81.

Sicilia A, Arregui I, Gallego M, Cabezas B and Cuesta S (2002) A systematic review of powered vs manual toothbrushes in periodontal cause-related therapy. *J Clin Periodontol* 29(Suppl 3), 39–54.

Sild E, Bernardi F, Caldari R, Carnevale G and Milano F (1987a) An assessment of pocket depth in vitro with a computerized periodontal probe. *Int J Periodontics Restorative Dent* 7, 44–55.

Sild E, Bernardi F, Carnevale G and Milano F (1987b) Computerized periodontal probe with adjustable pressure. *Int J Periodontics Restorative Dent* 7, 53–62.

Steiner GG, Pearson JK and Ainamo J (1981) Changes of the marginal periodontium as a result of labial tooth movement in monkeys. *J Periodontol* 52, 314–320.

Sullivan HC and Atkins JH (1968) Free autogenous gingival grafts. 3. Utilization of grafts in the treatment of gingival recession. *Periodontics* 6, 152–160.

Takei HH, Han TJ, Carranza FA, Kenney EB and Lekovic V (1985) Flap technique for periodontal bone implants. Papilla preservation technique. *J Periodontol* 56(4), 204–210.

Tarnow DP, Magner AW and Fletcher P (1992) The effect of the distance from the contact point to the crest of bone on the presence or absence of the interproximal dental papilla. *J Periodontol* 63, 995–996.

Taylor GW (2001) Bidirectional interrelationships between diabetes and periodontal diseases: an epidemiologic perspective. *Ann Periodontol* 6, 99–112.

Thilander H, Thilander B and Persson G (1973) Treatment of impacted teeth by surgical exposure. A survey study. *Sven Tandlak Tidskr* 66, 519–525.

Tinti C, Vincenzi G, Cortellini P, Pini PG and Clauser C (1992) Guided tissue regeneration in the treatment of human facial recession. A 12-case report. *J Periodontol* 63, 554–560.

Tonetti MS (1998) Cigarette smoking and periodontal diseases: etiology and management of disease. *Ann Periodontol* 3, 88–101.

Tonetti MS, Cortellini P, Lang NP, Suvan JE, Adriaens P, Dubravec D, Fonzar A, Fourmousis I, Rasperini G, Rossi R, Silvestri M, Topoll H, Wallkamm B and Zybutz M (2004) Clinical outcomes following treatment of human intrabony defects with GTR/bone replacement material or access flap alone. A multicenter randomized controlled clinical trial. *J Clin Periodontol* 31, 770–776.

Turkkahraman H, Sayin MO, Bozkurt FY, Yetkin Z, Kaya S and Onal S (2005) Archwire ligation techniques, microbial colonization, and periodontal status in orthodontically treated patients. *Angle Orthod* 75, 231–236.

Vanarsdall RL and Corn H (1977) Soft-tissue management of labially positioned unerupted teeth. *Am J Orthod* 72, 53–64.

Wennstrom JL (1994) *Muco-Gingival Surgery from Proceedings of the 1st European Workshop on Periodontology*. Quintessence.

Wennstrom JL, Lindhe J, Sinclair F and Thilander B (1987) Some periodontal tissue reactions to orthodontic tooth movement in monkeys. *J Clin Periodontol* 14, 121–129.

Wilson TG Jr (1996a) Supportive periodontal treatment introduction – definition, extent of need, therapeutic objectives, frequency and efficacy. *Periodontol 2000* 12, 11–15.

Wilson TG Jr (1996b) Compliance and its role in periodontal therapy. *Periodontol 2000* 12, 16–23.

Wisth PJ, Norderval K and Booe OE (1976) Comparison of two surgical methods in combined surgical-orthodontic correction of impacted maxillary canines. *Acta Odontol Scand* 34, 53–57.

Zachrisson BU (1997) Orthodontics and periodontics. In Lindhe J, Karring T and Lang NP (eds) *Clinical Periodontology and Implant Dentistry*, 4th edn. Oxford: Blackwell Munksgaard.

Zambon JJ (1996) Periodontal diseases: microbial factors. *Ann Periodontol* 1, 879–925.

14

Prosthetically Guided Orthodontic Strategies

Arturo Imbelloni, Cesare Luzi

Introduction

The objectives of orthodontic therapy are to establish a good occlusion, enhance the health of the periodontium and improve dental and facial aesthetics. In the latest years, the interrelationships between orthodontics, periodontics and prosthodontics to achieve a good biologic, functional and aesthetic result have become more and more important, leading to interdisciplinary treatment planning and therapies.

In the last decades, orthodontists have experienced a significant increase in the number of adult patients in their practices, either referred by the general practitioners or self-referred seeking orthodontic treatment. Adults have many different problems compared to growing patients, and especially the presence of two signs that become more frequent with ageing, tooth wear and periodontal problems. These characteristics make therapy more challenging. At the same time, our image of the value of teeth in current society also has changed. Even though chewing is still important for the public, nowadays the focus has greatly shifted towards aesthetics.

In this view, the dentists' primary objective is still the health of the patients and their teeth, but this trend towards a heightened awareness of appearance has challenged dentistry to look at dental aesthetics in a more organised and systematic manner. Moreover, some dentitions simply cannot be restored to an improved aesthetic appearance without the assistance of several different dental disciplines, and for this reason, today, every dental practitioner must have a thorough understanding of the roles of these various disciplines in achieving the best possible results when dealing the adult patient with high aesthetic demands. In order to satisfy the people's desire to look better, the joint effort of the formerly independent disciplines of orthodontics, periodontics and restorative dentistry may allow to meet this request, with the most conservative and biologically sound treatment plan.

The interdisciplinary team approach accounts for integrated therapeutic tools which improve the final outcome, provided that the diagnosis was correct and the sequence and the execution were proper.

Orthodontics has become fundamental in some cases in which a pure prosthetic therapy cannot offer a conclusive or ideal solution. Orthodontic techniques have thereby developed according to the new needs of treatment with the increasing age of patients, thus contributing to the birth of a

Adult Orthodontics, Second Edition. Edited by Birte Melsen and Cesare Luzi.
© 2022 John Wiley & Sons Ltd. Published 2022 by John Wiley & Sons Ltd.
Companion Website: http://www.wiley.com/go/melsen-adult-orthodontics

new interdisciplinary approach. The objective of the pre-prosthetic orthodontic treatment is to change the position of teeth in such a way that a prosthodontic treatment is made possible, simplified and performed with an improved outcome and minimally invasive procedures.

The purpose of this chapter of the book is to provide the reader with a systematic method of evaluating and treating patients who may benefit from an interdisciplinary orthodontic and restorative therapy.

Interdisciplinary treatment planning: orthodontics in periodontal prosthesis

In a 25-year retrospective, Amsterdam defined periodontal prosthesis as 'Those surgical and restorative endeavors that are absolutely essential in the treatment of advanced periodontal disease. Whereas this is specifically referred to the treatment of the dentition mutilated by the ravages of periodontal disease, in general, its basic concepts, principles, and techniques may be effectively employed in the restoration of any tooth or teeth in the natural dentition' (Amsterdam 1974).

Forty-seven years after the publication of that monograph, its basic principles associated with interdisciplinary therapy are still valid. Periodontal prosthesis is a clinically tested interdisciplinary perspective that offers a timeless blueprint to sequencing treatment planning and therapy. Innovative techniques and new products, coupled with well-established principles, facilitate site development for any restoration, ranging from the single crown to pontics or implant-supported restorations (Salama et al. 1998).

Blueprint to sequencing treatment planning: 'The execution of any well-organized and conceived treatment plan must occur in a preferred, orderly sequence to restore proper form and function to the system. The sequence in all cases should include the elimination or control of all inflammation, caries, periodontal and occlusal pathology and then the elimination of the deformities contributing to or created by the disease process' (Amsterdam 1974).

Lessons from periodontal prosthesis:

1. A comprehensive interdisciplinary perspective is necessary for both diagnosis and treatment planning.
2. Through a systematic and sequential stage of site development, it is possible to create the foundation for long-term predictable periodontal, occlusal, restorative and aesthetic success.
3. Test, re-evaluate and alter case-design decisions in the provisional restoration as predicated upon the patient's aesthetic needs, the occlusal aspect and the presence of inflammation prior to entering the final restorative and subsequent maintenance phases (Salama et al. 1998).

Orthodontic therapy plays a primary role in periodontal prosthesis interdisciplinary perspective, since it allows to correct anomalies and to enhance the final outcome; the periodontal prosthesis protocol includes an orthodontic phase that may be effectively employed not only in the treatment of advanced periodontal disease, but also in the restoration of any tooth or teeth in the natural dentition.

Predictable aesthetic outcomes resulting from interdisciplinary treatment approaches have traditionally represented elusive goals. This may be partially due to the level of complexity that is associated with these clinical scenarios (Lee and Jun 2002). In addition, it may be a result of the inadequate interaction between the specialists involved (Roblee 1994).

The recruitment of specialists per se does not have an additive effect on the desired aesthetic outcome. The preservation of aesthetics through multidisciplinary therapy requires the development of the clinical team into a cohesive therapeutic network supported by the establishment of a clinically relevant aesthetic template (Lee and Jun 2002).

Before starting the treatment of a new patient, the first steps are carried out to establish the treatment objectives. In growing patients with non-restored complete dentitions, orthodontic treatment objectives tend to be idealistic. Most orthodontists are trapped into applying these same idealistic treatment objectives to adult patients with missing teeth, abraded teeth, old restorations or other restorative and periodontal complications. This approach may not be appropriate for the ortho–perio–restorative patient. For these patients, it is important to establish realistic, not idealistic, treatment objectives. Realistic treatment objectives generally should be economically, occlusally, periodontally and restoratively realistic (Kokich and Spear 1997).

For instance, in case of a patient with a stable non-ideal occlusal scheme, no symptoms, good function and need of a combined orthodontic-prosthodontic treatment to correct a deep overbite, the orthodontist may leave the posterior occlusion unaltered while correcting the position only in the anterior section. In adults, the dental history and the restorative requirements play an important role in determining the final occlusion.

Some patients might need adjunctive periodontal therapy and/or orthognathic surgery beyond the orthodontic–prosthodontic combined approach; this increasing number of specialists involved augmenting the complexity of the treatment, thereby requiring their interaction along the treatment path. Consequently, the team has to design the specific treatment plan and the corresponding treatment sequence. The latter will be recorded by one of the clinicians (Kokich and Spear 1997).

A copy of the treatment sequence should be given to the each of the participating dentists and to the patient. Then, at any time during treatment, any of team members can review the sequence, determine his/her point of interaction and feel secure that the plan is proceeding properly. In addition, the patient is aware of the pathway towards completing treatment. The importance of this step in interdisciplinary treatment cannot be overemphasised (Kokich and Kokich 2005).

When a combined orthodontic–prosthodontic therapy is required, even for expert clinicians it may be difficult to visualise at baseline the final result. An excellent tool that helps to establish the final occlusal and restorative result in complex cases is a diagnostic wax setup; the modified casts can be further adjusted to foresee the ultimate plan by waxing up the teeth to be restored. Nowadays, an alternative to this procedure is the digital orthodontic setup; although digital tools have demonstrated to be effective and accurate (Barreto et al. 2016), and therefore a viable alternative to manual setups, the possibility of realistically 'touching and viewing three-dimensionally' the final outcome by means of a manual setup makes this solution still preferred by many clinicians and patients.

The utilisation of techniques that allow the intraoral testing of the restorative proposal constitutes the most valuable resource to clinically validate the aesthetic blueprint; several options can be used for this purpose: direct trial composite restorations, composite mock-ups, removable aesthetic templates or provisional restorations. Aesthetic treatment objectives can be clinically refined and accurately represented to the patient only by trial in an in vivo environment (Lee and Jun 2000). Surgical guides and therapeutic templates are also developed, providing a mechanism for the specialists to intraoperatively verify compliance with the initial project.

Prosthodontic indications for orthodontic therapy

A. Paralleling abutment teeth for a fixed bridge or partial denture.
B. Movements to prepare the edentulous space for proper implant or pontic size.
C. Extrusion for tooth preservation or site development.
D. Preventing pulpal involvement in tooth preparation.
E. Allowing for adequate thickness of restorative materials on teeth.
F. Re-establishing proper posterior occlusal plane.
G. Re-establishing proper anterior guidance.
H. Enhancing the aesthetic result.

Our classification of the prosthodontic indications for orthodontic therapy is a modification of Marks' classification (Marks 1980).

Pre-prosthodontic orthodontics

In recent years, a new trend has emerged that will not likely be reversed: the movement towards a more conservative approach to dental therapy; this trend is here to stay, as the patient, when given a choice, will always seek out more conservative alternatives. In the world of medicine, there are numerous examples of this steady migration towards less invasive procedures; dentistry is undoubtedly following the same path (Dennis 2010).

Minimally invasive dentistry is the application of 'a systematic respect for the original tissue'. This implies that the dental profession recognises that an artefact is of less biological value than the original healthy tissue (Ericson 2004).

The best way to improve the longevity of any restorative procedure is to delay treatment as long as possible, provided the delay is not negatively influencing the outcome or health of the patient.

This trend towards a more conservative approach has become reliable thanks to the development of two major breakthroughs in the dental field: adhesion and osseointegration. In the treatment of adult patients, these techniques move the restorative treatment to higher standards, especially when applied in conjunction with the 'orthodontic-improved' approach, which brings to a harmonious distribution of the edentulous spaces.

In the non-restored growing patient, orthodontic positioning of teeth follows idealistic criteria. However, in the orthodontic–restorative patient, it may not be prudent to position teeth ideally. If restorations are planned for the patient, it may be advantageous to position teeth to facilitate this restorative treatment. Specific restorations require different types of tooth positioning (Kokich and Kokich 2005).

Although orthodontic therapy is primarily utilised to improve tooth position and interarch relationships, its effects on osseous architecture and soft tissue remodelling may be advantageously applied in the treatment of periodontally compromised dentitions.

Furthermore, orthodontically induced bone remodelling may also be utilised for the development of future implant sites (Salama and Salama 1993).

Tarnow et al. studied the vertical relationship between the proximal contact and the underlying osseous crest. The presence or absence of the interproximal papilla was determined visually prior to probing. If there was no space visible apical to the contact point, the papilla was deemed present. They showed that papillae were present 100% of the time whenever the distance between the proximal contact and the osseous crest was up to 5 mm, while the greater was that distance, the lower was the chance for a complete filling of the space (Tarnow et al. 1992). The only successful way to predictably regenerate, up to a certain extent, gingival papillae is by closing the diastema by orthodontic or restorative therapy, in order to create the missing contact point; there are no surgical approaches able to achieve the same goal.

In the following pages, the prosthetic indications to orthodontic treatment will be described through a series of clinical cases.

Paralleling abutment teeth for a fixed bridge or partial denture

Several conditions cause misalignment of teeth in adults; besides untreated malocclusions, a major reason is tooth extraction due to caries or periodontal disease.

In case of advanced periodontitis, patients often present compromised periodontal attachment and missing one or more posterior teeth (the most frequently extracted are first molars), which cause a shift of the occlusal function towards the anterior sextant with consequent secondary occlusal trauma. Anterior teeth cannot stand this functional increase in presence of a compromised periodontal support, while the spaces corresponding to the extraction sites cause the posterior teeth to drift; the result is the so-called 'posterior bite collapse', represented by flaring and overeruption of anterior teeth, alteration of the posterior plane of occlusion with inclination of tooth axis and overeruption of posterior teeth towards the opposing edentulous areas. Furthermore, this results in the creation of uneven marginal ridge relations and adjacent cementoenamel junction levels, and concomitant unlevelled bony crests.

These events create an environment where the self-protective capacity of the teeth is compromised, resulting in the development of angular bony crests, frequently a precursor to infrabony pocket formation and posterior interproximal caries.

The treatment of these patients is most challenging and can benefit from the work of an interdisciplinary team. The sequence of treatment will be the following:

1. Initial periodontal therapy (causal therapy).
2. Re-evaluation.
3. Periodontal surgery (when indicated).
4. Orthodontic treatment.
5. Temporisation.
6. Prosthetic treatment.

This order can be slightly changed depending on the individual situation; in the represented patient for instance (Figures 14.1–14.5), following periodontal surgery (Figure 14.6) and the subsequent healing, a first set of temporaries was initially delivered only on the lower

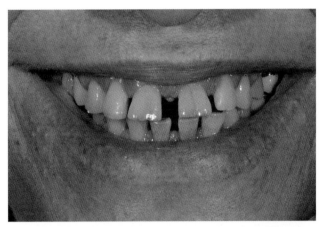
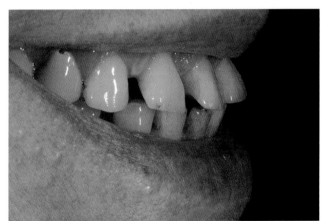
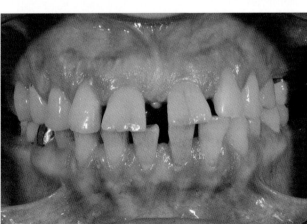
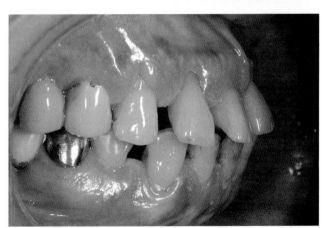
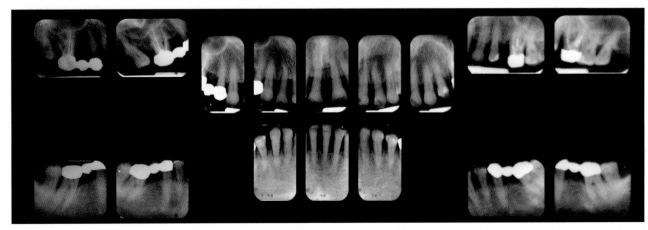

Figs. 14.1–14.5 A 60-year-old female patient presented anterior teeth flaring without posterior bite collapse; Full mouth series of periapical radiographs (FRX) showed advanced loss of bone support: the diagnosis was generalised chronic periodontitis with secondary trauma from occlusion.

posteriors: a Lucia Jig was inserted to move the mandible in centric relation (CR) (slightly posterior to the centric occlusion) and increase the vertical dimension of occlusion (VDO), thus gaining the necessary palatal space to retrude the upper anterior sextant (Figure 14.7).

Orthodontic treatment had a duration of 9 months and was performed with lingual appliances (Figures 14.8–14.10) and skeletal anchorage. Four miniscrews were inserted (two on the posterior palate and two on the mandibular posterior buccal interdental sites) and used as anchorage to retract the anterior segments and reduce the flaring. For the upper incisors, a stiff segment of rectangular 0.019 × 0.025-inch stainless-steel wire with bilateral power arms was used in order to reduce the tipping by generating a line of action of the orthodontic force closer to the CR of the group of teeth (Figures 14.11–14.13).

On completion of the orthodontic phase (Figure 14.14), a second set of temporaries was placed on the upper and lower arches to retain the final teeth position and to test the patient's function and aesthetics. The treatment plan was designed to splint all teeth because of a high chance of relapse due to the presence of secondary occlusal trauma. In this case, orthodontic therapy gives the further advantage of

avoiding root canal therapies and post and cores on anterior abutments (Figure 14.15) by correcting the axis of teeth; by retracting them, at tooth preparation stage, there was no invasion of the endodontic space, and proper function and aesthetics were established (Figures 14.16 and 14.17).

Movements to prepare the edentulous space for proper implant or pontic size

The objective of the pre-prosthetic orthodontic treatment is to change the position of teeth to enhance the results of prosthodontic treatment.

Adults may have edentulous spaces due to previous extractions, most of the time for caries or periodontitis; consequently, when patients do not start a dental therapy, misaligned teeth become a common feature. The space left after tooth removal tends to be occupied by proximal teeth which move towards the space, limiting a possible restorative solution over time, and teeth of the opposing arch which overerupt again reducing the vertical space available for restoration.

The possible treatment option is either to close the residual spaces or move teeth apart and align them to enhance prosthetic solutions.

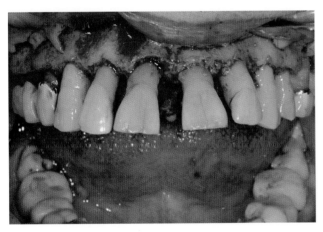

Fig. 14.6 Periodontal surgery was performed on all quadrants after full-mouth scaling and root planning. Here, full upper-arch pocket elimination and minor osseous resective surgery are shown (periodontist: Arturo Imbelloni).

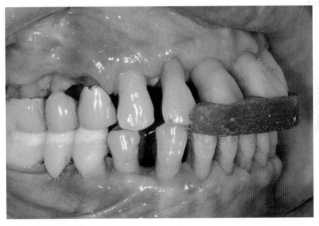

Fig. 14.7 A Lucia Jig was inserted to move the mandible in centric relation (CR) position at an increased vertical dimension of occlusion (VDO), thus gaining the palatal space to retrude the upper anterior sextant.

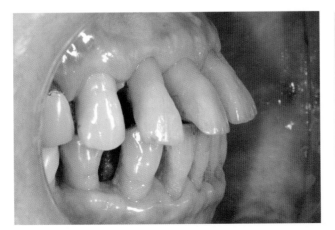

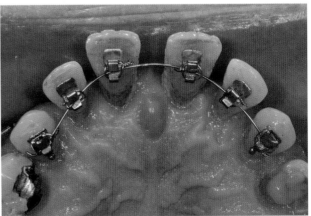

Figs. 14.8–14.14 The use of lingual brackets and skeletal anchorage. The upper and lower flared anterior teeth were retracted anchored to four miniscrews, two were inserted in the palate and two in the buccal aspect of the mandible. Diastemas were closed.

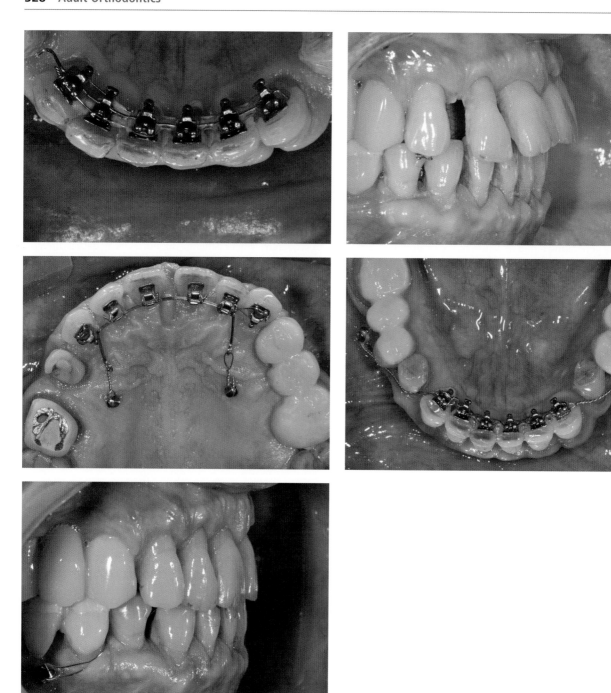

Figs. 14.8–14.14 (*Continued*)

In case of space opening, pre-prosthetic orthodontics is applied to create ideal space for a pontic of either a conventional bridge or a resin-bonded bridge, or for an implant-supported crown; the objective will be achieved by intrusion of the opposing tooth or teeth and/or uprighting of the teeth proximal to the edentulous area.

The therapeutic challenge is higher when creating the right space for an implant-supported restoration, since there is the need to obtain room not only at the crown level, as in case of a pontic, but also at the root level for the fixture, by making the adjacent roots parallel with a homogenous interradicular space. Thus, radiographs must be taken at the finishing phase;

in case the roots are too close together, an implant cannot be placed; hence, an orthodontic correction of the axis of the two teeth is a must when proceeding with implant surgery.

In case of a single implant, the distance between an implant and a tooth should not be less than 1.5 mm (Grunder et al. 2005), thus the required minimal mesiodistal space for a 4.0 mm implant is 7.0 mm. A strong correlation was found between bone loss at adjacent teeth and the horizontal distance fixture-tooth; with decreasing distance the bone loss increased, especially in the upper incisor region, and this will, in turn, cause a reduction or loss of the interproximal papilla (Esposito et al. 1993).

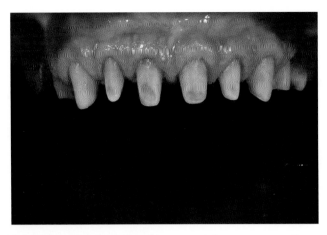

Fig. 14.15 Teeth were prepared with a feather-edge finish line: this approach is more conservative compared to a chamfer preparation and is more indicated for long 'periodontal' teeth.

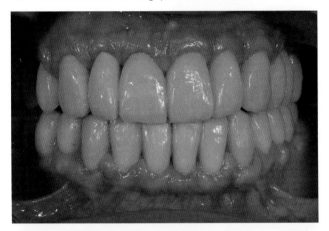

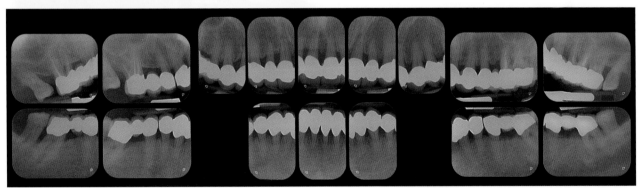

Figs. 14.16 and **14.17** Upper and lower fixed partial dentures (FPD) were delivered, splinting teeth in sections: incisors were splinted to posterior teeth in order to avoid the high chance of relapse in a patient like this with reduced periodontal support (lab technician: Roberto Iafrate).

The 1.5-mm-wide crater will also appear on the buccal side of the implant head. Therefore, to avoid losing bone height, the bone thickness should be at least 2 mm, preferably 4 mm (Spray et al. 2000).

If this amount of bone is not available, part of the buccal bone plate will be lost after remodelling, with the consequence of a high risk of soft-tissue recession.

Figures 14.18–14.21 display the case of a partially edentulous adult patient presenting different problems on the upper left and lower right quadrants.

On the left side, the loss of the clinical crowns of the upper premolars and the loss of the first lower molar originated compensatory overeruption of teeth 3.5 and 2.6; consequently, an insufficient interocclusal space was left.

On the right lower side, the loss of the clinical crown of the tooth 4.4 and the loss of tooth 4.6 jeopardised the correct restoration of the quadrant.

Orthodontic mechanics relying on skeletal anchorage were used in the second quadrant for molar intrusion (Figure 14.22) and in the fourth quadrant for space closure (Figure 14.23) in

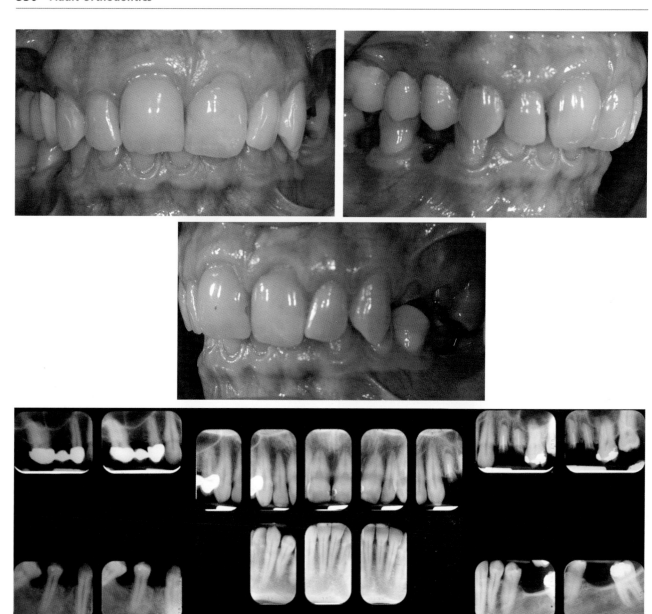

Figs. 14.18–14.21 A partially edentulous adult female patient presenting problems on different quadrants: on the left side, loss of the clinical crowns of the upper premolars and the loss of the first lower molar with the compensatory overeruption of teeth 2.6 and 3.5; on the right lower side, the loss of the clinical crown of tooth 4.4 and the loss of tooth 4.6 jeopardised the space distribution of the quadrant.

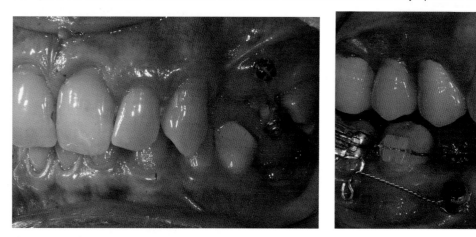

Figs. 14.22 and **14.23** Orthodontic intrusion of the upper left molar and mesialisation of the lower right molar. In both quadrants, orthodontic miniscrews served as anchorage.

order to obtain adequate interocclusal and mesiodistal spaces for rehabilitation.

On the second quadrant, after tooth extraction, the consequent ridge collapse required bone augmentation (by ridge-expansion technique) necessary to place two dental implants (Figures 14.24–14.26).

On the forth quadrant, both spaces proximal to tooth 4.5 were managed, closing the distal one and optimising the mesial one in order to better position a dental implant (Figure 14.27).

Extrusion for tooth preservation or site development

Studies have shown that eruption in the presence of gingival inflammation reduces bleeding on probing, decreases pocket depth and even causes the formation of new bone at the alveolar crest as teeth erupt, with no occlusal factor present and while controls remain unchanged (Van Venrooy and Vanarsdall 1987).

Eruption or uprighting of molars without scaling and root planing in human patients has been shown to reduce the number of pathogenic bacteria (Vanarsdall and Hamlin 1987).

During clinical treatment, however, inflammation always should be controlled to ensure that the supracrestal connective tissue remains healthy (Vanarsdall et al. 2016).

Orthodontic extrusion of an individual tooth is used for: correction of isolated periodontal osseous lesions, treating conditions that cause insufficient clinical crown exposure

and post-extraction implant-site development. In this chapter, the orthodontic–restorative interrelationship is discussed; hence, the second and third conditions are addressed.

Insufficient clinical crown exposure

Insufficient clinical crown exposure is related to six clinical conditions:

1. Subgingival caries.
2. Subgingival fracture.

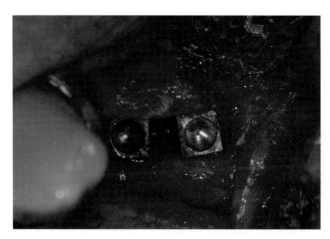

Fig. 14.24 After the extraction of both upper left premolar roots, the consequent ridge collapse required bone augmentation prior to place two implant fixtures: a ridge expansion technique was applied (periodontist: Arturo Imbelloni).

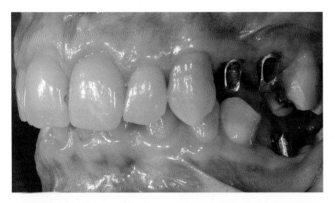

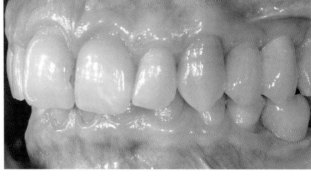

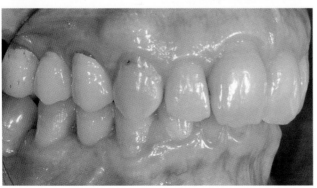

Figs. 14.25–14.27 Porcelain fused to metal (PFM) crowns were delivered on implants 2.4, 2.5, 3.6 and 4.4, while space left after extraction of tooth 4.6 was orthodontically closed by mesialising and uprighting tooth 4.7 (lab technician: Alberto Imbruglia).

3. Root perforation.
4. External resorption.
5. Altered passive eruption.
6. Restorative needs (ferrule effect).

The following treatment options are necessary to save or improve the prognosis of teeth in case of insufficient clinical crown exposure:

1. Orthodontic extrusion.
2. Crown lengthening.
3. Orthodontic extrusion followed by crown lengthening.

In case periodontal surgery ostectomy will result in extremely long clinical crowns and significantly weakened periodontal support of the treated and proximal teeth, orthodontic forced eruption may be chosen. Orthodontic treatment in these cases aims to rapidly extrude the tooth, without allowing time for remodelling of the bone and soft tissues surrounding the cervical portion of the root, thereby

exposing the necessary amount of sound tooth structure for the prosthodontist's safe intervention. If clinical crown volume is sufficient, orthodontic bracketing will be applied; if tooth structure is not enough, the endodontic space can be used (Figures 14.28–14.30) and elastic traction is applied through the coronal hook of a provisional post which is temporarily cemented (Figure 14.31). Because these teeth will eventually require a definitive post and core, the fabricated wire eyelet must be retrievable without causing damage to the tooth structure.

If a rapid movement is performed with a periodic circumferential fiberotomy, bone is prevented from following the erupted root (Pontoriero et al. 1987). The periodontal ligament fibers dictate alveolar bone formation and position; therefore, severing supracrestal connective tissue fibers, as the tooth rapidly erupts out of the socket, results in the exposure of sound tooth structure, with limited change of position of the alveolar crest and the free gingival margin.

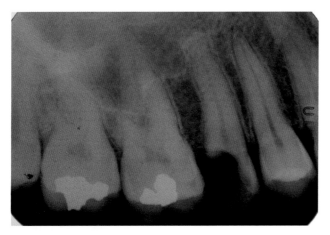 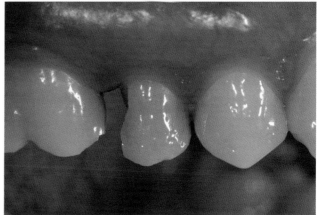

Figs. 14.28 and **14.29** A 36-year-old female patient presented a large decay over tooth #15 that involved the whole crown up to the bone level. She was extremely motivated to save this tooth if possible.

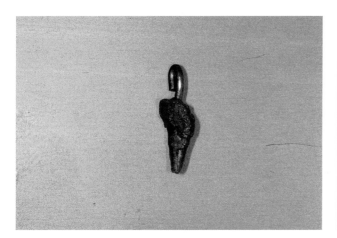 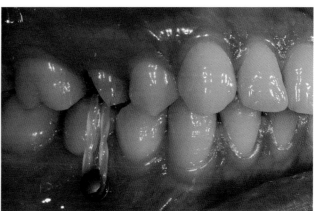

Fig. 14.30 After root canal therapy (RCT), a provisional post was fabricated to allow root extrusion: the author used a paper clip relined with GC Pattern Resin and cemented with temporary cement.

Fig. 14.31 Orthodontic forced eruption following circumferential fibrotomy. A miniscrew was inserted in the buccal aspect of the mandible and a full-time inter-maxillary elastomeric traction (6.5 oz) was used to extrude the root of the tooth.

On the contrary, if the movement is slow, bone follows and the gingival margin will be positioned more occlusally than proximal teeth, leaving nearly unaltered the exposed tooth structure; a crown-lengthening procedure is thus needed to uncover a sufficient part of root to achieve proper ferrule for the final restoration (Figures 14.32–14.35).

When the movement in occlusal direction has been completed, the tooth must be stabilised for 4–6 months to prevent re-intrusion due to the stretching of periodontal fibers that need time to adapt to the new tooth position. The tooth is now ready for restoration (Figure 14.36); the main problem to solve at this stage is the increased distance between the extruded and the adjacent roots, due to the narrower diameter of erupted single rooted teeth. This space needs to be partially reduced by overcontouring the fabricated crown; the alternative method, possible only if the entire arch is bracketed, consists in moving the interested roots to reduce the mesiodistal available space for the restoration. The final result of the presented case is displayed in Figures 14.37 and 14.38.

Implant site development

Slow controlled orthodontic tooth movement causes the entire attachment apparatus to shift in unison with the tooth (Reitan 1967).

There are cases when a compromised tooth cannot survive and the clinician has two options. The first is tooth extraction, and, to avoid major bone resorption, ridge preservation techniques may be employed to allow adequate implant insertion. The second is orthodontic tooth extrusion in order to generate or preserve bone, followed by a period of stabilisation; consequently, tooth will be extracted, and finally an immediate or a delayed implant may be inserted in the developed extraction site.

This second option involving orthodontic treatment is described with the following clinical case. An adult patient presented a hopeless tooth 2.1 with external root resorption and LEO (Figures 14.39 and 14.40) due to a trauma from a motorcycle accident at the age of 15; two root canal treatments and internal bleaching were later done over the years before coming to our attention.

The decision was taken to do an apicectomy first to allow apical bone growth and maturation, so that later a slow extrusion of the tooth could be safely performed to enhance implant-site development (Korayem et al. 2008; Somar et al. 2016). The upper arch was completely bonded and progressive extrusion bends on tooth 2.1 were incorporated in a 0.018-inch stainless-steel wire during a 6-month period until 5 mm of slow forced eruption was obtained following the long axis of the tooth (Figures 14.41–14.43).

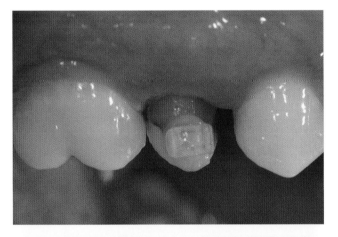
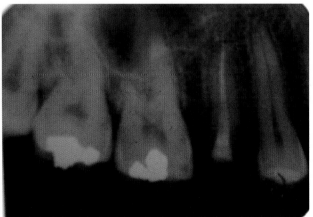
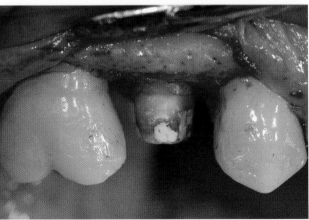
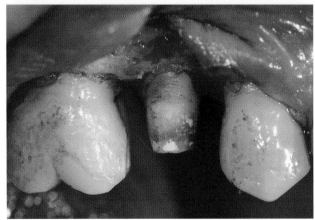

Figs. 14.32–14.35 Although the orthodontic movement was rapid, partially bone and the gingival margin shifted more occlusally than proximal teeth; a crown-lengthening procedure was thus needed to uncover part of tooth to achieve proper ferrule for the final restoration (periodontist: Arturo Imbelloni).

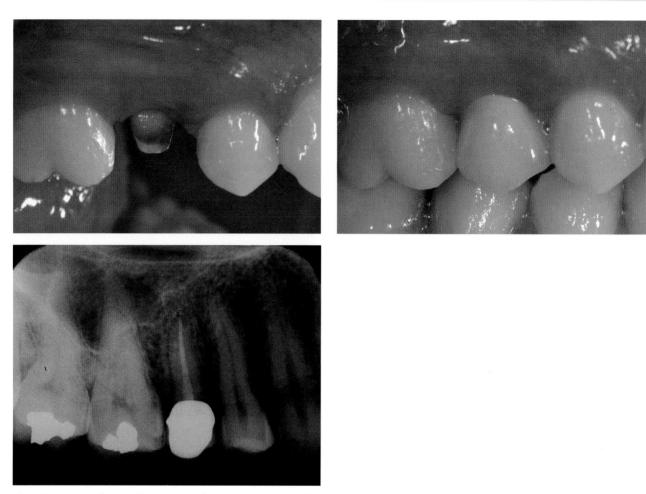

Figs. 14.36–14.38 The tooth was ready for restoration, even if roots are always narrower after extrusion: therefore, the increased distance with the proximal teeth may be compensated by increasing the convexity of the emergence profile of the zirconium ceramic crown (lab technician: Alberto Imbruglia).

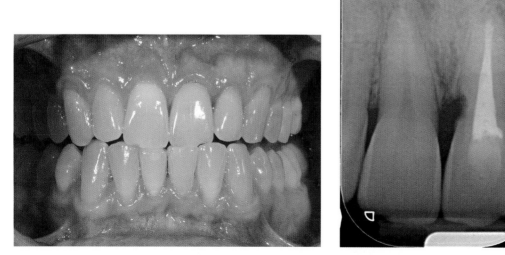

Figs. 14.39 and **14.40** A 52-year-old male patient presented a hopeless tooth 2.1 with external root resorption and a lesion of endodontic origin (LEO) due to a trauma from a motorcycle accident at the age of 15. Two subsequent RCTs and an internal bleaching were later done over the years before coming to our attention. The apicectomy was done by the endodontist (Cristiano Fabiani) to allow apical bone growth; then, after 3 months of maturation of the new tissue, orthodontic therapy began.

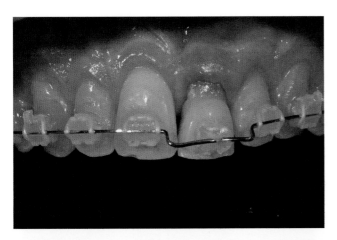
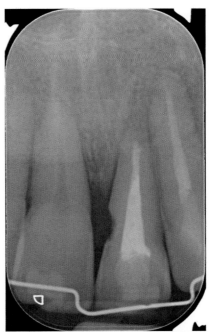
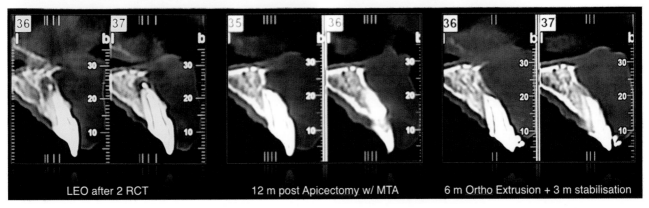

LEO after 2 RCT 12 m post Apicectomy w/ MTA 6 m Ortho Extrusion + 3 m stabilisation

Figs. 14.41–14.43 Orthodontics forced eruption with buccal fixed appliances. The slow and progressive extrusion aimed to migrate occlusally hard and soft tissues together with the tooth, for implant site development.

After three months of retention, at the extraction appointment, an immediate implant was inserted (Figures 14.44–14.46) with temporary post and core and crown; to prevent excessive occlusal load, the provisional was adjusted not to meet the opposing teeth (Figure 14.47).

The final ceramic crown preserved the adequate function and aesthetics of the original tooth while based on sound and healthy biologic tissues (Figure 14.48).

Preventing pulpal involvement in tooth preparation

In adults, teeth are not properly aligned for several reasons: altered natural eruption, adaptation to traumatic occlusion, tooth extraction with consequent migration of proximal and opposing teeth, worn clinical crowns due to parafunctional habits or iatrogenic causes.

When teeth are overerupted or horizontally inclined, patients may benefit from orthodontic alignment, especially if teeth must be restored; there are two clinical scenarios in which tooth repositioning helps to prevent root canal treatment.

(1) If one or more adjacent teeth are overerupted, the orthodontist can intrude them either with a sectional or a comprehensive therapy. This movement has two beneficial effects: creates enough interocclusal space necessary to restore the opposing tooth area, and, doing so, avoids the preparation of the occlusal part of the intruded teeth which, in many cases, should otherwise be root-canaled (Figures 14.49–14.51).

(2) When teeth are severely horizontally inclined, often because of advanced periodontal disease. This pathology may be characterised by the above-mentioned

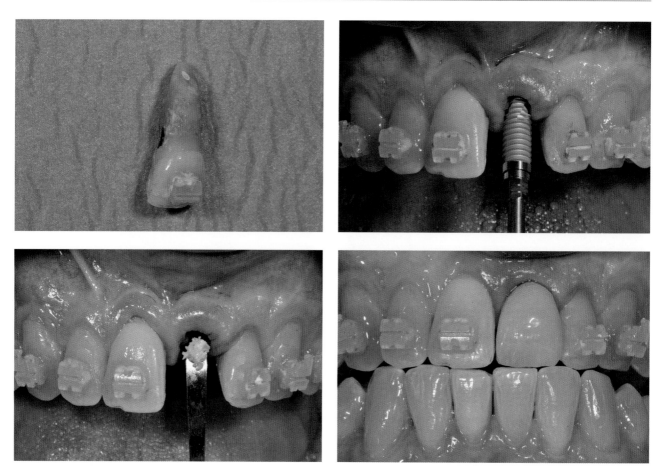

Figs. 14.44–14.47 After 3 months of retention, the tooth was extracted and an immediate implant was inserted with the temporary post and core and crown; to prevent excessive occlusal load, the provisional was adjusted not to meet the opposing teeth (periodontist: Arturo Imbelloni).

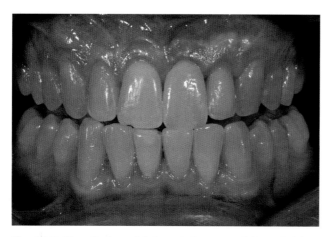

Fig. 14.48 The final well-integrated crown (lab technician: Alberto Imbruglia).

condition named 'posterior bite collapse', identified by flaring and overeruption of anterior teeth and alteration of the posterior plane of occlusion with inclination of teeth axis and overeruption of posteriors towards the opposing edentulous areas. Multidisciplinary treatment of these complex cases aims to re-establish a

physiological increased VDO in order to gain interocclusal space to align posteriors and retruded anteriors; thereby, if abutments need to be prepared for a full crown, endodontic treatment will not be necessary, since they can be moved to an ideal position, so that prosthetic reduction will not violate the pulp chamber.

Allowing for adequate thickness of restorative materials on teeth to be restored

Tooth wear is one of the greatest challenges for clinicians and its incidence is continuously increasing, particularly in the young age (Van't Spijker et al. 2009). It can be due to several causes such as occlusal problems, parafunction, chemical erosion, habits. (Grippo et al. 2004).

In orthodontic treatment of adult patients, tooth form is a common problem. As in the case of malformed teeth, it is always easier to correct the tooth form prior to the completion of orthodontics. Nevertheless, if this is not accomplished, the orthodontist will level the arches, aligning the incisal edges of the worn teeth and leaving the patient with the options of having periodontal crown lengthening or living with short teeth. A far more appropriate treatment

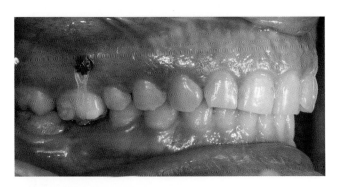
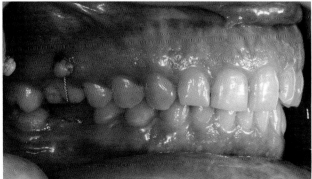
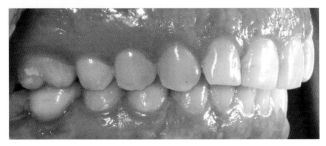

Figs. 14.49–14.51 Minimally invasive orthodontic intrusion of posterior teeth using miniscrews as anchorage.

is to correct the length of the worn teeth temporarily before or during the orthodontic treatment. This results in level arches with correctly positioned and sized teeth (Spear 2009)

The blueprint of the therapy is created by an orthodontic setup and a diagnostic wax-up. The worn teeth are cut from the setup and waxed to planned length, and then they are placed back in the setup in the established end position of treatment and become the guide for treatment.

In general, worn teeth are lengthened during orthodontics, since they are in contact with the opponents, due to continuous compensatory eruption and interocclusal space does not exist to lengthen prior to orthodontics; the clinician's responsibility is to help the patient not to have a compromised look, during the decompensation phase.

The orthodontist first creates space by intruding overerupted teeth, and then sends the patient to the restorative dentist for temporary restoration. In this way, the provisional restorations are built to fill the interocclusal space created, in order not to jeopardise patients' social life.

The goal of the orthodontist at this stage is to 'think pink' and level the gingival margins, considering them the reference (Kois 1994). Once the new gingival architecture has been finalised, the next step of the treatment becomes the final restoration (Figures 14.52–14.54). The orthodontist is responsible for the position of teeth, while shape and dimensions are in the hands of the restorative dentist.

The following adult patient presented generalised tooth wear as a result of a combination of erosion, due to gastroesophageal reflux, and attrition, due to parafunctional habits (Figures 14.55–14.57). First, an indirect transparent mock-up was made from the laboratory wax-up and tried in

to help visualising the final result. Second, orthodontic treatment with a continuous wire technique was undertaken in order to reduce the overbite by intrusion of both the upper and lower anterior sextants (Figure 14.58); the possibility of performing minimally invasive prosthetic techniques is related to the ability to achieve ideal tooth position with orthodontics (Figure 14.59).

Third, minor odontoplasty was performed to remove major undercuts, unsupported enamel edges and sharp angles (Figure 14.60); provisionals were not delivered, since tooth structure was left basically intact. Fourth, subgingival cervical palatal enamel was built up in composite (then prepared and finished supragingivally) for deep margin elevation, to allow isolation of the operatory field for adhesive procedures. Fifth, mock-up (Figure 14.61) followed by delivery of 6 upper anterior additive feldspathic veneers (Figure 14.62), restoring both buccal and palatal surfaces, was performed by adhesive cementation (Figures 14.63 and 14.64). Occlusal adjustment and a maxillary night guard completed the sequence of treatment.

Re-establishing proper posterior occlusal plane

In healthy individuals, functional masticatory stability is based on the concept of 'mutually protected occlusion'. For clarification purposes, the dentition is divided into two parts, the anterior group and the posterior group; when in function each group protects the other. During mandibular movements, anterior teeth serve the dentition by providing adequate anterior guidance, thus discluding the posteriors, while in maximum intercuspation, posterior teeth serve the dentition by creating stable posterior interdigitation to support the occlusal vertical dimension and protect the

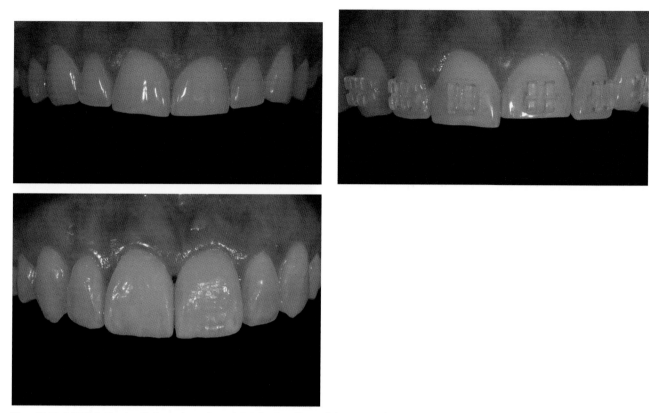

Figs. 14.52–14.54 Orthodontic intrusion of tooth 2.1 for levelling of the gingival margins. Following orthodontic tooth movement and 12-week stabilisation period, the anterior teeth received 6 upper anterior additive feldspathic veneers in order to achieve different goals: designing a harmonious incisal level of the entire sextant, restoring the lost tooth structure because of parafunctional habits (in particular on tooth 2.1) and fulfilling the patient's desire for a pleasant smile.

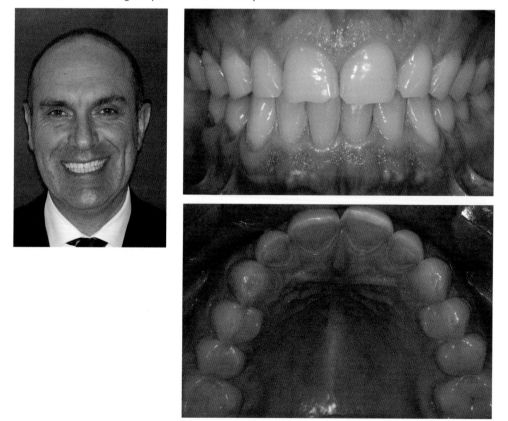

Figs. 14.55–14.57 The following 49-year-old male patient presented generalised tooth wear as a result of a combination of erosion, due to gastroesophageal reflux, and attrition, due to parafunctional habits.

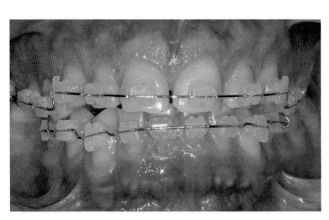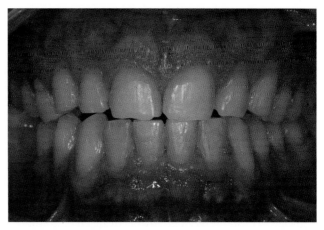

Figs. 14.58 and **14.59** Orthodontics intrusion of the upper and lower anterior segments to generate anterior space for prosthetic rehabilitation.

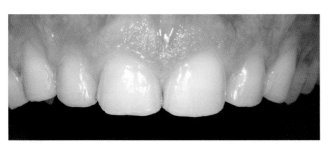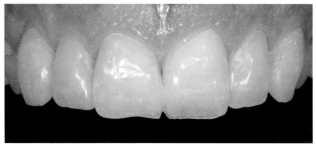

Fig. 14.60 Minor odontoplasty was performed to remove major undercuts, unsupported enamel edges and sharp angles; provisionals were not delivered, since tooth structure was left basically intact.

Fig. 14.61 Mock-up.

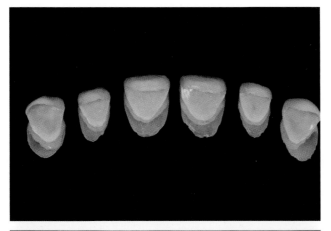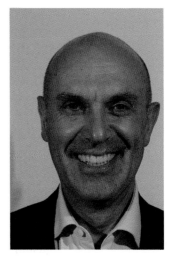

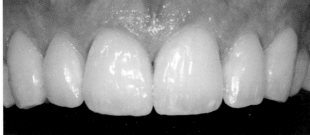

Figs. 14.62–14.64 Six upper anterior additive feldspathic veneers were delivered by adhesive cementation, restoring both buccal and palatal surfaces (lab technician: Roberto Iafrate).

maxillary anterior teeth from horizontally directed forces. This is how the dentition can be spared from horizontal overload and excessive wear.

The adult dentition may present situations where occlusal stability is lacking and its prognosis in the long term is in question. Functional balance may be jeopardised by caries, periodontal disease and occlusal trauma, with further detrimental consequences such as apical pathology, missing teeth, collapsed teeth, drifting teeth, etc.

The occlusal vertical dimension is supported by the posterior occlusion; however, with posterior tooth loss, the forces of occlusion remain on the anterior teeth. This will have a significant impact on their long-term function and viability (Starr 2001). In case of advanced periodontal disease with posterior bite collapse, the restoration of form and function is more difficult. The target of the therapy is to build a harmonic masticatory system by re-establishing proper posterior occlusal plane and anterior guidance, developed in concert with the posterior cusp height.

The anterior guidance, as a determinant of posterior occlusal form, must be perfected before occlusal contours can be finalised (Dawson 1989). On the other hand, if the patient is not affected by periodontal disease and tooth loss is caused by caries, the interdisciplinary treatment is less demanding, since periodontal support is efficient.

Re-establishing incisal guidance

Together with centric relation, anterior guidance is the most important assessment that must be made when restoring an occlusion, both in orthodontic and in restorative treatments. Failure to properly establish the correct guidance is a major cause of post-treatment instability. Anterior guidance is the dynamic relationship between lower and upper anterior teeth through all ranges of function (Dawson 1989). It is determined by the contour of the palatal surfaces of the upper teeth and the incisal edges of lower anterior teeth, the position of the anterior teeth and interarch and intraarch relationship. Therefore, it is linked to vertical and horizontal overlaps of anterior teeth.

- Overbite: the maxillary anterior group should demonstrate 0.5–3.0 mm of vertical overlap.
- Overjet: the maxillary anterior group should demonstrate 0.5–3.0 mm sagittal overlap.

The contour and position of upper and lower anterior teeth are so critical that an error of less than a millimetre in incisal edge location can be felt as a problem to some patients.

Dawson states that: 'If the condylar path does not dictate the anterior guidance, it should be clear that the anterior guidance cannot be determined on an articulator regardless of how perfectly the condylar path is duplicated. It is a separate entity and must be determined in the mouth where the determinants of anterior tooth position can be observed in function' (Dawson 1989).

When anterior teeth must be restored and the anterior relationship is correct, it is possible to duplicate it with acrylic resin by making a customised anterior guide table, which can be used with any coordinated articulator.

However, there are two pathologic conditions, such as posterior bite collapse and tooth wear, that necessitate a change of the existing anterior guidance; these problems cannot be corrected by duplicating the anterior guidance, but rather they require the restoration of a proper dental contour, different from the altered one. The multidisciplinary therapy can enhance the final outcome with orthodontic treatment.

The first, posterior bite collapse, is a clinical syndrome result of periodontal disease; this can lead to the extraction of one or more posterior teeth with the consequent loss of posterior occlusal support and the potential breakdown of the functional protective capacity of the entire dentition, often resulting in further tooth loss, increasing mobility, flaring of the anterior teeth and loss of occlusal vertical dimension. In this case, orthodontic therapy aims to correct the occlusal plane and to retract and intrude the flared anterior teeth, to make space for restorations, thus avoiding pulpal involvement.

In the second condition, tooth wear, orthodontic therapy aims to expand and intrude the extruded upper anterior sextant, and to intrude and align the worn lower anterior teeth to make space for additional restorations without pulpal involvement.

An adult patient presenting this last problem is illustrated here (Figures 14.65–14.67); he showed signs of attrition (which is wear from teeth rubbing against each other during mandibular movements) of the lower incisors in a deep bite relationship due to a restricted envelop of function and parafunctional habits, contraction of the posterior sextants of both arches, diastemas in the anterior region of the maxilla and highly dischromic teeth.

According to our protocol, an indirect transparent mock-up was made from the laboratory wax-up and tried in to help visualising the final result. Orthodontic mechanics with fixed appliances aimed to redistribute spaces in the upper arch (Figure 14.68) and intrude the lower front teeth in order to increase the overjet and decrease the overbite, allowing for adequate thickness of the prosthetic materials.

Minor odontoplasty consisting in minor removal of enamel at selected locations was employed, for a truly conservative approach that highly preserves natural tooth structure (Figure 14.69); therefore, provisionals could be avoided. 20 upper and lower additional feldspathic veneers were delivered, 12 veneers on the buccal and incisal surfaces of the anteriors allowed to restore proper function and aesthetics, while 8 veneers covering just the buccal surfaces of the premolars were applied to enhance the final aesthetic result.

In this case, cementing 20 additional veneers was a long-lasting procedure, and more time was necessary to

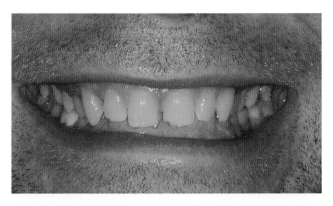

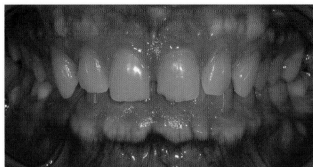

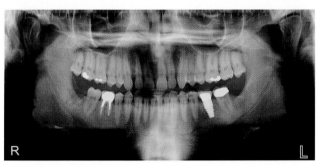

Figs. 14.65–14.67 An 43-year-old male patient presented: signs of attrition of the lower incisors in a deep bite relationship due to a restricted envelope of function and parafunctional habits, contraction of the posterior sextants of both arches, diastemas in the anterior region of the maxilla and highly dischromic teeth.

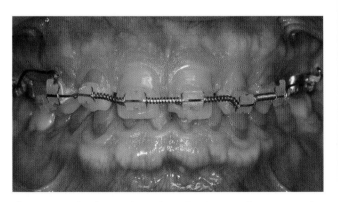

Fig. 14.68 Orthodontics buccal mechanics to adjust spaces for prosthetic rehabilitation.

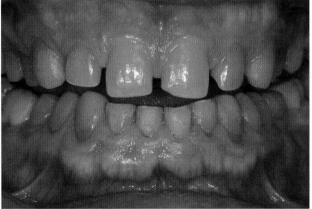

Fig. 14.69 Minor odontoplasty, consisting in minor removal of enamel at selected locations, was employed, for a truly conservative approach that highly preserves natural tooth structure.

thoroughly adjust the occlusion in order to avoid premature fractures of the restorations (Figures 14.70–14.72); this phase of the treatment is very important, especially in a case like this where the patient had gone through orthodontic treatment with consequent change of the original occlusal relationship. An upper night guard was delivered to protect teeth and restorations from the adverse effects of uncontrolled nocturnal parafunctional habits.

A second early appointment allowed careful finishing and polishing of the veneers margins; this is the only phase of the treatment that occasionally required local anaesthesia,

since the margins of the restorations were adjacent to the marginal gingiva in some areas and the rotatory instruments could slightly hurt it.

Thoroughly finished and polished additional feldspathic veneers achieve optimal periodontal integration (Figure 14.73).

Enhancing the aesthetic result

The marginal gingival contour of the upper anterior sextant is paramount for the smile appearance (Kokich 1997). The physiologic gingival architecture has been described as

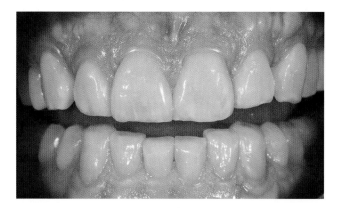

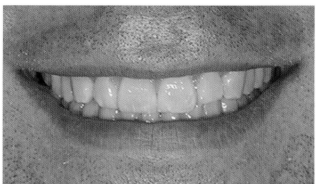

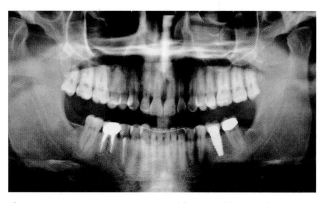

Figs. 14.70–14.72 Twenty upper and lower additional feldspathic veneers were adhesively cemented: 12 veneers on the buccal and incisal surfaces of the anteriors allowed to restore proper function and aesthetics, while 8 veneers covering just the buccal surfaces of the premolars were applied to enhance the final aesthetic result (lab technician: Roberto Iafrate).

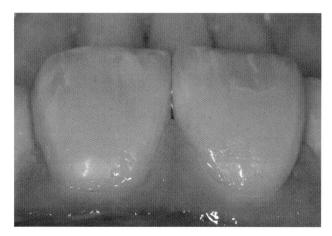

Fig. 14.73 Thoroughly finished and polished additional feldspathic veneers achieve optimal periodontal integration.

having a scalloped contour (Prichard 1961) which follows the course of the cementum–enamel junction. The healthy festooned gingival margin is affected by the degree of concavity and convexity of the tooth surface and by the individual biotype; the more convex is the root, the more scalloped is the gingival margin.

Some patients show gingival margin discrepancies caused by altered natural tooth eruption, delayed migration of the gingival margins (altered passive eruption), abrasion of the incisal edges and tooth extraction with consequent migration of proximal teeth.

To make the right therapeutical decision, in case of apparent discrepancy, it is necessary to evaluate four criteria (Kokich and Spear 1997):

1. The relationship between the gingival margin of the maxillary central incisor and the patient's lip line during smile.
2. The labial sulcular depths of the two central incisors.
3. The relationship between the shortest central incisor and the adjacent lateral incisors.
4. The abrasion of the incisal edges.

The following case describes a combined orthodontic–prosthetic approach to a patient requiring aesthetic improvement of her smile and dentition (Figures 14.74 and 14.75). The patient presented several anomalies of the anterior sextants: crowding, asymmetric microdontia of the upper lateral incisors, some teeth were rotated and the gingival margin contour was uneven. Her desire was to improve the overall appearance of her smile without 'grinding' her teeth; to achieve this goal, a multidisciplinary treatment was proposed including orthodontics to obtain alignment and improve the 'pink aesthetics', and additional veneers to improve the 'white aesthetics'.

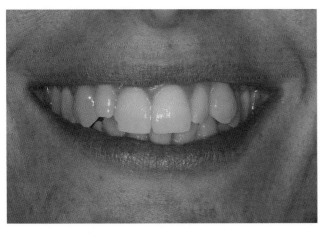
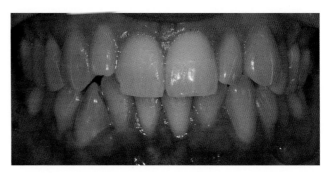

Figs. 14.74 and **14.75** This 36-year-old female patient presented several anomalies of the anterior sextants: crowding, asymmetric microdontia of the upper lateral incisors, some teeth were rotated and the gingival margin contour was uneven. Her desire was to improve the overall appearance of her smile without 'grinding' her teeth.

The problems list included:

– Crowding on both arches.
– Microdontia of maxillary lateral incisors.
– Thin gingival biotype.
– High-angle vertical pattern.
– Lip incompetence.
– Relapse of earlier adolescent orthodontic arch-expansion treatment.

The orthodontic treatment lasted 24 months and was performed with the extraction of four first premolars, alignment of the dental arches and space closure and finishing (Figures 14.76–14.78).

One of the specific goals was to align the outline of the gingival margins extruding the two upper laterals and to finish positioning them in mesial contact with the two centrals (Figures 14.79 and 14.80); at the end of this phase, two removable Essix-type retainers were immediately delivered while waiting for the prosthetic treatment. This arrangement gives a natural emergence profile at the mesial aspect of the lateral incisors, while the distal diastema will later be closed with two partial additional feldspathic veneers (Figure 14.81) for each side, one on the lateral and one on the canine; a fifth one was cemented to restore the distoincisal angle of the upper right central.

Dental and gingival architecture is now harmonious: the orthodontist prepared the ground to the prosthodontist levelling the gingival margins and aligning anterior teeth, therefore, enhancing a very conservative restorative approach; consequently the prosthodontist, in synergy with the ceramist, was able to build proper tooth shape that further allowed both vertical and horizontal papillary growth to fill the interproximal spaces (Figure 14.82) (Tarnow et al. 1992). The additional veneers made with feldspathic ceramic, the material recognised to have the best optical properties among all ceramics, contributed to achieve a natural aesthetic result (Figures 14.83 and 14.84).

The final prosthetic treatment of the above-described clinical cases was executed either by preparing teeth for conventional crowns and fixed partial dentures or leaving tooth structure intact, or nearly intact, to receive additional feldspathic ceramic veneers; in the latter case, the reader can refer to the quoted article for the description of the corresponding clinical steps (Imbelloni et al. 2019).

Role of temporisation in interdisciplinary treatment

The goals for a temporary restoration in routine crown and bridge treatments are to protect the tooth, provide an occlusal stop, maintain interproximal contact and ensure gingival health through proper fit and contour, usually for few weeks before being replaced by the final restoration (Amsterdam and Fox 1959; Yuodelis and Faucher 1980).

In complex interdisciplinary care, the role of temporisation is very different, since they become the main stability key factor in the treatment process and may be in place several months or, in some cases, years, due to the necessity to ensure a good quality of life to the patients while they go through tooth extraction, periodontal surgery, implant surgery or orthodontics (Chiche 1994; Amet and Phinney 1995; Christensen 1996; Donovan and Cho 1999).

There is not a strict timing protocol for temporisation in case of interdisciplinary therapy; the possible guidelines are based on the individual situation of the patient:

(A) When patient is missing teeth and function is jeopardised, when old crowns are present with recurrent caries that cannot be accessed without their removal, when an existing fixed prosthesis is present and the patient requires ridge augmentation or desires an implant, in all these cases, temporisation will be the first step after emergency treatment; it plays the role of testing function, maintenance and aesthetic satisfaction.

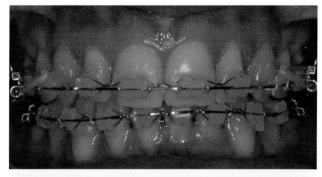

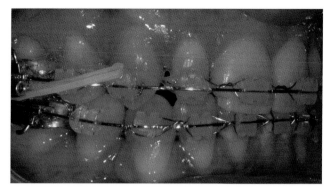

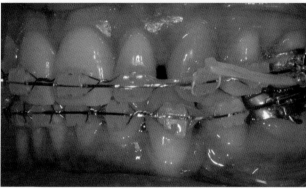

Figs. 14.76–14.78 Orthodontic finishing following space closure. Four first premolars were extracted.

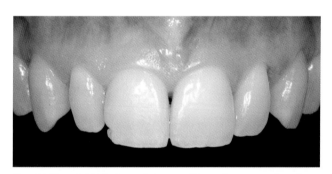

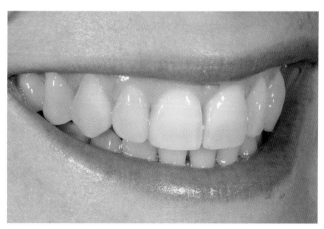

Figs. 14.79 and **14.80** One of the specific goals was to align the outline of the gingival margins extruding the two upper laterals and to finish positioning them in mesial contact with the two centrals.

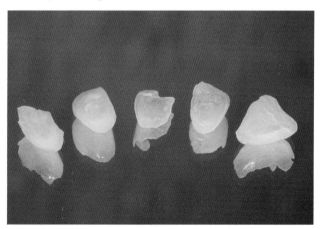

Fig. 14.81 Five upper anterior partial additive feldspathic veneers were delivered by adhesive cementation: 2 for each side, on the distal half of the laterals and on the mesial half of the canines; the 5th one was cemented to restore the disto-incisal angle of the upper right central (lab technician: Roberto Iafrate).

Fig. 14.82 The newly built proper tooth shape caused both vertical and horizontal papillary growth to fill the interproximal spaces between laterals and canines.

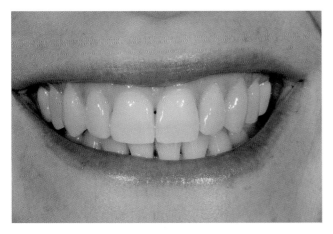 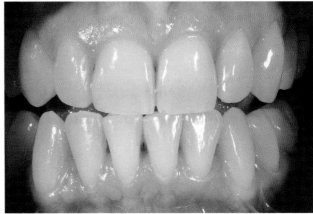

Figs. 14.83 and **14.84** The additional veneers made with feldspathic ceramic, the material recognised to have the best optical properties among all ceramics, contributed to achieve a natural aesthetic result.

(B) When there is periodontal disease, temporisation follows re-evaluation after initial periodontal therapy; subsequently, the patient's response to hygiene instructions and subgingival scaling gives to the team the necessary information to evaluate single abutments' stability and the capacity to maintain the future restorative work in time.

(C) When the treatment is more complex and the patient must face orthodontic treatment, it is safer to temporise once periodontal surgery has healed and orthodontics has been completed. The exceptions to this general rule are when the temporary pontic structure is used to extrude teeth and when damaged teeth without an existing crown are present; in these cases, it is better to restore those teeth and place a provisional before periodontal surgery and/or orthodontic therapy begin. Further reasons to place temporaries prior to orthodontics or surgery are when there are problems in tooth form (Vanarsdall 1989; Kokich and Spear 1997; Kokich 2001).

These may be localised developmental problems (e.g., peg-shaped lateral incisors), functional in nature (e.g., severe wear), or the result of developmental problems that affect all the teeth (e.g., amelogenesis imperfecta). If orthodontics or periodontal surgery is contemplated and the tooth form is not correct, improving the shape of the teeth prior to surgery or orthodontics may be beneficial.

The laboratory wax-up is utilised as a basis for the fabrication of a temporary restoration. In case of treatments not involving orthodontic therapy, the aesthetic outcome is pre-established in the wax-up that is processed into acrylic to produce the provisional prosthesis; this may be utilised as a guide during adjunctive treatment procedures.

On the other hand, multidisciplinary cases requiring significant orthodontic therapy may present an exception, since it may not be possible to predict extensive changes in tooth position with sufficient accuracy to warrant the development of the provisional prosthesis directly from the diagnostic wax setup.

Following intraoral placement, the provisional is gradually modified until all the objectives required in the final restoration have been achieved (Chiche 1990), thus it becomes the template from which the outline of the definitive prosthesis will be realised.

Prosthodontic finalisation

The clinical reference for multidisciplinary cases is the position of the gingival margins of anterior teeth. This aesthetic landmark can be changed either by periodontics or orthodontic therapies, where the latter gives a more conservative option to preserve residual tooth structure and attached gingiva; on the other hand, when orthodontic extrusion is performed, depending on the orthodontic technique used, it is often necessary to refine the final gingival margin position by means of a crown-lengthening procedure. When this is completed by the periodontist, the team must follow the tissue positional changes in order to decide the correct timing for the prosthodontist to take the final impression and finalise the treatment.

Pontoriero and Carnevale have shown that, in case of circumferential resection surgery with an apically positioned flap, the tissue level can take up to 12 months to mature (i.e., the duration of the study); furthermore, they have suggested that thick periodontal biotypes have a greater and longer-lasting coronal regrowth compared to thin biotypes and also that tissue maturation appeared to be influenced by individual variations in the healing response (Pontoriero and Carnevale 2001).

Consequently, it is advisable to monitor these patients, especially in the interproximal areas where regrowth is greater (Smith et al. 1980; Kaldhal et al. 1996).

The orthodontist must request input from the prosthodontist during the finishing stage for final tooth positioning; certainly, teamwork better flows when the two specialists work in the same office. The joint effort makes the orthodontist better understand the space requirements associated with different restorations, and the prosthodontist learns about the different therapeutic options orthodontic therapy can give to his work.

Once the orthodontist has completed soft-tissue positioning in accordance with the prosthodontist's opinion, the latter will study and test in the patient's mouth the correct incisal edge position. At this stage, the patient may present different situations to be restored: spacing in case of narrower teeth (i.e., lateral incisors), short clinical crowns in case of overerupted worn teeth, etc. In some of these cases, patients wear temporary composite restorations which have been adapted step by step during orthodontic treatment. Hence, it becomes necessary to finally test the incisal edge position using direct trial composite restorations, composite mock-ups, removable aesthetic templates or temporaries. As previously stated, aesthetic treatment objectives can be clinically refined and accurately represented to the patient only by trial in an in vivo environment (Lee and Jun 2000).

Using a removable overlay appliance to identify the aesthetic position of the incisal edge is less accurate. Instead, it is much more predictable to lengthen the teeth temporarily with a fixed restoration to evaluate the aesthetic and functional success of the new incisal edge position, and then copy this result by taking an impression of the arch.

Finally, a category of restoration congruent with the previously established functional and aesthetic objectives must be selected.

Complex orthodontic–prosthetic cases with advanced periodontal involvement including secondary occlusal trauma require splinting, and this is most predictably accomplished with the use of porcelain-fused-to-metal prostheses (Amsterdam 1974).

Thanks to research and development in all areas of dentistry, today we have the ability to offer our patients healthy, natural-looking, metal-free restorative solutions. The advancements in ceramics give us the opportunity to replace tooth structure in a manner that reflects the original anatomy of our patients' teeth. The development and improvements in adhesive dentistry offer functional and aesthetically pleasing restorative procedures with less or no-demolition procedures.

While in conventional prosthodontics dental reinforcement is achieved at the expense of the intact dental structure, using various types of partial or total coverage, in additive restorative dentistry it is achieved thanks to maximum preservation of the intact dental structure, using either composite direct restorations or ceramic adhesive restorations.

Tooth preparation for ceramic veneers removes 3–30% of the coronal tooth structure by weight, while that for all-ceramic and metal–ceramic crowns removes 63–72% (Edelhoff and Sorensen 2002a, 2002b).

Particularly when the colour is correct and there is only the need to change the form, tooth reduction can be avoided. The advantage of additional veneers (or non-prep veneers) is that teeth are not reduced, and adhesion is performed fully on enamel (if teeth are virgin and there is no dentin exposed) giving a predictable result that will last in time; adhesion, in fact, is universally accepted as being reliable particularly on enamel, the more enamel is left, the better it is (Gurel et al. 2013). The disadvantage is that, especially in case of feldspathic additional veneers, this is not an easy procedure and requires both the ceramist and the clinician during try-in to be very careful in handling these extremely thin restorations (in some area, the veneers can be only 0.1-mm thick).

In conclusion, it is the combination of orthodontics and additive prosthodontics that offers to the patients the most conservative and aesthetically pleasing results.

While proper diagnosis and treatment planning as well as precise execution of the treatment are important for the interdisciplinary approach, it is the good communication and collaboration among the specialists that is the key to the success of the final outcome.

References

Amet EM and Phinney TL (1995) Fixed provisional restorations for extended prosthodontic treatment. *J Oral Implantol* 21, 201–206.

Amsterdam M (1974) Periodontal prosthesis. Twenty-five years in retrospect. *Alpha Omegan* 67(3), 8–52.

Amsterdam M and Fox L (1959) Provisional splinting: principals and techniques. *Dent Clin North Am* 4, 73–99.

Barreto MS, Faber J, Vogel CJ and Araujo TM (2016) Reliability of digital orthodontic setups. *Angle Orthod* Mar;86(2), 255–259.

Chiche G (1990) Improving marginal adaptation of provisional restorations. *Quint Int* 21(4), 325–329.

Chiche GJ (1994) Provisional restorations in anterior procedures. *Dent Today* 13, 32, 34–37.

Christensen GJ (1996) Provisional restorations for fixed prosthodontics. *J Am Dent Assoc* 127, 249–252.

Dawson PE (1989) *Evaluation, Diagnosis and Treatment of Occlusal Problems*, 2nd edn. St Louis: Mosby. 274–297.

Dennis W (2010) "No-Prep" veneers. *Inside Dentistry* 6(8).

Donovan TE and Cho GC (1999) Diagnostic provisional restorations in restorative dentistry: the blueprint for success. *J Can Dent Assoc* 65, 272–275.

Edelhoff D and Sorensen JA (2002a) Tooth structure removal associated with various preparation designs for anterior teeth. *J Prosthet Dent* 87(5), 503–509.

Edelhoff D and Sorensen JA (2002b) Tooth structure removal associated with various preparation designs for posterior teeth. *Int J Periodontics Restorative Dent* 22(3), 241–249.

Ericson D (2004) What is minimally invasive dentistry? *Oral Health Prev Dent* 2(Suppl 1), 287–292.

Esposito M, Ekestubbe A and Grondahl K (1993) Radiological evaluation of marginal bone loss at tooth surfaces facing single Brånemark implants. *Clin Oral Implants Res* 4, 151–157.

Grippo JO, Simring M and Schreiner S (2004) Attrition, abrasion, corrosion, and abfraction revisited: a new perspective on tooth surface lesions. *J Am Dent Assoc* 135(8), 1109–1118.

Grunder U, Gracis S and Capelli M (2005) Influence of the 3-D bone-to-implant relationship on esthetics. *IJPRD* 25(2), 113–119.

Gurel G, Sesma N, Calamita MA, Coachman C, and Morimoto S. (2013) Influence of enamel preservation on failure rates of porcelain laminate veneers. *Int J Periodontics Restorative Dent* 33(1), 31–39.

Imbelloni A, Iafrate R and Luzi C (2019) Noninvasive interdisciplinary treatment of a dischromic partially worn dentition. *Quintessence Int* 50, 294–304.

Kaldhal WB, Kalkwarf KL, Patil KD, Molvar MP and Dyer JK (1996) Long-term evaluation of periodontal therapy. I. Response to 4 therapeutic modalities. *JP* 67, 93–102.

Kois JC (1994) Altering gingival levels: the restorative connection part I. biologic variables. *J Esthet Dent* 6(1), 3–9.

Kokich V and Spear F (1997) Guidelines for managing the orthodontic-restorative patient. *Semin Orthod* 3, 3–20.

Kokich VG (2001) Managing orthodontic-restorative treatment for the adolescent patient. In McNamara JA Jr (ed.) *Orthodontics and Dentofacial Orthopedics*. Ann Arbor, MI: Needham Press, Inc.

Kokich VG (1997) Esthetics and vertical tooth position: the orthodontic possibilities. *Compend Contin Educ Dent* Dec;18(12), 1225–1231.

Kokich VG and Kokich VO (2005) *In Ravindra Nanda: Biomechanic and Esthetic Strategies in Clinical Orthodontics*. Philadelphia: Elsevier Saunders.

Korayem M, Flores-Mir C, Nassar U and Olfert K (2008) Implant site development by orthodontic extrusion. A systematic review. *Angle Orthod* Jul;78(4), 752–760.

Lee EA and Jun SK (2000) Achieving aesthetic excellence through an outcome-based restorative treatment rationale. *Pract Periodont Aesthet Dent* 12(7), 641–648.

Lee EA and Jun SK (2002) Aesthetic design preservation in multidisciplinary therapy: philosophy and clinical execution. *Pract Proced Aesthet Dent* 14(7), 561–569.

Marks MH (1980) Tooth movement in periodontal therapy. In Goldman HM and Cohen DW (eds.) *Periodontal Therapy*. Mosby, St Louis, 6th edition, 564–627.

Pontoriero R and Carnevale G (2001) Surgical crown lengthening: a 12-month clinical wound healing study. *JP* 72, 841–848.

Pontoriero R, Celenza F Jr, Ricci G and Carnevale G (1987) Rapid extrusion with fiber resection: a combined orthodontic-periodontic treatment modality. *Int J Periodontics Restorative Dent* 7, 30–43.

Prichard J (1961) Gingivoplasty, gingivectomy and osseous surgery. *J Periodontol* 10, 275–282.

Reitan K (1967) Clinical and histologic observations on tooth movement during and after orthodontic treatment. *Am J Orthod* 53, 721–745.

Roblee RD (1994) *Interdisciplinary Dentofacial Therapy: A Comprehensive Approach to Optimal Patient Care*. Carol Stream, IL: Quintessence Publishing.

Salama H, Garber DA, Salama MA, Adar P and Rosenberg ES (1998) 50 years of interdisciplinary site development: lessons and guidelines from periodontal prosthesis. *J Esth Dent* 10(3), 149–156.

Salama H and Salama MA (1993) The role of orthodontic extrusive remodeling in the enhancement of soft and hard tissue profiles prior to implant placement: a systematic approach to the management of extraction site defects. *Int J Periodont Rest Dent* 13(4), 312–333.

Smith DH, Ammons WF Jr and van Belle G (1980) A longitudinal study of periodontal status comparing osseous recontouring with flap curettage. I. Results after 6 months. *JP* 51, 367–375.

Somar M, Mohadeb JV and Huang C (2016) Predictability of orthodontic forced eruption in developing an implant site: a systematic review. *J Clin Orthod* Aug;50(8), 485–492.

Spear F (2009) The role of temporisation in interdisciplinary periodontal and orthodontic treatment. *International Dentistry SA* 11(3), 6–16.

Spray RJ, Black CG, Morris HF and Ochi S (2000) The influence of bone thickness on facial marginal bone response: stage 1 placement through stage 2 uncovering. *Ann Periodontol* 5, 119–128.

Starr NL (2001) The distal extension case: an alternative restorative design for implant prosthetics. *Int J Periodontics Restorative Dent* 21, 61–67.

Tarnow DP, Magner AW and Fletcher P (1992) The effect of the distance from the contact point to the crest of bone on the presence or absence of the interproximal dental papilla. *J Periodontol* 63(12), 995–996.

Vanarsdall RL (1989) Orthodontics. Provisional restorations and appliances. *Dent Clin North Am* 33, 479–496.

Vanarsdall RL Jr., Blasi I, Jr., Secchi AG (2016) Periodontal–Orthodontic Interrelationships. In Graber, Vanarsdall, Vig, and Huang (eds.) *Orthodontics: Current Principles and Techniques*. Elsevier Saunders, Philadelphia, 621–668.

Vanarsdall RL and Hamlin J (1987) The effects of molar uprighting on the microbiological flora of the periodontium. Thesis. Philadelphia: University of Pennsylvania.

Van't Spijker A, Rodriguez JM, Kreulen CM, Bronkhorst EM, Barlett DW and Creugers NH (2009) Prevalence of tooth wear in adults. *Int J Prosthodont* 22(1), 35–42.

Van Venrooy JR and Vanarsdall RL (1987) Tooth eruption: correlation of histologic and radiographic findings in the animal model with clinical and radiographic findings in humans. *Int J Adult Orthodon Orthognath Surg* 2(4), 235–247.

Yuodelis RA and Faucher R (1980) Provisional restorations: an integrated approach to periodontics and restorative dentistry. *Dent Clin North Am* 24, 285–303.

15

Patients with Temporomandibular Joint (TMJ) Problems

Birte Melsen

Orthodontics and dysfunction

The relationship between orthodontic and functional problems has been the focus of many studies. A PubMed search with the keywords 'malocclusion' and 'temporomandibular dysfunction' (TMD) resulted in 1664 references, and 1253 references were registered under the keywords orthodontics and TMD, but a search for randomised controlled trials reduced the number of published papers to 65. This reflected the fact that most papers were case reports and several questions remain unanswered. Does malocclusion lead to craniomandibular disorder? Does orthodontic treatment play a role in the treatment of craniomandibular disorders? In other words, can TMD be considered an indication for orthodontic treatment?

The relationship between craniomandibular disorders and malocclusion is rated highly by some authors, while others claim that the presence of a malocclusion has no impact on the risk of TMD (Luther 2007a, 2007b). One explanation for this discrepancy is the difference between morphological occlusion and functional occlusion. The patient in Figure 15.1 with a Class I occlusion complained of muscle pain and tension headache. When the patient was given a flat occlusal splint, her occlusion changed from neutral occlusion to distal occlusion. She clearly had a dual bite and an electromyographic examination demonstrated significantly higher muscle activity in the contact position than in the position in which the patient was occluding when she was asked to bite together. Radiographs, taken in the two different occlusion positions, verified that the mandibular condyles were displaced forwards and downwards when the patient was occluding in Class I intercuspation and were centred when she attempted the retruded contact position. The fact that patients are generally registered in maximum intercuspation, which does not necessarily represent a mandibular position that is in harmony with the functional occlusion, may be a confounding factor when assessing the correlation between occlusion and TMD (Tallgren et al. 1979).

The above-mentioned example illustrates but one of the methodological problems which may contribute to the conflicting notions regarding malocclusion and oral function. As the functional deviation may be related to the deterioration of the dentition, adult patients with TMD should be asked to explain their version of the development of the problem. This also applies to all aspects of oral function such as parafunctions and bruxism.

Whereas the general relationship between occlusion and TMD is controversial, there is general agreement that misarticulation is more frequent in patients with certain types of malocclusion, such as excessive overjet, lateral crossbite and anterior open bite (Johnson and Sandy 1999; Pahkala and Qvarnstrom 2002). Misarticulation can be evaluated subjectively by the orthodontist, by a speech therapist (Laine 1992) or objectively by an electro-acoustic sound analysis (Mehnert 1987). In cases in which misarticulation is diagnosed, speech training rarely helps the patient unless the morphology does allow for normal function. Mastication can be evaluated either subjectively by asking the patient to explain the problem or objectively by asking the patient to chew on a standard object (Huggare and Skindhoj 1997).

Adult Orthodontics, Second Edition. Edited by Birte Melsen and Cesare Luzi.
© 2022 John Wiley & Sons Ltd. Published 2022 by John Wiley & Sons Ltd.
Companion Website: http://www.wiley.com/go/melsen-adult-orthodontics

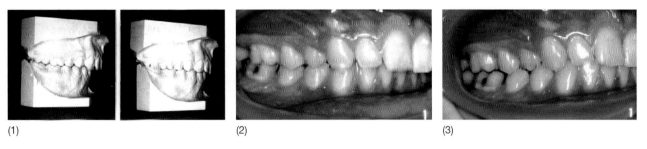

(1)   (2)   (3)

Fig. 15.1 (1) Study casts in two different occlusion positions. The cast on the right side displays the spontaneous occlusion observed when the patient is asked to bite together, and that to the left displays the posterior contact position that occurs after a period of wearing a flat splint. (2) and (3) Clinical views of the same situations.

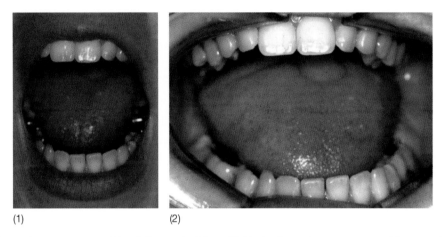

(1)   (2)

Fig. 15.2 (1) Normal opening movement with midlines coinciding. (2) Limited opening movement with more deviation towards the left side.

Lip activity during swallowing and the presence or absence of tooth contact during swallowing can be evaluated clinically. Cinefluorography studies have been used to describe the tongue movement and its adaptation to morphology (Hiiemae and Palmer 2003; Kawamura et al. 2003).

Analysis of jaw movement and palpation of muscles should precede the analysis of the occlusion, as detailed knowledge of the occlusion may bias the registration of the signs and symptoms of TMD. The muscles included in the examination are usually the temporal, masseter, digastric and the pterygoid muscles. Jaw movement can be evaluated clinically or registered by means of jaw-tracking equipment (Simonet and Clayton 1981; Piehslinger et al. 1991). It should be recorded whether the opening movement is symmetrical and smooth, asymmetrical or irregular, and the presence of any sounds and clicking should be noted. If clicking is present, it should be noted whether it occurs at the same spot during opening and closing. Clicking during opening may reflect an anterior disc displacement. The click occurs when the condyle is repositioned on to the disc and the click during closing occurs when the condyle slips off the disc again (disc displacement with reduction). The click therefore does not occur at the same spot during opening and closing. In a patient in whom the click is at the same spot during opening and closure of the mouth, it is most

likely a symptom of a disc that is ankylosed to the articular eminence of the joint fossa (Bumann and Lotzmann 2002).

The range of lateral movements and protrusion should likewise be noted. A limitation especially in protrusion may be a sign of a permanently forwards displaced disc. In the case of a midline discrepancy, this may either be reduced or increased by opening (Figure 15.2). In the patient with a skeletal asymmetry, the asymmetry will increase during opening, and the mandible will deviate towards the short side or to the side with the least translation. If the midline is centred during maximum opening, this is a sign of a forced bite and closure can proceed in two different ways: either starting with symmetrical closure until the initial tooth contact position is reached, after which deviation towards maximal intercuspation takes place; or closure that proceeds towards a midline discrepancy in a smooth manner. In the first case, the sensory input from the primary contact is still present and the midline discrepancy can most likely be corrected by removal of the primary contact. In the latter case, the neuromuscular pattern has adapted to the malocclusion and the parasympathetic input from the occlusion should be removed before the structural position of the mandible can be established. This can be done with a flat occlusal splint. The importance of determining the condylar position in the orthodontic diagnosis has been underlined by several authors (Gianelly 1989; Roth 1995; Johnson and Sandy 1999; Cordray 2002).

Controversy in the literature regarding TMD and occlusion

The controversies regarding the relationship between occlusion and TMD may be related to the design of the studies as well as the reproducibility and validity of the parameters. In addition, the specificity and the sensitivity of the applied methods may have an impact. The methods used to establish the presence of a TMD have involved questionnaires, clinical analyses and instrumental analyses. The result of questionnaires and the clinical analyses are both subject to fluctuation over time, since the cause of TMD is generally being accepted as multifactorial (Dworkin and LeResche (1992)) (see Chapter 16).

The reproducibility of jaw tracking, however, has proved to be very high when computerised methods are used. Kimmel et al. (1986) performed axiographic and sirognathographic analyses in young adults with normal occlusion who had never had temporomandibular joint (TMJ) symptoms and had clinically normal opening capacity. In 7 of the 30 test subjects, the axiographic registrations indicated internal derangement in one or both joints and six were confirmed by the sirognathographic registration. Repeated examinations gave identical results, indicating good reproducibility but low specificity, as there were a large number of positive findings in healthy persons. The sensitivity was, on the other hand, good, as clinical findings were always confirmed by the jaw-tracking method.

Instrumental methods can thus be used to follow the development of the pathology in a joint, but not as a diagnostic tool. The validity of the condylar movement could also be questioned, as the sensor moving was not localised to the condyle and it is doubtful whether a patient is able to perform natural movement of the mandible with the tray in the mouth (Figure 15.3). In the case of sirognathography, a small magnet was glued to the lower incisors and the displacement of the magnet during mandibular movement was picked up in a magnetic field generated by an appliance placed adjacent to the cheeks of the patient (Figure 15.3). Without doubt, the advantage of both methods is that the results can be presented in a digital form or graphically in all three planes of space, whereby changes occurring over a period of treatment or development of a disease can be followed (Figure. 15.3). When jaw tracking was used to study the influence of occlusion on condylar movement patterns, it was refuted that there was a correlation between occlusion and joint pathology, as clinically healthy patients were diagnosed as having internal derangement.

The parameters reflecting occlusion may also influence the result of studies relating occlusion to TMD. Normally, the morphological occlusion is expressed using Angle classification or selected features such as overjet > 6 mm, overbite > 5 mm, etc. Gianniri et al. (1991) performed a study with the purpose of analysing the relationship between occlusion and TMD. Based on systematic screening, 30 16-year-old individuals with significant subjective symptoms and clinical signs of TMD were matched with individuals of the same age, gender and with identical occlusion, and no symptoms and signs according to the form filled in by the community dentistry team. In addition to the parameters reflecting TMD and occlusion, the distribution, number and intensity of occlusal contacts were noted by means of a photo-occlusal method. The study demonstrated that although the occlusion was registered as identical, both the distribution and intensity of the occlusal contacts differed between the two groups. In the population without symptoms, the occlusal contacts were distributed symmetrically, whereas they were asymmetrically distributed in the group with symptoms. In addition, the intensity of the occlusal contacts when evaluated by photo-occlusion differed. The intensity of individual occlusal contact was significantly higher in the group with symptoms than in the healthy group. This indicates that the method by which the occlusion is registered influences the results of the studies evaluating the relationship between occlusion and TMD.

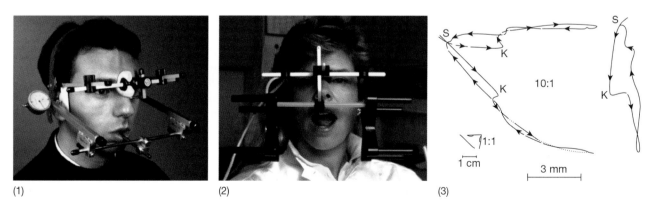

(1) (2) (3)

Fig. 15.3 Jaw-tracking devices. (1) Classic axiograph. (2) In sirognathography, the movement of a small magnet glued to the lower incisors is followed in three planes of space. (3) Enlarged image obtained by the jaw-tracking device revealing that the clicking is related to a medial displacement of the condyle.

Treatment and TMD

Treatment of TMD can focus on the patient as a whole (see Chapter 16), on the joint or on the occlusion. Regarding treatments focusing directly on the joint, intra-articular surgery or lavage has been performed as well as intra-articular injections of various substances (Dolwick 2007). Bertolami et al. (1993) divided 120 patients with TMD into two groups, one of which had injections of 1% sodium hyaluronate in physiological saline and the other only physiological saline. The result was clearly in favour of the sodium hyaluronate group, both when evaluated by the Helkimo index and with a visual analogue scale used for the level of pain and noise during movement. Glucocorticoid injections have been recommended (Kopp et al. 1985, 1987) in spite of the detrimental effect discussed already by Chandler and Wright in 1958 (Chandler and Wright 1958). The long-term results of glucocorticosteroid injections were evaluated as positive in 16 out of 19 patients examined. However, the results of the 8-year follow-up may not necessarily solely represent the effect of the cortisone injection (Wenneberg et al. 1991).

Whether orthodontics plays a role in treatment of patients with TMD depends on the probability that changing the occlusion will have an impact on the symptoms. This can be evaluated by the use of a splint. These splints may be soft or hard, balanced flat, repositioning or stabilising splints. Comparisons of the results of treatment with splints clearly reflect the multifactorial character of TMD. Several studies (Table 15.1) have demonstrated that the type of appliance or splint used was not important. All splints were associated with a positive response with regard to the level of pain, whereas clicking was less influenced. Most studies have reported short-term results, but the few long-term follow-up studies that have been reported have demonstrated that the effect is not permanent in most cases, although the best long-term results seemed to be related to the repositioning splints. A significant effect in the short term was also seen in the control groups and had an obvious influence on the conclusions of such studies. A meta-analysis focusing on the treatment of disc dislocation with reduction confirmed that a repositioning splint was significantly more effective than a flat splint in reduction of both pain and clicking (Santacatterina et al. 1998). However, it could be argued that sample size in all the included studies was limited.

The importance of elucidating the aetiology of the pain before deciding on the therapy was confirmed in a clinical randomised study. Raphael and Marbach (2001) randomly divided 63 women into a group with a balanced splint and a group with a palatal splint with no occlusal interference. They found that the patients with localised pain experienced pain relief with the balanced splint, whereas the patients with widespread pain did not respond to either splint. The lack of differentiation of patients with widespread and localised pain in most studies doubtless also contributes to the explanation of the controversies regarding TMD and occlusion.

In the case of an anterior disc displacement, the hours in which a splint is worn daily also influences the result. Davies and Gray (1997a, 1997b) studied 70 patients diagnosed with an anterior disc displacement and assigned them randomly to nightwear, daywear or full-time wear of a repositioning splint. Among the patients using their splint full-time, a significantly higher percentage had improvement compared with either nighttime or daytime wear. When repeating the study, this time with a stabilising splint, the result was even better and again full-time wear was the most efficient.

Splint therapy, if leading to a successful result, must be followed by the establishment of an occlusion corresponding to the mandibular position in which the patient is symptom-free for a longer period. The following possibilities are then available: (a) equilibration; (b) conservative restorative therapy; (c) major occlusal rehabilitation; (d) orthodontics combined with options (a), (b) or (c) or (e) orthognathic surgery combined with any of the other therapies. Independent of the type of treatment, the main issue is that the mandibular position is maintained and that it represents the correct condyle–fossa relationship.

Occlusal adjustments should not be done before the mandibular position is established. The malocclusion

Table 15.1 Treatment success

Author	Splint type	Number of patients	Success rate (pain)		Success rate (click)	
			Initially	Later	Initially	Later
Carraro and Caffesse (1978)	Flat	170	37%	45%		
Okeson et al. (1982)	Flat	33	85%			
Lundh et al. (1988a)	Reposition	20	95%		95%	26%
	Flat	21	60%		25%	0
	No treatment	223	0%		25%	0
Moloney and Howard (1986)	Reposition	241			70%	36%
Lundh et al. (1988b)	Onlay	15	82%	82%	82%	
Okeson (1988)	Reposition	40	80%	55%	80%	25%
Ghafari et al. (1988)	Reposition	13	38%		38%	
	Physiotherapy	44	59%		59%	
	Control	15	33%		33%	
Lous (1978)	Pivot	60	72%		72%	

presented by the patient with TMD at the first visit may not be the one that has to be treated if the habitual occlusion is the result of a forced bite. As an example, the patient in Figure 15.4 has an edge-to-edge incisal relationship, a crossbite on the right side and a lower midline discrepancy of about 3 mm to the right. Following the splint therapy and several adjustments of the splint, the malocclusion changed character. Displacement of the condyle in an upwards and forwards direction took place leaving the patient with an open bite and midline discrepancy of about the same magnitude as before, but this was now the malocclusion to be treated.

The importance of the distribution of occlusal contacts mentioned in the earlier text is supported by a randomised controlled study in which half of a group of orthodontically treated patients were equilibrated following orthodontics and the other half were not. The equilibrated group had significantly fewer patients with TMD after treatment than the control group (Karjalainen et al. 1997).

Treatment of clicking joints

Patients seek orthodontic treatment not only for resolution or reduction in pain but also with a desire to get rid of a click in the joint (Figure 15.5).

However, the possibility of treating a functional disturbance in TMD is also a matter of controversy, especially the treatment of a clicking joint. Some authors claim that clicking can be treated, while others refrain from treatment. Roberts et al. (1988) reported that in 72 patients with a clicking joint only 53 could be ascribed to a disc displacement with reduction and only these had a chance of being treated. Ronquillo et al. (1988) found that 72 out of 142 patients were candidates for repositioning. Among the factors mentioned to have an influence are age; sex; general health; social status; psychological profile; education; dental care; parafunction and facial morphology.

In the patient presenting with a click of the joint as the primary problem, it should be verified whether the click can be treated with changes to the occlusion before embarking on an orthodontic treatment which may not solve the problem. The patient in Figure 15.5 complained about a very loud click, which interfered with her social life. A flat splint did not result in any change in the mandibular posture, but after having tested the resilience of the joint, it was decided to attempt distraction of the condyle out of the fossa using onlays on the posterior part of the splint. This led to disappearance of the clicking and a repositioning splint was cemented in the lower arch, while the midline was corrected by extraction of the first upper right premolar and retraction of the canine into a neutral occlusion. Following correction of the upper arch, a retention splint that kept the condylar position was inserted in the upper arch and in the lower arch, the molars and premolars were extruded with cantilevers and the lower anterior teeth were proclined and intruded while the splint thickness was gradually reduced. The necessary occlusal rehabilitation was indicated by the composite onlays left in the lower arch after treatment.

Orthodontic treatment of patients with TMD

Although orthodontics has been accused of generating TMD, no valid studies support this statement (Gianelly 1989). The prevalence of functional disturbance in a population treated with orthodontics is reported as both reduced and unaltered (Henrikson and Nilner 2003; Luther 2007a). Case reports documented both curing and development of TMD as a result of orthodontic treatments (Reynders 1990).

Orthodontic treatment of patients with TMD, with a few exceptions, should only be initiated when the structural position of the mandible, where the muscles and joint function are in physiological harmony, has been established.

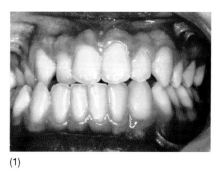 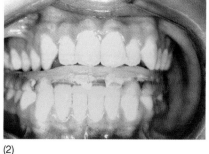 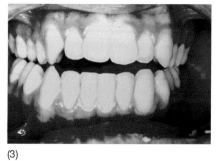

(1) (2) (3)

Fig. 15.4 (1) Patient with head-on occlusion, crossbite on the right side and a midline discrepancy. (2) As the patient had severe muscle tenderness especially of the temporal and the pterygoid muscles, she was given a flat balanced splint in the anticipation of a relocation of the midline. This did not happen, but after a short period, the bite started opening and acrylic onlays were added to the splint to maintain a balanced occlusal contact. (3) When the treatment was stopped, the patient had developed significant bite opening. The midline discrepancy was still present, but the patient had no muscle tension when the splint was worn. In order to establish an occlusion with the condyles maintained in this position, combined orthognathic surgery and orthodontic treatment was required.

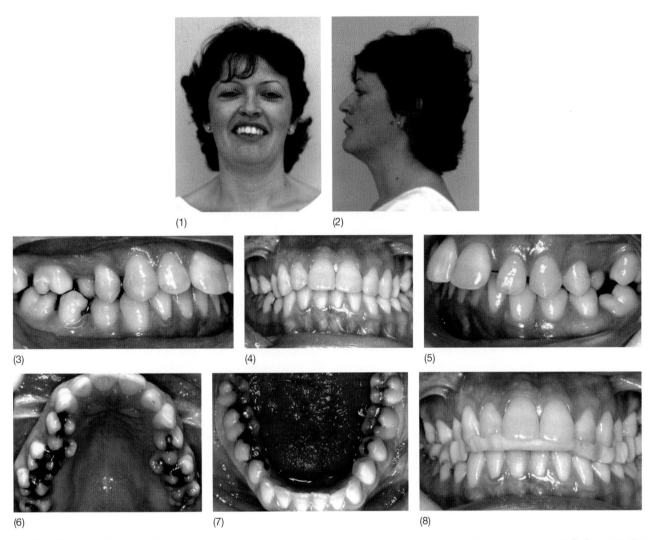

Fig. 15.5 (1) and (2) Patient with severe clicking that interfered with her social life. An axiographic examination revealed an anterior and medial disc displacement relative to the left condyle. The click occurred when the condyle was passing the compressed posterior rim of the disc, whereas during the sliding away of the condyle from the disc on closure, the click could be registered but not heard. (3)–(7) Intraoral images before treatment. Three molars had been extracted and the second upper premolars were rotated 180°. The canine relationship was distal on the right side and neutral on the left side, and the upper midline was 2 mm to the left of the facial midline. The patient had increased overjet and overbite with palatal impingement. (8) A flat fully balanced splint was inserted in the lower jaw for full-time use. As there was no change in the mandibular position in the sagittal and transverse planes, a downwards distraction of the condyle within the fossa was attempted by increasing the thickness of the posterior part of the splint. (9)–(12) The distraction splint was fabricated from a thin, fully balanced splint. Aluminium foil of thickness corresponding to the amount of distraction desired was added in the housing of the articulator. A posterior open bite was thereby generated and filled with composite, whereby the condyle would be lowered corresponding to the thickness of the aluminium foil. It is important that the foil is not thicker than the resilience of the joint, that is, the capacity of the condyle to be lowered within the fossa. The click disappeared with this treatment and the splint was modified into a repositioning splint. (13) and (14) The overjet and the midline discrepancy were corrected by extraction of a right upper premolar. While the space was being closed, the mandibular position was maintained by the splint in the lower jaw. (15) and (16) Following space closure, the upper midline coincided with the lower, which was also in harmony with the facial midline. As a result of the condylar distraction, an open bite developed in the posterior region. This was corrected by cantilever mechanics applying a combination of uprighting and extrusive forces on the second molars and desired proclination of the lower incisors. The same procedure was used to extrude the premolars. (17)–(24) Following treatment, small onlays were left in the lower arch in order to indicate where occlusal rehabilitation was necessary. (25)–(28) Five years post treatment. Although the patient did not undergo full rehabilitation, the occlusion was stable with no more clicking affecting the patient's social life. A follow-up axiography could not confirm whether the disc had been repositioned; it is more likely the distance between the bottom of the fossa and the condyle generated by the distraction-prevented compression of the posterior margin of the disc.

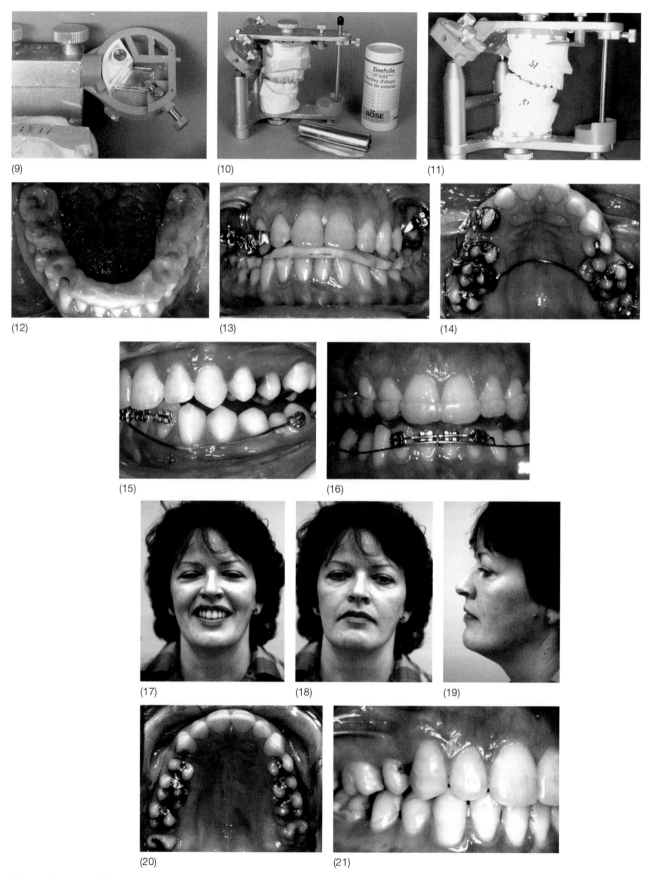

(9)

(10)

(11)

(12)

(13)

(14)

(15)

(16)

(17)

(18)

(19)

(20)

(21)

Fig. 15.5 (*Continued*)

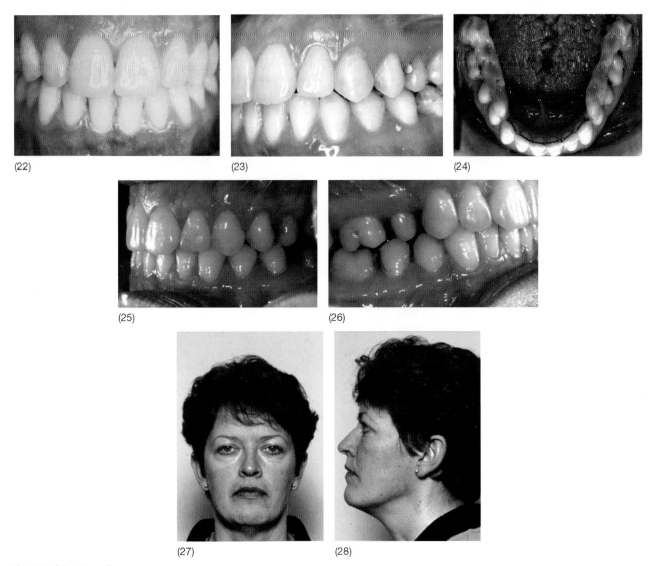

(22)   (23)   (24)

(25)   (26)

(27)   (28)

Fig. 15.5 *(Continued)*

In some cases, this position cannot be found until after initial orthodontic treatment for relieving occlusal interferences. This applies to patients with retroclined incisors, in whom the mandible is forced posteriorly (Figure 15.6). Abrasion facets on the incisors will often indicate if this is the case. If the bite is also very deep, the splint necessary to release the forced bite will often be unacceptably high, and although relieved from symptoms from the joint, the patients may experience muscle symptoms indicating the lack of acceptance of the bite height. Therefore, the mandibular position in these patients cannot be established until after proclination and possible intrusion of the guiding teeth. This may also apply to lateral deep bite (see Chapter 8, Case 2 on the companion website at www.wiley.com/go/melsen).

Having established the desired mandibular position, the main goal is to maintain this position and therefore it is frequently necessary to treat one arch at a time (Figure 15.7).

The type of appliance chosen for the treatment is not crucial as long as it can be used to establish an occlusion compatible with the correct mandibular position. The young woman in Figure 15.8 had developed severe symptoms after orthodontic treatment. The questionnaire indicated that she had severe pain in both joints and several sore muscles (Table 15.2). She presented with a midline discrepancy, but midline was centred during maximal opening. She seemed to be satisfied with her occlusion, as the incisors that were aligned crowding had been the main cause for seeking orthodontic treatment initially. The lower right premolar was missing and the space had been closed, and a scissors bite had developed in the right side. An axiographic analysis revealed normal movement in the right joint, whereas very limited rotational movement only was occurring on the left side. The tomograms of the joints showed that the right condyle was in posterior location, whereas the left

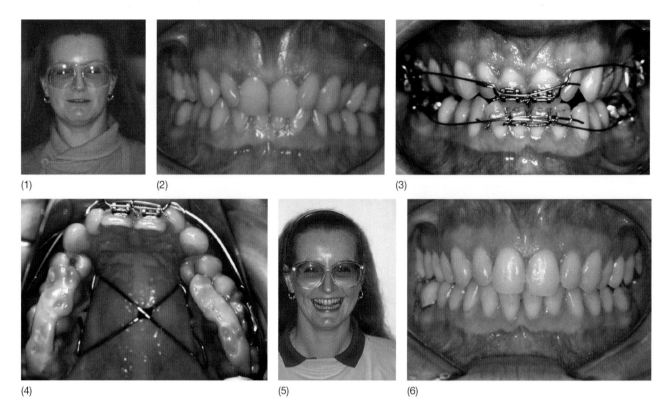

Fig. 15.6 Patient with posterior forced bite and severe tension headache. (1) and (2) Before treatment. The occlusion was characterised by retroclined incisors and a deep bite. Both upper and lower incisors exhibited abrasion facets, reflecting a posterior forced bite, which was also confirmed by the clinical examination. (3) and (4) Bite opening with occlusal onlays and a utility-shaped base arch for intrusion and proclination of the upper incisors. During this bite opening, and proclination of the incisors and canines, the mandible came forward spontaneously. The structural position of the mandible was maintained by onlays bonded to the occlusal surfaces. (5) and (6) Patient following treatment.

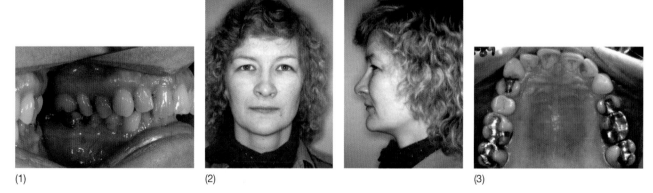

Fig. 15.7 (1)–(4) This patient had one upper premolar on the right side and one lower premolar on the left side extracted in relation to prior orthodontic treatment. Following the treatment, the patient had developed severe TMD. She had tinnitus, globus sensation and severe pain in the left condylar area. (3) and (4) As a result of the unilateral extraction, both arches were asymmetrical at the beginning of the treatment. (5) Occlusion before treatment (6 and 7). The patient was fitted with a splint, with which she was symptom-free. (8) Panoramic radiograph demonstrating symmetrical condyles. (9–13) Appliance used in the upper jaw for space opening in the region of the extracted premolar on the left side. During this part of the treatment, the mandibular position was maintained with a splint in the lower jaw. (14) Once the upper arch had been treated, a splint was made for the upper arch and space opening was performed in the lower jaw with a cantilever extending from the right to the left side. (15)–(20) Post-treatment situation.

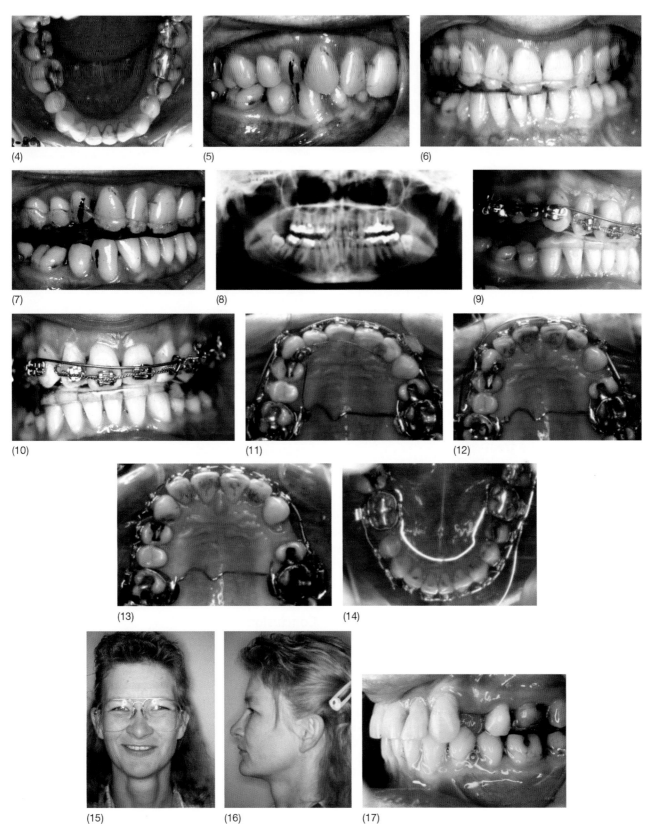

(4)

(5)

(6)

(7)

(8)

(9)

(10)

(11)

(12)

(13)

(14)

(15)

(16)

(17)

Fig. 15.7 (*Continued*)

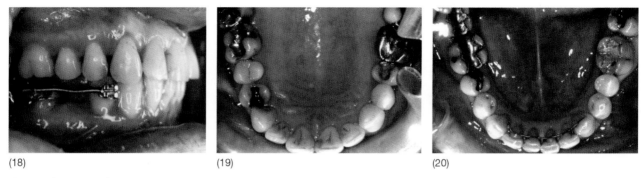

(18)   (19)   (20)

Fig. 15.7 (Continued)

condyle was centrally placed. With an open mouth, however, it was obvious that no translation occurred on the left side. On the contrary, the left condyle was displaced more dorsally during opening, while the right condyle was translating downwards and forwards. The patient was provided with a splint with built-in distraction of the condyle on the left side and the coordination of the two arches was initiated with Crozat appliance (Herrmann 1987; Baranko 1993).

Organisation of the treatment

Based on the above-mentioned considerations, the following treatment approach is suggested. The establishment of centric relation may need the assistance of physiotherapist and it is advisable to request a pain specialist to determine whether orthodontic treatment will be beneficial. In the case of severe muscle tension, physiotherapy eventually supplemented by medication may be recommended (see Chapter 16). In the cases of forced bite and deep bite, it may be difficult to establish the correct vertical and sagittal positions and the mandible and the structural position will be found only during treatment, when the teeth leading to the forced bite have been displaced. Occlusal coverage, which is gradually removed along with the proclination of the upper and lower incisors, is preferred in these cases (Figure 15.6).

Once the mandibular position is established, it should be maintained during treatment. Therefore, orthodontic treatment often has to be done in one jaw at a time, while maintaining the position with a bonded splint. Following orthodontic treatment, occlusal rehabilitation will be required in most cases to adapt the teeth to the new

Table 15.2 Muscle findings for the patient in Figure 15.8.

Muscle group	Findings	
	Right	Left
Anterior temporal	xxx	xxx
Medial temporal	xx	xxx
Posterior temporal		
Lateral pterygoid	xxx	xxx
Masseter	xx	xxx
Medial pterygoid	xxx	xxx
Digastric	xx	xxx
Suprahyoid		
Infrahyoid	x	x
Sternocleidomastoid		

x = mild pain; xx = middle pain; xxx = severe pain.

occlusion. Restorations carried out before orthodontics should be made as temporaries and should help maintain the repositioning of the mandible, in order to maintain the mandible in one position.

Conclusion

The unresolved conflict between those who deny any significance of occlusion in the aetiology of TMD and those who assign major importance to occlusion still exists. The conflict can to a large extent be explained by the methods used in the published studies. Numerous case reports have demonstrated that orthodontics can be an integrated part of treatment of TMD. However, if the orthodontic treatment results in an occlusion that is not in concordance with centric relation, it may also have a detrimental effect.

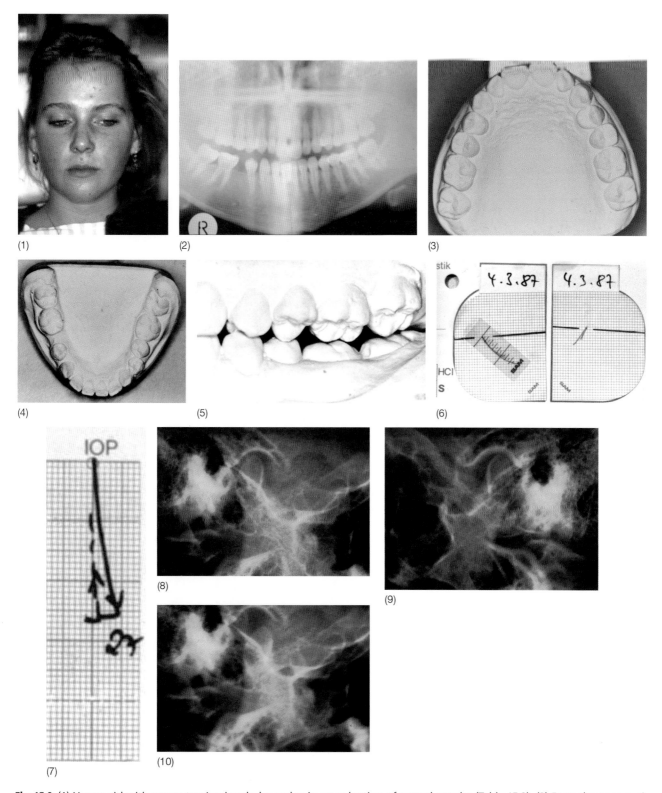

Fig. 15.8 (1) Young girl with severe tension headache and pain on palpation of several muscles (Table 15.2). (2) From the panoramic radiograph, it can be seen that the second lower premolar was missing on the right side. The space in the region of the missing tooth had been partially closed as part of earlier orthodontic correction of crowding in the lower arch. (3)–(5) The study casts demonstrated a transverse discrepancy and scissors bite on the left side involving the second premolar and both molars. (6) and (7) Jaw tracking demonstrated decreased translation of the left condyle. (8) and (9) Tomograms of the temporomandibular joints demonstrated that both condyles were placed in the upper posterior part of the fossa. (10) and (11) During mouth-opening, normal movement was seen on the right side, whereas the mobility of the left condyle was limited to a slight downwards movement. (12)–(15) A repositioning splint was used to re-establish symmetrical condylar positions and the appliance used for this was a combination of the repositioning splint and Crozat appliance. (16)–(18) The appliance in place in the mouth. (19)–(21) Progress obtained with the appliance. (22) At this stage, the treatment could be finished with a fixed appliance, without influencing the intermaxillary position.

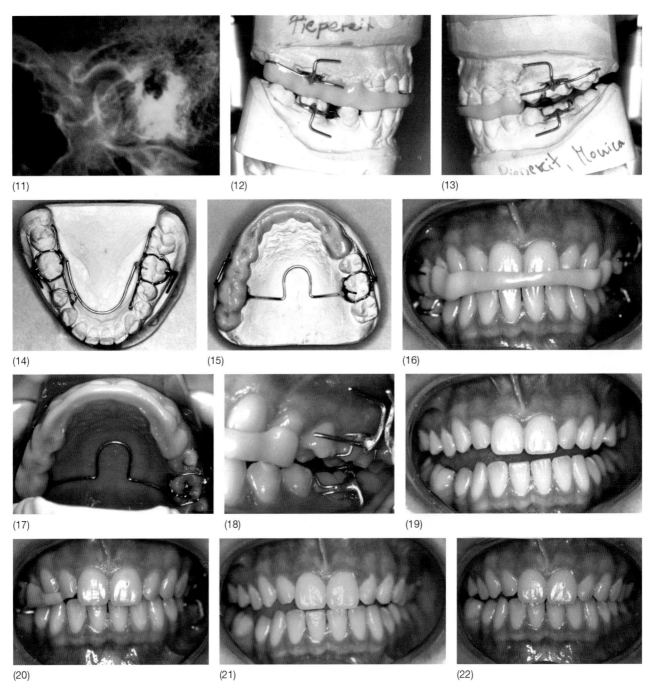

(11) (12) (13)
(14) (15) (16)
(17) (18) (19)
(20) (21) (22)

Fig. 15.8 (*Continued*)

References

Baranko JG (1993) Crozat therapy for orthopedic gnathology. *J Am Acad Gnathol Orthop* 10, 5–8, 13.

Bertolami CN, Gay T, Clark GT, Rendell J, Shetty V, Liu C and Swann DA (1993) Use of sodium hyaluronate in treating temporomandibular joint disorders: a randomized, double-blind, placebo-controlled clinical trial. *J Oral Maxillofac Surg* 51, 232–242.

Bumann A and Lotzmann U (2002) *TMJ Disorders and Orofacial Pain. The Role of Dentistry in a Multidisciplinary Diagnostic Approach.* Stuttgart: Thieme.

Carraro JJ and Caffesse RG (1978) Effect of occlusal splints on TMJ symptomatology. *J Prosthet Dent* 40(5), 563–566.

Chandler GN and Wright V (1958) Deleterious effect of intra-articular hydrocortisone. *Lancet* 2, 661–663.

Cordray FE (2002) The importance of the seated condylar position in orthodontic correction. *Quintessence Int* 33, 284–293.

Davies SJ and Gray RJ (1997a) The pattern of splint usage in the management of two common temporomandibular disorders. Part III: long-term follow-up in an assessment of splint therapy in the management of disc displacement with reduction and pain dysfunction syndrome. *Br Dent J* 183, 279–283.

Davies SJ and Gray RJ (1997b) The pattern of splint usage in the management of two common temporomandibular disorders. Part I: the anterior repositioning splint in the treatment of disc displacement with reduction. *Br Dent J* 183, 199–203.

Dolwick MF (2007) Temporomandibular joint surgery for internal derangement. *Dent Clin North Am* 51, 195–viii.

Dworkin SF and LeResche L (1992) Research diagnostic criteria for temporomandibular disorders: review, criteria examinations and specifications, critique. *J Craniomandib Disord* 6, 301–355.

Ghafari J, Clark RE, Shofer FS and Berman PH (1988) Dental and occlusal characteristics of children with neuromuscular disease. *Am J Orthod Dentofacial Orthop* 93(2), 126–132.

Gianelly AA (1989) Orthodontics, condylar position, and TMJ status. *Am J Orthod Dentofacial Orthop* 95, 521–523.

Gianniri AI, Melsen B, Nielsen L and Athanasiou AE (1991) Occlusal contacts in maximum intercuspation and craniomandibular dysfunction in 16- to 17-year-old adolescents. *J Oral Rehabil* 18, 49–59.

Henrikson T and Nilner M (2003) Temporomandibular disorders, occlusion and orthodontic treatment. *J Orthod* 30, 129–137.

Herrmann C (1987) Possibilities of the Crozat method – report of results. *Fortschr Kieferorthop* 48, 340–346.

Hiiemae KM and Palmer JB (2003) Tongue movements in feeding and speech. *Crit Rev Oral Biol Med* 14, 413–429.

Huggare J and Skindhoj B (1997) A new method for assessing masticatory performance: a feasibility and reproducibility study. *J Oral Rehabil* 24, 490–495.

Johnson NC and Sandy JR (1999) Tooth position and speech–is there a relationship? *Angle Orthod* 69, 306–310.

Karjalainen M, Le BY, Jamsa T and Karjalainen S (1997) Prevention of temporomandibular disorder-related signs and symptoms in orthodontically treated adolescents. A 3-year follow-up of a prospective randomized trial. *Acta Odontol Scand* 55, 319–324.

Kawamura M, Nojima K, Nishii Y and Yamaguchi H (2003) A cineradiographic study of deglutitive tongue movement in patients with anterior open bite. *Bull Tokyo Dent Coll* 44, 133–139.

Kimmel FP, Athanasiou AE and Melsen B (1986) The evaluation of the function of the stomatognathic system using combination of 3-dimensional axiography, sirognathography, electromyography and photo-occlusion. *Orthod Fr* 57(Pt 2), 593–604.

Kopp S, Carlsson GE, Haraldson T and Wenneberg B (1987) Long-term effect of intra-articular injections of sodium hyaluronate and corticosteroid on temporomandibular joint arthritis. *J Oral Maxillofac Surg* 45, 929–935.

Kopp S, Wenneberg B, Haraldson T and Carlsson GE (1985) The short-term effect of intra-articular injections of sodium hyaluronate and corticosteroid on temporomandibular joint pain and dysfunction. *J Oral Maxillofac Surg* 43, 429–435.

Laine T (1992) Malocclusion traits and articulatory components of speech. *Eur J Orthod* 14, 302–309.

Lous I (1978) Treatment of TMJ syndrome by pivots. *J Prosthet Dent* 40(2), 179–182.

Lundh H, Westesson PL, Jisander S and Eriksson L (1988b) Disk-repositioning onlays in the treatment of temporomandibular joint disk displacement: comparison with a flat occlusal splint and with no treatment. *Oral Surg Oral Med Oral Pathol* 66(2), 155–162.

Lundh H, Westesson PL, Rune B and Selvik G (1988a) Changes in mandibular position during treatment with disk-repositioning onlays: a roentgen stereophotogrammetric study. *Oral Surg Oral Med Oral Pathol* 65(6), 657–662.

Luther F (2007a) TMD and occlusion part I. Damned it we do? Occlusion: the interface of dentistry and orthodontics. *Br Dent J* 202, E2–E9.

Luther F (2007b) TMD and occlusion part II. Damned it we don't? Functional occlusal problems: TMD epidemiology in a wider context. *Br Dent J* 202, E3–E9.

Mehnert T (1987) Investigations on the relation of dysgnathias and S-sound pronunciation. *J Oral Rehabil* 14, 95–103.

Moloney F and Howard JA (1986) Internal derangements of the temporomandibular joint. III. Anterior repositioning splint therapy. *Aust Dent J* 31(1), 30–39.

Okeson JP (1988) Long-term treatment of disk-interference disorders of the temporomandibular joint with anterior repositioning occlusal splints. *J Prosthet Dent* 60(5), 611–616.

Okeson JP, Kemper JT and Moody PM (1982) A study of the use of occlusion splints in the treatment of acute and chronic patients with craniomandibular disorders. *J Prosthet Dent* 48(6), 708–712.

Pahkala RH and Qvarnstrom MJ (2002) Mandibular movement capacity in 19-year-olds with and without articulatory speech disorders. *Acta Odontol Scand* 60, 341–345.

Piehslinger E, Celar AG, Celar RM and Slavicek R (1991) Computerized axiography: principles and methods. *J Craniomandib Pract* 9, 344–355.

Raphael KG and Marbach JJ (2001) Widespread pain and the effectiveness of oral splints in myofascial face pain. *J Am Dent Assoc* 132, 305–316.

Reynders RM (1990) Orthodontics and temporomandibular disorders: a review of the literature (1966–1988). *Am J Orthod Dentofacial Orthop* 97, 463–471.

Roberts CA, Katzberg RW, Tallents RH, Espeland MA and Handelman SL (1988) Correlation of clinical parameters to the arthrographic depiction of temporomandibular joint internal derangements. *Oral Surg Oral Med Oral Pathol* 66, 32–36.

Ronquillo HI, Guay J, Tallents RH, Katzberg R, Murphy W and Proskin H (1988) Comparison of condyle-fossa relationships with unsuccessful protrusive splint therapy. *J Craniomandib Disord* 2, 178–180.

Roth RH (1995) Occlusion and condylar position. *Am J Orthod Dentofacial Orthop* 107, 315–318.

Santacatterina A, Paoli M, Peretta R, Bambace A and Beltrame A (1998) A comparison between horizontal splint and repositioning splint in the treatment of 'disc dislocation with reduction'. Literature meta-analysis. *J Oral Rehabil* 25, 81–88.

Simonet PF and Clayton JA (1981) Influence of TMJ dysfunction on Bennett movement as recorded by a modified pantograph. Part III: progress report on the clinical study. *J Prosthet Dent* 46, 652–661.

Tallgren A, Melsen B and Hansen MA (1979) An electromyographic and roentgen cephalometric study of occlusal morphofunctional disharmony in children. *Am J Orthod* 76, 394–409.

Wenneberg B, Kopp S and Grondahl HG (1991) Long-term effect of intra-articular injections of a glucocorticosteroid into the TMJ: a clinical and radiographic 8-year follow-up. *J Craniomandib Disord* 5, 11–18.

16

Patients with Temporomandibular Disorders

Peter Svensson, Fernando G. Exposto

Introduction

Essentially, there are two distinct views on how orthodontics and temporomandibular disorders (TMD) relate to each other: A traditional view holds that abnormal occlusal traits impinge on the function of the jaw muscles and the temporomandibular joint (TMJ), leading to 'dysfunctional' movements and abnormal muscle recruitment which then cause pain in the overloaded tissue. From this, a logical approach will be to correct the malocclusion, for example, by orthodontic means. The second and opposite view challenges this relationship and basically disconnects occlusal traits from any relationship to TMD pain problems. Can both views be wrong or right? Controversies should not be clouded by personal beliefs, emotions, traditions or professional politics, but rather resolved by critical examination of the evidence in favour of or against the hypothesis. The present chapter is an attempt briefly to summarise what is known about TMD pain problems with implications for orthodontics, and also

to point out significant questions and issues which may not be answered or guided by the highest level of evidence yet, but where patient-based concerns and clinical experience must be used in the prudent management of individual patients.

Classification and epidemiology

The definition and terminology of TMD pain continues to be debated even more than six decades after Costen's original description of a pain syndrome involving the TMJ. Problems with pain and soreness in the jaw muscles, noises such as clicking and crepitation in the TMJ and difficulties in moving the jaw – usually restrictions in opening capacity – as well as signs of dental attrition and oral habits with tooth grinding or tooth clenching have in the past been lumped into many different categories and labelled various names such as 'myofascial pain dysfunction', 'temporomandibular joint dysfunction' 'craniomandibular disorders', 'oromandibular disorders' and bruxism. Different disciplines and professional groups tend to favour their own classification systems, which basically are based on clusters of different signs and symptoms. This may seem a trivial point, but nonetheless also important because the many different classification systems have contributed to difficulties to make comparisons between studies and have hampered the communication between clinicians and researchers. There is therefore an urgent need to apply a common universal classification system for TMD problems. Although the pathophysiological mechanisms may not be sufficiently understood at this point in time (see later) and there may be no perfect way to classify TMD pain, a non-hierarchical classification scheme based on operationalised and systematic criteria has been developed and extensively tested for reliability and validity (Dworkin and LeResche 1992; Pehling

Adult Orthodontics, Second Edition. Edited by Birte Melsen and Cesare Luzi.
© 2022 John Wiley & Sons Ltd. Published 2022 by John Wiley & Sons Ltd.
Companion Website: http://www.wiley.com/go/melsen-adult-orthodontics

et al. 2002; John et al. 2005). These Research Diagnostic Criteria (RDC/TMD) have indeed been a starting point for international collaborations and new clinical research in TMD pain, and can also rationally be applied in daily clinical practice. In 2014, the RDC/TMD was upgraded to the Diagnostic Criteria for Temporomandibular Disorders (DC/TMD) (Schiffman et al. 2014a), and in 2020, all orofacial pain conditions were classified in the International Classification of Orofacial Pain (ICOP 2020). The ICOP divides the most common TMD such as myofascial pain and joint pain into primary and secondary as well as including non-TMD pain conditions such as dental, oral mucosal, salivary and jaw bone pain, orofacial pain due to lesion or disease of the cranial nerves, orofacial pain resembling presentation of primary headaches and idiopathic orofacial pain. Non-painful TMD such as disc displacement with and without reduction as well as subluxation can be diagnosed according to the DC/TMD (Schiffman et al. 2014a). Less common TMD such as ankylosis, systemic arthritides and idiopathic condylar resorption can be diagnosed according to the expanded version of the DC/TMD (Peck et al. 2014). The lack of generally accepted diagnostic criteria across disciplines for TMD is most likely the reason why epidemiology surveys have provided quite different estimates of prevalence and incidence (Carlsson and LeResche 1995; LeResche 1997).

The descriptive epidemiology has indicated that between 3% and 19% of the population will qualify for a TMD pain diagnosis (LeResche 1997; Drangsholt and LeResche 1999; Jussila et al. 2017). Few studies have tried to separate TMJ pain from myofascial TMD pain, but the latter appears to be less prevalent than the former (Drangsholt and LeResche 1999); however, a study using the DC/TMD found that the prevalence for myalgia and arthralgia was quite similar, around 5% (Jussila et al. 2017). Most studies have found that TMD pain is 1.5–2 times more prevalent in women. However, it is critical to distinguish between the number of TMD cases presenting in the clinic and the number of TMD cases in the community because treatment-seeking patterns and use of health services may bias a biological sex difference (Warren and Fried 2001; Svensson and Sessle 2004). In addition, the Orofacial Pain: Prospective Evaluation and Risk Assessment (OPPERA) studies found that TMD is more prevalent in women than men. However, the incidence was the same for both genders (Slade et al. 2011, 2013). This means that gender most likely plays a role in the persistence of TMD pain and less so in its initiation. The prevalence of TMD across the lifetime is still debated, but there seems to be a peak around 20–45 years for women, although also elderly people may suffer from TMD pain (Riley et al. 1998; Schmitter et al. 2005a; Slade et al. 2013). For some types of TMD problems such as degenerative joint disease (DJD), there seems to be an increase over the lifespan. There are a few good studies on the incidence of TMD problems (i.e., number of new TMD cases per time unit usually per year). There is some evidence that the incidence is in the range of 2–4% with the persistent types being around 0.1% (Drangsholt and LeResche 1999). The OPPERA study is the most extensive study on the incidence of TMD as well as on the risk factors that can lead to painful TMD incidence and/or persistence. In the study, the incidence of painful TMD was 3.9% (Slade et al. 2013) with 2% of cases being persistent (Slade et al. 2016). Knowledge about the epidemiology of TMD is essential for clinicians to have in mind because it also provides clues about the natural progression of the disorder. Some longitudinal studies have shown substantial variations in the time course of myofascial TMD (Rammelsberg et al. 2003) with 31% being persistent over a 5-year period, 33% being remittent and 36% recurring. Asymptomatic clicks in the TMJ (disc displacement with reduction – DDwR) are very common (10–35%) (Kononen et al. 1996; LeResche 1997), but have been shown very rarely to progress to disc displacement without reduction (DDwoR), in fact none of the 114 adolescents that were followed over a 9-year period progressed from DDwR to DDwoR (Kononen et al. 1996). Interestingly, this study indicated major fluctuation also in the presence and absence of a DDwR, so that only 2% of the examined population had a consistent click at all examination points during the 9-year study period (Kononen et al. 1996). This strongly indicates that asymptomatic DDwR should be managed by conservative techniques. Other studies have shown that patients with combined diagnosis of DDwR and arthralgia may have a higher risk to progress to a DDwoR (Lundh et al. 1987; Sato et al. 2003). Careful considerations of the treatment options are mandatory in this situation, but generally the least invasive technique should be chosen, since the long-term outcome of more extensive procedures including prosthodontics, orthodontics and surgery is highly questionable (see later).

It is a common clinical experience that ethnical and cultural factors may influence the presentation of TMD problems. However, so far these issues have not received much attention even though it appears that psychological status and pain-related disability (Axis II findings) are more likely to vary between races and ethnic groups than the physical TMD status (Axis I findings) (Moore and Brødsgaard 1999; Plesh et al. 2005; Reiter et al. 2006). Interestingly, the OPPERA study found that the rate of TMD was 52% greater in African Americans than Caucasians (Slade et al. 2016). Estimates from current studies suggest that 3–4% of the Western population may demand management of a TMD problem (Magnusson et al. 2002), making this type of functional problem significant to consider in contemporary oral rehabilitation.

Diagnostic procedures

Axis I

At this stage, it is appropriate to consider in more details the proposed DC/TMD questionnaires and examination form. Readers can find a complete manual of the procedures on the Internet address https://ubwp.buffalo.edu/rdc-tmdinternational and can download the questionnaires and examination forms for free.

For a quick and reliable assessment of painful TMD, the DC/TMD recommends the use of the TMD Pain Screener, which is a 6-item questionnaire (Gonzalez et al. 2011). Another validated questionnaire that allows for a painful TMD diagnosis is the 3Q/TMD (Lövgren et al. 2017). Even though these questionnaires do not allow for a specific TMD diagnosis to be made, they can be used by clinicians who are not trained in the DC/TMD or who do not have time to do the examination to assess if the patient needs to be referred to a colleague with orofacial pain training.

For an experienced examiner, the physical examination of the patient for potential TMD problems may take no more than 10–12 minutes. The specific items in the examination form may not differ substantially from other forms except that the conditions, for example, how the patient is sitting, exactly where the palpation is done, how much pressure is applied, how many times the open–close movements are repeated, have all been carefully described and should be followed exactly by the examiner in order to obtain an accurate and reliable outcome. This may require training and calibration, and recent studies have highlighted the importance of calibration and recalibration (Schmitter et al. 2005b; List et al. 2006). Training videos are also available on the DC/TMD Internet site and the interested readers are referred to this. The strength of the DC/TMD is that specific diagnostic algorithms have been developed. For example, to establish a painful diagnosis, the DC/TMD requires a positive answer to questions 1 and 2 of the DC/TMD symptom questionnaire, as well as examiner confirmation of pain location and familiar pain provoked by either jaw opening or palpation of the masticatory muscles and/or TMJ. The novelty is the addition of the concept of familiar pain, which allows confirmation that the provoked pain is the same the patient experiences in their daily life and not just due to excessive pressure applied during palpation. In addition, palpation force and duration have been standardised. Regarding force, the masseter and temporalis muscles should be palpated with 1 kg, whereas the TMJ, lateral pterygoid area, temporalis tendon, submandibular region and posterior mandibular region should be palpated with 0.5 kg. Regarding duration, for the diagnoses of myofascial or TMJ pain, the palpation should be done for 2 seconds, whereas for the diagnosis of referred pain, the palpation should be done for 5 seconds.

Thus, the DC/TMD system uses stringent and well-characterised criteria for the most usual types of *manifest* TMD problems, and the extensive translation to many languages helps to disseminate the system so that both researchers in the field and clinicians treating patients can benefit from a consensus on the terminology. This is predicted to have major impact on the future understanding of TMD pathophysiology and etiological factors as well as management strategies.

Assessment of pain

Pain is one of the main characteristics of many of the different types of TMD (myofascial TMD pain and TMJ arthralgias) and needs to be evaluated carefully. It is important to note that the DC/TMD questionnaire and examination form also include quantitative measures of the perceived pain intensity using rating scales such as the numerical rating scales (NRS) and visual analogue scales (VAS). Because a simple VAS may not capture the entire complexity of a patient's pain experience, it has been suggested that a composite measure such as the characteristic pain intensity (CPI), derived from the first 3 questions of the Graded Chronic Pain Scale (GCPS), which is the average of the present, worst and average pain in the last time period, is used. Additional VAS scores can provide useful information on both the perceived intensity and unpleasantness of clinical pain conditions because pain intensity mainly reflects the sensory-discriminative component of pain, whereas unpleasantness provides information on the hedonic character of pain, that is, the affective and emotional dimensions of pain. Clinical studies on persistent TMD pain generally indicate that the average pain level measured on a 10-cm VAS with the jaws at rest ranges between 3 cm and 5 cm (Svensson and Graven-Nielsen 2001), probably representing 'moderate' pain levels (Collins et al. 1997). The perceived pain intensity of TMD patients is often fluctuating and there can be significant differences between the lowest, the highest and the average pain VAS scores during a week (Maixner et al. 1998) and even between different facial sites (Carlson et al. 1998). Therefore, the use of pain diaries can be helpful to estimate the pain, since the perceived pain intensity of TMD patients can change over time simply due to regression to the mean (Whitney and Von Korff 1992). The use of pain diaries is for example a cornerstone in the evaluation of headache patients, and the International Headache Society (ICHD-3 2018) classification uses the intensity dimension of the headache to separate between migraine, which is labelled as 'strong pain', and tension-type headache, which more often is described as 'moderate pain'. It is obvious that many internal as well as external factors can affect the VAS scores of perceived pain intensity in the clinic. Nevertheless, subjective reports of pain are the yardstick of pain measurement (Gracely 2006). Continued efforts should be made to distinguish between the perceived pain intensity in the different TMD subgroups. It should be noted that a DC/TMD Axis I version for children and adolescents has been proposed (Rongo et al. 2021) and there are also pain scales available for children with good evidence that these can be reliably used and provide clinically meaningful data (McGrath and Unruh 2006).

In addition to the intensity of pain, the quality of pain should receive attention. The usual way to describe persistent TMD pain is a 'deep', 'dull' 'ache' sometimes with a 'boring', 'pressing' or 'tightening' type of pain (Okeson 2005). This is in contrast to the superficial types of pain (skin and mucosa) being described as 'pricking' and 'burning', or neuropathic types of pain described as 'electrical-like', paroxsymal or 'sharp' and 'burning'. In order to identify the quality of pain, checklists with adjectives are useful. The McGill Pain Questionnaire (MPQ) was originally introduced as an attempt to provide a detailed description of the quality of pain (Melzack 1975), and has since then become one of the most used pain questionnaires (Melzack and Katz 2006). Several studies have examined the validity of the structure of the MPQ, and, generally, it has an acceptable sensitivity, specificity and reliability. In addition to the qualitative description of pain, the MPQ also provides quantitative measures of the different dimensions of pain, that is, pain rating indices of the sensory, affective, evaluative and miscellaneous dimensions of pain can be calculated.

In a sample of 200 patients with persistent facial pain including TMD pain, Türp et al. (1997) found that the words 'aching', 'tight', 'throbbing', 'tender', 'exhausting', 'nagging', 'sharp' and 'tiring' were used by more than 30% of the population. The choice of 'radiating' (26%) and 'pressing' (22%) seems rather specific for TMD pain conditions compared to other pain conditions (Türp et al. 1997). Patients with myofascial TMD pain also frequently choose 'annoying' (Stohler and Lund 1995). The quality of pain appears to be markedly different between patients with myofascial TMD pain and pain in the TMJ (Mongini and Italiano 2001). It is unclear whether this difference can be explained by neurobiological factors such as activation of different nociceptive fibres in the muscle and joint tissue or may be due to higher-order cognitive–emotional differences. Thus, there are certain words which seem to be specifically related to the description of persistent TMD pain, but no word is on the other hand pathognomonic for this pain condition in a similar way that 'pulsating' has been tied to migraine and 'pressing' and 'tightening' to tension-type headache (ICHD-3 2018).

Pain from deep structures (muscle, joint, tendon, ligaments, etc.) is frequently described as diffuse and difficult to locate precisely in contrast to superficial types of pain (Mense 1993; Svensson and Sessle 2004). Thus, the perceived localisation of deep pain may be quite different from the original source of pain. This can also cause problems when TMJ pain must be differentiated from myofascial TMD pain. Pain located to the source of pain is termed local pain, whereas pain felt in a different region and/or structure away from source of pain is termed referred pain. The International Association for the Study of Pain (IASP) task force on taxonomy has not provided any official definition of referred pain, but in the orofacial region, referred pain has been described as pain in other structures and completely separated from the local pain areas (Stohler and Lund 1994). However, the validity of this definition has not been established and there could be a time- or intensity-dependent relationship between local pain in the masticatory muscles, referral of pain and spreading of pain (Svensson and Arendt-Nielsen 2000). Studies have shown that referred

pain can be elicited by palpation of the masticatory muscles of healthy individuals. It was shown that the longer the muscle is palpated, and the more intense the pain caused during palpation, the higher the chances of causing referred pain (Exposto et al. 2018; Masuda et al. 2018). These findings need to be studied in more detail in healthy controls as well as TMD patients. From a practical point of view, the DC/TMD emphasises that the examiner points to the TMJ and jaw muscles in order to help the patient determine the source of the pain. TMJ pain is similar to myofascial TMD pain based on both a patient report of ongoing pain in the TMJ or pain on opening or on excursion in addition to familiar pain on palpation. However, other functional tests (e.g., joint play, compression and provocation tests) could in the future prove to be a valuable addition to distinguish between TMJ arthralgia and myofascial TMD pain (Bumann and Lotzmann 2002).

Pain drawings made by the patients are simple, but yet useful tools to illustrate the localisation and extent of pain areas in general. Pain drawings administered on a systematic basis to patients with pain complaints in the craniofacial region have revealed that only about 20% have pain confined to this region, whereas 66% have widespread pain outside the craniofacial and cervical regions (Türp et al. 1998). Information on these concomitant sites of pain in other parts of the body is important because they could indicate comorbidity or involvement of more widespread pathophysiological mechanisms in some patients with TMD pain (Dao et al. 1997; John et al. 2003). Alternatively, the reports of pain outside the craniofacial region could to some extent be due to referral of pain (see later). In any case, the DC/TMD recommends the use of drawings of the head and face as well as a general map of other possible pain conditions in the body. Figure 16.1 shows an example of these maps applied to patients with different RDC/TMD diagnoses as well as tension-type headache for a comparison.

In summary, the key points for the diagnostic TMD procedure are to obtain information on the pain intensity using VAS or similar rating scales, and to evaluate pain quality and pain distribution using MPQ or similar instruments. The physical examination can reliably and rationally be performed by the DC/TMD.

Axis II

In addition to the operationalised criteria for the clinical examination of the jaw muscles and TMJs, which form the basis for the so-called Axis I or physical diagnosis, the DC/TMD system is remarkable in the sense that it also provides a tool to examine the consequences of pain-related disability and psychosocial distress (Axis II) (Table 16.1). Most clinicians dealing with TMD patients have experienced these psychological alterations, for example, patients seem to be depressed and with many other complaints, and will unfortunately often label such patients as 'psychogenic' or chronic pain patients. Nevertheless, the current view on persistent

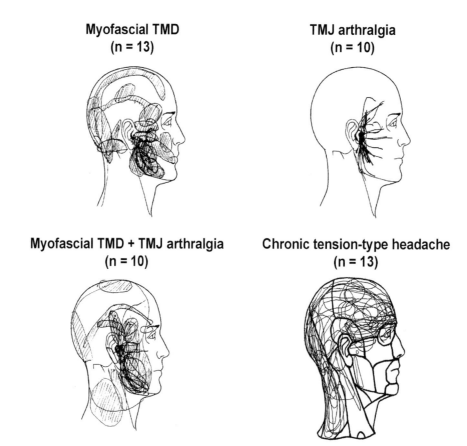

Fig. 16.1 Patient-derived pain drawings showing characteristic patterns in patients with myofascial TMD pain, TMJ, arthralgia, combined myofascial TMD pain and TMJ arthralgia and chronic tension-type headache. Note the difference between the presentation of the TMD pain and tension-type headache.

pain conditions including TMD pain problems suggests that these psychological and behavioural changes could be secondary to a long period with pain and not necessarily the cause of the pain. In most cases, it will also be impossible to identify an exact cause–effect relationship and it may be more prudent to accept that pain as defined by the IASP has emotional and cognitive–behavioural components. The DC/TMD offers the possibility for clinicians not specifically trained in clinical psychology to evaluate the amount of psychosocial distress on the second axis in the diagnostic system. Thus, the CPI (see in the earlier text) is linked to a disability score based on specific questions in the history form (Table 16.1). Based on the CPI and disability points, a 0–4 graded chronic pain scale is created (Table 16.1). The rule of thumb is that dentists in primary care should be trained to diagnose and manage graded chronic pain scale groups 1 and 2 patients, whereas specialist training and collaboration with general physicians, psychologists, psychiatrists, pain specialists and pain clinics can be recommended for groups 3 and 4 patients. It is important to realise early the involvement of psychosocial issues and adjust treatment plan and prognosis accordingly and not view psychosocial issues as a last resort when conventional therapy has failed.

There is clear evidence that recognition of pain-related disability and psychosocial factors plays an important role for outcome of management and prognosis (Dworkin et al. 2002a, 2002b; Turner and Dworkin 2004).

In addition to the GCPS and the pain drawing that have already been discussed, the DC/TMD recommends several other tools that can be used for either screening or a comprehensive assessment. The recommended tools are the Jaw Functional Limitation Scale (JFLS) to assess jaw limitation, the Patient Health Questionnaire (PHQ) 4, 9 and 15 to assess distress, depression and somatic symptoms, respectively, the Generalized Anxiety Disorder (GAD-7) questionnaire to assess anxiety and the Oral Behavior Checklist (OBC) to assess parafunction. Details Axis II instruments can be found in Table 16.1. This approach with early characterisation of the pain not only in a somatic manner (Axis I) but also in a more comprehensive biopsychosocial way (Suvinen et al. 2005) should be the yardstick for modern oral rehabilitation. It needs to be said that oral rehabilitation must be viewed as more than the physical reconstruction of the occlusion, but clearly also involves other biomedical and psychological approaches to bring or restore to a normal or optimal state of health.

Table 16.1 Overview on Axis I and II diagnoses based on the International Classification of Orofacial Pain (ICOP).

Axis I

ICOP TMD diagnoses

Myofascial orofacial pain

    Primary myofascial orofacial pain

        Acute primary myofascial orofacial pain

        Chronic primary myofascial orofacial pain

    Secondary myofascial orofacial pain

        Myofascial orofacial pain attributed to tendonitis

        Myofascial orofacial pain attributed to myositis

        Myofascial orofacial pain attributed to muscle spasm

Temporomandibular joint (TMJ) pain

    Primary TMJ pain

        Acute primary TMJ pain

        Chronic primary TMJ pain

    Secondary TMJ pain

        TMJ pain attributed to arthritis

        TMJ pain attributed to disc displacement

        TMJ pain attributed to degenerative joint disease

        TMJ pain attributed to subluxation

DC/TMD diagnoses

Disc displacement with reduction

Disc displacement with reduction with intermittent locking

Disc displacement without reduction with limited opening

Disc displacement without reduction without limited opening

Degenerative joint disease

Subluxation

Axis II

Pain-related disability and psychological status

I. Graded chronic pain scale score

    a. Grade 0 = no TMD pain in the prior 6 months

    b. Grade I = low disability – low-intensity pain

    c. Grade II = low disability – high-intensity pain

    d. Grade III = high disability – moderately limiting

    e. Grade IV = high disability – severely limiting

Other recommended instruments

    Jaw limitation – JFLS

    Distress – PHQ-4

    Depression – PHQ-9

    Anxiety – GAD-7

    Physical symptoms – PHQ-15

    Parafunction – OBC

JFLS = Jaw Functional Limitation Scale; PHQ = Patient Health Questionnaire; GAD = Generalized Anxiety Disorder; OBC = Oral Behavior Checklist

Table 16.2 Overview on reported risk factors for TMD pain divided into presumed predisposing, initiating and perpetuating factors.

Predisposing factors (Bair et al. 2013; Slade et al. 2013)

Comorbid pain conditions

Depression/somatisation

Bruxism/oral parafunctions

Sleep quality

Nonspecific orofacial symptoms **(fatigue, tiredness, etc.)**

Perceived limited mouth opening in the last month

Initiating factor (Sharma et al. 2019)

Incident jaw injury

Perpetuating factors (Meloto et al. 2019)

Female gender

Comorbid pain conditions

High pain intensity, frequency and duration in the previous month

Pain modified by chewing hard or tough food

Associated factors (Drangsholt and LeResche 1999; Manfredini et al. 2017)

Generalised joint hypermobility

Occlusal variables

    CR to ICP slide

    Mediotrusive interference

CR = centric relation; ICP = intercuspal contact position

indicate the probability that TMD pain and the factors are related. A stringent view on these risk factors has suggested that very few of the assumed and often clinically believed etiological factors actually meet the criteria for a statistical relationship (Table 16.2). It must also be noted that although these factors meet or are close to meet the statistical criteria, they do not necessarily indicate a straightforward cause-and-effect relationship, which is exemplified by the risk factor depression that conceivably could be an effect of persistent TMD pain rather than its cause.

The OPPERA studies have shown some interesting risk factors that can contribute differentially to the initiation and perpetuation of TMD and confirm that TMD is a multifactorial disorder. A summary of these risk factors can be found in Table 16.2.

In particular, occlusal factors have been subject to an overheated and emotional discussion and continue to be within the dental community. A small number of occlusal factors (Table 16.2) appear to be weakly associated with TMD, but for many clinicians, it is a surprise not to find more occlusal parameters on the list. Again, it must be remembered that a change in occlusion could occur as an effect of an underlying pathology (e.g., DJD leading to an anterior open bite). In particular, many clinicians are surprised not to see the deep bite as a significant risk factor because the conventional view has been that deep bite may lead to a posterior displacement of the mandible leading to TMJ clicking and degeneration associated with TMJ

Risk factors and aetiology

Modern epidemiology is far more advanced than a basic description of the prevalence and incidence of TMD symptoms and can also be used as an analytic tool. This line of research has helped identify a number of factors likely to be related to TMD pain. These factors are termed risk factors to arthralgia and myofascial TMD pain. This view would at first glance seem to gain support from a study where 320 persons were followed over 20 years and where deep bite was a significant risk factor (odds ratio 12.5) for dysfunctional problems (Carlsson et al. 2002). However, a careful reading of the conclusion shows that although there was a significant correlation between deep bite and some signs and symptoms of TMD, the study could not demonstrate that deep bite was a risk factor for clinically diagnosed TMD pain. In support of this conclusion, another study showed in 3033 persons that deep bite and anterior open bite were not associated with the cardinal signs and symptoms of TMD, that is, pain, limited opening capacity and joint sounds/noises (John et al. 2002). The current view is that dental occlusion plays only a minor, if any, role for development and maintenance of TMD pain (Pullinger et al. 1993; McNamara et al. 1995; Seligman and Pullinger 2000; Gesch et al. 2004, 2005). A recent systematic review showed that only centric relation to maximum intercuspation slide and mediotrusive interferences were associated with TMD in a robust number of studies (Manfredini et al. 2017). However, it is not known if these occlusal features are the cause or the result of TMD. A challenge for future research is to operationalise and better quantify functional aspects of occlusion, since reproducibility and validity of most occlusal examination procedures are poor to modest (Baba et al. 2000). A search for a single etiological factor in the occlusion, however, is not warranted (Green 2001), but a better understanding of how dental occlusion and function and other neurobiological/neuromuscular and psychosocial risk factors interact may still be relevant for a complete understanding of orofacial musculoskeletal pain and other localised symptoms from the masticatory system in a few and select number of TMD patients.

From an orthodontic perspective, several studies have suggested that orthodontic treatment can neither cause nor prevent most types of TMD (e.g., Egermark et al. 2003; Henriksson and Nilner 2003; Koh and Robinson 2003; Molin et al. 2004), which clearly must be appreciated when the indications for orthodontics are considered (see other chapters).

Pathophysiology

The exact pathophysiology of TMD pain is not known given the fact that multiple factors related to anatomical, psychological–psychosocial, genetic and neurobiological components seem to be involved (De Boever and Carlsson 1994; Slade et al. 2013). Thus, TMD may be viewed from a population basis as a multifactorial condition which in the individual patient actually means an idiopathic pain condition (Green 2001; Svensson and Sessle 2004; Svensson and Kumar 2016). Nevertheless, there are several studies in progress to outline some of the potential underlying

mechanisms in TMD pain and these will be described briefly in the following paragraphs. For a more detailed review of orofacial pain mechanisms, the reader is referred to recent reviews (Svensson and Sessle 2004; Benoliel et al. 2013; Svensson et al. 2015).

One of the most prominent features of painful TMDs is the report of pain on palpation of jaw muscles or TMJ. Several studies have indeed reported lower pressure pain thresholds in the jaw muscles of patients with TMD pain compared to normal subjects (Reid et al. 1994; Svensson et al. 1995, 2001; Maixner et al. 1998). The pathophysiological mechanism responsible for lower pain thresholds in deep tissues could be a sensitisation of peripheral nociceptors. Animal data have documented that deep noxious inputs cause sensitisation of the peripheral receptors (Berberich et al. 1988; Schaible 2006). Thus, endogenous substances released by tissue trauma such as bradykinin, serotonin, prostaglandins, adrenaline and hypoxia in addition to the excitatory amino acid glutamate lower the mechanical threshold of nociceptors into the innocuous range making weak stimuli able to excite nociceptors and elicit pain (Mense 1993; Cairns et al. 2001, 2003; Graven-Nielsen and Mense 2001). Furthermore, experimental myositis in animals is associated with an increased density of substance P and nerve growth factor (NGF) immunoreactive nerve fibres, which could contribute to the peripheral sensitisation process (Reinert et al. 1998; McMahon et al. 2006). Clinical studies have confirmed an increase of algogenic substances in the masseter muscle of TMD patients when compared to healthy controls such as glutamate, IL-6, IL-13 and serotonin, as well as an upregulation of serotonin receptors (Castrillon et al. 2010; Christidis et al. 2014; Louca Jounger et al. 2017). In the TMJ, a series of studies have suggested correlations between levels of serotonin, tumour necrosis factor alpha, interleukin beta and prostaglandin E2 and lower pressure pain thresholds as indices of hyperalgesia/allodynia in the TMJ (Kopp 2001).

Although peripheral sensitisation may contribute to deep tissue hyperalgesia, there is substantial evidence that sensitisation of higher-order neurons in the spinal cord or brainstem is also involved in the pathophysiological process (Hu et al. 1992; Mense 1993; Ren and Dubner 1999; Sessle 2000; Schaible 2006). The neuropharmacology of central sensitisation has been described in detail and particularly the N-methyl-D-aspartate (NMDA) and neurokinin-1 receptors and regulation of nitric oxide may play a crucial role for hyperexcitability and spontaneous hyperactivity (Mense et al. 1997; Woolf and Salter 2006). Such sites therefore also become a logical target for pharmacological treatment of orofacial musculoskeletal pain conditions. Interestingly, recent studies in animals and humans have shown that peripheral administration of the NMDA antagonist ketamine is able to block afferent discharges and pain and prevent sensitisation providing further evidence that also peripheral glutamate receptors could be involved in the pathophysiology of deep pain conditions (Cairns et al. 2003, 2006).

A yet open question regarding the lowered pressure pain thresholds in TMD patients is how site-specific and localised are these changes? A number of reports have indicated lower pressure pain thresholds outside the orofacial region (Malow et al. 1980; Maixner et al. 1998; Svensson et al. 2001). Subsequently, it has been speculated that this generalised deep hyperalgesia could be caused by dysfunction of endogenous inhibitory control systems similar to the observations of generalised hyperalgesia in tension-type headache patients (Langemark et al. 1989; Bendtsen and Treede 2005) and fibromyalgia patients (Lautenbacher et al. 1994). In the normal somatosensory system, descending inhibitory control and segmentally organised inhibitory mechanisms could partly compensate the peripheral and central sensitisation (Le Bars et al. 1979; Arendt-Nielsen et al. 1998). Animal studies have indeed suggested that deep noxious stimulation effectively can trigger these inhibitory systems and inhibit nociceptive activity in spinal dorsal horn or brainstem neurons (Gjerstad et al. 1999). On the other hand, brainstem structures such as the ventral nucleus reticularis gigantocellularis may have coincident descending inhibitory and facilitatory effects on the development of hyperexcitability in spinal dorsal horn neurons (Wei et al. 1999; Dickenson et al. 2005). Imbalance between such opposing descending modulating systems could be of importance for the variability of deep sensitivity.

Patients with myofascial TMD pain have also been found to have hyperalgesic responses to segmental as well as extra-segmental application of thermal heat, although this may less often be a clinical problem (Maixner et al. 1998). It was argued that sensitised thermoreceptors were unlikely to explain this finding because the heat detection thresholds were unchanged. Instead, it was suggested that integrative mechanisms in the central nervous system participated because of an augmented temporal summation of thermal stimuli on the hand (Maixner et al. 1998). Temporal summation mechanisms and wind-up phenomena in central neurons could be strongly related to the development of central hyperexcitability (Woolf and Salter 2006). This indicates that patients with persistent TMD pain are in a state of generalised central hyperexcitability, which also has been suggested for patients with fibromyalgia (Sörensen et al. 1998). Thus, in the patients who have generalised hyperalgesia to superficial stimuli outside the local pain area, it is unlikely that peripheral sensitisation and sensitisation of second-order neurons in the trigeminal sensory nuclear complex in the brainstem can explain the findings. A generalised hyperexcitability of central nociceptive processing in TMD patients has recently been indicated by the finding of more pronounced temporal summation of pain and greater after-sensations following repetitive painful mechanical stimulation of the fingers versus control subjects (Sarlani et al. 2004). Dysfunction of the nociceptive system is also implicated by the finding of suppression of cortical responses and brainstem reflexes elicited by painful laser stimulation of the skin in TMD patients (Romaniello et al. 2003) (Figure 16.2). Furthermore, ischaemic pain models and less effective activation of endogenous pain-inhibitory systems indicate that TMD patients may have increased pain sensitivity at remote sites (arm) (Kashima et al. 1999). In particular, female TMD patients appear unable effectively to engage the normal pain-inhibitory systems (Zubieta et al. 2002), and it has been suggested that opioid receptor desensitisation and/or downregulation could be involved (Bragdon et al. 2002). From a more psychological point of view, it has been

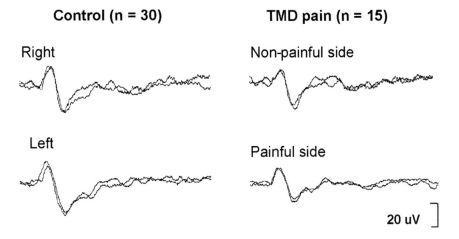

Control (n = 30)

Right

Left

TMD pain (n = 15)

Non-painful side

Painful side

20 uV

Fig. 16.2 Illustration of cortical laser-evoked potentials (LEPs) in healthy control subjects and TMD pain patients. The tracings show the electroencephalographic responses to a brief laser stimulus applied to the orofacial region. The amplitude of the LEPs is significantly attenuated in the TMD patients both on the painful and non-painful sides suggesting a dysfunction of the trigeminal nociceptive system. Modified from Romaniello et al. (2003).

suggested that depression and somatisation are associated with different measures of experimental pain in TMD patients. Thus, somatisation may be related to more attentional and perceptual measures of clinically relevant pain, while depression may be related to more behavioural measures of pain (Sherman et al. 2004). Recently, catechol-O-methyltransferase (COMT) activity has been linked to experimental pain sensitivity, and it appears that the three major haplotypes which determine COMT activity in humans are inversely correlated with pain sensitivity and the risk of developing TMD (Zubieta et al. 2003; Stohler 2004; Diatchenko et al. 2005). However, in the OPPERA study, no single nucleotide polymorphism was directly associated with TMD onset and only 5 were linked to TMD onset through an intermediary phenotype such as non-specific orofacial symptoms and heat pain temporal summation (Smith et al. 2013). Together, this could indicate that there are different subgroups of TMD patients. Clinical studies have confirmed this with some patients showing mainly peripheral involvement and other showing both peripheral and central involvement (Pfau et al. 2009; Moana-Filho and Herrero Babiloni 2018). Specifically, some patients show hyperexcitability of central nociceptive processing, others show a less effective activation of endogenous pain-inhibitory systems and others show both.

Sensitisation can probably also occur at higher levels in the central nervous system and it has been suggested that the ascending reticular formation could be involved (Maixner et al. 1995). First, there are projections from dorsal horn and brainstem neurons via the spinoreticular/trigeminoreticular tract (Willis and Coggeshall 1991). Secondly, the many nuclear groups in the brainstem and basal forebrain areas project to other brain areas related to a wide range of functions such as regulation of sensory perception, emotional responses, arousal, endocrine responses, somatomotor output and autonomic function (Maixner et al. 1995). It was suggested that disinhibition of the ascending reticular formation would be consistent with a generalised hyperalgesia as well as the many psychological, sensory, motor, autonomic and neuroendocrine changes often observed in TMD pain patients (Maixner et al. 1995, 1998). The activity of the ascending reticular formation is normally under the control of peripheral baroreceptor afferent input, and a dysfunction of the regulatory systems could be involved in persistent myofascial TMD pain (Maixner et al. 1997). An alternative, but not mutually exclusive explanation for the generalised hyperalgesia could be an interaction between NGF (Stohler 1997) and variations in female hormones such as estrogen (Sherman and LeResche 2006). Such an interaction with upregulation of NGF could probably explain both the widespread nature of deep pain and hyperalgesia (McMahon et al. 2006) and the female preponderance among patients with persistent jaw-muscle pain (Stohler 1997; Drangsholt and LeResche 1999). The sequence of events could be initiated by acute muscle

inflammation (Reinert et al. 1998; McMahon et al. 2006) and/or long-term sensitisation of nociceptive afferent fibres (Svensson et al. 2003; Mann et al. 2006), but the long-term effects of NGF on pain and hyperalgesia are still not known (McMahon et al. 2006). Furthermore, the common complaint of pain in the orofacial region can at this moment only be hypothesised to be related to the rich innervation of the trigeminal tissues, the prominent representation in the somatosensory cortex and the frequent use of the masticatory system (Maixner et al. 1995; Sessle 2000).

Finally, the various theories on referred pain mechanisms have been reviewed recently (Graven-Nielsen and Arendt-Nielsen 2003). There is general agreement that the diffuse nature and poor localisation of muscle pain is related to the central convergence of afferent fibres onto common central neurons because this feature will in effect reduce the spatial resolution of somatosensory information. Several studies in the orofacial region (Sessle et al. 1986; Sessle 2000; Takeshita et al. 2001) have shown that nociceptive afferents from muscles, joints, skin and viscera converge onto common projection neurons. It is nevertheless not clear why muscle or joint pain can be referred to the skin, whereas the reverse is seldom encountered. Differences between cutaneous and muscular nociceptive afferents in terms of somatotopic organisation, sizes of receptive fields and laminar distribution of their terminals may explain the predominant referral of muscle pain (Dubner 1995; Svensson and Sessle 2004). Other mechanisms than central convergence are also likely be involved in the expression of referred pain, since there is normally a time delay between the onset of local and referred pain (Graven-Nielsen and Arendt-Nielsen 2003). One possibility is that the nociceptive barrage from muscle tissue opens up latent connections, that is, a form of central divergence. Thus, myositis-induced input from muscle nociceptors could lead to an expansion of the responding neuron population in the spinal cord or brainstem (Mense et al. 1997). The synaptic connections between neurons that originally had no effective drive from the myositis-induced muscle may now become effective. The neurobiology subserving such mechanisms is probably related to central sensitisation of second-order neurons and the development of hyperexcitability.

In summary, spontaneous pain and stimulus-evoked pain (e.g., pain on palpation) responses in TMD pain patients have been fairly well characterised in the last two decades, but there is a continued need to use systematic descriptions and standardised quantitative psychophysical measures in larger and well-defined subgroups of TMD patients. This clinical information should then be paired with data obtained from animal and human experimental models of TMD pain in order to further elucidate the involved pain mechanisms. The most prominent pain mechanisms appear to be sensitisation of the primary afferent fibres and central sensitisation phenomena of the second-order neuron in the trigeminal sensory nuclear complex in the brainstem, but also imbalances between the endogenous pain regulatory systems with certain sex-related and genetic contributions.

Taking into consideration the many potential risk factors and the complexity of the pathophysiological mechanisms underlying TMD pain, it has been suggested that stochastic interactions between multiple risk factors may help explain the trajectories of pain in individual patients (Svensson and Kumar 2016). Further studies will be needed to translate this concept into clinical practice, but it may be important for clinicians to keep in mind that simple and monocausal explanatory models for TMD pain belong to a long gone era.

Management

When the underlying mechanisms and etiology of TMD pain are only partly known (see previous paragraphs), it becomes difficult to perform causal therapy and cure the pain and dysfunction. Instead, a more realistic goal will most often be to alleviate TMD pain and restore function. Thus, the management strategies for TMD pain follow the same principles of management of other musculoskeletal pain conditions, that is, there can be physical, pharmacological and psychological oriented strategies (Table 16.3). Furthermore, decision algorithms have been developed and tested in clinical practice in order to ensure a systematic and least-invasive approach to TMD pain (Clark 1996). The different strategies will be covered briefly in the following paragraphs. There are several recent updates on the management of TMD pain (e.g., Okeson 2005; Schindler and Svensson 2006; Häggman-Henrikson et al. 2017) and the reader is referred to these for a more in-depth discussion. It should be noted here that there is hierarchy of evidence ranging from meta-analysis and systematic critical reviews to randomised control clinical trials and open case studies to expert opinions. The decision of management needs to be based on the best available evidence and on clinical experience when there is a lack of controlled clinical trials to guide the decision.

Physical management

It is a common clinical experience that various physical strategies can be effective for management of the different types of TMD pain (Figure 16.3). Unfortunately, it has been much more difficult to support this with proper research data adhering to randomised controlled trial (RCT) principles. Critical reviews and meta-analysis have, however, started to appear to evaluate the claimed efficacy of the procedures (Table 16.3) (Michelotti et al. 2005; List and Axelsson 2010; Aggarwal et al. 2019). Most conclusions state that there may be a significant reduction in perceived pain intensity following the intervention (e.g., acupuncture, biofeedback, splints, etc.), but that there may only be marginal or even no difference when the active treatment is compared to a placebo control (Feine and Lund 1997). Thus, the specificity of many of the proposed treatments appears to be remarkably low. While it is difficult to find an optimal placebo control for massage or acupuncture, etc., it is nevertheless necessary to include some form of control treatment which generates the some amount of expectancy for the patients and which is comparable in terms of number and intensity of treatment sessions (Marbach and Raphael 1996).

Oral splints have also been used extensively for management or even for 'curing' TMD pain. This was to a large extent based on assumptions related to the importance of structural deviations in the occlusion (malocclusion) and problems with alignment of the condyle–disc complex in the temporal fossa, which could be detected following the use of a splint, and later fixed by rehabilitation of the occlusion, for example, by orthodontics. These views and ideas have been challenged in the last decade and no longer appear to be valid. For example, a landmark study failed to show significant differences between a flat oral splint and a

Table 16.3 Overview on management modalities for TMD pain.

Physical[a,b,c,d,e]	Pharmacological[f,g,h]	Psychological[i,j]
Stretch therapy	Topical NSAIDs	Information
Jaw exercises	NSAIDs	Counselling
Massage	Acetaminophen	Education
Ultrasound	Glucocorticosteroids	Stress management
Soft laser	Muscle relaxants	Biofeedback
Heat/cold	Benzodiazepines	Relaxation
Transcutaneous	Tricyclic antidepressants	Cognitive–behavioural
Electrical Stimulation (TENS)	Opioids	Psychotherapy
Acupuncture	Botulinum toxin	
Oral splints		

Possible strategies for non-surgical management of temporomandibular disorders. Several reviews, but relatively few meta-analyses on the efficacy are available.
[a]Feine and Lund (1997), [b]Ernest and White (1999), [c]Crider and Glaros (1999), [d]Forssell and Kalso (2004), [e]Michelotti et al. (2005), [f]Dionne (1997), [g]List et al. (2003), [h]Schindler and Svensson (2006), [i]Sherman and Turk (2001), [j]Suvinen et al. (2005).

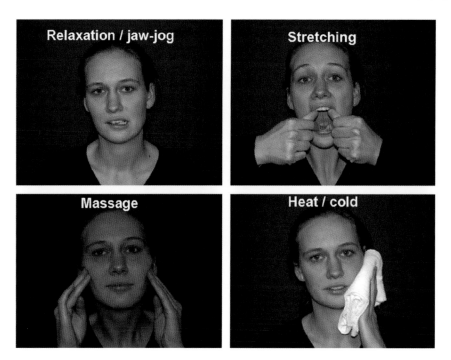

Fig. 16.3 Physical therapy should include a 'self-care' exercise programme with conscious relaxation of the jaw and gentle small movements up and down and sidewards (jaw jogging), stretching, massage and application of either heat or cold.

placebo splint in the perceived pain intensity of myofascial TMD pain (Dao et al. 1994). Later, some differences were reported between the flat oral splint and placebo splint when TMJ arthralgia and myofascial TMD were treated (Ekberg et al. 1998; Ekberg and Nilner 2006). Patients with widespread myofascial pain complaints throughout the body including the orofacial region seem to demonstrate a similar degree of pain relief following the use of flat and placebo splints, whereas patients with myofascial pain only in the orofacial region have more effect from a flat oral splint (Raphael and Marbach 2001). Recent meta-analyses concluded that oral splints appear to be of some benefit in the treatment of TMD pain especially in the short term, but more and well-designed controlled studies are needed (Al-Ani et al. 2004; Forssell and Kalso 2004; Kuzmanovic et al. 2017). The mode of action of the oral splints has certainly not been clearly demonstrated (Dao and Lavigne 1998), and it may so far be helpful to continue to think of oral splints as 'oral crutches'. There have been attempts to calculate the 'number needed to treat' (NNT) values (i.e., the number of patients that should be treated in order to obtain 1 patient with at least 50% pain relief) for oral splints. The available NNT estimates range between 3 and 4 for management of myofascial TMD patients and around 5 and 6 for TMJ arthralgia patients (Forssell and Kalso 2004) suggesting a moderate efficacy of oral splints. Very recently, another controlled study compared the conventional hard splint with a soft splint and a usual self-care-based treatment approach (Truelove et al. 2006). This study failed to show

any significant differences between the three different treatment groups and all patients improved over time, which suggests that oral splints are not essential in the management of most TMD patients and that low-cost non-splint self-care therapy should be considered as an initial step in the management.

Finally, it should be noted that oral splints may still be useful when major occlusal rehabilitation is required (e.g., orthodontics, extensive prosthodontic treatment, etc.) and when the structural position needs to be defined due to lack of sufficient occlusal support, but it should be emphasised that this is a very different situation and has very little to do with management or prevention of TMD problems (Koh and Robinson 2003).

Pharmacological management

Several reviews have discussed the possibilities for pharmacological intervention in TMD pain (DeNucci et al. 1996; Dionne 1997; Fricton and Schiffman 2001; List et al. 2003; Häggman-Henrikson et al. 2017). However, there are surprising few randomised controlled trials on the management of TMD pain and very few studies which have separated the various subtypes of TMD pain.

Nonsteroidal anti-inflammatory drugs (NSAIDs) such as ibuprofen in combination with diazepam have been shown to provide significantly better pain relief compared to ibuprofen alone and placebo in myofascial TMD pain patients (Singer and Dionne 1997). However, naproxen (500 mg twice a day) is significantly better than celecoxib (100 mg twice a day) and placebo for management of TMJ arthralgia (Ta and Dionne 2004). A short-acting benzodiazepine (Triazolam) has also been shown to improve sleep, but failed to provide significant pain relief in myofascial TMD patients (DeNucci et al. 1998). Cyclobenzaprine (a muscle relaxant) has been shown to have minor, but significant effect on jaw-muscle pain upon awakening (Herman et al. 2002), and it has been suggested that flupirtine (another muscle relaxant) with its additional effects on potassium channels and membrane-stabilising actions may be useful in management of myofascial TMD pain (Schindler and Svensson 2006). A combination of paracetamol, codeine and doxylamine succinate (antihistamine) provided significantly greater pain relief than placebo in another study on mixed TMD patients (Gerschman et al. 1984). In addition, low doses of tricyclic antidepressants (TCA) have been shown to provide significantly better pain relief than placebo (Sharav et al. 1987). Open studies have later supported the usefulness of TCAs and gabapentin in the management of persistent TMD pain (Plesh et al. 2000; Haviv et al. 2015). Intra-articular morphine (0.1–1.0 mg) administered as a single dose has been shown to increase the pressure pain thresholds and mouth-opening capacity and reduces the VAS pain intensity. However, the clinical relevance of these findings was not impressive (List et al. 2001). The use of botulinum toxin for myofascial TMD pain cannot at present be recommended due to inconclusive evidence (Nixdorf et al. 2002; von Lindern et al. 2003; Thambar et al. 2020). There is clearly a need for more research before firm recommendations of specific pharmacological procedures in the management of TMD pain conditions can be given, since there is only scattered, reliable information on the efficacy of most of the suggested drugs (Table 16.3).

Psychological management

Systematic studies on the efficacy of psychological management of TMD pain are rather scarce. It has been demonstrated that a combination of biofeedback and stress management and oral splints provide a significant and long-lasting pain relief in TMD pain patients (Turk et al. 1993; Rudy et al. 1995). There is also good evidence that self-care instructions and monitoring can provide at least as good pain relief as usual dental approaches to TMD pain, and that in more severely affected patients the inclusion of comprehensive care provided by a clinical psychologist will provide a significant advantage compared to the usual dental treatment (Dworkin et al. 2002a, 2002b). It appears to be important to tailor the treatment to each individual patient and not consider psychological interventions of TMD pain as a treatment of last resort, but rather use it concurrent with biomedical/dental treatments (Sherman and Turk 2001). Recently, it was shown that a brief cognitive–behavioural treatment programme was indeed able significantly to reduce catastrophising, increase perceived control over pain and improve activity interferences and jaw-use limitations (Turner et al. 2005). Further research is also needed in order to clearly define advantages

with combinations of psychological–behavioural management and other treatment modalities.

Surgical management

In some selected cases with persistent pain in the TMJ and restrictions in movements, which have not responded adequately to conservative treatment, it has been recommended to use surgical approaches to alleviate the symptoms. The procedures range from irrigation of the upper joint space of the TMJ (arthrocentesis), direct inspection, lysis and lavage (arthroscopy) to positional changes in the condyle (e.g., modified condylotomy) or removal of the disc (discectomy). It is a clear trend that irrespective of the specific procedure the success rate (decreased pain and improved jaw opening) is close to 80% or more (Fridrich et al. 1996; Hall et al. 2000; Murakami et al. 2000; Holmlund et al. 2001; Ethunandan and Wilson 2006). Most of the studies have an open design and have for various reasons not included randomisation or placebo controls, thus many open questions remain about the efficacy of these procedures. Therefore, it may be important also to look at the natural course of the disorders affecting the TMJ. Symptomatic disc displacement without reduction appears to have a beneficial prognosis, since about 75% are free of symptoms or have improved and only 25% remain to have problems after 2½ years (Kurita et al. 1998). Few studies have directly compared the efficacy of the available surgical procedures (Barkin and Weinberg 2000; Sanroman 2004). A review has suggested that there was no scientific evidence yet to support a major advantage of the surgical procedures (arthrocentesis and arthroscopy) versus physical therapy (Kropmans et al. 1999). The indications for surgical management of pain problems in the TMJ need very careful considerations, since the relation between mechanical distortions and pain is not fully understood. More comparative and controlled studies with long-term follow-ups are needed to make evidence-based decisions on when and what kind of TMJ surgery should be recommended for specific subtypes of pain problems in the TMJ. One study clearly demonstrated in an RCT study design with a 5-year follow-up period that patients with magnetic resonance imaging (MRI)-confirmed TMJ closed lock had similar clinical effects of medical management, non-surgical rehabilitation, arthroscopic surgery and arthroplasty, and therefore non-surgical conservative approaches should be used before considering TMJ surgeries (Schiffman et al. 2014b).

Summary

This review has sought to highlight some recent clinical and experimental findings in the intriguing and challenging field of TMD. It is unlikely that epidemiological studies alone or in vitro experiments alone will be able to answer the questions posed in the beginning of this chapter. A combination of the basic sciences, human experimental pain studies and clinical trials in TMD patients continues to seem to be a logical strategy to synthesise information and further improve the diagnostic classification and clinical management of TMD pain. At present, there seems to be enough scientific information on the putative etiological factors and underlying pain mechanisms to allow the formulation of researchable hypothesis and to provide initial guidelines for the management approaches to TMD. There is an urgent need for the dental profession to acknowledge that 'oral rehabilitation' of TMD patients does not always mean 'occlusal rehabilitation'. This is the most profound shift in paradigm over the last couple of decades and it seems reasonable and justified based on the available information to consider 'occlusal problems' and 'TMD problems' separately for the benefits of our patients.

References

Aggarwal VR, Fu Y, Main CJ and Wu J (2019) The effectiveness of self-management interventions in adults with chronic orofacial pain: a systematic review, meta-analysis and meta-regression. *Eur J Pain*. May; 23(5), 849–865. doi: 10.1002/ejp.1358. Epub 2019 Feb 7.

Al-Ani MZ, Davies SJ, Gray RJ, Sloan P and Glenny AM (2004) Stabilisation splint therapy for temporomandibular pain dysfunction syndrome. *Cochrane Database Syst Rev* 1, CD002778. doi: 10.1002/14651858. CD002778.pub2. PMID: 14973990.

Arendt-Nielsen L, Graven-Nielsen T and Drewes AM (1998) Referred pain and hyperalgesia related to muscle and visceral pain. *IASP Newsletter* 3–5.

Baba K, Tsukiyama Y and Clark GT (2000) Reliability, validity, and utility of various occlusal measurement methods and techniques. *J Prosthet Dent* 83, 83–89.

Bair E, Ohrbach R, Fillingim RB, Greenspan JD, Dubner R, Diatchenko L, Helgeson E, Knott C, Maixner W, Slade GD (2013) Multivariable modeling of phenotypic risk factors for first-onset TMD: the OPPERA prospective cohort study. *J Pain*. Dec; 14(12 Suppl), T102-15. doi: 10.1016/j.jpain.2013.09.003. PMID: 24275218; PMCID: PMC4036699.

Barkin S and Weinberg S (2000) Internal derangements of the temporomandibular joint: the role of arthroscopic surgery and arthrocentesis. *J Can Dent Assoc* 66, 199–203.

Bendtsen L and Treede RD (2005) Sensitization of myofascial pain pathways in tension-type headaches. In Olesen J, Goadsby PJ, Ramadan N, Tfelt-Hansen P and Welch KM (eds) *The Headaches*, 3 edn, pp. 635–639. Philadelphia: Lippincott Williams Wilkins.

Benoliel R, Svensson P and Eliav E (2013) Pathophysiology of persistent masticatory myofascial pain. In Green CS and Laskin DM (eds) *Treatment of Temporomandibular Disorders: Bridging the Gap between Advances in Basic Research and Clinical Patient Management*, pp. 17–32. Quintessence, Chicago, USA.

Berberich P, Hoheisel U and Mense S (1988) Effects of carrageenan-induced myositis on the discharge properties of group III and IV muscle receptors in the cat. *J Neurophysiol* 59, 1395–1409.

Bragdon EE, Light KC, Costello NL, Sigurdsson A, Bunting S, Bhalang K and Maixner W (2002) Group differences in pain modulation: pain-free women compared to pain-free men and to women with TMD. *Pain* 96, 227–237.

Bumann A and Lotzmann U (2002) *TMJ Disorders and Orofacial Pain. The Role of Dentistry in a Multidisciplinary Diagnostic Approach*. Stuttgart: Thieme.

Cairns BE, Hu JW, Arendt-Nielsen L, Sessle BJ and Svensson P (2001) Sex-related differences in human pain perception and rat afferent discharge evoked by injection of glutamate into the masseter muscle. *J Neurophysiol* 86, 782–791.

Cairns BE, Svensson P, Wang K, Castrillon E, Hupfeld S, Sessle BJ and Arendt-Nielsen L (2006) Ketamine attenuates glutamate-induced mechanical sensitization of the masseter muscle in human males. *Exp Brain Res* 169, 467–472.

Cairns BE, Svensson P, Wang K, Hupfeld S, Graven-Nielsen T, Sessle BJ, Berde CB and Arendt-Nielsen L (2003) Activation of peripheral NMDA receptors contributes to human pain and rat afferent discharges evoked by injection of glutamate into the masseter muscle. *J Neurophysiol* 90, 2098–2105.

Carlson CR, Reid KI, Curran SL, Studts J, Okeson JP, Falace D, Nitz A and Bertrand PM (1998) Psychological and physiological parameters of masticatory muscle pain. *Pain* 76, 297–307.

Carlsson GE, Egermark I and Magnusson T (2002) Predictors of signs and symptoms of temporomandibular disorders: a 20-year follow-up study from childhood to adulthood. *Acta Odontol Scand* 60, 180–185.

Carlsson GE and LeResche L (1995) Epidemiology of temporomandibular disorders. In Sessle BJ, Bryant PS and Dionne RA (eds) *Progress in Pain Research and Management*, pp. 211–226. Seattle: IASP Press.

Castrillon EE, Ernberg M, Cairns BE, Wang K, Sessle BJ, Arendt-Nielsen L and Svensson P (2010) Interstitial glutamate concentration is elevated in the masseter muscle of myofascial temporomandibular disorder patients. *J Orofac Pain* 24(4), 350–360.

Christidis N, Kang I, Cairns BE, Kumar U, Dong X, Rosen A, Kopp S and Ernberg M (2014) Expression of 5-HT3 receptors and TTX resistant sodium channels (Na(V)1.8) on muscle nerve fibers in pain-free humans and patients with chronic myofascial temporomandibular disorders. *J Headache Pain* 15, 63.

Clark GT (1996) A diagnosis and treatment algorithm for common TM disorders. *J Jpn Prosthodont Soc* 40, 1029–1043.

Collins SL, Moore RA and McQuay HJ (1997) The visual analogue pain intensity scale: what is moderate pain in millimeters? *Pain* 72, 95–97.

Crider AB and Glaros AG (1999) A meta-analysis of EMG biofeedback treatment of temporomandibular disorders. *J Orofac Pain* 13, 29–37.

Dao TTT and Lavigne GJ (1998) Oral splints: the cruthches for temporomandibular disorders and bruxism. *Crit Rev Oral Biol Med* 9, 345–361.

Dao TTT, Lavigne GJ, Charbonneau A, Feine JS and Lund JP (1994) The efficacy of oral splints in the treatment of myofascial pain of the jaw muscles: a controlled clinical trial. *Pain* 56, 85–94.

Dao TTT, Reynolds WJ and Tenenbaum HC (1997) Comorbidity between myofascial pain of the masticatory muscles and fibromyalgia. *J Orofac Pain* 11, 232–241.

De Boever JA and Carlsson GE (1994) Etiology and differential diagnosis. In Zarb GA, Carlsson GE, Sessle BJ and Mohl ND (eds) *Temporomandibular Joint and Masticatory Muscle Disorders*, pp. 171–187. Copenhagen: Munksgaard.

DeNucci DJ, Dionne RA and Dubner R (1996) Identifying a neurobiologic basis for drug theraphy in TMDs. *J Am Dent Assoc* 127, 581–593.

DeNucci DJ, Sobiski C and Dionne RA (1998) Triazolam improves sleep but fails to alter pain in TMD patients. *J Orofac Pain* 12, 116–123.

Diatchenko L, Slade GD, Nackley AG, Bhalang K, Sigurdsson A, Belfer I, Goldman D, Xu K, Shabalina SA, Shagin D, Max MB, Makarov SS and Maixner W (2005) Genetic basis for individual variations in pain perception and the development of a chronic pain condition. *Hum Mol Genet* 14, 135–143.

Dickenson AH, Bee LA and Suzuki R (2005) Pains, gains, and midbrains. *Proc Natl Acad Sci USA* 102, 17885–17886.

Dionne RA (1997) Pharmacologic treatments for temporomandibular disorders. *Oral Surg Oral Med Oral Pathol Oral Radiol Endod* 83, 134–142.

Drangsholt M and LeResche L (1999) Temporomandibular disorder pain. In Crombie IK, Croft PR, Linton SJ, LeResche L and Von Korff M (eds) *Epidemiology of Pain*, pp. 203–233. Seattle: IASP Press.

Dubner R (1995) Hyperalgesia in response to injury to cutaneous and deep tissues. In Fricton JR and Dubner R (eds) *Orofacial Pain and Temporomandibular Disorders. Advances in Pain Research and Therapy*, vol 21, pp. 61–71. New York: Raven Press.

Dworkin SF and LeResche L (1992) Research diagnostic criteria for temporomandibular disorders: review, criteria, examinations and specifications, critique. *J Craniomandib Disord Facial Oral Pain* 6, 301–355.

Dworkin SF, Turner JA, Mancl L, Wilson L, Massoth D, Huggins KH, LeResche L and Truelove E (2002a) A randomized clinical trial of a tailored comprehensive care treatment program for temporomandibular disorders. *J Orofac Pain* 16, 259–276.

Dworkin SF, Huggins KH, Wilson L, Mancl L, Turner J, Massoth D, LeResche L and Truelove E (2002b) A randomized clinical trial using research diagnostic criteria for temporomandibular disorders -axis II to target clinic cases for a tailored self-care TMD treatment program. *J Orofac Pain* 16, 48–63.

Egermark I, Magnusson T and Carlsson GE (2003) A 20-year follow-up of signs and symptoms of temporomandibular disorders and malocclusions in subjects with and without orthodontic treatment in childhood. *Angle Orthod* 73, 109–115.

Ekberg EC, Nilner M. Treatment outcome of short and long-term appliance therapy in patients with TMD of myogenous origin and tension-type headache. *J Oral Rehabil.* 2006 Oct; 33(10):713 21. doi: 10.1111/j.1365-2842.2006.01659.x. PMID: 16938099

Ekberg EC, Vallon D and Nilner M (1998) Occlusal appliance therapy in patients with temporomandibular disorders. A double-blind controlled study in a short-term perspective. *Acta Odont Scand* 56, 122–128.

Ernst E and White AR (1999) Acupuncture as a treatment for temporomandibular joint dysfunction: a systematic review of randomised trials. *Arch Otolaryngol Head Neck Surg* 125, 269–272.

Ethunandan M and Wilson AW (2006) Temporomandibular joint arthrocentesis – more questions than answers? *J Oral Maxillofac Surg* 64, 952–955.

Exposto FG, Masuda M, Castrillon EE and Svensson P (2018) Effects of nerve growth factor experimentally-induced craniofacial muscle sensitization on referred pain frequency and number of headache days: a double-blind, randomized placebo-controlled study. *Cephalalgia* 0(0), 0333102418758481.

Feine JS and Lund JP (1997) An assessment of the efficacy of physical therapy and physical modalities for the control of chronic musculoskeletal pain. *Pain* 71, 5–23.

Forssell H and Kalso E (2004) Application of principles of evidence-based medicine to occlusal treatment for temporomandibular disorders: are there lessons to be learned? *J Orofac Pain* 18, 9–22.

Fricton JR and Schiffman E (2001) Management of masticatory myalgia and arthralgia. In Lund JP, Lavigne GJ, Dubner R and Sessle BJ (eds) *Orofacial Pain: From Basic Science to Clinical Management*, pp. 235–248. Chicago: Quintessence Book.

Fridrich KL, Wise JM and Zeitler DL (1996) Prospective comparison of arthroscopy and arthrocentesis for temporomandibular joint disorders. *J Oral Maxillofac Surg* 54, 816–820.

Gerschman JA, Reade PD and Burrows GD (1984) Evaluation of a proprietary analgesic/antihistamine in the management of pain associated with temporomandibular joint pain dysfunction syndrome. *Aus Dent J* 29, 300–304.

Gesch D, Bernhardt O, Kocher T, John U, Hensel E and Alte D (2004) Association of malocclusion and functional occlusion with signs of temporomandibular disorders in adults: results of the population-based study of health in Pomerania. *Angle Orthod* 74, 512–520.

Gesch D, Bernhardt O, Mack F, John U, Kocher T and Alte D (2005) Association of malocclusion and functional occlusion with subjective symptoms of TMD in adults: results of the Study of Health in Pomerania (SHIP). *Angle Orthod* 75, 183–190.

Gjerstad J, Tjølsen A, Svendsen F and Hole K (1999) Inhibition of evoked C-fibre responses in the dorsal horn after contralateral intramuscular injection of capsaicin involves activation of descending pathways. *Pain* 80, 413–418.

Gonzalez YM, Schiffman E, Gordon SM, Seago B, Truelove EL, Slade G and Ohrbach R (2011) Development of a brief and effective temporomandibular disorder pain screening questionnaire: reliability and validity. *J Am Dent Assoc* 142(10), 1183–1191.

Gracely RH (2006) Studies of pain in human subjects. In McMahon SB and Koltzenburg M (eds) *Wall and Melzack´s Textbook of Pain*, pp. 267–289. Elsevier Churchill Livingstone, Philadelphia, PA.

Graven-Nielsen T and Arendt-Nielsen L (2003) Induction and assessment of muscle pain, referred pain, and muscular hyperalgesia. *Curr Pain Headache Rep* 7, 443–451.

Graven-Nielsen T and Mense S (2001) The peripheral apparatus of muscle pain: evidence from animal and human studies. *Clin J Pain* 17, 2–10.

Green CS (2001) The etiology of temporomandibular disorders: implications for treatment. *J Orofac Pain* 15, 93–105.

Häggman-Henrikson B, Alstergren P, Davidson T, Högestätt ED, Östlund P, Tranaeus S, Vitols S and List T (2017) Pharmacological treatment of oro-facial pain – health technology assessment including a systematic review with network meta-analysis. *J Oral Rehabil* 44(10), 800–826.

Hall HD, Navarro EZ and Gibbs SJ (2000) Prospective study of modified condylotomy for treatment of nonreducing disk displacement. *Oral Surg Oral Med Oral Pathol Oral Radiol Endod* 89, 147–158.

Haviv Y, Rettman A, Aframian D, Sharav Y and Benoliel R (2015) Myofascial pain: an open study on the pharmacotherapeutic response to stepped treatment with tricyclic antidepressants and gabapentin. *J Oral Facial Pain Headache* 29(2), 144–151.

Headache Classification Comittee of the International Headache Society (2018) The International Classification of Headache Disorders, 3rd edition (ICHD-3). *Cephalalgia* 38, 1–211.

Henrikson T and Nilner M (2003) Temporomandibular disorders, occlusion and orthodontic treatment. *J Orthod* 30, 129–137.

Herman CR, Schiffman EL, Look JO and Rindal DB (2002) The effectiveness of adding pharmacologic treatment with clonazepam or cyclobenzaprine to patient education and self-care for the treatment of jaw pain upon awakening: a randomized clinical trial. *J Orofac Pain* 16, 64–70.

Holmlund AB, Axelsson S and Gynther GW (2001) A comparison of discectomy and arthroscopic lysis and lavage for the treatment of chronic closed lock of the temporomandibular joint: a randomized outcome study. *J Oral Maxillofac Surg* 59, 972–977.

Hu JW, Sessle BJ, Raboisson P, Dallel R and Woda A (1992) Stimulation of craniofacial muscle afferents induces prolonged facilitatory effects in trigeminal nociceptive brain-stem neurons. *Pain* 48, 53–60.

John MT, Dworkin SF and Mancl LA (2005) Reliability of clinical temporomandibular disorder diagnoses. *Pain* 118, 61–69.

John MT, Hirsch C, Drangsholt MT, Mancl LA and Setz JM (2002) Overbite and overjet are not related to self-report of temporomandibular disorder symptoms. *J Dent Res* 81, 164–169.

John MT, Miglioretti DL, LeResche L, Von Korff M and Critchlow CW (2003) Widespread pain as a risk factor for dysfunctional temporomandibular disorder pain. *Pain* 102, 257–263.

Jussila P, Kiviahde H, Napankangas R, Pakkila J, Pesonen P, Sipila K, Pirttiniemi P and Raustia A (2017) Prevalence of temporomandibular disorders in the Northern Finland Birth Cohort 1966. *J Oral Facial Pain Headache* 31(2), 159–164.

Kashima K, Rahman OI, Sakoda S and Shiba R (1999) Increased pain sensitivity of the upper extremities of TMD patients with myalgia to experimentally-evoked noxious stimulation: possibility of worsened endogenous opioid systems. *Cranio* 17, 241–246.

Koh H and Robinson PG (2003) Occlusal adjustment for treating and preventing temporomandibular joint disorders. *Cochrane Database Syst Rev* 1, CD003812. doi: 10.1002/14651858.CD003812. PMID: 12535488.

Kononen M, Waltimo A and Nystrom M (1996) Does clicking in adolescence lead to painful temporomandibular joint locking? *Lancet* 347, 1080–1081.

Kopp S (2001) Neuroendocrine, immune, and local responses related to temporomandibular disorders. *J Orofac Pain* 15, 9–28.

Kropmans JB, Dijkstra PU, Stegenga B and De Bont LGM (1999) Therapeutic outcome assessment in permanent joint disc displacement. *J Oral Rehabil* 26, 357–363.

Kurita H, Westesson P-L, Yasa H, Toyama M, Machida J and Ogi N (1998) Natural course of untreated symptomatic temporomandibular joint disc displacement without reduction. *J Dent Res* 77, 361–365.

Kuzmanovic Pficer J, Dodic S, Lazic V, Trajkovic G, Milic N and Milicic B (2017) Occlusal stabilization splint for patients with temporomandibular disorders: meta-analysis of short and long term effects. *PLoS One* 12(2), e0171296.

Langemark M, Jensen K, Jensen TS and Olesen J (1989) Pressure pain thresholds and thermal nociceptive thresholds in chronic tension-type headache. *Pain* 38, 203–210.

Lautenbacher S, Rollman GB and McCain GA (1994) Multi-method assessment of experimental and clinical pain in patients with fibromyalgia. *Pain* 59, 45–53.

Le Bars D, Dickenson AH and Besson J-M (1979) Diffuse noxious inhibitory controls (DNIC). I. Effects on dorsal horn convergent neurones in the rat. *Pain* 6, 283–304.

LeResche L (1997) Epidemiology of temporomandibular disorders: implications for the investigation of etiologic factors. *Crit Rev Oral Biol Med* 8, 291–305.

List T and Axelsson S (2010) Management of TMD: evidence from systematic reviews and meta-analyses. *J Oral Rehabil* 37(6), 430–451.

List T, Axelsson S and Leijon G (2003) Pharmacologic interventions in the treatment of temporomandibular disorders, atypical facial pain, and burning mouth syndrome. A qualitative systematic review. *J Orofac Pain* 17, 301–310.

List T, John MT, Dworkin SF and Svensson P (2006) Recalibration improves inter-examiner reliability of TMD examination. *Acta Odontol Scand* 64, 146–152.

List T, Tegelberg K, Haraldson T and Isacsson G (2001) Intra-articular morphine as analgesic in temporomandibular joint arthralgia/osteoarthritis. *Pain* 94, 275–282.

Louca Jounger S, Christidis N, Svensson P, List T and Ernberg M (2017) Increased levels of intramuscular cytokines in patients with jaw muscle pain. *J Headache Pain* 18(1), 30.

Lövgren A, Marklund S, Visscher CM, Lobbezoo F, Haggman-Henrikson B and Wanman A (2017) Outcome of three screening questions for temporomandibular disorders (3Q/TMD) on clinical decision-making. *J Oral Rehabil* 44(8), 573–579.

Lundh H, Westesson PL and Kopp S (1987) A three-year follow-up of patients with reciprocal temporomandibular joint clicking. *Oral Surg Oral Med Oral Pathol* 63, 530–553.

Magnusson T, Egermark I and Carlsson GE (2002) Treatment received, treatment demand, and treatment need for temporomandibular disorders in 35-year-old subjects. *Cranio* 20, 11–17.

Maixner W, Fillingim R, Booker D and Sigurdsson A (1995) Sensitivity of patients with painful temporomandibular disorders to experimentally evoked pain. *Pain* 63, 341–351.

Maixner W, Fillingim R, Sigurdsson A, Kincaid S and Silva S (1998) Sensitivity of patients with painful temporomandibular disorders to experimentally evoked pain: evidence for altered temporal summation of pain. *Pain* 76, 71–81.

Maixner W, Fillingim RB, Kincaid S, Sigurdsson A and Harris MB (1997) Relationship between pain sensitivity and resting arterial blood pressure in patients with painful temporomandibular disorders. *Psychosom Med* 59, 503–511.

Malow RM, Grimm L and Olson RE (1980) Differences in pain perception between myofascial pain dysfunction patients and normal subjects: a signal detection analysis. *J Psychosom Res* 24, 303–309.

Manfredini D, Lombardo L and Siciliani G (2017) Temporomandibular disorders and dental occlusion. A systematic review of association studies: end of an era? *J Oral Rehabil* 44(11), 908–923.

Mann MK, Dong X, Svensson P and Cairns BE (2006) Influence of intramuscular nerve growth factor injection on the response properties of rat masseter muscle afferent fibers. *J Orofac Pain* Fall; 20(4), 325–336. PMID: 17190031. (In press).

Marbach JJ and Raphael KG (1996) Treatment of orofacial pain using evidence-based medicine: the case for intraoral appliances. In Campbell JN (ed.) *Pain 1996 – An Updated Review. Refresher Course Syllabus*, pp. 413–422. Seattle: IASP Press.

Masuda M, Iida T, Exposto FG, Baad-Hansen L, Kawara M, Komiyama O and Svensson P (2018) Referred pain and sensations evoked by standardized palpation of the masseter muscle in healthy participants. *J Oral Facial Pain Headache* Mar 21; 32(2), 159–166. doi: 10.11607/ofph.2019. Epub ahead of print. PMID: 29561916.

McGrath PJ and Unruh AM (2006) Measurement and assessment of paediatric pain. In McMahon SB and Koltzenburg M (eds) *Wall and Melzack´s Textbook of Pain*, pp. 305–315. Elsevier Churchill Livingstone.

McMahon SB, Bennett DLH and Bevan S (2006) Inflammatory mediators and modulators of pain. In McMahon SB and Koltzenburg M (eds) *Wall and Melzack´s Textbook of Pain*, pp. 49–72. Elsevier Churchill Livingstone.

McNamara JA Jr, Seligman DA and Okeson JP (1995) Occlusion, orthodontic treatment, and temporomandibular disorders: a review. *J Orofac Pain* 9, 73–90.

Meloto CB, Slade GD, Lichtenwalter RN, Bair E, Rathnayaka N, Diatchenko L, Greenspan JD, Maixner W, Fillingim RB, Ohrbach R (2019) Clinical predictors of persistent temporomandibular disorder in people with first-onset temporomandibular disorder: A prospective case-control study. *J Am Dent Assoc.* Jul; 150(7):572–581.e10. doi: 10.1016/j.adaj.2019.03.023. PMID: 31248483.

Melzack R (1975) The McGill Pain Questionnaire: major properties and scoring methods. *Pain* 1, 277–300.

Melzack R and Katz J (2006) Pain assessment in adult patients. In McMahon SB and Koltzenburg M (eds) *Wall and Melzack´s Textbook of Pain*, pp. 291–304. Elsevier Churchill Livingstone.

Mense S (1993) Nociception from skeletal muscle in relation to clinical muscle pain. *Pain* 54, 241–289.

Mense S, Hoheisel U, Kaske A and Reinert A (1997) Muscle pain: basic mechanisms and clinical correlates. In Jensen TS, Turner JA and Wiesenfeld-Hallin Z (eds) *Proceedings of the 8th World Congress on Pain. Progress in Pain Research and Management*, vol 8, pp. 479–496. Seattle: IASP Press.

Michelotti A, de Wijer A, Steenks M and Farella M (2005) Home-exercise regimes for the management of non-specific temporomandibular disorders. *J Oral Rehabil* 32, 779–785.

Moana-Filho EJ and Herrero Babiloni A (2018) Endogenous pain modulation in chronic TMD: derivation of pain modulation profiles and assessment of its relationship with clinical characteristics. *J Oral Rehabil.* Nov 22. PMID: 30388304.

Moana-Filho EJ, Herrero Babiloni A (2019) Endogenous pain modulation in chronic temporomandibular disorders: Derivation of pain modulation profiles and assessment of its relationship with clinical characteristics. *J Oral Rehabil.* Mar; 46(3),219–232. doi: 10.1111/joor.12745.

Mohlin BO, Derweduwen K, Pilley R, Kingdon A, Shaw WC and Kenealy P (2004) Malocclusion and temporomandibular disorder: a comparison of adolescents with moderate to severe dysfunction with those without signs and symptoms of temporomandibular disorder and their further development to 30 years of age. *Angle Orthod* 74, 319–327.

Mongini F and Italiano M (2001) TMJ disorders and myogenic facial pain: a discriminative analysis using the McGill Pain Questionnaire. *Pain* 91, 323–330.

Moore R and Brødsgaard I (1999) Cross-cultural investigations of pain. In Crombie IK (ed.) *Epidemiology of Pain*, pp. 53–80. Seattle: IASP Press.

Murakami K, Segami N, Okamoto M, Yamamura I, Takahashi K and Tsuboi Y (2000) Outcome of arthroscopic surgery for internal derangement of the temporomandibular joint: long-term results covering 10 years. *J Craniomaxillofac Surg* 28, 264–271.

Nixdorf DR, Heo G and Major PW (2002) Randomized controlled trial of botulinum toxin A for chronic myogenous orofacial pain. *Pain* 99, 465–473.

Okeson JP (2005) *Bell's Orofacial Pains*. Chicago: Quintessence.

Peck CC, Goulet JP, Lobbezoo F, Schiffman EL, Alstergren P, Anderson GC, de Leeuw R, Jensen R, Michelotti A, Ohrbach R, Petersson A and List T (2014) Expanding the taxonomy of the diagnostic criteria for temporomandibular disorders. *J Oral Rehabil* 41(1), 2–23.

Pehling J, Schiffman E, Look J, Shaefer J, Lenton P and Fricton J (2002) Interexaminer reliability and clinical validity of the temporomandibular index: a new outcome measure for temporomandibular disorders. *J Orofac Pain* 16, 296–304.

Pfau DB, Rolke R, Nickel R, Treede RD and Daublaender M (2009) Somatosensory profiles in subgroups of patients with myogenic temporomandibular disorders and Fibromyalgia Syndrome. *Pain* 147(1–3), 72–83.

Plesh O, Curtis D, Levine J and McCall WD Jr (2000) Amitriptyline treatment of chronic pain in patients with temporomandibular disorders. *J Oral Rehabil* 27, 834–841.

Plesh O, Sinisi SE, Crawford PB and Gansky SA (2005) Diagnoses based on the research diagnostic criteria for temporomandibular disorders in a biracial population of young women. *J Orofac Pain* 19, 65–75.

Pullinger AG, Seligman DA and Gornbein JA (1993) A multiple logistic regression analysis of the risk and relative odds of temporomandibular disorders as a function of common occlusal features. *J Dent Res* 72, 968–979.

Rammelsberg P, LeResche L, Dworkin S and Mancl L (2003) Longitudinal outcome of temporomandibular disorders: a 5-year epidemiologic study of muscle disorders defined by research diagnostic criteria for temporomandibular disorders. *J Orofac Pain* 17, 9–20.

Raphael KG and Marbach JJ (2001) Widespread pain and the effectiveness of oral splints in myofascial face pain. *J Am Dent Assoc* 132, 305–316.

Reid KI, Gracely RH and Dubner RA (1994) The influence of time, facial side, and location on pain-pressure thresholds in chronic myogenous temporomandibular disorder. *J Orofac Pain* 8, 258–265.

Reinert A, Kaske A and Mense S (1998) Inflammation-induced increase in the density of neuropeptide-immunoreactive nerve endings in rat skeletal muscle. *Exp Brain Res* 121, 174–180.

Reiter S, Eli I, Gavish A and Winocur E (2006) Ethnic differences in temporomandibular disorders between Jewish and Arab populations in Israel according to RDC/TMD evaluation. *J Orofac Pain* 20, 36–42.

Ren K and Dubner R (1999) Central nervous system plasticity and persistent pain. *J Orofac Pain* 13, 155–163.

Riley JL, Gilbert GH and Heft MW (1998) Orofacial pain symptom prevalence: selective sex differences in the elderly? *Pain* 76, 97–104.

Romaniello A, Cruccu G, Frisardi G, Arendt-Nielsen L and Svensson P (2003) Assessment of nociceptive trigeminal pathways by laser-evoked potentials and laser silent periods in patients with painful temporomandibular disorders. *Pain* 103, 31–39.

Rongo R, Ekberg E, Nilsson IM, Al-Khotani A, Alstergren P, Conti PCR, Durham J, Goulet JP, Hirsch C, Kalaykova SI, Kapos FP, Komiyama O, Koutris M, List T, Lobbezoo F, Ohrbach R, Peck CC,

Restrepo C, Rodrigues MJ, Sharma S, Svensson P, Visscher CM, Wahlund K, Michelotti A (2021) Diagnostic criteria for temporomandibular disorders (DC/TMD) for children and adolescents: An international Delphi study-Part 1-Development of Axis I. *J Oral Rehabil* 48(7), 836–845.

Rudy TE, Turk DC, Kubinski JA and Zaki HS (1995) Differential treatment responses of TMD patients as a function of psychological characteristics. *Pain* 61, 103–112.

Sanroman JF (2004) Closed lock (MRI fixed disc): a comparison of arthrocentesis and arthroscopy *Int J Oral Maxillofac Surg* 33, 344–348.

Sarlani E, Grace EG, Reynolds MA and Greenspan JD (2004) Evidence for up-regulated central nociceptive processing in patients with masticatory myofascial pain. *J Orofac Pain* 18, 41–55.

Sato S, Goto S, Nasu F and Motegi K (2003) Natural course of disc displacement with reduction of the temporomandibular joint: changes in clinical signs and symptoms. *J Oral Maxillofac Surg* 61, 32–34.

Schaible HG (2006) Basic mechanisms of deep somatic tissue. In McMahon SB and Koltzenburg M (eds) *Wall and Melzack´s Textbook of Pain*, pp. 621–634. Elsevier Churchill Livingstone.

Schiffman E, Ohrbach R, Truelove E, Look J, Anderson G, Goulet JP, List T, Svensson P, Gonzalez Y, Lobbezoo F, Michelotti A, Brooks SL, Ceusters W, Drangsholt M, Ettlin D, Gaul C, Goldberg LJ, Haythornthwaite JA, Hollender L, Jensen R, John MT, De Laat A, De Leeuw R, Maixner W, Van Der Meulen M, Murray GM, Nixdorf DR, Palla S, Petersson A, Pionchon P, Smith B, Visscher CM, Zakrzewska J and Dworkin SF (2014a) Diagnostic Criteria for Temporomandibular Disorders (DC/TMD) for clinical and research applications: recommendations of the International RDC/TMD consortium network* and orofacial pain special interest group. *J Oral Facial Pain Headache* 28(1), 6–27.

Schiffman EL, Velly AM, Look JO et al (2014b) Effects of four treatment strategies for temporomandibular joint closed lock. *Int J Oral Maxillofac Surg* 43(2), 217–226. doi: 10.1016/j.ijom.2013.07.744

Schindler H and Svensson P (2006) Myofascial TMD pain – pathophysiology – management. In Türp JC, Sommer C and Hugger A (eds) *Orofacial Pain. Integration of Research into Clinical Management*. Karger.

Schmitter M, Ohlmann B, John MT, Hirsch C and Rammelsberg P (2005b) Research diagnostic criteria for temporomandibular disorders: a calibration and reliability study. *Cranio* 23, 212–218.

Schmitter M, Rammelsberg P and Hassel A (2005a) The prevalence of signs and symptoms of temporomandibular disorders in very old subjects. *J Oral Rehabil* 32, 467–473.

Seligman DA and Pullinger AG (2000) Analysis of occlusal variables, dental attrition, and age for distinguishing healthy controls from female patients with intracapsular temporomandibular disorders. *J Prosthet Dent* 83, 76–82.

Sessle BJ (2000) Acute and chronic craniofacial pain: brainstem mechanisms of nociceptive transmission and neuroplasticity, and their clinical correlates. *Crit Rev Oral Biol Med* 11, 57–91.

Sessle BJ, Hu JW, Amano N and Zhong G (1986) Convergence of cutaneous, tooth pulp, visceral, neck and muscle afferents onto nociceptive and non-nociceptive neurones in trigeminal subnucleus caudalis (medullary dorsal horn) and its implication for referred pain. *Pain* 27, 219–235.

Sharav Y, Singer E, Schmidt E, Dionne RA and Dubner R (1987) The analgesic effect of amitriptyline on chronic facial pain. *Pain* 31, 199–209.

Sharma S, Wactawski-Wende J, LaMonte MJ, Zhao J, Slade GD, Bair E, Greenspan JD, Fillingim RB, Maixner W, Ohrbach R (2019) Incident injury is strongly associated with subsequent incident temporomandibular disorder: results from the OPPERA study. *Pain*. Jul;160(7), 1551–1561. doi: 10.1097/j.pain.0000000000001554. PMID: 30883525; PMCID: PMC6586508.

Sherman JJ and LeResche L (2006) Does experimental pain response vary across the menstrual cycle? A methodological review. *Am J Physiol Regul Integr Comp Physiol* 291, R245–56.

Sherman JJ, LeResche L, Huggins KH, Mancl LA, Sage JC and Dworkin SF (2004) The relationship of somatization and depression to experimental pain response in women with temporomandibular disorders. *Psychosom Med* 66, 852–860.

Sherman JJ and Turk DC (2001) Nonpharmacologic approaches to the management of myofascial temporomandibular disorders. *Curr Pain Headache Rep* 5, 421–431.

Singer E and Dionne R (1997) A controlled evaluation of ibuprofen and diazepam for chronic orofacial muscle pain. *J Orofac Pain* 11, 139–146.

Slade GD, Bair E, By K, Mulkey F, Baraian C, Rothwell R, Reynolds M, Miller V, Gonzalez Y, Gordon S, Ribeiro-Dasilva M, Lim PF, Greenspan JD, Dubner R, Fillingim RB, Diatchenko L, Maixner W, Dampier D, Knott C and Ohrbach R (2011) Study methods, recruitment, sociodemographic findings, and demographic representativeness in the OPPERA study. *J Pain* 12(11 Suppl), T12–T26.

Slade GD, Fillingim RB, Sanders AE, Bair E, Greenspan JD, Ohrbach R, Dubner R, Diatchenko L, Smith SB, Knott C and Maixner W (2013) Summary of findings from the OPPERA prospective cohort study of incidence of first-onset temporomandibular disorder: implications and future directions. *J Pain* 14(12 Suppl), T116–124.

Slade GD, Ohrbach R, Greenspan JD, Fillingim RB, Bair E, Sanders AE, Dubner R, Diatchenko L, Meloto CB, Smith S and Maixner W (2016) Painful temporomandibular disorder: decade of discovery from OPPERA studies. *J Dent Res*. Sep; 95(10), 1084–1092. doi: 10.1177/0022034516653743. Epub 2016 Jun 23. PMID: 27339423; PMCID: PMC5004239.

Smith SB, Mir E, Bair E, Slade GD, Dubner R, Fillingim RB, Greenspan JD, Ohrbach R, Knott C, Weir B, Maixner W and Diatchenko L (2013) Genetic variants associated with development of TMD and its intermediate phenotypes: the genetic architecture of TMD in the OPPERA prospective cohort study. *J Pain: Official Journal of the American Pain Society* 14(12 Suppl), T91–101.e101–103.

Sörensen J, Graven-Nielsen T, Henriksson K-G, Bengtsson M and Arendt-Nielsen L (1998) Hyperexcitability in fibromyalgia. *J Rheumatol* 25, 152–155.

Stohler CS (1997) Masticatory myalgias. Emphasis on the nerve growth factor – estrogen link. *Pain Forum* 6, 176–180.

Stohler CS (2004) Taking stock: from chasing occlusal contacts to vulnerability alleles. *Orthod Craniofac Res* 7, 157–161.

Stohler CS and Lund JP (1994) Effects of noxious stimulation of the jaw muscles on the sensory experience of volunteer human subjects. In Stohler CS and Carlson DS (eds) *Biological & Psychological Aspects of Orofacial Pain*. Craniofacial Growth Series 29. Center for Human Growth and Development, 55–73. Ann Arbor: The University of Michigan.

Stohler CS and Lund JP (1995) Psychophysical and orofacial motor responses to muscle pain – validation and utility of an experimental model. In Morimoto T, Matsuya T and Takada K (eds) *Brain and Oral Function*, pp. 227–237. Amsterdam: Elsevier.

Suvinen TI, Reade PC, Kemppainen P, Kononen M and Dworkin SF (2005) Review of aetiological concepts of temporomandibular pain disorders: towards a biopsychosocial model for integration of physical disorder factors with psychological and psychosocial illness impact factors. *Eur J Pain* 9, 613–633.

Svensson P and Arendt-Nielsen L (2000) Clinical and experimental aspects of temporomandibular disorders. *Cur Rev Pain* 4, 158–165.

Svensson P, Arendt-Nielsen L, Nielsen H and Larsen JK (1995) Effect of chronic and experimental jaw muscle pain on pressure-pain thresholds and stimulus-response curves. *J Orofac Pain* 9, 347–356.

Svensson P, Cairns BE, Wang K and Arendt-Nielsen L (2003) Injection of nerve growth factor into human masseter muscle evokes long-lasting mechanical allodynia and hyperalgesia. *Pain* 104, 241–247.

Svensson P and Graven-Nielsen T (2001) Craniofacial muscle pain: review of mechanisms and clinical manifestations. *J Orofac Pain* 15, 117–145.

Svensson P and Kumar A (2016) Assessment of risk factors for oro-facial pain and recent developments in classification: implications for management. *J Oral Rehabil* 43(12), 977–989. doi: 10.1111/joor.12447

Svensson P, List T and Hector G (2001) Analysis of stimulus-evoked pain in patients with myofascial temporomandibular pain disorders. *Pain* 92, 399–409.

Svensson P and Sessle BJ (2004) Orofacial pain. In Miles TS, Nauntofte B and Svensson P (eds) *Clinical Oral Physiology*, pp. 93–139. Quintessence.

Svensson P, Sharav Y and Benoliel R (2015) Myalgia, myofascial pain, tension-type headaches, and fibromyalgia. In Sharav Y and Benoliel R (eds) *Orofacial Pain and Headache*, pp. 195–256. Quintessence Publishing Co, Inc.

Ta LE and Dionne RA (2004) Treatment of painful temporomandibular joints with a cyclooxygenase-2 inhibitor: a randomized placebo-controlled comparison of celecoxib to naproxen. *Pain* 111, 13–21.

Takeshita S, Hirata H and Bereiter DA (2001) Intensity coding by TMJ-responsive neurons in superficial laminae of caudal medullary dorsal horn of the rat. *J Neurophysiol* 86, 2393–2404.

Thambar S, Kulkarni S, Armstrong S and Nikolarakos D (2020) Botulinum toxin in the management of temporomandibular disorders: a systematic review. *Br J Oral Maxillofac Surg.* Jun; 58(5), 508–519. doi: 10.1016/j.bjoms.2020.02.007. Epub 2020 Mar 3. PMID: 32143934.

The ICOP classification committee (2020) International Classification of Orofacial Pain, 1st edition (ICOP). *Cephalalgia* Feb;40(2), 129–221. doi: 10.1177/0333102419893823. PMID: 32103673.

Truelove E, Huggins KH, Mancl L and Dworkin SF (2006) The efficacy of traditional, low-cost and nonsplint therapies for temporomandibular disorder: a randomized controlled trial. *J Am Dent Assoc* 137, 1099–1107.

Turk DC, Zaki HS and Rudy TE (1993) Effects of intraoral appliance and biofeedback/stress management alone and in combination in treating pain and depression in patients with temporomandibular disorders. *J Prothet Dent* 70, 158–164.

Turner JA and Dworkin SF (2004) Screening for psychosocial risk factors in patients with chronic orofacial pain: recent advances. *J Am Dent Assoc* 135, 1119–1125.

Turner JA, Mancl L and Aaron LA (2005) Brief cognitive-behavioral therapy for temporomandibular disorder pain: effects on daily electronic outcome and process measures. *Pain* 117, 377–387.

Türp JC, Kowalski CJ, O´Leary NO and Stohler CS (1998) Pain maps from facial pain patients indicate a broad pain geography. *J Dent Res* 77, 1465–1472.

Türp JC, Kowalski CJ and Stohler CS (1997) Pain descriptors characteristic of persistent facial pain. *J Orofac Pain* 11, 285–290.

Von Lindern JJ, Niederhagen B, Berge S and Appel T (2003) Type A botulinum toxin in the treatment of chronic facial pain associated with masticatory hyperactivity. *J Oral Maxillofac Surg* 61, 774–778.

Warren MP and Fried JL (2001) Temporomandibular disorders and hormones in women. *Cells Tissues Organs* 169, 187–192.

Wei F, Dubner R and Ren K (1999) Nucleus reticularis gigantocellularis and nucleus raphe magnus in the brain stem exert opposite effects on behavioral hyperalgesia and spinal Fos protein expression after peripheral inflammation. *Pain* 80, 127–141.

Whitney CW and Von Korff M (1992) Regression to the mean in treated versus untreated chronic pain. *Pain* 50, 281–285.

Willis WD and Coggeshall RE (1991) *Sensory Mechanisms of the Spinal Cord.* New York: Plenum Press.

Woolf CJ and Salter MW (2006) Plasticity and pain: role of the dorsal horn. In McMahon SB and Koltzenburg M (eds) *Wall and Melzack´s Textbook of Pain*, pp. 91–106. Elsevier Churchill Livingstone.

Zubieta JK, Heitzeg MM, Smith YR, Bueller JA, Xu K, Xu Y, Koeppe RA, Stohler CS and Goldman D (2003) COMT val158met genotype affects mu-opioid neurotransmitter responses to a pain stressor. *Science* 299, 1240–1243.

Zubieta JK, Smith YR, Bueller JA, Xu Y, Kilbourn MR, Jewett DM, Meyer CR, Koeppe RA and Stohler CS (2002) mu-opioid receptor-mediated antinociceptive responses differ in men and women. *J Neurosci* 22, 5100–5107.

17

Clear Aligners and Their Role in Orthodontics

Sonil Kalia, Reginald Mietke, Birte Melsen

History of aligners

The origin of aligner treatment can be traced back nearly one hundred years to the invention of the 'Flex-O-Tite' removable gum massaging appliance by Orrin Remensnyder in 1925 (Remensnyder 1926). The invention was intended for use in treating periodontal disease, but it was recognised by Dr Remensnyder that the teeth actually moved slightly during its use. Kesling (1945) took this concept further with the invention of the tooth 'positioner' with the purpose of achieving 'final artistic positioning and retention' after treatment with fixed appliances; the positioner was made of an elastic vulcanite plastic. When the patient chewed on the appliance, the bite force would be applied to the teeth with the intention of repositioning the crowns to a better occlusion. Doctors sometimes use tooth positioners today and Kesling stated that 'major tooth movements could be accomplished with a series of positioners by changing the teeth on the setup slightly as treatment progresses'. This describes the concept of aligner treatment. In 1964, Dr Henry Nahoum (1964) created the dental contour appliance by thermoforming a plastic sheet over a plaster model. A jeweller's saw or disc was used to separate the teeth to be moved from the plaster model, and wax was used to reposition them to thermoform the next aligner for treatment. The contour appliance functions by 'exerting pressure until the teeth attain their predetermined positions'. The magnitude of the pressure and force systems applied to the teeth was unknown. The main assumption in the design of the appliance was that tooth positions fabricated in the appliance would determine and control the movements of the teeth. The appliance was shown to be more effective in contraction of the arch than expansion of the arch. In 1993, Sheridan et al. developed the Essix retainer, but also developed a series of thermoformed plastic overlays similar to those fabricated by Nahoum (1964). The force applied to the teeth could be modified in two ways: (1) spot thermoforming by using a heated plier developed by Dr Hilliard to create a dimple in the plastic that would contact the tooth and cause the plastic to bow, hence applying force to the tooth, and (2) placing a mound of composite on the tooth surface and allowing the plastic to contact it. It is important to first create a space between the other side of the tooth and the aligner, into which the tooth can move. Without space, no movement can take place. Using these techniques, the Essix appliance can be designed to affect mild-to-moderate tooth movements. The force system applied to the teeth is however essentially unknown.

Clear aligners are produced from thermoplastic material and can be characterised as the ones fabricated via manual setup and the ones using a CAD/CAM technology to design and produce aligners. The latter have one concept in common, that is, the desired position of the tooth is used to fabricate the appliance. It is assumed that, given time, the tooth will reposition until it aligns with its desired position in the appliance. This can be called a 'displacement-driven approach' and is used in some of the aligners on the market. However, the fundamental concept of using the appliance to control force applied to the teeth and controlling which teeth move and which do not move is missing. Planning and control of the active and reactive groups of teeth are imperative to control treatment and achieve the desired outcome; this is attempted with the 'force-driven approach' used in the best-known aligner system: Invisalign®.

Difference between aligner treatments and conventional orthodontic treatments

The biggest difference between the treatment with fixed appliances and treatment with aligners is that most aligner treatments are planned from the first to the last movement in all possible detail. In contrast to fixed appliances, the sequence, the direction and the amount of any tooth movement can only be changed by a mid-treatment correction if during treatment there is a severe discrepancy between what is planned and what is occurring. This may seem to be disadvantageous, but can also be considered a challenge. The visualisation of the anticipated outcome of a treatment with fixed appliances was accomplished by using occlusograms (Melsen 2012), a standard study model setup, or, as in the case of aligners, by a virtual setup.

When determining the final position of the teeth on the proposed setup, the doctor must also evaluate the final occlusal contacts and in some instances occlusal interferences have to be removed clinically. Most aligner companies are dividing the treatment in stage-by-stage progression of tooth movements from the initial position of the teeth to the final position of the teeth. Orthodontic biomechanics should govern the principle of staging. The disadvantage of aligner therapy is that once approved and manufactured, aligners cannot be changed, and consequently new aligners have to be manufactured if the treatment doesn't track and lead to the desired result. One company Orthocaps® tries to alleviate this problem by phasing the amount of aligners during treatment.

What types of patients are seeking aligner treatments?

Some patients may arrive in an orthodontic office with the request to be treated with an invisible appliance. In this situation, they can be offered lingual appliances or aligner therapy. It is fundamental that the doctor, before embarking on treatment with a particular treatment modality, understands the patient's expectations from the treatment. Some patients are only interested in a 'quick fix', where they just want the front 'social 6' teeth corrected with no consideration of the occlusion, etc. The 'pros and cons' of the treatment being offered must be discussed with the patient and the different options explained. The treatment offered must also be in the best interest of the patient and the doctor must follow the orthodontic principles for a successful treatment result that is compatible with normal function.

Pre-treatment considerations

As is the norm with treating with fixed appliances, the use of aligners requires just as much information given to the patient regarding hygiene and compliance.

Aligner therapy is orthodontics with just a different appliance system. Therefore, consultation, record collection, documentation of existing problems and treatment goals should follow standard orthodontic procedures.

Diagnosis and treatment planning are essential to every patient case and aligner treatment is no exception to this basic rule. The doctor has to appropriately examine, diagnose and determine the best treatment plan for the patient, and also outline any unavoidable compromises due to degeneration of the dentition. As most treatments with clear aligners are so far carried out on adult patients, the treatment goal can be limited due to marginal bone loss, tooth wear or extensive restorative work and the patient has to be informed that restorative work may be needed following the aligner treatment. In patients with crowding, one might consider interproximal reduction (IPR) if the amount of necessary expansion and proclination is not providing the necessary space (see Chapter 18).

Most aligner companies fabricate all the aligners required from beginning to end, while others divide the treatment into stages.

As with all orthodontic treatments, a full mouth examination has to be carried out noting all the pertinent observations (see Chapter 2) and the following records are needed:

- Photographs (extra oral: frontal (at rest/smiling) and profile; intraoral: frontal, left/right lateral, maxillary/mandibular occlusal).
- Radiographs (panoramic or periapical, optional: cephalogram).
- Digital 3D scan/or vinyl polysiloxane impressions (maxillary, mandibular) plus bite registration.
- Completed treatment form.

The accurate images of the teeth of the upper and lower arches as well as the bite of the patient are the necessary input for the fabrication of aligners. This information can be obtained by intra-oral scanning or a polyvinyl siloxane impression of the teeth. This is used to create a 'virtual patient' in the software. A computer code then determines the positions of the teeth in final occlusion and calculates the total movements needed of each tooth from the beginning to the end of treatment. Finally, it divides the movement of each tooth into smaller movements corresponding to the displacement between aligners (0.10–0.33 mm) and alters the progression of these movements to minimise interferences that may occur during the treatment.

What has to be evaluated before the aligners are produced?

In relation to most of the aligner companies, a virtual setup will be presented for evaluation, inspection and possible acceptance. The first step of the evaluation should ensure that the morphology of all teeth and the occlusion reflect the correct intraoral situation. An improper occlusion of the virtual model can indicate an impression/scan failure.

The orthodontist should then compare his/her treatment plan including any annotated remarks with the virtual treatment plan. There may be differences either because the IT technician overlooked some information or realised during the virtual setup that interferences, which could impede the progress of treatment, were present and therefore altered the treatment plan. If the treatment plan has to be modified, the proposal is rejected. It is then altered until it is acceptable to the orthodontist and the patient. Acceptance will be followed by a description of the necessary attachments and recommended interproximal enamel reduction.

In relation to both force-driven and displacement-driven aligners, preformed attachments or auxiliaries will be added by indirect bonding technique and preplaced in a transfer tray before the first aligner.

This approach is a complete proactive planning of treatment, not reactive orthodontics as has been practised for decades. Upon acceptance of the treatment plan, the aligners are thermoformed and delivered to the respective dental offices.

Force-driven or displacement-driven aligners?

As the demand and need for aesthetic orthodontic treatment alternatives have grown, aligners have secured a firm place in the orthodontic repertoire. However, the inherent disadvantages associated with the use of removable appliances such as aligners for orthodontic tooth movement pose great challenges in improving their efficacy. Invisalign® represents the force-driven approach, whereas the Orthocaps® system is an effort to utilise the displacement-driven system.

A short presentation of two aligner systems is presented in the following text.

Invisalign®

Biomechanical basis

The Invisalign® system in 1997 claimed that when planned correctly it could achieve desirable treatment results in relation to a majority of malocclusions. Invisalign® is a force-driven system. The basis was that once the desired tooth displacements are determined, there is only one force system that can generate this movement (Burstone 1981). To describe a force system, information about three points is needed: (1) the point of application of the force, (2) the direction of the force and (3) the magnitude of the force. When focusing on tooth displacement, the force system necessary should be defined in relation to the centre of resistance of the tooth or groups of teeth. The displacement generated by a removable appliance, as an aligner will, generally results from the contact with the crown and thus be a tipping type of movement. The contact between aligner wall and tooth will not be able to generate a specific force system, but with the Invisalign® system, not only action and reaction forces can be controlled, but also the type of movement generated. The aligner has no contact with the tooth, but only with special attachments bonded indirectly to the teeth with the attachment template. These attachments are designed so that the contact with the aligner will result in the correct displacement. Figure 17.1 demonstrates a special attachment designed, so that the force from the aligner acts perpendicular to the active surface and generates an extrusion and a distal displacement. In the direction of the tooth displacement, the aligner has room around it to allow the tooth to move while the contact is tight to the anchorage unit, hence differentiating between the active and reactive units.

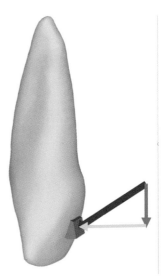

Fig. 17.1 The optimised extrusion attachment is positioned and oriented such that the aligner is able to apply force to the flat active surface of the attachment. The extrusive component of the force effectively extrudes the tooth.

As the contacts delivered from the aligner are limited to the crown of the tooth via the attachment, this can, when be combined with forces from the so-called Power Ridges®, generate the moment-to-force ratio necessary for a root movement similar to the torque included in a prescription bracket. The power ridge is a specific shape of the aligner that results in the development of the force system necessary to control the lingual movement of the root, as it applies a lingual pressure near the incisal edge whereby the needed moment-to-force ratio for root movement is produced (Figures 17.2 and 17.3).

Smart features

The Invisalign® system is marketed as a combination of three 'Smart' parts: SmartForce® feature, SmartTrack® material and SmartStage® technology. All parts work together to control tooth movement during treatment and attain a predictable treatment outcome.

SmartForce® feature

In contrast to most aligners that have contact between the aligners and the teeth in the Invisalign® system, the aligner has no contact with the crown of the tooth, but only to specially designed attachments. Once the tooth movements are determined, the necessary line of action of the force can be defined and the 'optimised attachments' produced. The attachments are shaped so that the contact with aligner will create a desired force perpendicular to the active surface. The Power Ridges® feature, which is a special part of the aligner that, together with the attachments, supports lingual displacement of the root. To the SmartForce® feature belong also special attachments and aligner configuration used for the generation of angulation, rotation and correction of vertical problems (Figures 17.4–17.6).

Power Ridges® feature

The Power Ridges® feature is designed to generate lingual root torque to anterior teeth by applying two forces to the crown of a tooth (Figure 17.2). The ClinCheck™ treatment plan may show a tooth which from beginning to end of treatment requires a lingual root movement. The Power

Ridges® feature is an intentional change to the shape of the aligner, which results in applying the needed force system (Figure 17.3(1),(2)). The Power Ridges® feature causes the buccal aspect of the aligner to bow outwards and act as a spring. It applies the concentrated lingual force F1 to the tooth. This force alone would cause the tooth to tip lingually.

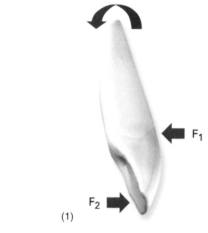

(1)

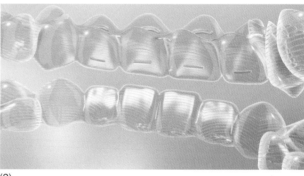

(2)

Fig. 17.2 (1) The aligner with two power ridges is shown. The shape of the aligner is not the shape of the tooth to apply the two forces necessary for the lingual root torque movement. (2) The force system required to achieve lingual root torque is shown. The aligner applies both forces. The M/F ratio of the resultant force and total moment are correct to control the inclination change of the tooth with a lingual movement of the root.

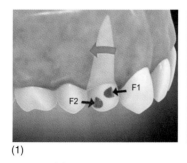

(1)

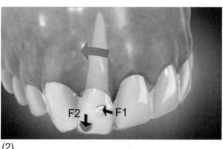

(2)

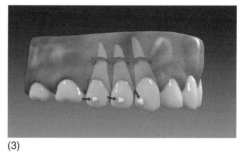

(3)

Fig. 17.3 (1)–(3) Three methods of controlling a second-order movement of the canine are shown. The two forces are applied on the two attachments in the first image. The distal force is applied to the pressure points on the buccal and lingual aspects of the aligner. The force on the attachment provides for the counter-moment to control the tooth movement.

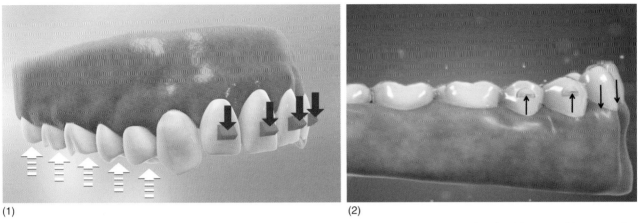

(1)   (2)

Fig. 17.4 (1) The shape of the aligner is modified, so it applies equal force to the upper anterior dentition to achieve anterior extrusion as a unit. (2) The force system applied to the mandibular arch in the treatment of a deep bite is shown.

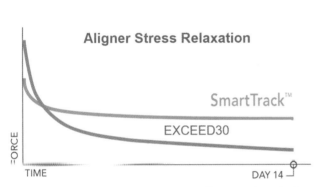

Fig. 17.5 Aligners comprising SmartTrack® material apply low constant force and lower force upon insertion than Exceed30 material.

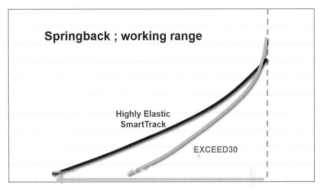

Fig. 17.6 The springback and working range of an aligner comprising SmartTrack® material are much greater than that of Exceed30. Orthodontic force is being applied throughout a greater range of movement in each aligner.

However, the bowing of the aligner on the buccal aspect results in pulling on the lingual aspect also applying force F2. The Power Ridges® feature is designed to apply F1 larger in magnitude than F2, and hence the resultant force is lingual.

Optimised second-order root control

As the thermoformed aligner does not contact these facets of the tooth, optimised root control attachments are designed to address this situation (Figure 17.3). The images show three methods by which the correct force system for a root distal angulation change may be applied to the tooth. In Figure 17.3(1), two attachments are shown under pressure by the aligner, resulting in a tipping. In Figure 17.3(2), a pressure point from the aligner to the tooth is adding to the necessary force system. The last suggestion is to position the attachment, so that the root will be displaced with respect to the crown.

Invisalign® treatment of vertical discrepancies

In relation to correction of vertical problems, all forces for extrusion or intrusion of anterior teeth are done via optimised attachments with very low forces, while the forces acting on the posterior teeth are also depending on contact between aligner and the teeth (Figure 17.6).

SmartTrack® material

The second part of the three 'Smart' features is the 'SmartTrack® material' that deals with the force level and describes how new development of composite materials has improved the maintenance of the force level. Within fixed appliances, the development of the wire materials has made it possible to lower the force without changing the dimension and to maintain the force level without adding to the wire length. An equivalent development has taken place within the composite materials used for aligners.

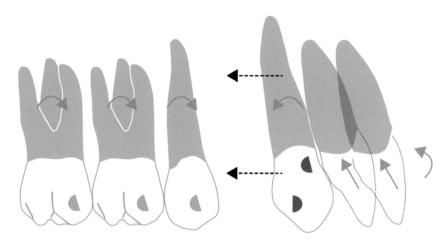

Fig. 17.7 The force system applied by the Invisalign aligner to achieve extraction space closure with maximum anchorage is shown.

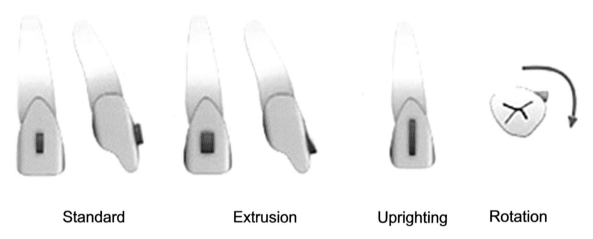

Standard   Extrusion   Uprighting   Rotation

Fig. 17.8 These attachments are an adjunct to the tooth movements desired and are robust. The design is specially developed to achieve the desired movement necessary.

The superior ability of SmartTrack® material is to apply low more constant force, and demonstrate high elasticity and resilience enabling it to achieve more consistent movement during each stage of treatment. SmartTrack® material comprises polyurethane and copolyester materials. One of the benefits of SmartTrack® material over the previous Invisalign® material, Exceed30, is shown in Figure 17.7. The SmartTrack® material displays an almost constant force. Also, the working range (Figure 17.8) is improved with the newly developed material. In fact, the material can move more than that is needed for each stage of treatment.

Finally, it has been verified that the stiffness of the new material is such that it can provide better anchorage than a 0.021 × 0.025-inch stainless-steel wire inserted in the posterior segment.

SmartStage® technology

A last and essential part of the system is SmartStage® technology. SmartStage® technology is the optimised progression

of tooth movements developed to improve predictability and reduce unwanted interferences during treatment. SmartStage® technology is the answer to the questions: Which tooth moves when in treatment? How does one control the movement of the active segment and minimise any unwanted movement of the anchorage? This is the main issue of rational mechanics (see Chapter 7).

Seeing a tooth distalise in the virtual software does not mean it will occur, not without the proper anchorage reinforcement. Anchorage control needs to be considered by the clinician during the treatment planning and then applied clinically during treatment in conjunction with the clear aligner treatment.

The advantage of SmartStage® technology compared to sliding mechanics where tipping and uprighting alternate is that the force system developed by the combination of contacts between aligner and optimised attachments and contacts between special designs of the aligner and teeth thereby reduces the amount of jiggling and perhaps lowers the treatment time.

Table 17.1 The Orthocaps Standard Polymer Sequence (OSPS) is used to simulate the same process that occurs when one uses different wires in orthodontics. In conventional orthodontics, the initial wires are flexible with memory and elastic, then moving onto stiffer wires as the teeth align. The forces are therefore increased, and this is also simulated in that different polymers are used for the different stages within the Orthocaps aligner journey.

Force levels	Day	Night	Recommendations
Light force	DLP 460/SLP 600	DLP 800*	*First phase/Vertical movements/ Excessive crowding/ Periodontal bone loss.*
Medium force	DLP 460/SLP 800*	DLP 1000*	*Subsequent phase/Expansion/ Alteration in arch form/ Inter-maxillary elastics.*
Heavy force	DLP 580*/SLP 1000*	DLP 1000*/DLP 580*	*Last phase/Refinement phase/ Over correction/Root movement/ Uprighting/Torque/ Limited movement.*
Retention	SLP 800*	SLP 800*/SLP 1000*	*Retention/Relapse treatment which requires movement less than 2 mm.*
	Can be used with inter-maxillary elastics.	*Can be used with inter-maxillary elastics.*	

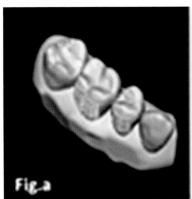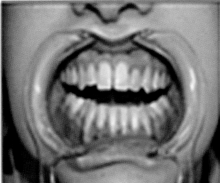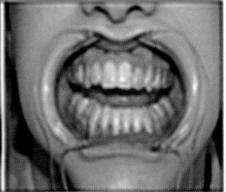

Fig. 17.9 (1) CAD model of the friction pads on two teeth. They are on the teeth with a transfer tray supplied and already loaded with the pads within them. (2) With the aligner placed, (3) they are hardly noticeable, as can be seen from the photo.

The latest development of Invisalign® technology labelled G6 focus on how the company handles the treatment of first premolar extraction and maximum anchorage. One of the features introduced is the application of power arms for application of a sagittal force close to the centre of resistance and temporary anchorage devices (TADs) for insurance of the anchorage.

Orthocaps®

A representative of the displacement-driven system is the Orthocaps® aligner marketed as the 'TwinAligner®'.

Accepting that aligner–tooth interface is mechanically less efficient in transmitting orthodontic forces than systems based on brackets and wires is being addressed by Orthocaps® in several ways.

Pre-aligner treatment auxiliaries

Appliances for distalisation, expansion and constriction can be used before the initial use of aligners. Examples include such appliances as the Beneslider™, Wilson lingual arch, quad helix, hyrax expander and transpalatal arches.

Aligner polymer sequencing

As many of the other available clear aligners, Orthocaps® developed a patented material: the aligner polymer sequencing (Orthocaps Standard Polymer Sequence, OSPS) to select forces delivered at different phases of treatment (Table 17.1).

Improving the contact between aligner and teeth with auxiliaries

To overcome the disadvantage of aligner–tooth interface being mechanically less efficient in transmitting orthodontic forces than systems based on brackets and wires that transmit the forces effectively, the Orthocaps® aligners incorporate features that enable the aligners to have a good grip on the teeth by maximising the surface contact with the teeth to be moved. The company aims at the delivery of a force system that controls both forces and moments in all 3 planes of space without loss in force level and change in direction during usage (Khan 2009, 2014). Patients treated with Orthocaps therefore have auxiliaries placed in the transfer tray ready for indirect bonding (Figure 17.8). It maybe 'friction pads' in order to increase the friction between the inner aligner surface and the tooth and special attachments to help certain tooth movements to occur (Figure 17.9).

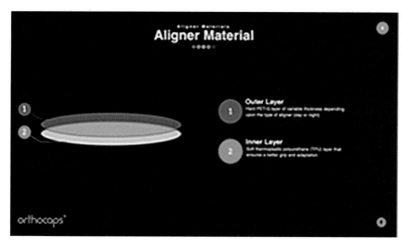

Fig. 17.10 This describes the makeup of the dual-layered aligner material used for the Orthocaps aligners. The thicknesses can be varied as described in Table 17.1 for the OSPS sequencing.

The quality of the force is ensured by the tight fit, and the constancy is obtained by the use of materials with different elasticity. Each aligner is composed of two materials, an inner more elastic, adaptive core and an outer stiffer shell (Figure 17.10). This dual-layered plastic system ensures the application of optimal forces. High-pressure thermoforming techniques also facilitate flow of the inner aligner layer into the interdental areas, thereby increasing the aligner–tooth contact. In fact, the inner core material is also slightly 'sticky', thereby gaining better adaptivity and grip.

Dividing the treatment in phases

In relation to fixed-appliance orthodontic treatments, the progress of treatment will be monitored at every appointment. This is not possible in relation to treatment with aligners, as the clinician merely can assess the fit of the aligner and cannot influence the course of the treatment. To address this and to assess the progress, Orthocaps® treatments are split into phases. For the first phase, there is a choice, but normally 8 aligners are sent, and when the last aligner is used, a new scan or impression is carried out. The company then carries out a detailed superimposition of the treatment result compared with the desired result to see if it is on track. Any deviations are noted in a 'treatment evaluation report' and then the next set of aligners are sent addressing these issues. This then follows a principle of continuous treatment monitoring and tracking.

A certain number of aligners (range between 8 and 12) are initially sent in the first phase. The clinician chooses the number of aligners for the first phase. Usually, for difficult cases, fewer aligners are used in the first phase so as to evaluate the treatment progression more frequently. This approach leads to a more controlled treatment progression and may lead to shorter treatment times. This feature is exclusive to Orthocaps. Figure 17.11 shows an example of the report that is sent at the evaluation.

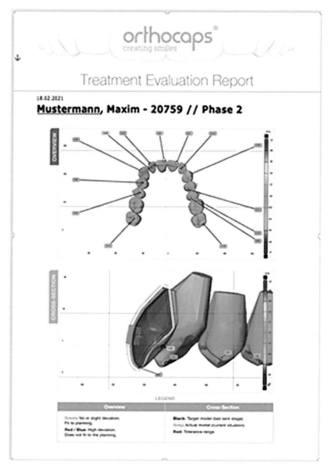

Fig. 17.11 Evaluation report: this illustration is just of the upper teeth. The evaluation report will cover all the teeth being treated. The superimpositions are carried out and the deviations noted and described. Green = no or slight deviation for the original tooth movements planned. Red/blue = high deviation, therefore not going to plan. This is a good way of monitoring treatment progress and addressing any issues early. The aligners then manufactured for this phase 2 will address any issues that have been highlighted.

Hybrid aligner treatment

All aligners are characterised by a difficulty of achieving targeted and constant orthodontic forces throughout the treatment. Attachments are therefore essential to transmit the right forces to correct the malpositions.

An important difference between the force-driven Invisalign® – where the forces necessary for specific displacements are generated by specially designed attachments – and Orthocaps® is that Orthocaps® combines fixed appliances with the aligners to produce the displacements impossible to obtain with the aligner alone, that is, hybrid aligner treatment (HAT). The HAT allows for concomitant use of two conceptually and mechanically different appliances, through which an effective treatment can lead to better clinical results (Khan 2014). The exact times, modalities and use of the common lingual fixed auxiliaries should be determined in the treatment plan. The HAT is composed of segments of lingual appliances that are indirectly bonded to the lingual tooth surfaces while the aligner is used. The displacement of teeth will be controlled by the fixed segments while the aligner maintains the anchorage. The teeth to be displaced are moved within the special cavities or movement channels within the aligner in a targeted manner. Virtual brackets and wires are part of the treatment plan according to this concept, and the sequential movement that should be achieved by the aligner and the planned movement induced by the fixed partial appliances are synchronised using computer technology. The planned movement of the teeth can be mapped and simulated using 3D tracking.

An example of a case using HAT where the position of the teeth prior to aligner treatment and placement of the auxiliaries in order to accelerate the treatment process and derotate the canines and further treatment process up to the end result is shown in Figure 17.12(1)–(8).

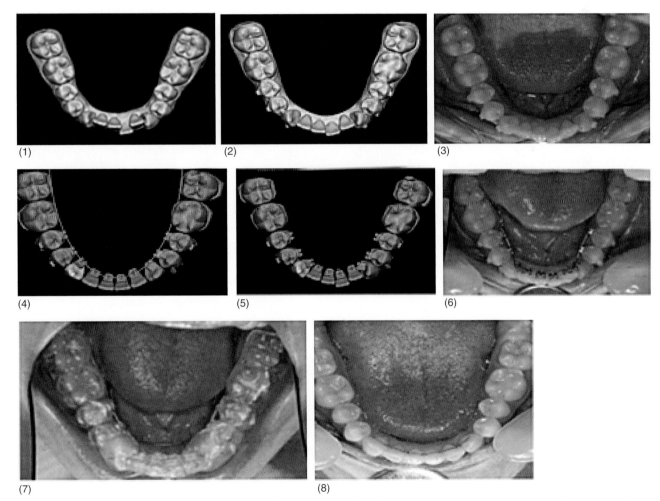

(1) (2) (3)

(4) (5) (6)

(7) (8)

Fig. 17.12 (1) Hybrid aligner treatment (HAT) shows the starting position of the teeth prior to placement of attachments for aligner treatment. (2) and (3) show the attachments placed virtually and on the teeth; this situation is prior to placement of the auxiliaries in order to accelerate the treatment process and derotate the canines and further treatment process up to the end result. (4) The virtual end result setup with the lingual brackets and wire in situ. (5) The virtual setup of the original position of the teeth with the brackets. (6) With an indirect bonding tray, the brackets are fitted with the wire. (7) The aligners are fitted over the lingual segmental arch. (8) Finished result.

Post-aligner treatment auxiliaries

In cases where root uprighting is necessary after space closure with aligners, as in extraction cases, the lingual sectional HAT system can be used for root uprighting (Figures 17.13 and 17.14).

Orthocaps® BiteMaintainer

A constant use of aligners may interfere with lateral occlusal contacts for which the interdigitation would benefit from equilibration of the occlusion. If the occlusion interdigitation is insufficient, then Orthocaps® recommends the use of a BiteMaintainer to achieve a tight and functional occlusion. The Orthocaps® BiteMaintainer is a type of positioning device made from dental silicone. A lateral cephalogram and a bite registration in centric occlusion are needed. The BiteMaintainer is then modelled in a CAD software according to the localisation of the mandibular hinge axis (Figure 17.15). The BiteMaintainer can be used as a retention device and a finishing device.

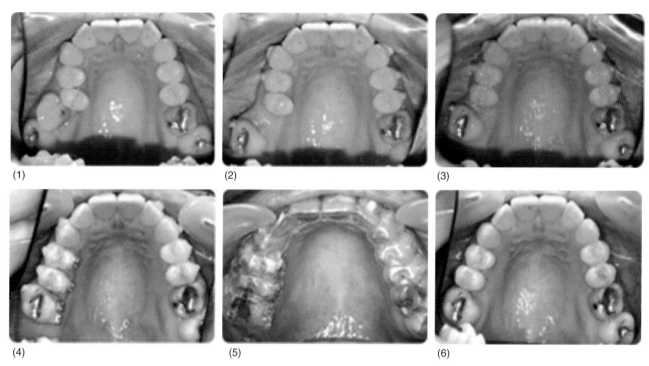

(1) (2) (3)

(4) (5) (6)

Fig. 17.13 (1) The 16 needed extraction due to its poor state. (2) Attachments placed and aligner treatment commenced. (3) The closing of the extraction space near completion. (4) After the extraction space is closed, the uprighting of the root of the 17 needs addressing. The HAT sectional lingual appliance is bonded with 2 brackets placed onto the tooth 17 to create a moment for pure root uprighting when the wire is placed. (5) The aligner is placed over the teeth to counteract any side effects of the sectional lingual appliance. (6) Finished result.

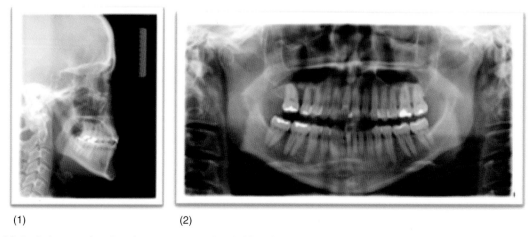

(1) (2)

Fig. 17.14 (1) Cephalogram showing the 17 root uprighted. (2) orthopantomogram (OPT) also showing the 17 root uprighted after concomitant aligner and HAT treatment.

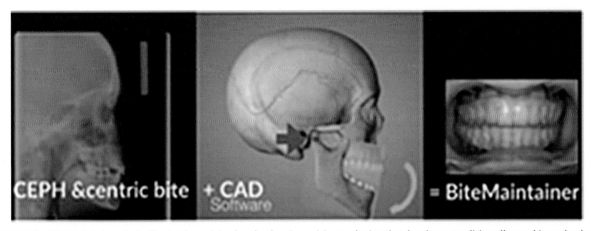

Fig. 17.15 The BiteMaintainer is similar to the original orthodontic positioner device that has been traditionally used in orthodontics. (1) Orthocaps just requires a lateral cephalogram in a centric bite position, and (2) then with their sophisticated CAD software, they can simulate the hinge movement (as in a hinge articulator), and (3) therefore allow the BiteMaintainer to be made as can be seen in the mouth.

Studies on treatment efficacy and efficiency of aligner

The number of companies delivering clear aligner in 2020 is close to 40 and the number of publications registered with the keyword 'clear aligner' is more than 100 per year, mostly case reports. No independent studies on the efficacy of aligner systems such as Orthocaps™, ClearCorrect, ClearPath, Orthero, K Line and Cligner have so far been performed. The clinical studies to date have mainly focused on the one aligner system, which has dominated the market since 1999, namely, Invisalign®. Differences in the treatment results between the different systems mentioned could be expected, since there are significant differences in the respective concepts, workflows and materials used. The assessments of results obtained with Invisalign® and fixed appliances do, on the other hand, apply to all removable thermoplastic appliances.

The papers cited in the following text are chosen based on how often they have been cited. Djeu et al. (2005) was one of the first to compare the results of 48 Invisalign®-treated cases with 48 similar patients treated with fixed appliances. When applying the grading system developed by the American Board of Orthodontics, the success rate with Invisalign® was 27% lower than the success rate with fixed appliances. The aligner system was, on the other hand, shown to have advantages in the closure of small gaps and anterior tooth rotations. Phan and Ling (2007) corroborated these findings when they claimed that Invisalign® appliance could be used with limitations in patients with simple malocclusions, but that perfect results of complicated malocclusions were easier to achieve with fixed appliances. They also described that a combination of aligners with fixed appliances could shorten treatment duration and improve the results. Kravitz et al. (2009) came to the same conclusion when they showed that the mean accuracy of

tooth movements with Invisalign® was 47.1% of that obtained with fixed appliances. The least accurate movement was extrusion of the maxillary central incisors (18.3%) and the mandibular central incisors (24.5%). Accuracy decreased significantly with rotations of more than 15°. According to Simon et al. (2014), the mean success of tooth movement with Invisalign® was 59%. The mean accuracy of incisor torque was 42%. Premolar derotation showed the lowest accuracy of approximately 40%. Distalisation of the maxillary molars was achieved in 87% of cases. The extent of the planned movements and the staging had a significant influence on the treatment result.

Several reviews (Rossini et al. 2015; Galan-Lopez L et al. 2019; Tamer et al. 2019) described the main concept founding the basis for the aligners and cited the results obtained by aligners in a number of studies. All the reviews agree that Invisalign® is a suitable and effective method for closure of minor gaps, lingual constriction and correction of anterior rotation, but this system alone was not able to correct anteroposterior discrepancies, occlusal contacts, extrusions and rotations of more than 15°. Shortened treatment duration and chair time in mild-to-moderate cases appear to be the only significant conclusions based on the results from the effectiveness of clear aligners over conventional systems that are supported by the current evidence.

Weir (2017), a faithful user of Invisalign®, published a survey of at the time 27 different available clear aligners, and presented a table classifying treatment results of different malocclusion traits obtained with aligners alone as either predictable, moderate or difficult. His results were in agreement with the above-mentioned reviews.

Recently, Papageorgiou et al. (2020) also published a systematic review comparing treatment outcome obtained with aligners and fixed appliances. They claimed that previous reviews of clinical studies were biased for various reasons and therefore decided to assess only evidence derived from randomised clinical trials. They found that independent of the method used for evaluation, peer assessment rating (PAR) index (Richmond et al. (1992), discrepancy index (Cangialosi et al. 2004) or American Board of Orthodontics Objective Grading System, the results obtained with fixed appliances were better than those observed following aligner treatment. However, the differences were only significant in relation to root movement and rotations. There was an extreme variability in all the assessed variables, but in summary the results were worse with aligners than with fixed appliances.

In studies regarding root resorption, Li et al. (2020) found significantly less apical root resorption in patients treated with Invisalign® than in patients treated with fixed appliance. This could most likely be described to the fact that less jiggling is taking place in relation to the aligner treatment, as each aligner is prescribed for a specific goal.

With respect to decalcification, a recent randomised clinical trial demonstrated that the type of decalcifications varied, as the aligner-treated patients exhibited large but shallow white spot lesions than the patients with fixed appliance that showed smaller but more severe decalcification (Albhaisi et al 2020).

The validity of the studies comparing aligners with fixed appliances is questionable, as the description of the selection of the cases treated with fixed appliances might be biased. A comparison with the ClinCheck™ might be considered more valid.

Sheldon Peck, Secretary Emeritus of the Edward H. Angle Society of Orthodontists, just before passing away, philosophised over the impact of aligners on present orthodontics and reported how aligner treatments are carried out without any contact between patient and doctor and are often administered by dental hygienists. He concluded that trained orthodontics should demand more from our profession (Peck 2021).

What role will the aligners play in the future?

In 2018, the Journal of Clinical Orthodontics (JCO) dedicated the December volume to aligners and described the most known 13 aligners being used at that particular time. The 'Aligner Corner' provided information on each of the aligners and also reported the number of patients treated by each of the different aligner systems ranging from 'thousands to more than 6 million', the latter by Invisalign®. In January 2021, the JCO was again dedicated to aligners, this time some of the cases were treated with a combination of fixed appliances and aligners, the fixed appliances being preferentially used as enhancement of anchorage occasionally combined with TADs.

Crooked teeth and unsatisfactory aesthetics are leading to an increasing number of adult individuals seeking treatments for straightening of their teeth and aligners seem to be a fascinating solution for many of them. There will,

however, be a difference between the treatments being offered with or without professional support and this is where patient information is essential for the patient to be able to differentiate between a professionally or a company-recommended treatment.

The assessment of the efficacy of aligner treatments has been carried out either by comparing identical groups of patients treated by aligners and fixed appliances or by comparing the completed result with the predicted result in the ClinCheck™ (Haouili et al. 2020), both methods are however characterised by an important bias. The problem, and the reason, why not all treatments can be solved by aligners is that the total treatment has to be carried out with one initial planning, where the desired movement is divided into small steps based on the original morphology of the teeth, and consequently the original estimate of the centre of resistance. The centre of resistance is however changing during the tooth/teeth displacement (Cattaneo et al. 2005). Another reason is that the individual parts of the treatment do not necessarily follow the sequence indicated by the aligner. Extrusion will, for example, occur before and easier than intrusion and the resistance to movement may vary with the bone quality being in the different parts of the alveolar wall. This variance during treatment cannot be taken into consideration in the production of the aligners. Whereas the force system delivered by a fixed appliance can be monitored and adjusted accordingly when the displacement occurring is not the one predicted, this cannot be the case with aligners for which reason a second phase of aligners is often needed. This is to some degree taken into consideration by the Orthocaps® system where the treatment is broken down into stages. There is, however, even when we take these weaknesses into consideration, the fact that the aligners are less detrimental than many companies' guided fixed appliances. Aligners have a defined treatment goal, and with a straight-wire appliance, there is no control of where the arches are ending up in the face.

The aligners are here to stay both as a single appliance and probably increasingly as part of a hybrid appliance combined with fixed appliances, TADs or repositioning splints. The computer-aided treatment (CAT) system, and other aligner systems marketed directly to the public without intervention of professionals, will also be part of daily orthodontics and of the ever-increasing cosmetic industry. It will not always bring the result we as professionals desire, but to minimise the damage that may possibly be the result, patient information is essential to highlight the differences between a professionally supported treatment and one without. We may not all like tattoos or botox injections, but they are as similar in concept as the non-dental-guided orthodontics and most likely here to stay.

Direct-to-consumer orthodontics (DTCO) was studied on 1441 subjects (Bous et al. 2021); 83% of the participants have considered pursuing orthodontic treatment to some extent. Twenty-three per cent reported that they would highly likely choose DTCO products. Convenience was the greatest benefit of DTCOs, followed by cost. The conclusions were that the majority of participants seemed to perceive DTCOs as a viable alternative for seeking orthodontic care. The study highlights the fact that orthodontists and their constituent organisations may consider more robust awareness and advocacy campaigns in order to educate the population about the benefits of pursuing treatment with a trained orthodontist. This issue was also discussed in an editorial in American Journal of Orthodontics and Dentofacial Orthopedics (AJO-DO, 2021) by Hyun Park who discussed do-it-yourself (DIY) treatments and focused on the harm a DIY treatment can do, and concluded that 'collectively we need to implement patient-centric solutions to overcome the barriers that lead to the DIY orthodontic revolution, access to care and cost of orthodontic treatment by a licensed professional'.

Conclusion

Aligners are here to stay, but the benefit of aligners can only be obtained with the same level of knowledge of orthodontic problem listing and biomechanics as when working with fixed appliances. It is therefore a misunderstanding when dentists without this knowledge treat cases with aligners which may lead to solutions that are not compatible with normal function and therefore not maintainable. An automobile maybe fast and good-looking, but should not be driven without a driver's licence, as this maybe a risk for all involved. Buying the equipment does not solve the problem.

It is also imperative that we as a profession educate the public about the level and knowledge of service we offer to allow the public to be able to choose the quality of service they desire.

References

Albhaisi Z, Al-Khateeb SN and Abu Alhaija ES (2020) Enamel demineralization during clear aligner orthodontic treatment compared with fixed appliance therapy, evaluated with quantitative light-induced fluorescence: a randomized clinical trial. *Am J Orthod Dentofacial Orthop* May;157(5), 594–601.

Bous RM, Apostolopoulos K and Valiathan M (2021) When convenience trumps quality of care: a population-based survey on direct to consumer orthodontics. *Am J Orthod Dentofacial Orthop* May;159(5), e411–e422.

Burstone CJ (1981) Variable-modulus orthodontics. *Am J Orthod* 80, 1–16.

Buschang PH, Shaw SG, Ross M, Crosby D and Campbell PM (2014) Comparative time Bous RM, Apostolopoulos K, Valiathan M. When convenience trumps quality of care: A population-based survey on direct to consumer orthodontics. Am J Orthod Dentofacial Orthop. 2021 May;159(5):e411-e422. doi: 10.1016/j.ajodo.2020.10.025. Epub 2021 Feb 27. PMID: 33648802 efficiency of aligner therapy and conventional edgewise braces. *Angle Orthod* 84 P, 391–396.

Bous RM, Apostolopoulos K, Valiathan M. (2021) When convenience trumps quality of care: A population-based survey on direct to consumer

orthodontics. *Am J Orthod Dentofacial Orthop.* May; 159(5), e411-e422. doi.10.1016/j.ajodo.2020.10.025. Epub 2021 Feb 27. PMID: 33648802.

Cattaneo PM, Dalstra M and Melsen B (2005) The finite element method: a tool to study orthodontic tooth movement. *J Dent Res* 84(5), 428–433.

Christiansen R and Burstone C (1969) Centers of rotation within the periodontal space. *Am J Orthod* 55, 353–369.

Djeu G, Shelton C and Maganzini A (2005) Outcome assessment of Invisalign and traditional orthodontics treatment compared with the American board of orthodontics objective grading system. *Am J Orthod Dentofacial Orthop* 128, 292–298.

Galan-Lopez L, Barcia-Gonzalez J, Plasencia E. (2019) A systematic review of the accuracy and efficiency of dental movements with Invisalign®. *Korean J Orthod.* May; 49(3), 140–149. doi:10.4041/kjod.2019.49.3.140. Epub 2019 May 21. PMID: 31149604; PMCID: PMC6533182.

Haouili N, Kravitz ND, Vaid NR, Ferguson DJ and Makki L (2020) Has Invisalign improved? A prospective follow-up study on the efficacy of tooth movement with Invisalign? *Am J Orthod Dentofacial Orthop* 158(3), 420–425.

Hart A, Taft L and Greenberg S (1992) The effectiveness of differential moments in establishing and maintaining anchorage. *Am J Orthod* 102, 434–442.

Kesling HD (1945) The philosophy of the tooth-position appliance. *J Dent Res* 31(6), 297–304.

Khan W. (2009) Kieferorthopädische Behandlungen mit einem neuen Twin-Aligner-System (Orthocaps®) [Orthodontic Treatment Using a New Twin Aligner System (Orthocaps®)]. *Inf Orthod Kieferorthop* 2009; 41, 175–182.

Khan W (2014) Nouveaux concepts de traitement par aligneurs: le système Orthocaps [New concepts in aligner therapy with the orthocaps system]. *Orthod Fr* Sep;85(3), 253–264. French. doi:10.1051/orthodfr/2014011. Epub 2014 Aug 28. PMID: 25158748.

Kravitz ND, Kusnoto B, BeGole E, Obrez A and Agran B (2009) How well does Invisalign work? A prospective follow-up study on the efficacy of tooth movement with Invisalign. *Am J Orthod Dentofac Orthop* 135, 27–35.

Li Y, Deng S, Mei L, Li Z, Zhang X, Yang C and Li Y (2020) Prevalence and severity of apical root resorption during orthodontic treatment with clear aligners and fixed appliances: a cone beam computed tomography stud. *Prog Orthod* Jan 6;21(1), 1.

Nahoum H (1964) The vacuum-formed dental contour appliance. *N Y State Dent J* 9, 385–390.

Papageorgiou SN, Koletsi D, Iliadi A, Peltomaki T and Eliades T (2020) Treatment outcome with orthodontic aligners and fixed appliances: a systematic review with meta-analysis. *Eur J Orthod* 42(3), 331–343.

Park HP (2021) A licensed orthodontist versus do-it-yourself orthodontics. *Am J Orthod Dentofacial Orthop* 157(5), 591–592.

Phan X and Ling PH (2007) Clinical limitations of Invisalign. *J Can Dent Assoc* 73(3), 263–266.

Remensnyder O (1926) A gum-massaging appliance in the treatment of pyorrhoea. *Dent Cosmos* 28, 381–384.

Richmond S, Shaw WC, O'Brien KD, Buchanan IB, Jones R, Stephens CD, Roberts CT and Andrews M (1992) The development of the PAR Index (Peer Assessment Rating): reliability and validity. *Eur J Orthod* Apr;14(2), 125–139.

Rossini G, Parrini S, Castrflorio T, Deregibus A and Debermardi C (2015) Efficacy of clear aligners in controlling orthodontic tooth movement. *Angle Orthod* 85, 881–889.

Sheridan J, LeDoux W and McMinn R (1993) Essix retainers; fabrication and supervision for permanent retention. *J Clin Ortho* 27, 37–45.

Simon M, Keilig L, Schwarze J, Jung B and Bourauel C (2014) Treatment outcome and efficacy of an aligner technique – regarding incisor torque, premolar derotation and molar distalization. *BMC Oral Health* 14, 68. Published online 2014 Jun 11. doi:10.1186/1472-6831-14-68

Smith R and Burstone C (1984) Mechanics of tooth movement. *Am J Orthod* 85, 294–307.

Tamer I, Öztas E and Marsan G (2019) Orthodontic treatment with clear aligners and the scientific reality behind their marketing: a literature review. *Turk J Orthod* 32(4), 241–246.

Weir T (2017) Aligners in orthodontic treatment. *Aus Den J* 62, 58–62.

18

Progressive Slenderising Technique

Dr Pablo Echarri, Emma Vila Mancho

Definition and objectives

Slenderising refers to the mechanical reduction of the dental interproximal enamel layer, which is carried out in order to re-shape the contact area and decrease the mesiodistal diameter of the teeth to facilitate alignment. Compared with extractions, slenderising allows removal of only the required amount of tooth material without decreasing the vertical dimension or adversely affecting the profile through retraction of the incisors, and it also avoids other side effects of the space closure.

The ratio between the enamel loss and space gain is 1:1, that is, for each millimetre of slenderising, 1 mm of space is gained. The orthodontist can maintain anchorage during the treatment, if he or she wants to use this space for achieving the orthodontic objectives.

The objectives of slenderising include:

- Correction of dentoalveolar discrepancies.
- Treatment of tooth-size discrepancy between the upper and lower teeth (Bolton discrepancy).

Adult Orthodontics, Second Edition. Edited by Birte Melsen and Cesare Luzi.
© 2022 John Wiley & Sons Ltd. Published 2022 by John Wiley & Sons Ltd.
Companion Website: http://www.wiley.com/go/melsen-adult-orthodontics

- Adjustment of interdental contact point to the papilla shape.
- Increasing the interdental contact surface in order to contribute to better stability of corrected rotations
- Improving the occlusion by allowing the tooth cusps of a dental arch to occlude into the interdental embrasures and grooves of the antagonist teeth.
- Correction of asymmetries in order to improve aesthetics.

Ballard (1944) described this technique for the first time in 1944. Other authors have since contributed to its development (Sheridan 1997).

Anthropological justification of slenderising

Black published a text in 1902 on teeth anatomy in which he referred to the natural interproximal abrasion of the teeth as natural slenderising. Begg (1954) and Murphy (1964) studied occlusions of Aborigines presenting interproximal wear, losing up to 14–15 mm of tooth material during their whole life as a consequence of non-refined diets and the absence of crowding. The studies confirmed that slenderising was necessary in order to increase stability, and part of an adaptation system, which consists of:

- Passive tooth eruption to compensate for occlusal wear: the tooth erupts until it makes contact with the antagonist, and in that way it maintains the occlusion and vertical dimension.
- Spontaneous mesial migration to compensate for interproximal wear: this preserves the interdental contact points.
- Formation of the secondary dentine to maintain a constant thickness of hard tissue between the dental pulp and the exterior of the tooth.
- Increased density as well as accelerated remineralisation of enamel in the more abraded zones.

These defence mechanisms, which do not affect reproductive ability or longevity (Begg 1954), are still evident today, but the teeth do not get as worn because they are used only for chewing and the food consistency is much softer than it was in the Stone Age. These dental mechanisms are similar to hair or nail growth.

Harry Sicher (1953), speaking about the attrition of teeth, said that it is possible that wear of teeth has a positive function, and questioned whether nature sacrifices tooth substance to achieve an increase in function. Peck and Peck (1972) discovered the relation between tooth size, mesiodistal and labiolingual widths of the inferior incisors and the degree of crowding (PI index). Betteridge (1981) also found a relationship between tooth size and degree of crowding (BI index).

These facts can be considered an anthropological base for the practice of current techniques of slenderising.

Influence of slenderising on dental plaque, caries and periodontal disease

A comparison of crowded or rotated teeth with teeth aligned after slenderising demonstrates that accumulation of the bacterial plaque is reduced and hygiene is facilitated following alignment. As far as the relation between slenderising and caries is concerned, studies carried out by cardiologists (Brudevold et al. 1982; El-Mangoury et al. 1991) reveal that dental grinding provokes a defence reaction that creates the nucleation zones for accelerated remineralisation. Within a few minutes, the saliva starts to neutralise affected zones and a remineralisation process can be demonstrated 1 hour later. At the beginning, the process is very fast, but then it slows down and is completed within 9 months. At the end, the enamel is as resistant to caries as it was prior to slenderising.

As far as the relation between slenderising and periodontal diseases is concerned, periodontal defects should be taken into consideration along with the risk–benefit balance between the effect of bacterial plaque accumulating periodontal pockets and risk factors of each patient. Tooth shape and the anatomy of the interproximal contact points, among other factors, influence the development of periodontal diseases. When the contact points are correctly established, toothbrushing and self-cleaning become easier, thus minimising the food impaction, and at the same time, the contact points protect the interdental papilla. The prevalence of intraosseous defects is minor in aligned teeth with good contact points (Heins and Wieder 1986). Also, Nielsen et al. (1980), Tal (1984) and Heins et al. (1988) highlighted the importance of the inter-radicular width in the creation of interdental septum defects.

Even if we carry out slenderising on already aligned teeth, the interdental septum thickness is reduced when closing the spaces, but the periodontal status is improved according to Betteridge (1976, 1979). Out of 17 cases of slenderising, he found that 14 had an improved gingival inflammation index; Boese (1980a, 1980b) did not find any significant difference in the alveolar crest height when comparing radiographs of 40 patients before and after slenderising. Crain and Sheridan (1990) also did not find any significant differences in the gingival index 3–5 years after the end of the treatment in 151 interproximal surfaces treated with slenderising. In all these studies, the enamel reduction was no more than 0.5 mm per proximal surface.

Figure 18.1 presents the case of a 29-year-old female patient with crowding in the lower arch, crossbite of the lower right canine and a midline deviation. She was treated with fixed appliances and slenderising in the lower arch. The initial panoramic and intraoral views after slenderisation and reproximation demonstrate the health of the interdental septum.

Obviously, it is important to avoid gingival injury while carrying out slenderising. This can be accomplished with brass-wire protectors or using Dr Sheridan's safe-tipped burs

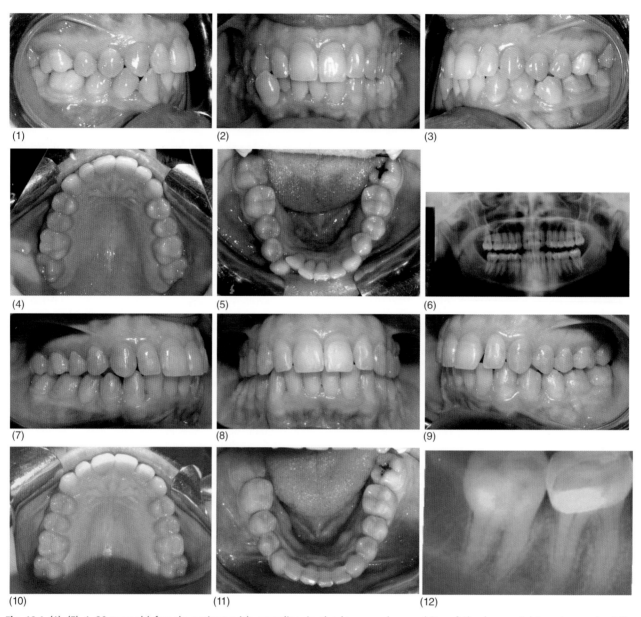

Fig. 18.1 (1)–(5) A 29-year-old female patient with crowding in the lower arch, crossbite of the lower right canine and midline deviation. Intraoral photographs showing the status before treatment. (6) Initial panoramic X-ray. (7)–(11) Final results. Intraoral X-rays after slenderising and reproximation: (12) lower right molars; (13) lower right canine; (14) lower incisors; (15) lower left canine and (16) lower left molars.

(Raintree Essix), or Ortho-Strips files (Intensiv), or Orthocare strip files (Dentacare, Swiss Dental). The safe-tipped burs have inert tips that do not cause any damage to the gingival tissues, while Orthocare and Ortho-Strips files are made in such a way that they can only cut hard but not soft tissues.

Indications

Crowding

Slenderising is a technique for the treatment of minor crowding, but an experienced orthodontist also can treat moderate crowding cases.

Bolton discrepancies

The upper and lower canine-to-canine and upper and lower molar-to-molar Bolton indices indicate where slenderising might be undertaken to improve the occlusion. Bolton determined that the relation between the upper and lower molar-to-molar tooth size is 91.3 ± 1.91 (Figure 18.2(1)) and that the canine-to-canine relation is 77.2 ± 1.65 (Figure 18.2(2)). If a '12' Bolton index is achieved, a molar Class I relationship is obtained, and if the '6' Bolton index is achieved, a canine Class I relationship is obtained. If the patient presents a Bolton discrepancy, it is necessary to compensate for this discrepancy by slenderising.

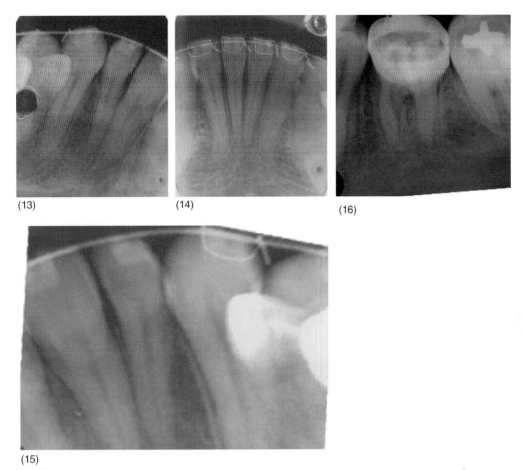

(13)   (14)   (16)

(15)

Fig. 18.1 (*Continued*)

Triangular and 'barrel' tooth shapes

According to Bennett and McLaughlin (1997), we can distinguish three main tooth shapes: rectangular, triangular and barrel-shaped teeth (Figure 18.2(3)). Tooth shape has great importance in orthodontic treatment. The rectangular shape allows a wide and stable contact point without visible interdental spaces. The triangular shape allows a reduced and very occlusal or incisal contact point with 'black gingival triangles' (Figure 18.3). Barrel-shaped teeth have a reduced contact point in the middle with apparent embrasures at the incisal level.

It is possible that spaces due to triangular or barrel-shaped teeth spaces are not obvious at the beginning of the treatment due to presence of crowding or rotations. The patient in Figure 18.3 had crowding of triangular teeth without interdental spaces. Alignment of the teeth led to development of 'black gingival triangles'. It is important to inform the patient about this fact before starting the treatment and to include a solution for this problem in the treatment plan. If the dentoalveolar discrepancy is negative, slenderising and reproximation can solve the problem, but if the discrepancy is positive, some aesthetic restorations may be necessary (Figure 18.4).

If the crown has a triangular shape, the distance between the bone crest and the contact point is relatively large. In these cases, the interproximal papilla tends to be absent. Tarnow et al. (1992) demonstrated that if the distance from the contact point to the interdental bone crest is 5 mm or less, the papilla is present in 100% of the cases. If this distance is 6 mm, the papilla is found in 56% of the cases, and if it is 7 mm or more, the papilla is present only in 27% or less (Figure 18.5(1)). Therefore, he recommended that the distance between the bone crest and the top of the papilla should be 4.5 mm (Figure 18.5(2)).

Black gingival triangles do not always appear due to an increase in the distance between the contact point and the bone crest. According to Bennett and McLaughlin (1997) (Figure 18.6), a black gingival triangle can appear as a consequence of a bracket malpositioning with respect to tooth inclination. In this case, the bracket position should be corrected and slenderising should not be carried out. In

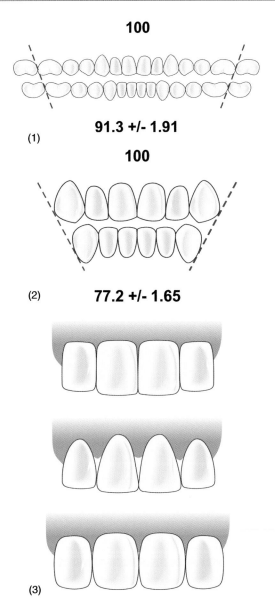

Fig. 18.2 (1) Molar-to-molar Bolton index (12 teeth). (2) Canine-to-canine Bolton index (6 teeth). (3) Tooth shapes according to Bennett and McLaughlin (1997): rectangular, triangular and barrel-shaped teeth.

these cases, an 'occlusal black triangle' can be observed on the other side of the tooth and the periapical X-ray will show that the roots are not parallel.

There is no relation between dental shape and the enamel thickness (Figure 18.7), therefore the amount of possible slenderising does not depend on the dental shape; however, minimal grinding of triangular and barrel-shaped teeth will generate considerable space in the dental arch. According to Andrews (1989), if the teeth are tipped mesiodistally, they occupy more space in the dental arch than teeth in a more vertical position, but Bennett and McLaughlin (1997) emphasise that this fact is truer for rectangular teeth than for other tooth shapes (Figure 18.8). This is why significant tooth uprighting as a solution for a mild negative discrepancy is possible only in rectangular teeth.

According to Steiner, incisal protrusion allows us to obtain double space, that is, the discrepancy is reduced by 2 mm for every 1 mm of protrusion. According to Bennett and McLaughlin (1997), increasing the torque without protrusion also permits the orthodontist to gain 1 mm for every 5° of increased palatal root torque (Figure 18.9(1)).

Macrodontia

Dental shape does not have any influence on the enamel thickness (Figure 18.7), but it is aesthetically more advisable to perform slenderising on macrodontic rather than on microdontic teeth. The 'golden proportion' described by Ricketts (1989), between upper central incisors and lateral incisors, can serve as a guide.

Over-extended crowns and fillings

In such cases, slenderising is indicated to obtain normal tooth shape and dimensions (Figure 18.9(2)).

Bilateral dental asymmetries

Slenderising, veneers and crowns are often indicated in order to compensate for dental asymmetries, especially in the upper anterior region.

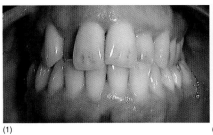
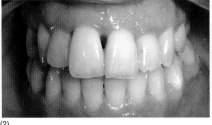
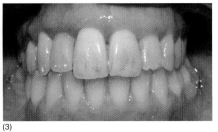

Fig. 18.3 (1) Patient with crowding and triangular-shaped teeth. (2) After alignment with lingual brackets, the 'black gingival triangles' appeared due to the triangular shape of the teeth. (3) Final result after slenderising and reproximation (no black gingival triangles).

Adult patient (narrowed pulp chambers)

Adults have narrower pulp chambers, so slenderising can be carried out with less risk of compromising dental sensibility than in young patients.

Low caries index

Slenderising should only be carried out in patients with a low caries index, in order to avoid increase in susceptibility.

Good oral hygiene – low bacterial plaque index

Slenderising is recommended only in patients with good oral hygiene, in order to avoid the risk of caries.

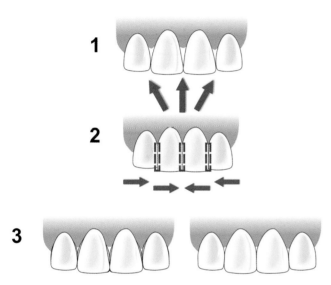

Fig. 18.4 (1) Scheme of a case with 'black gingival triangles' due to the triangular teeth. (2) Cases with negative dentoalveolar discrepancy are treated with slenderising and reproximation. (3) Cases with positive dentoalveolar discrepancy are treated with aesthetic restorations.

Multiple rotations, in order to achieve better stability

In patients who present with multiple rotations, slenderising can result in wider interproximal contact areas, which makes the tooth position more stable with respect to the risk of relapse (Figure 18.9(3)).

Cases treated with lower incisor extraction

These cases need to be compensated by upper canine-to-canine slenderising in order to improve overjet and achieve Class I canine occlusion.

Patients who are given the treatment information and who gave their consent for slenderising

Patients should be informed about the treatment that is going to be carried out and they should give their written consent. It is very important to use a slenderising chart (Figure 18.10) to note down which contact points have been slenderised and give a copy of the chart to the patient or inform the family dentist, to avoid repeating the procedure in areas previously slenderised.

Contraindications

- Patients who do not consent to slenderising.
- High caries index.
- Poor oral hygiene: high bacterial plaque index.
- Rectangular-shaped teeth.
- Young patient (large pulpal chambers).
- Hyper-sensible patient.
- Enamel hypoplasia, dentine hypoplasia, etc.
- Interproximally abraded teeth.

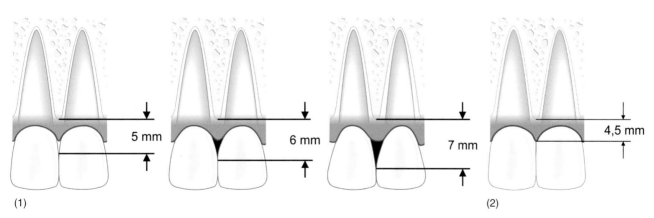

(1) (2)

Fig. 18.5 (1) Tarnow et al. (1992) evaluated the relationship between the distance from the interdental contact point to the bone crest and the presence or absence of 'black gingival triangles'. (2) The height of the interdental papilla should be 4.5 mm.

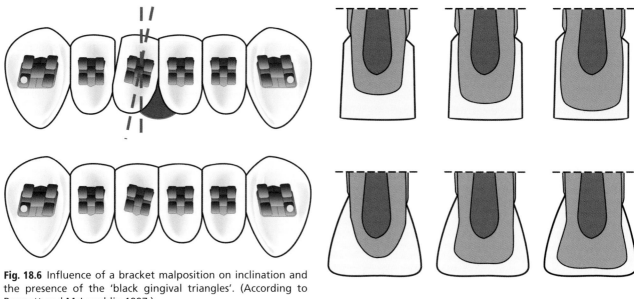

Fig. 18.6 Influence of a bracket malposition on inclination and the presence of the 'black gingival triangles'. (According to Bennett and McLaughlin 1997.)

Fig. 18.7 Triangular, 'barrel-shaped' and rectangular teeth with different sizes and different thicknesses of the enamel layer.

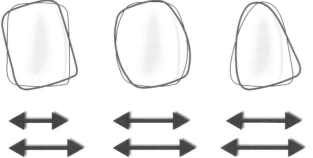

Fig. 18.8 Only the rectangular shape has an important influence on the space occupied by a tooth in the dental arch, in relation to its inclination. (According to Bennett and McLaughlin 1997.)

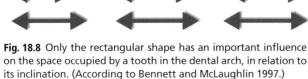

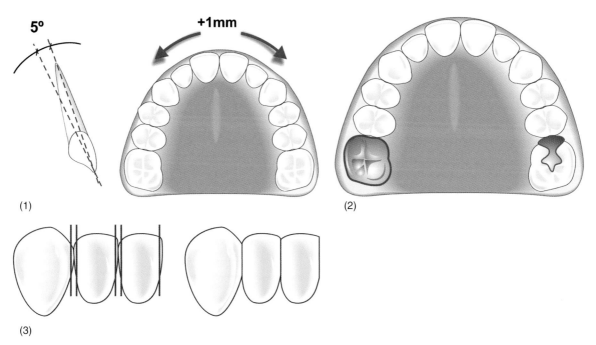

Fig. 18.9 (1) A 5° torque increase without protrusion allows increase of 1 mm of space in the arch (Bennett and McLaughlin 1997). (2) Over-extended crowns and fillings. (3) With slenderising and reproximation, the contact point comes closer to the crest of the interdental septum. (According to Bennett and McLaughlin 1997.)

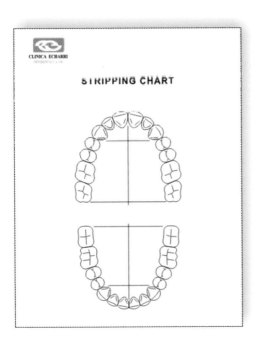

Fig. 18.10 Clinical slenderising chart.

Advantages of slenderising

Minimising the need for extractions and their consequences

The consequences of extraction orthodontic therapy are:

- Difficulties in extraction space closure due to loss of archwire control.
- Difficulties in root paralleling next to extraction sites.
- Extraction cases present the need for greater anchorage reinforcement than slenderising cases, although anchorage is fundamental to the slenderising technique.
- Possibility of the space re-opening (relapse), especially in adult patients.

Less loss of tooth material

Slenderising causes less tooth volume loss than extractions. Normally, when carrying out the extraction, the tooth volume removed is greater than it is actually necessary, but the excess space must be closed. On the other hand, in slenderising cases, only the quantity necessary for alignment is removed.

Smaller tooth movements

With the progressive slenderising technique, tooth movements required are smaller than in extraction cases.

Less treatment time

Slenderising treatments are shorter, although more frequent appointments are required during the process of progressive slenderising.

Less root resorption risk

With smaller tooth movements and shorter treatment times, the risk of root resorption is reduced.

Greater stability

Contact points transformed into contact areas are more stable and provide greater control of rotation. This also eliminates the risk of re-opening of the extraction space.

With lower incisor size reduction, the risk of late lower incisor crowding and rotations is also reduced.

Better aesthetics

By using the 'artistic grinding' slenderising, black gingival triangles are avoided, positioning the contact point at 5 mm from the bone crest; tooth asymmetries can be compensated, and at the same time tooth shape can be improved.

For better aesthetics:

- In the anterior group, incisors and canines, asymmetries should be compensated and midlines should be centred (Figure 18.11(1)).
- In premolars and molars, the cusps should remain untouched for intercuspation (Figure 18.11(2)).
- Slenderising should be carried out in such a way that the vertex of the interdental papilla and the contact point remain in the same perpendicular line to the occlusal plane (Figure 18.11(3)), because if this is not the case, the teeth will look as if they were not inclined as they should be (Figure 18.11(4)).
- Slenderising should be carried out in such a way that the interproximal contact point remains at the distance of 4.5–5 mm from the tip of the alveolar crest to assure that black gingival triangles will not be visible due to the presence of the dental papilla. The bone crest height is determined by probing and radiographic examination (Figure 18.12).

How much enamel can be stripped?

The enamel thickness studies of Hudson (1956), Gillings and Buonocore (1961) and Shillingburg and Grace (1973) allow us to draw the following conclusions:

- The minimal enamel thickness, and not the average values, must be taken into account when determining the enamel quantity that is going to be removed, since it is not possible to know which teeth present minimal thickness.
- There is no relation between the tooth size and the thickness of the enamel layer, thus, macrodontic teeth should not be stripped more than microdontic teeth, although it is better to carry out slenderising on macrodontic teeth due to aesthetics.
- There is no relation between the tooth shape and the thickness of the enamel layer, thus the shape of a tooth cannot dictate how much enamel can be stripped.
- The enamel is slightly thicker in the contact point and the thickness gradually decreases towards the cementoenamel junction. Therefore, it is very important to

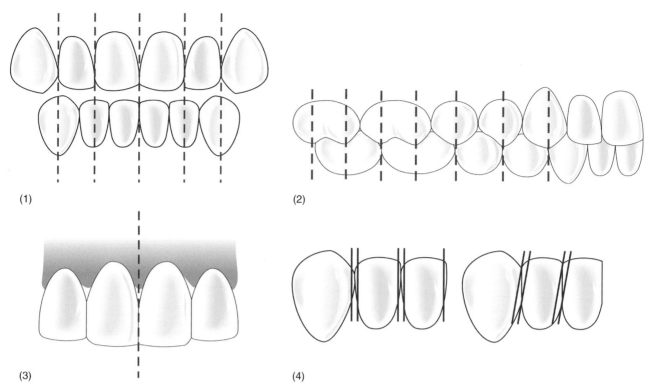

(1)   (2)

(3)   (4)

Fig. 18.11 (1) Slenderising from canine to canine is carried out to improve the midline and the dental symmetry. (2) Slenderising in the posterior teeth is carried out to improve the occlusion. (3) The vertex of the dental papilla and the contact point must be in the same vertical line. (4) If the vertex of the dental papilla and the contact point are not in the same vertical line, there is an illusion of faulty inclination.

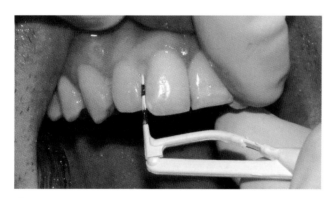

Fig. 18.12 Measuring the distance from the alveolar bone crest to the contact area.

reduce the enamel layer only up to the level of the contact point.

- The enamel thickness is slightly lesser on distal than on mesial surfaces. In upper canines and lower second premolars, these differences are more significant. The exception is the upper lateral incisors, where distal enamel thickness is slightly greater than the mesial. This must be taken into account before slenderising.
- It is important to know how much enamel can be grinded so as to decide between extraction and non-extraction treatments. Boese (1980a, 1980b) recommends slenderising up to half of the enamel layer thickness (Figure 18.7). Berrer (1975) claims that lower incisors can be stripped to gain 4 mm, which corresponds to 0.5 mm of slenderising per proximal surface of the lower incisors. Paskow (1970) allows slenderising between 0.25 mm and 0.37 mm. Hudson (1956) suggests 0.20 mm for central incisors, 0.25 mm for the laterals and 0.30 mm for the lower canines, which gives a total of 3 mm for the whole lower anterior group. Tuverson (1980) claims that it is possible to grind 0.3 mm per proximal surface of the lower incisors, and 0.4 mm of the canines, which means in total an elimination of 4 mm enamel in the anterior group. Alexander (1986) permits only 0.25 mm for all the teeth and Sheridan (1985) argues for 0.8 mm slenderising per surface of posterior teeth and 0.25 mm in the anterior teeth, gaining in total some 8.9 mm.

The studies have shown that in non-abraded teeth, the enamel layer at the level of the contact points has a minimum 1 mm thickness, except the lower incisors, where it is 0.6 mm. This allows the orthodontist to grind half of the layer: 0.5 mm on mesial or distal surface of all teeth, except the lower incisors where 0.3 mm can be removed.

Special considerations

When planning slenderising, the orthodontist must consider the amount of physiological abrasion that a patient presents (contact points or areas) (Figure 18.13). If the interproximal teeth are abraded, slenderising is not recommended. The distal contact point of the upper canines and contact point of the upper lateral incisors are a little bit less due to the thickness of the enamel layer.

Slenderising should not be performed before indirect bonding. The teeth may move while the bracket transfer tray is being fabricated, and the tray might not fit, leading to inaccuracies in bracket positioning. Anchorage can be lost and with it the obtained space. Slenderising should also not be performed on rotated teeth without previous separation. Slenderising is done in different zones, which is difficult; though files with one-sided abrasive coating are used, it is difficult to avoid damaging the labial or lingual tooth surface. As mentioned in the earlier text, the author recommends separating the teeth before performing slenderising.

Separating the teeth before carrying out slenderising can avoid excessive reduction, and shaping and polishing are also easier. Slenderising should be performed under irrigation and no anaesthesia. Only half of the thickness of the enamel layer should be removed. If the orthodontist does not use the Dentacare System, gingival protective gear should be used instead to avoid damaging the gingival margin. The distance between the alveolar crest tip and the contact point should be measured with a periodontal probe before carrying out slenderising. It should be 5 mm, to assure the presence of the interdental papilla.

Progressive slenderising technique provides for minimal anchorage loss. If a group of teeth is slenderised at the same appointment, anchorage control is more difficult to achieve. The cuspal positions in occlusion should be taken into consideration while performing slenderising of posterior teeth. The occlusion must be controlled in order to provide correct intercuspation between both dental arches and to achieve the correct occlusion. Bilateral symmetry and the positions of the midlines should also be taken into

consideration while performing slenderising of anterior teeth.

As already mentioned in the earlier text, when carrying out slenderising, the vertex of interdental papilla and the contact point should be aligned in the same vertical perpendicular to the occlusal plane.

Instrumentation for slenderising

The following instruments may be used:

- Stainless-steel strips.
- Burs.
- Discs.
- Intensiv System.
- Dentacare System.
- Echarri PST Set (Scheu-Dental).
- Measuring instruments and gauges.

Stainless-steel strips

These are polishing strips (Figure 18.14(1)) that are mounted on different systems. In the early days of slenderising, they were the sole instrument used for this purpose. Abrasive strips are available with abrasive coating on one or both sides and in different abrasion grades.

Burs

The most frequently used burs are tungsten carbide burs, thin diamond burs (Figure 18.14(2)) or air rotor slenderising (ARS) system burs, developed by Dr Sheridan, also called safe-tipped burs, made of diamond and with an inert tip (Raintree Essix).

Discs

Obviously, this system produces the greatest abrasion, but it must be used with protection gear to avoid possible damage. Due to the type of abrasion produced, this method cannot be recommended.

Intensiv System for slenderising

This system was developed at the University of Zurich by Professor Van Waes and Professor Matter. The Intensiv Ortho-Strips System Set (Figure 18.14(3)) has five diamond files with abrasive coating on both sides, in sizes of 90 μm (thickness 0.408 mm), 60 μm (0.364 mm), 40 μm (0.159 mm), 25 μm (0.128 mm) and 15 μm (0.111 mm). These exclusively fabricated diamond files can be used for stripping the enamel without the risk of cutting the soft tissues: gingiva, lips or tongue. The flexibility of the files (up to 45°) allows shaping of the tooth surfaces. The file breaks as a security system if there is any major deflection. The files are used with W&H Synea head with oscillation of 0.8 mm. The thread of the contra-angle head allows placing the saw in any position and moving it in a 360° arc.

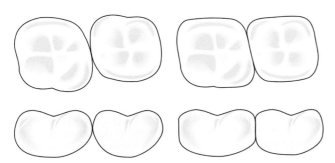

Fig. 18.13 Normal evolution of the contact point increases the area of contact area into a contact surface.

Dentacare System

Dentacare offers the Orthocare Set (Figure 18.14(4)) with the same size files as Intensiv. They use the same contra-angle handpiece but with some improvements: they last longer, and are colour-coded files with one or both sides having abrasive coating and perforations to increase cooling during usage. Dentacare also offers Proxocare Set, with files of 120 μm (green), 90 μm (grey), 40 μm (red) and 15 μm (yellow).

Echarri PST Set

The Echarri PST Set includes: the 5 files and the measuring gauges.

- Green – the 90 μm file (to be used on crowns or fillings).
- Grey – the 60 μm file.
- Red – the 40 μm file.
- White – the 25 μm file.
- Yellow – the 10 μm file.

The Green, Grey, Red and Yellow files are perforated to maintain a lower temperature during the process of slenderising, but the Yellow one not for a better polishing and finishing.

Measuring instruments and gauges

For better control of the amount of enamel stripped, it is necessary to measure the space between the teeth before and after performing slenderising. The space-measuring gauge (Figure 18.15(1)) and the incremental interproximal gauge (Raintree Essix Inc.) (Figure 18.15(2)) are instruments designed to do this.

The author uses Orthocare Set, which consists of 60 μm, 25 μm and 15 μm files for slenderising of all teeth, except for the upper lateral incisors and lower incisors. For these teeth, the author uses 40 μm, 25 μm and 15 μm files. The author also uses the Proxocare Set for slenderising contouring. These are sets of oscillating files, with one or both sides with abrasive coating with different abrasion grades. Dr Emma Vila and the author carried out a comparative study of the different instruments for slenderising using human teeth, using scanning electron microscopy (SEM) to determine its effect on enamel. In this study, the researchers compared stainless-steel strips, diamond burs, tungsten burs, the Ortho-Strips System and the Orthocare System. In the previous studies, neither Ortho-Strips System nor Orthocare System was included.

In 1989, Radlanski et al. (1989a, 1989b) carried out an SEM study that demonstrated that the finishing strips cannot eliminate the deep furrows which are the result of prior slenderising with stainless-steel strips. Jost-Brinkmann et al. (1991) published an SEM study of the primary teeth, which demonstrated that the smooth surfaces can be achieved after slenderising and that both rotating and oscillating polishing procedures are good for obtaining a smooth surface. Piacentini and Sfondrini (1996) recommended a tungsten bur and a polishing soft disc to obtain smooth surfaces. Zhong et al. (2000) recommended the use of diamond-coated disc and Sof-Lex XT disc for polishing to obtain a smooth surface.

Lucchese et al. (2001) compared the effect of various slenderising techniques on enamel surfaces and found that the least roughness is achieved by the use of a tungsten carbide bur followed by finishing with fine and super-fine

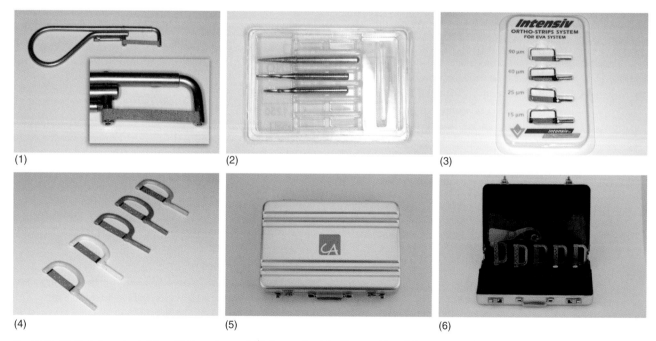

Fig. 18.14 (1) Stainless-steel strips. (2) Tungsten carbide bur and a thin diamond bur. (3) Intensiv Ortho-Strips System Set. (4) Dentacare's Orthocare System. (5) Echarri PST Set. (6) Echarri PST Set.

Sof-Lex discs. Rossouw and Tortorella (2003) recommended the use of acid-etching agents. These are convenient to obtain a smooth surface in combination with the mechanical aids. The unpublished study of Echarri and Vila (2021) showed that the unique, acceptable surfaces after slenderising are obtained with (Figure 18.15(3)):

- A tungsten bur used for less than 30 seconds.
- Ortho-Strips System and Orthocare System using files of 40 μm or 60 μm, and for polishing, files of 25 μm and 15 μm.
- Irrigating while using the files and rinsing generously between files to eliminate the enamel powder completely.
- Maintaining the handpiece in the same position and allowing the handpiece to guide its own in–out movement.

Together with Dr Vila and Dr Manchón, the author carried out a study using human teeth and the helical scanner (CT, CT Twin II Philips) to find out how much enamel is lost with the slenderising technique when using different instruments (Figure 18.16(1),(2); unpublished data, 2009).

The conclusions were:

- Tungsten burs used for 30 seconds leave a polished surface and remove 0.5 mm of enamel thickness. Therefore, tungsten burs can be used for slenderising upper central incisors, and upper and lower incisors, premolars and molars, but not the upper lateral incisors or lower incisors.
- Using the Ortho Strips and Orthocare systems:
  - File 60 μm used for 60 seconds removes 0.5 mm of the enamel thickness.
  - File 40 μm used for 30 seconds removes 0.3 mm of the enamel thickness.
  - Files 25 μm and 15 μm used for 30 seconds each remove a measurable thickness of the enamel.

The conclusions of both studies were that to obtain a smooth surface of enamel and to remove the correct thickness of enamel, slenderising should be carried out in the following way:

- To remove 0.5 mm in the upper central incisors, upper and lower canines, premolars and molars, tungsten burs or the Ortho-Strips or Orthocare system can be used: file 60 μm for 60 seconds and files 25 μm or 15 μm for 30 seconds each.
- To remove 0.3 mm in the upper lateral incisors and the four lower incisors, the Ortho-Strips or Orthocare system can be used: file 40 μm for 30 seconds or the files 25 μm or 15 μm for 30 seconds each.

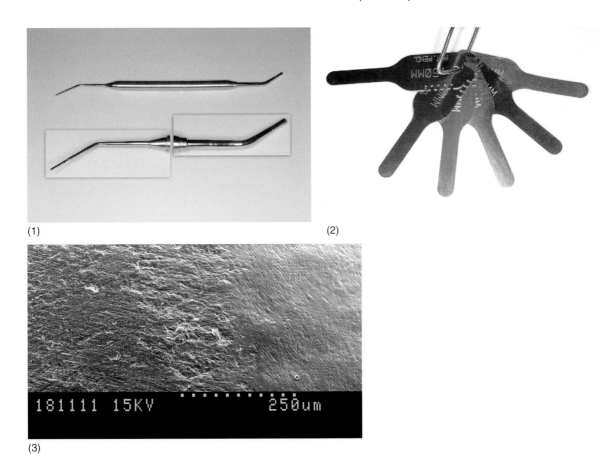

(1)   (2)

(3)

Fig. 18.15 (1) Space-measuring gauge. (2) The incremental interproximal gauge with which it is possible to measure a distance of 3.0–0.75 mm with a precision of 0.25 mm. (3) Scanning electron microscopic image of the enamel surface after using the Orthocare System 60 μm file, 25 μm file and 15 μm file, and enamel without any treatment.

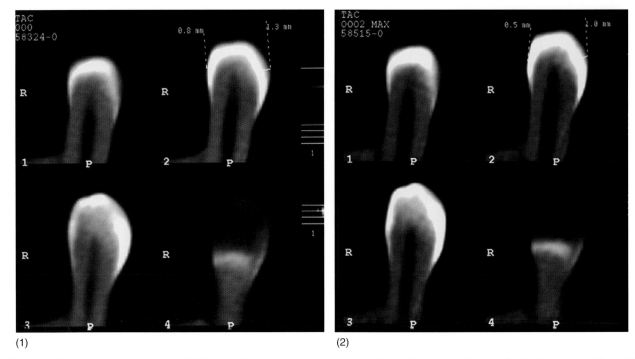

(1)   (2)

Fig. 18.16 (1) Computed tomography (CT) images before slenderising; enamel layer thickness: 1.3 mm. (2) CT after slenderising with files 40 μm, 25 μm and 15 μm; enamel layer thickness: 1.0 mm. Enamel loss was thus 0.3 mm.

By measuring the time of use of each file, the orthodontist will know how much enamel has been removed. Furthermore, the Ortho-Strips and Orthocare systems are safe for the soft tissues, that is, gingival papilla, tongue and lips. These systems can be used in patients undergoing orthodontic treatment with fixed or removable appliances (Figure 18.17).

Progressive slenderising technique

In 1987, Sheridan published an article in the *Journal of Clinical Orthodontics*, 'Air-Rotor Stripping Update', which explained the advantages of opening spaces and carrying out a sequential slenderising from posterior to anterior. In this paper, he recommended carrying out slenderising with tungsten and diamond burs with 0.020-inch wires to protect the gingival tissues and to open the spaces with coil springs.

Progressive slenderising (Echarri 2000a, 2000b) can be done in three ways:

- Total progressive slenderising (all teeth).
- Posterior slenderising (molars and premolars).
- Anterior slenderising (canines and incisors).

Depending on the case characteristics, especially the Bolton index, slenderising will be carried out in different zones.

Progressive slenderising is carried out:

- Before alignment, in order to avoid the following protrusion (the ligated archwire is passive).
- Starting from distal towards mesial.

- Simultaneously in both halves of an arch. If it is indicated in both jaws, it is also carried simultaneously, so the intercuspation can be kept under control.
- After separation of contact points, only the contact point area is stripped.
- Without anaesthesia.
- With irrigation and rinsing between the use of two files.
- With appropriate burs.
- Without protection, if Orthocare files are used. If not, then with protection.
- In order to maintain the anchorage control.
- In order to allow for alignment, levelling and rotation control of the teeth that require distalisation.

Slenderising is followed by polishing, in order not to leave rough surfaces. A fluoride varnish should be applied after slenderising (Duraphat, Colgate) and the patient should be encouraged to brush their teeth using toothpaste with high fluoride content (Fluodontil 1350, Sanofi-aventis).

Clinical procedure

Carry out direct or indirect bonding of the labial or lingual brackets and tubes (it is not advisable to use bands with slenderising) and a 0.016-inch stainless-steel coaxial round archwire, ligated without activation. Do not start slenderising before indirect bonding because this would reduce the bracket-positioning precision. Another option is to use a figure-of-eight ligature between first molars on the right and the left side. By using elastic separators between the first and second molars, the second molar will be moved 1 mm distally (Figure 18.18(1)). Usually, the separation is achieved

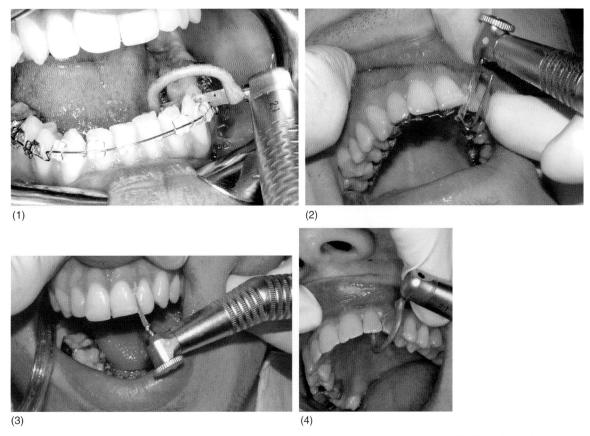

Fig. 18.17 (1) Orthocare System being used with labial brackets. (2) Slenderising in a patient with lingual brackets; Ortho-Strips System. (3) Slenderising in a patient with lingual brackets; Proxoshape system. (4) Orthocare System in combination with clear aligner treatment.

within 24–48 hours, but due to the way appointments are usually organised, it usually takes 1 week.

Carry out slenderising of the mesial surface of the second molar and the distal surface of the first molar (Figure 18.18(2)). If Ortho-Strips or Orthocare files are not being used, a brass wire can be used to protect the gingiva. The brass indicator wire depresses and protects the gingival tissues and it serves as a guide and support for a slenderising bur. Contour the margins of the stripped area with the Proxocare files (Figure 18.18(3)).

It is possible to use a continuous 0.016-inch archwire or a 0.016 × 0.016-inch stainless-steel sectional archwire. An omega loop inserted on the mesial side of the second molar tube enhances second molar anchorage, and a ligature between the omega loop and the second molar tube prevents the forward movement of the incisors. An elastic separator between the second premolar and the first molar is used to move the first molar towards distally (Figure 18.18(4)). Depending on the case, two elastic separators can be used simultaneously (Figure 18.18(5)).

Once the first molar has distalised, slenderising is carried out on the mesial surface of the first molar and the distal surface of the second premolar (Figure 18.18(6)). Insert a 'figure-of-eight' splinting ligature between the first molar and the second molar. Continue derotating rotated second

premolar rotations using elastomeric if necessary. Carry out distalisation of the second premolar with the elastic chain from the second premolar to the first molar (Figure 18.18(7)). Carry out slenderising of the distal surface of the second premolar and mesial surface of the first molar (Figure 18.18(8)). Move the first premolar distally with an elastic chain from this tooth to the second premolar, and maintain the anchorage with the figure-of-eight ligature from the second premolar to the second molar (Figure 18.18(9)). Proceed in the same way for the canine and incisors.

When posterior slenderising is to be carried out, the canines are the last teeth to be stripped. If anterior slenderising is to be carried out, begin by placing the elastic separator between the canine and the first premolar. For slenderising in the canine-to-canine region, an archwire with four omega loops is used (Figure 18.18(10)). That is, a 0.016-inch stainless-steel archwire with omega loops mesially to the second molar tubes and also mesial to the first premolar brackets is used to avoid anchorage loss.

While performing slenderising in the anterior segment, aesthetics, symmetry and midline discrepancies should be taken into account. Progressive slenderising requires 8–10 appointments in total, one every 15 days.

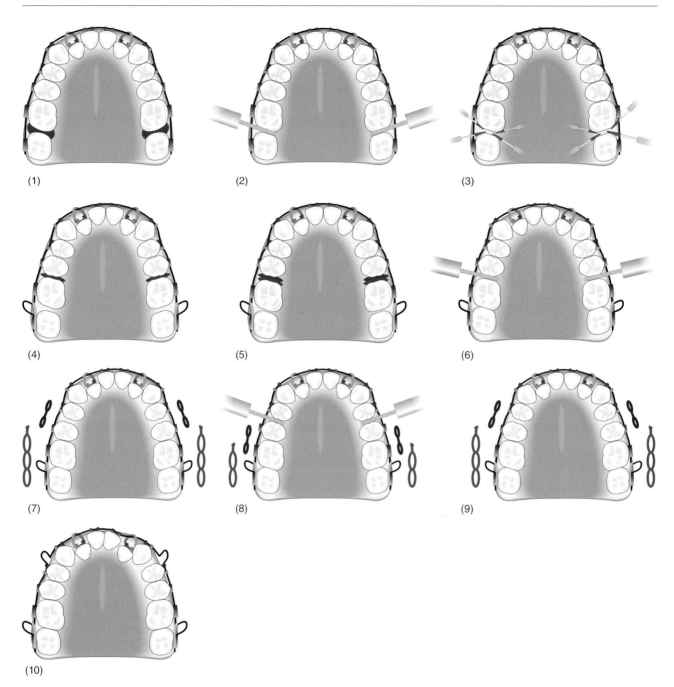

Fig. 18.18 Progressive slenderising technique. (1) Brackets bonding, passive 0.016-inch stainless-steel coaxial archwire and elastic separator between the first and second molar to move the second molar distally by 1 mm. (2) Slenderising the distal surface of the first molar, and of the mesial surface of the second molar, using Orthocare files. (3) Contouring the margins of the stripped area with the Proxocare files. (4) A 0.016-inch stainless-steel archwire with omega bends mesial to the second molar tube to avoid mesialisation. The archwire is ligated without activation. Elastic separators between the second premolar and the first molar to distalise the first molar. (5) If one elastic separator is not enough, complete the distalisation of the first molars by using two separators. (6) Slenderising the distal surface of the second premolar and the mesial surface of the first molar. (7) 'Figure-of-eight' ligature from the first molar to the second molar and elastic chain from the second premolar to the first molar. (8) Slenderising the distal surface of the first premolar and the mesial surface of the second premolar. (9) 'Figure-of-eight' ligature from the second molar to the second premolar and elastic chain from the first premolar to the second premolar. (10) Archwire with four omega loops.

Biomechanical archwire sequence

Labial slenderising technique

Slenderising archwire

- 0.016-inch stainless steel coaxial archwire or figure-of-eight ligature.
- 0.016 inch stainless-steel archwire with distal omega loops.

Carry out progressive slenderising.

Alignment, levelling and rotations

- 0.016-inch Ni–Ti.

Establishment of torque and arch shape

- Intermaxillary elastics (Class II and Class III) if needed.
- 0.016 × 0.022-inch stainless steel.
- Omega loops positioned mesially from the second molar tubes and ligated to these tubes.
- Sagittal and horizontal compensation curves.

Finishing archwire

- 0.018 × 0.025-inch stainless steel.
- Omega loops positioned mesial to the second molar tubes and ligated to these tubes.
- Sagittal and horizontal compensation curves.

Lingual slenderising technique

Slenderising archwire

- 0.0155-inch stainless-steel coaxial or figure-of-eight ligature.
- 0.016-inch stainless-steel archwire with distal omega loops.

Carry out progressive slenderising.

Alignment, levelling and rotations

- 0.016-inch Ni–Ti or 0.017 × 0.017-inch copper Ni–Ti.

Establishment of torque and arch shape

- 0.0175 × 0.0175-inch titanium molybdenum (TMA) with the cinch-back bend.

Establish the arch shape. Use intermaxillary elastics (Class II and Class III).

- 0.016 × 0.022-inch stainless steel.
- Omega loops positioned mesial to the second molar tubes and ligated to these tubes.
- Sagittal and horizontal compensation curves.

Finishing archwire

- 0.016-inch stainless steel.
- First- and second-order compensation bends
- Omega loops positioned mesial to the second molar tubes and ligated to these tubes.
- Sagittal and horizontal compensation curves.

The finishing archwire that the author uses for aesthetic finishing is a 0.016-inch stainless-steel archwire. First and second-order bends are incorporated for aesthetic finishing or to improve the occlusion instead of re-bonding, because it is easier in lingual technique. Omega loops mesial to the molar tubes are ligated to avoid space opening. This is more accurate than the cinch back used in the lingual technique. Sagittal (tip-back) and horizontal (toe-out) compensation curves are used to prevent the bowing effect.

Slenderising with aligners

The slenderising technique is very useful with the aligner technique. The author follows his technique (progressive stripping technique (PST) also with aligners).

The technique could be summarised in the following list:

1. Open spaces in between first bicuspids and canines and in the midline with an expansion aligner.
2. Carry out the stripping in the mesial surfaces of the central incisors, the distal surfaces of the canines and the mesial surfaces of the first bicuspids.
3. Then, move the teeth with the aligner to close the spaces between the central incisors and between the 1st bicuspids and the canines, opening spaces mesial and distal of the lateral incisors.
4. Carry out the stripping in the mesial surfaces of the canines, mesial and distal surfaces of the lateral incisors and distal surfaces of the central incisors.
5. Align, level and correct the rotations of the teeth and close the spaces.

The following case shows the process and planification of the technique:

The case is a young female patient with crowding in the lower incisors and canines and with Bolton '6' excess in the lower arch (Figures 18.18 and 18.19 initial records).

The digital planification is shown in Figures 18.19 and 18.20.

The process is shown in Figures 18.18–18.21 (phase 1); Figures 18.18–18.22 (phase 2) and Figures 18.18–18.23 (phase 3).

The final results can be observed in Figures 18.18–18.24.

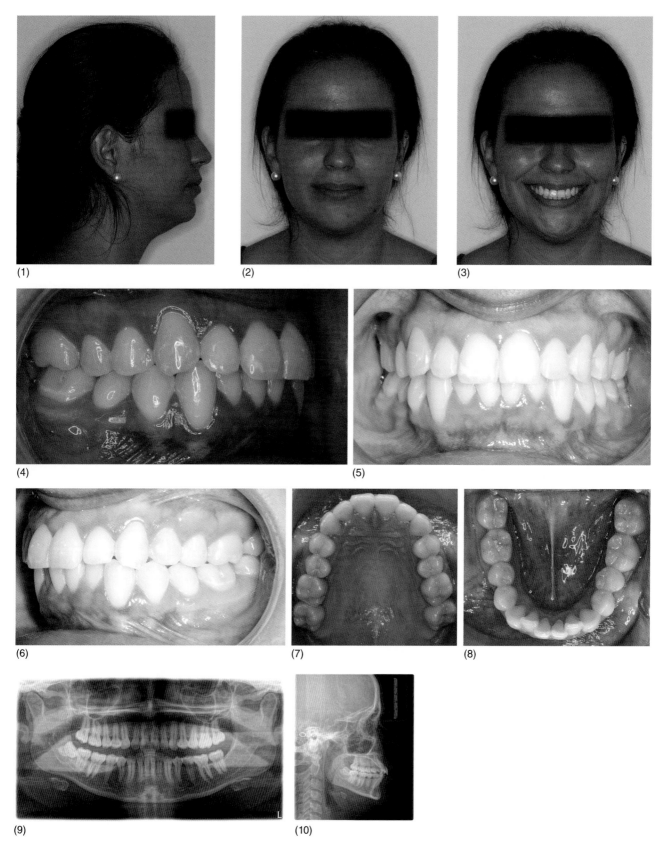

(1) (2) (3)

(4) (5)

(6) (7) (8)

(9) (10)

Fig. 18.19 Case report – slenderising and aligners. initial records.

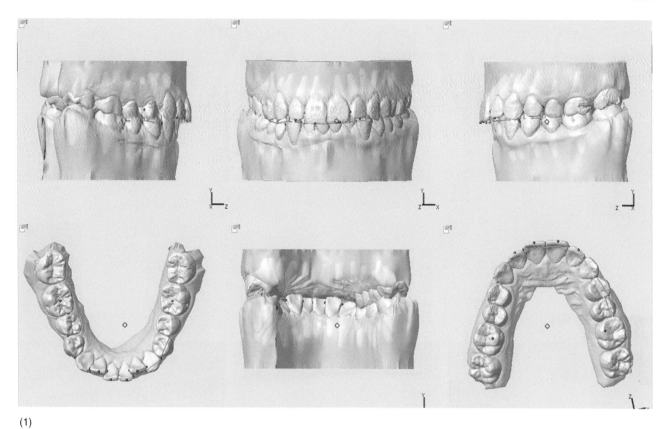

(1)

Análisis zona de soporte						
Variable	Descripción	Norma [ ]	Valor [ ]	Diff	Desviación	Verbal
SZrmax	Espacio Disponible Zona Soporte S	21,5mm	24,1mm	+2,6		
D SZrmax	Discrepancia Zona de Soporte Sup		2,6mm			
SZlmax	Espacio Disponible Zona de Soport	23,7mm	24,0mm	+0,2		
D SZlmax	Discrepancia Zona de Soporte Sup		0,2mm			
ASmax	Espacio Disponible Segmento Ante	32,9mm				
D ASmax	Discrepancia Segmento Anterior Su					
D max	Discrepancia Maxilar					
SZrmand	Espacio Disponible Zona Soporte Ir	23,5mm	22,7mm	-0,8		
D SZrmand	Discrepancia Zona de Soporte Inf.		-0,8mm			
SZlmand	Espacio Disponible Zona de Soport	23,6mm	22,5mm	-1,1		
D SZlmand	Discrepancia Zona de Soporte Inf.		-1,1mm			
ASmand	Espacio Disponible Segmento Ante	24,7mm				
D ASmand	Discrepancia Segmento Anterior In					
D mand	Discrepancia Mandibular					

(2)

Bolton - anterior						
Variable	Descripción	Norma [ ]	Valor [ ]	Diff	Desviación	Verbal
Smax	Suma de Dientes Antero Superiore		48,3mm			
Smand	Suma de Dientes Antero Inferiores	37,3mm	39,3mm	+2,0		
Indice	Proporción de los Dientes Anterior	77,2±0,2%	81,3%	+3,9	⬛	
Comentario			Dientes Antero Inferiores Relativamente Anchos			

(3)

Fig. 18.20 Case report – slenderising and aligners. digital planification.

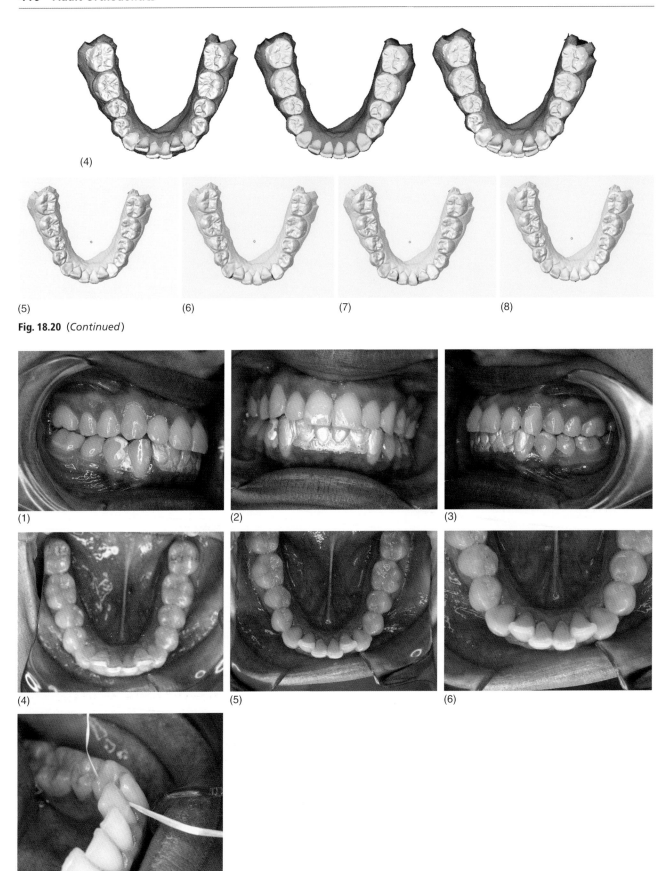

(4)

(5) (6) (7) (8)

Fig. 18.20 (*Continued*)

(1) (2) (3)

(4) (5) (6)

(7)

Fig. 18.21 Case report – slenderising and aligners. phase 1.

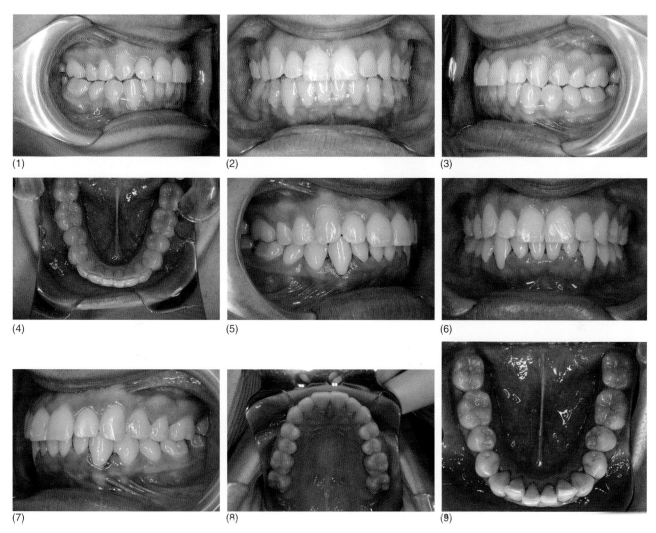

(1) (2) (3)

(4) (5) (6)

(7) (8) (9)

Fig. 18.22 Case report – slenderising and aligners. phase 2.

The design and planning of the slenderising and preventing risks in slenderising

The interproximal contact point is very important in the maintenance of the alignment of the dental arches. If there are crowding or rotations, the interproximal relationship is broken and normally the evolution goes to increase the crowding and/or the rotations (Aprile). Also, the interproximal contact point facilitates that the occlusal forces are transmitted to the dental arch. Each tooth supports the neighbouring teeth, and when this balance is broken, it provokes modification in the periodontal tissues. These contact points preserve the health of the dento-dental and supraseptal fibres (Figure 18.25). Immediately inside these fibres that contribute to the rapprochement of the teeth, and which are found at the base of the interdental papilla, the periodontal insertion is located, and hence is the importance of conservation (Aprile).

For this reason, it is very important that the orthodontists know the interproximal contact point from an anatomical point of view.

Normally, the contact point is in the occlusal third of the mesial and distal surfaces of all the teeth, but it depends on the dental shape. We recognise three main dental shapes: rectangular, triangular and 'barrel' shapes following Bennet and McLaughlin (Figure 18.2). In the rectangular teeth, the contact point is bigger and more gingival; in the triangular ones, is smaller and in a more incisal position and in the 'barrel-shaped' teeth, the contact point is in the middle third in the incisal–gingival sense.

In the anterior teeth, incisors and cuspids, the contact point is in the middle third in labiolingual sense, but in the posterior teeth, normally it is in the labial third (Aprile) (Figures 18.26 and 18.27).

The contact point can increase its surface and transform into an interproximal contact surface, ovoid in all cases but

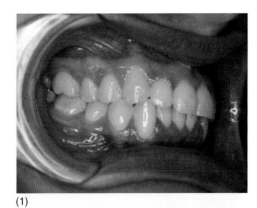

(1)

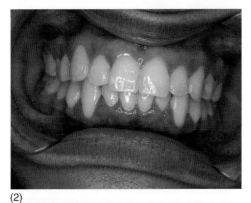

(2)

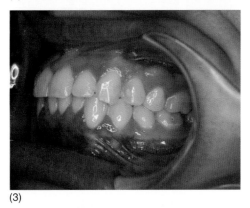

(3)

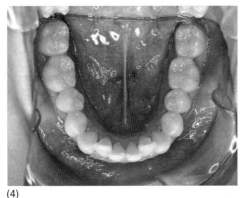

(4)

Fig. 18.23 Case report – slenderising and aligners. phase 3.

more vertical in anterior teeth and more horizontal in posterior teeth (Figure 18.28). According to Begg, the spontaneous mesial movement of the teeth is to compensate the abrasion of mesial and distal surfaces during the mastication of hard food.

Around the contact point, there are four spaces in the four possible directions: occlusal, gingival, labial and lingual (Figure 18.29). The occlusal space is called interdental sulcus, the gingival space is called the interdental space and the other two are the labial and lingual spaces (Aprile).

These spaces are very important during the mastication because the movement of the food is sliding over these surfaces (Figure 18.30).

The functions of the interproximal contact point are:

- Maintenance of the position of the teeth in the dental arch, avoiding crowding and rotations.
- Protection of the dental papilla and the dento-dental and supra-septal fibres.
- Avoid the food retention.
- Aesthetics.

According to Tarnow et al. (1992), interdental papilla in normal anatomic conditions is always 4.5 mm from the papilla vertex to the bone crest (Figure 18.5).

Therefore, if interproximal contact point is established 5 mm from the bone crest, the papilla is present in a 100% of cases. If the contact point is 6 mm from the bone crest, the papilla is present in only 56% of cases, and if the same distance is increased up to 7 mm or more, the papilla is present in only 27% of cases (Tarnow) (Figure 18.5).

Stripping and approximation allow the correction of gingival 'black triangles' because they fix the contact point to 5 mm from the bone crest.

Figure 18.4 shows the scheme of a case with 'black triangles' (1). If there is Bolton excess and crowding, 'black triangles' are corrected with stripping and approximation (2). If there were no Bolton discrepancy and crowding, an aesthetic reconstruction would be the best option (3) (Echarri).

Stripping and Bolton index

The Bolton index is the relation in the size of the upper and lower teeth. The Bolton index '12' takes into account from first molar to first molar and the Bolton index '6' takes into account from canine to canine measurements.

The Bolton index '12' norm is 91.3 ± 1.91 (Figure 18.2), and the Bolton index '6' is 77.2 ± 1.65 (Figure 18.2).

The following situations can be found:

- If Bolton index '12' is normal, it means that the case after the orthodontic treatment can be finished in molar Class I, and if Bolton index '6' is normal, the case can be

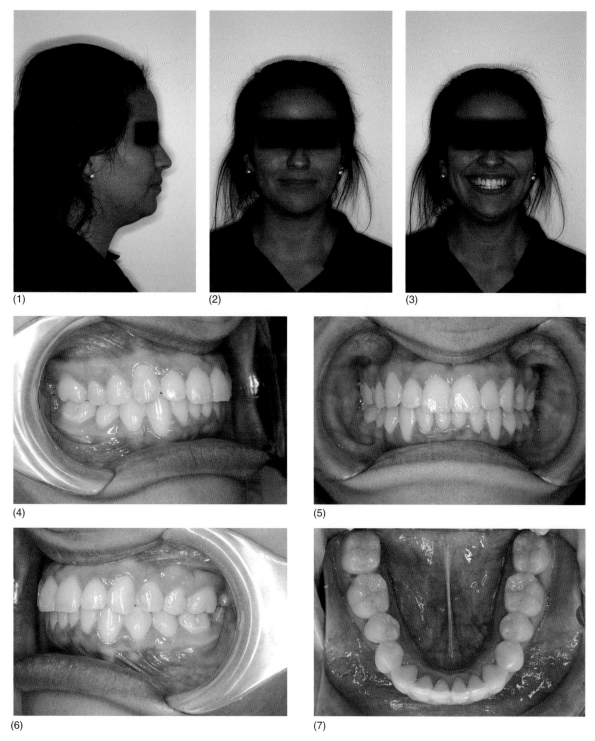

Fig. 18.24 Case report – slenderising and aligners. final.

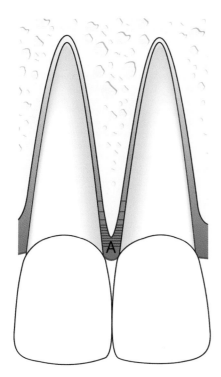

Fig. 18.25 Interdental fibres in the base of the papilla.

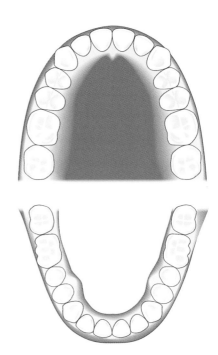

Fig. 18.27 Upper and lower arches and interproximal contact point.

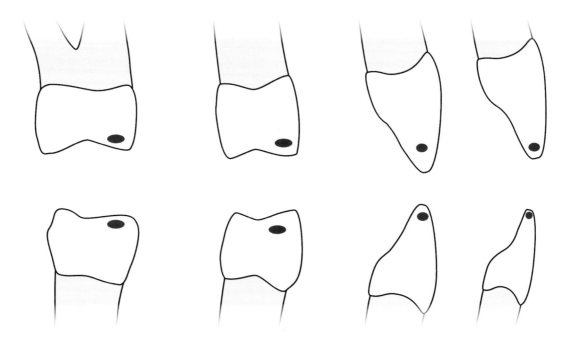

Fig. 18.26 Position of the interproximal contact point in different teeth.

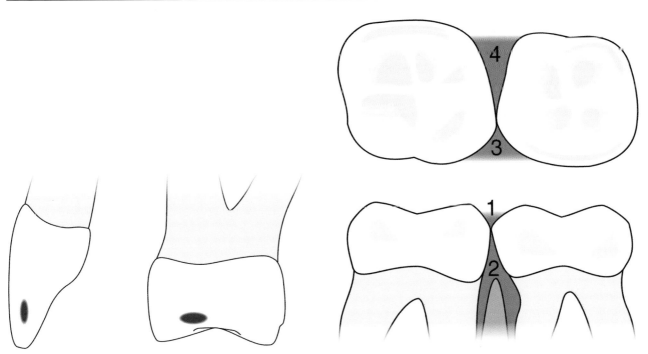

Fig. 18.28 Interproximal contact surface.

Fig. 18.29 Spaces around the interproximal contact point: (1) interdental sulcus; (2) interdental space; (3) labial space; (4) lingual space.

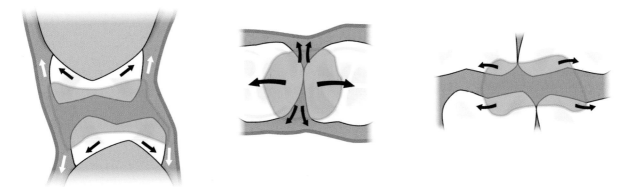

Fig. 18.30 Movement of the food during the mastication: (1) Mesial view: the food slides over the labial and lingual surfaces of the teeth (white arrows) and over the papilla (black arrows). (2) Occlusal view: the food slides over the occlusal sulcus to the occlusal surfaces of the teeth and the labial and lingual sulcus. (3) Labial view: circulation of the food. (Taken and modified from Aprile and Figún).

finished in canine Class I. This would be the ideal situation and in another words means that there is no size discrepancy between the teeth of the upper arch and the teeth of the lower arch considering all the teeth from the upper first molar to the upper first molar of the other side for the Bolton index '12' or having into account only the teeth from canine to canine for the Bolton index '6' (Figure 18.31).

- If there is Bolton index '12' excess of, for example, 4 mm, and there is also Bolton index '6' excess of 4 mm too, that is, both Bolton indexes have equal excess, a canine-to-canine stripping in maxilla should be carried out, because the Bolton index '6' is included into the Bolton index '12', meaning that the amount of excess corresponds exclusively to the anterior sector (Figure 18.32).

- If there is Bolton index '12' excess of, for example, 4 mm, and Bolton index '6' is normal, in this situation, the upper molars and bicuspids should be stripped, because the excess is located in the posterior sector (Figure 18.33).

- If there is Bolton index '12' excess of, for example, 4 mm, and there is also Bolton index '6' excess of, for example, 2 mm, that is, Bolton index '12' excess is higher than Bolton index '6' excess, total stripping in maxilla should be carried out. In this case, there is excess in both anterior and posterior sectors (Figure 18.34).

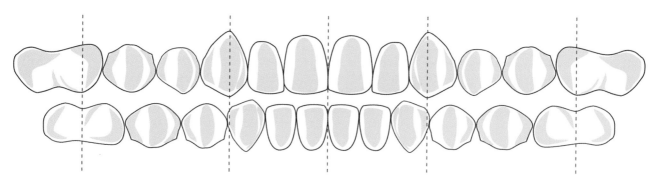

Fig. 18.31 Case without Bolton index discrepancy.

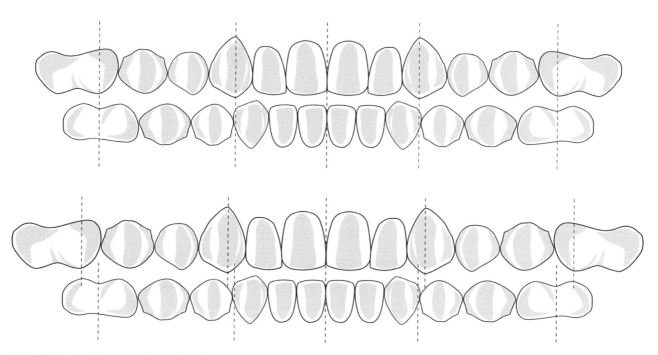

Fig. 18.32 Case with excess of maxilla Bolton index '12' and '6'.

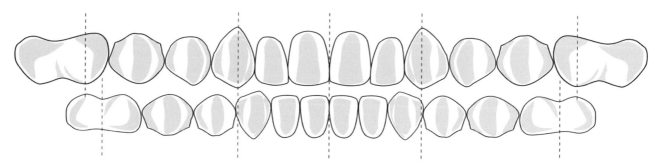

Fig. 18.33 Case with excess of maxilla Bolton index '12' and without Bolton index '6' discrepancy.

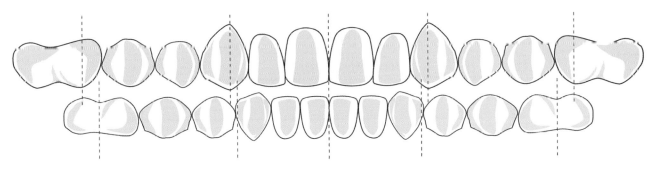

Fig. 18.34 Case with maxilla Bolton index '12' excess higher than Bolton index '6' excess.

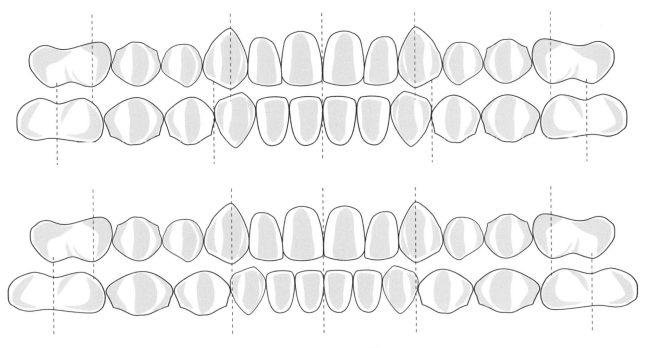

Fig. 18.35 Case with mandible Bolton index '12' excess and no Bolton index '6' excess.

- The same reasoning is applied to Bolton index excess in mandible (Figure 18.35).
- To sum up, it can be said that Bolton index indicates where the excess of dental size is located and consequently where the stripping should be carried out, and where not. If there is no Bolton index discrepancy, the stripping should be done in both arches in order to not modify the relationship of size between the upper and lower arches.

How much enamel can be worn out?

Anatomic studies reveal that the minimal thickness of an enamel layer in the contact point is 1 mm for all teeth except upper lateral incisors and four lower incisors. As most of authors accept the rule that says it is possible to wear half of the enamel layer, it is acceptable to wear:

- 0.5 mm on mesial and distal surfaces of upper central incisors, upper and lower cuspids, upper and lower bicuspids and upper and lower molars.
- 0.3 mm on mesial and distal surfaces of upper lateral incisors and four lower incisors.

Recommended values for stripping can be seen in Figure 18.36, and this figure shows a stripping chart in which the record is left about the stripping that has been already done. Also, the stripping chart (Figure 18.10) can be used for the stripping treatment plan.

	Central incisor		Lateral incisor		Canine		First bicuspid		Second bicuspid		First molar	
	mesial	distal	mesial	distal	mesial	distal	mesial	distal	mesial	distal	mesial	
Maxilla	0.5	0.5	0.3	0.3	0.5	0.5	0.5	0.5	0.5	0.5	0.5	
Inter-dental reduction	1.0		0.8		0.8		1.0		1.0		1.0	
Mandible	0.3	0.3	0.3	0.3	0.5	0.5	0.5	0.5	0.5	0.5	0.5	
Inter-dental reduction	0.6		0.6		0.8		1.0		1.0		1.0	

Fig. 18.36 Chart with the recommended stripping values.

Facial and dental midlines

The facial midline is determined by glabella, tip of the nose, upper labial philtrum, Cupid's arch centre and chin. Upper and lower dental midlines have to match among themselves and they have to match with facial midlines in an aesthetic ideal situation (Figure 18.37) (Jerrold and Johnston).

The goal of the treatment is to match the upper and lower dental midlines with the facial midline.

Teeth size

The teeth should be proportional among themselves and in relation to the patient's face. As Levin has demonstrated (Levin 1978), the so-called 'golden proportions'[9] (Figure 18.38) have always been a constant feature in the nature, art and design.

According to the 'golden proportion', the anterior teeth proportion from the frontal point of view should be:

- Upper central incisor – 1.618.
- Upper lateral incisor – 1.0.
- Upper canine – 0.618.

But, if absolute measures are taken into account, Sterrett et al. determined the recommended measurements (Figure 18.39).

The scheme in Figure 18.40 shows the recommended teeth shapes depending on sex, age and personality, according to Lombardi.

This measurements and proportions are useful when a decision has to be made on aesthetic retouches of the teeth, whether by stripping or by reconstruction (Kokich; Sarver and Echarri).

Design and planning of the stripping

For the design and planning of the stripping, it is necessary to take into account:

- Dentoalveolar discrepancy.
- Bolton indexes '12' and '6'.

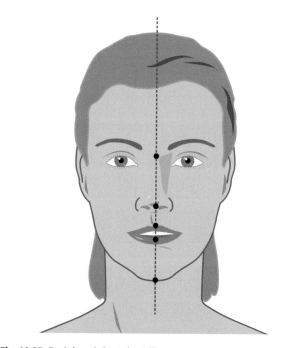

Fig. 18.37 Facial and dental midline.

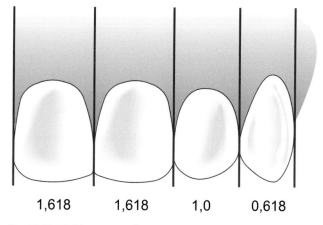

| 1,618 | 1,618 | 1,0 | 0,618 |

Fig. 18.38 'Golden proportion'.

Tooth	Height (male)	Height (female)	Width (male)	Width (female)
Central incisor	10.2	9.4	8.6	8.1
Lateral incisor	8.7	7.8	6.6	6.1
Canine	10.1	8.9	7.6	7.1

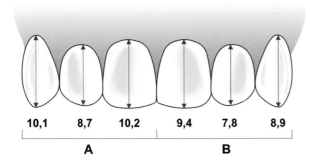

Fig. 18.39 Teeth size according to Sterrett.

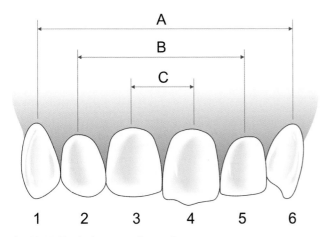

Fig. 18.40 Teeth size according to Sterrett.

- Position of the teeth in relationship of the facial midline.
- Upper and lower dental midline discrepancies.
- Shapes of the teeth.
- Dental size proportions.
- Dental asymmetries.
- Intercuspation.
- Distance of the contact point to the bone crest.
- If the teeth present a contact point or a contact surface.

When the interproximal relationship is a surface and not a point, it means that the teeth have suffered already an abrasion and this fact will limit the stripping possibilities. The stripping should be performed to meet all the goals if possible:

- Correct the crowding.
- Compensate the Bolton's discrepancies.

- Match the upper and lower midlines with the facial midface.
- Compensate the abnormal shapes of the teeth.
- Compensate the dental size proportions.
- Compensate the asymmetries of the teeth.
- Achieve the intercuspation of upper and lower teeth.
- Fix the interproximal contact point 5 mm far of the bone crest to achieve the presence of the papilla.
- Get a stable contact point of surface.

Progressive stripping technique

The PST recommends using the files of the PST kit to perform the stripping. It includes the following files:

- Green 90 µm file.
- Grey 60 µm file.
- Red 40 µm file.
- White 25 µm file.
- Yellow 15 µm file.

The upper central incisors and all cuspids, bicuspids and molars can be trimmed 0.5 mm, and for this purpose, we recommend to use (Echarri):

- File 60 µm during 60 seconds.
- File 25 µm during 30 seconds.
- File 15 µm during 30 seconds.

The upper lateral incisors and all lower incisors can be trimmed 0.3 mm, and for this purpose, we recommend to use (Echarri):

- File 40 µm during 30 seconds.
- File 25 µm during 30 seconds.
- File 15 µm during 30 seconds.

The teeth with prosthetic crowns or interproximal fillings often need to reshape the interproximal contact point and the dental size by using (Echarri):

- File 90 µm as much as necessary.
- File 25 µm during 30 seconds.
- File 15 µm during 30 seconds.

These files also have another advantage. These files can wear the hard tissues without damaging the soft tissues, and it is easier to limit the stripping to the contact point area using a file and not a bur.

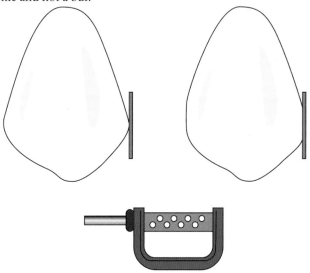

Fig. 18.41 Relationship of the stripping file with the contact point or contact surface.

Figure 18.41 shows how a flat file can wear only the most convex area of the mesial or distal dental surface, including the cases with an increased surface of contact point.

It is very important to position the files perpendicular to the occlusal plane and parallel to the dental axis to make a correct dental wear.

The PST recommends separating the teeth before the stripping to have a better access to the contact point area and to maintain the handpiece in one position allowing the file to make the stripping only by the movement of the handpiece and under irrigation (Echarri). Avoiding the circular movement of the handpiece, the resulting dental surface will be more polished.

Also, it is important to avoid the oscillating movement of the files in the vertical sense in order not to change the shape of the interdental space and the interdental sulcus (Figure 18.42). Increasing the interdental space, the possibility of gingival 'black triangles' will be also increased. And modifying the shape of the interdental sulcus, the circulation of the food during the mastication will be modified. Avoiding the horizontal oscillating movement of the files, the shapes of the labial and lingual spaces are preserved and the circulation of the food wouldn't change (Figure 18.43).

It is very important to design and plan the stripping properly to achieve all the goals of the treatment from an aesthetic and functional point of view. After the stripping treatment plan, it is very important to use the proper instrument as well as to follow a proper protocol.

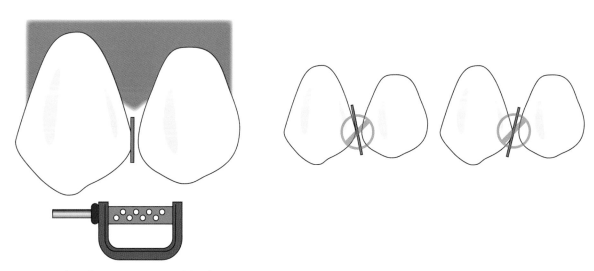

Fig. 18.42 Vertical oscillating movement of the file.

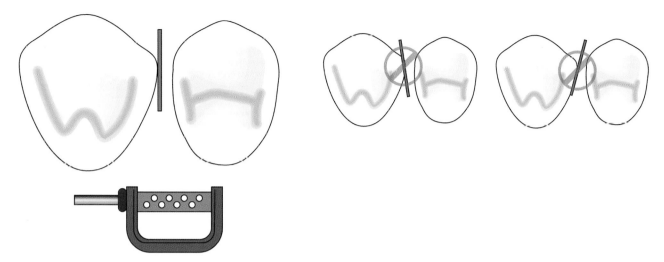

Fig. 18.43 Horizontal oscillating movement of the file.

Case reports

For more examples, see the cases on the companion website at www.wiley.com/go

References

Alexander RG (1986) 'Wick'. The Alexander discipline. In Engel GA (ed.) *Contemporary Concepts and Philosophies*. Glendora, CA: Ormco Corporation.

Andrews LF (1989) *Straight Wire. The Concept and Appliance*. Sand Diego, CA: LA Wells Co.

Aprile H and Figún ME (1960) *Anatomía odontológica*, Tercera edición. Buenos Aires, Argentina: Editorial El Ateneo.

Ballard ML (1944) Asymmetry in tooth size: a factor in the etiology, diagnosis, and treatment of malocclusion, *Angle Orthod* 14, 67–70.

Begg, P.R. (1954) Stone age man's dentition. *American Journal of Orthodontics* 40, 298-312, 373-383, 462-475, 517-531. doi:10.1016/0002-9416(54)90092-5.

Bennett JC and McLaughlin RP (1997) Consideraciones sobre la forma de la corona de los incisivos en el tratamiento ortodóncico. *Rev Esp Ortod* 27, 359–369.

Berrer HG (1975) Protecting the integrity of mandibular incisor position through keystoning procedure and spring retainer appliance. *J Clin Orthod* 9, 486–494.

Betteridge MA (1976) Index for measurement for lower labial segment crowding. *Br J Orthod* 3, 113–116.

Betteridge MA (1979) A method of treatment for incisor crowding. *Br J Orthod* 6, 43–48.

Betteridge MA (1981) The effects of interdental stripping on the labial segments evaluated one year out of retention. *Br J Orthod* 8, 193–197.

Black GV (1902) *Descriptive Anatomy of the Human Teeth*, 4th edn. Philadelphia, PA: SS White Dental.

Boese LR (1980a) Fiberotomy and reproximation without lower retention, nine years in retrospect, part I. *Angle Orthod* 50, 88–97.

Boese LR (1980b) Fiberotomy and reproximation without lower retention, nine years in retrospect, part II. *Angle Orthod* 50, 169–178.

Brudevold F, Tehrani A and Bakhos Y (1982) Intraoral mineralization of abraded dental enamel. *J Dent Res* 65, 456–459.

Crain G and Sheridan JJ (1990) Susceptibility to caries and periodontal disease after posterior air-rotor stripping. *J Clin Orthod* 24, 84–85.

Echarri P (2000a) Ortodoncia Lingual. Parte VI-A. Tratamiento sin extracciones. *Ortod Clín* 3(2), 86–93.

Echarri P (2000b) Ortodoncia Lingual. Parte VI-B. Tratamiento sin extracciones. *Ortod Clín* 3(3), 132–142.

Echarri P (2012) Ortodoncia en adultos. Enfoque actual. *Revista Ripano* 9(24), 18–24.

Echarri P and Vila E (2021) Tratamiento ortodóncico con stripping. En: Echarri P. Tratamiento sin extracciones Volumen III: Distalización y Stripping. Barcelona (España): Athenea Dental Institute, 383–435.

Echarri P (2013) *Clear Aligner*, 1st edn. Madrid, España: Ripano SA.

El-Mangoury NH, Moussa M, Mostafa Y and Girgis A (1991) In vivo remineralization after air-rotor stripping. *J Clin Orthod* 25, 75–78.

Gillings B and Buonocore M (1961) An investigation of enamel thickness in human lower incisor teeth. *J Dent Res* 40, 105–118.

Heins PJ, Thomas RG and Newton JW (1988) The relationship of interradicular width and alveolar bone loss. A radiometric study of periodontitis population. *J Periodontol* 59, 73–79.

Heins PJ and Wieder SM (1986) A histological study of the width and nature of interradicular spaces in human adult premolars and molars. *J Dent Res* 65, 948–951.

Hudson AR (1956) A study to the effects of mesiodistal reduction on mandibular anterior teeth. *Am J Orthod* 42, 615–624.

Jerrold L and Lowenstien LJ (1990) The midline: diagnosis and treatment. *Am J Orthod Dentofac Orthop* 97, 453–462.

Johnston CD, Burden DJ and Stevenson MR (1999) The influence of dental to facial midline discrepancies on dental attractiveness ratings. *Eur J Orthod* 21, 517–522.

Jost-Brinkmann PG, Otani H and Nakata M (1991) Surface condition of primary teeth after approximal grinding and polishing. *J Clin Pediatr Dent* 16(1), 41–45.

Kokich VO, Kiyah HA and Shapiro PA (1999) Comparing the perceptions of dentists and lay people to altered dental esthetics. *J Esthet Dent* 11, 311–324.

Levin EI (1978) Dental esthetics and golden proportion. *J Prosthet Dent* 40, 244–252.

Lucchese A, Porcú F and Dolci F (2001) Effects of various stripping techniques on surface enamel. *J Clin Orthod* 35, 691–695.

Murphy T. R. (1964) *Reduction of the Dental Arch By Approximal Attrition*. Journal, 1. London: British Dental Journal. (tDAR id: 113361).

Nielsen IM, Glavind L and Karring T (1980) Interproximal periodontal intrabony defects: prevalence, localization and ethiological factors. *J Clin Periodontol* 7, 187–198.

Paskow H (1970) Self-alignment following interproximal stripping. *Am J Orthod* 58, 240–249.

Peck H and Peck S (1972) An index for assessing tooth shape deviations as applied to the mandibular incisors. *Am J Orthod* 61, 384–401.

Piacentini C and Sfondrini G (1996) A scanning electron microscopy comparison of enamel polishing methods after air-rotor stripping. *Am J Orthod Dentofacial Orthop* 109, 57–63.

Radlanski RJ, Jager A and Zimmer B (1989a) Morphology of interdentally stripped enamel one year after treatment. *J Clin Orthod* 23, 748–750.

Radlanski RJ, Jager A, Zimmer B, Schwestka R and Bertzbach F (1989b) The results of scanning electron microscopy research on interdental stripping in vitro. *Fortschr Kieferorthop* 50(4), 276–284.

Ricketts RM (1989) *Provocations and Perceptions in Cranio-Facial Orthopedics. Dental Science and Facial Art, Vol. 1, Book1, Part 1,2.* Denver, CO: Rocky Mountains Orthodontics.

Ricketts RM (1995) The biologic significance of the divine proportion and Fibonacci series. *Am J Orthod* 81, 105–126.

Rossouw PE and Tortorellla A (2003) A pilot investigation of enamel reduction procedures. *J Can Dent Assoc* 69(6), 384–388.

Sarver DM and Ackerman MB (2005) Dynamic smile visualization and quantification and its impact on orthodontic diagnosis and treatment plan. In Romano R (ed.); Bichacho N. y Touati B associated editors. *The Art of Smile*, pp. 109–139. London (Great Britain): Quintessence Publishing.

Sheridan JJ (1985) Air-rotor stripping. *J Clin Orthod* 19, 43–59.

Sheridan JJ (1987) Air-rotor stripping update. *J Clin Orthod* 21, 781–788.

Sheridan JJ (1997) The physiologic rationale for air-rotor stripping. *J Clin Orthod* 31, 609–612.

Shillingburg HT and Grace CS (1973) Thickness of enamel and dentin. *J S Calif St Dent Assoc* 41, 33–52.

Sicher H (1953) The biology of attrition. *Oral Surg* 6, 406–412.

Tal H (1984) Relationship between the interproximal distance of roots and the prevalence of intraboney pockets. *J Periodontol* 55, 604–607.

Tarnow D, Margner WS and Fletcher P (1992) The effect of distance from the contact point to the crest of bone on the presence or absence of interproximal dental papilla. *J Periodontol* 63, 993–996.

Tuverson DL (1980) Anterior interocclusal relations: part I. *Am J Orthod* 75, 361–370.

Zhong M, Jost-Brinkmann PG, Zellmann M, Zellman S and Radlanski RJ (2000), Clinical evaluation of a new technique for interdental enamel reduction. *J Orofac Orthop* 61(6), 432–439.

19

Post-Treatment Maintenance

Birte Melsen, Sonil Kalia

Stability

Stability only exists post mortem. Indeed, retention is the most difficult problem in orthodontia – in fact, it is the main problem, as stated by Oppenheim in 1934 (1934). As long as we are alive, biological changes occur continuously. Changes in the dentition, the periodontal tissues and the occlusion will continue to occur whether or not an individual has had orthodontic treatment (Hopkins and Murphy 1971; Humerfelt and Slagsvold 1972; Sinclair and Little 1983; Harris and Behrents 1988; Dalstra et al. 2016). Growth and development in young individuals and the continuous age-related degeneration of the occlusion in adults result in clinically manifest occlusal adaptations. Stability of orthodontic treatment results, nevertheless, has been a frequently discussed topic (Little 1990; Kahl-Nieke 1996; Zachrisson 1997b; Shah et al. 2003; Littlewood et al. 2006). Based on many years' experience, Zachrisson (1997a) stated that long-term stability of alignment is highly variable and largely unpredictable. According to Zachrisson, the key to successful stability is paying more attention to finishing. Post-treatment changes are frequently perceived as relapse, but long-term observations of untreated individuals have demonstrated that untreated Class

II and Class III malocclusions tend to increase in severity, whereas Class I malocclusions seem to remain more stable (Harris and Behrents 1988). Nevertheless, orthodontists continue the search for the factors that may aid prediction of post-treatment changes. Only weak correlations have been found with treatment-related factors. When Little (1990) followed over 600 patients for more than 35 years, he found that neither pre-treatment variables nor treatment variables could be used to identify the patients who would show the largest post-treatment changes.

Post-treatment changes can be divided into two categories: the tendency of the teeth to move back towards their original position immediately after treatment; and the continuous development, related to growth in young patients and to the ageing process in adult individuals. Most studies focusing on stability of treatment results have not distinguished between the two types of changes.

Acceptance of the fact that post-treatment changes may occur has led orthodontists to focus on various retention regimens. In a Cochrane systematic review paper, Littlewood et al. (2006) made an attempt to evaluate the effectiveness of different retention strategies and concluded that there was insufficient research data on which clinicians could base their retention strategy. If absolute stability of the dentition is required, maintenance of the occlusion should be carried out independent of whether the patient has been orthodontically treated or not. With increasing age, the rate of change is influenced by both local and general factors (Riedel 1960, 1974; Hopkins and Murphy 1971; Humerfelt and Slagsvold 1972; Riedel and Brandt 1976; Little et al. 1981, 1988, 1990; Sinclair and Little 1983; Little and Riedel 1989; Melsen 1989; Little 1990; Riedel et al. 1992; Kahl-Nieke 1996). Yet, in spite of the lack of evidence and acceptance of post-treatment changes, orthodontists still desire stability, and show cases with occlusions that apparently have been stable over many years with or without previous orthodontic treatment.

Whereas several factors are known to contribute to changes within the dentition, predictors for a stable occlusion have not yet been identified. Patients with identical occlusions at a certain point in time may, years later, exhibit large differences in their occlusions. Untreated individuals experience changes in occlusion as part of natural development, whereas treated individuals experience changes that are a combination of relapse of tooth movements and ongoing development. Therefore, prior to commencing orthodontic treatment, the patient has to be informed of the need for maintenance of the treatment result from both biological and mechanical points of view (Kalia and Melsen 2001).

The immediate changes occurring after orthodontic treatment, when the teeth tend to return to their original positions, can be categorised under the term 'relapse'. The long-term changes reflecting the age-related degeneration of the dentition and occlusion should be called 'development' (Little et al. 1988; Little 1990). The maintenance of an orthodontic treatment result includes prevention of both short-term relapse and long-term developmental changes. Although age-related skeletal changes cannot be prevented, the rate of change can be influenced by general and local maintenance of the dentition. The local and general factors influencing the dentition have been discussed in detail in relation to the development of malocclusion (Chapter 2) and are still valid following rehabilitation of a deteriorated dentition (Graber 1966; Little et al. 1988). However, it is also important that the treatment result is compatible with normal function. Correction of anterior teeth for aesthetic reasons without taking the total occlusion into consideration can therefore rarely be maintained, and will be subject to continuous changes.

Biological maintenance

The maintenance of the treatment result comprises two aspects, neither of which can be neglected: biological maintenance and mechanical maintenance (Reitan 1951, 1954, 1967, 1969; Melsen 1991; Kahl-Nieke 1996). Mechanical

retention usually denotes orthodontic retention; however, biological maintenance of the dental and periodontal health is of equal if not more importance. Both types of maintenance should be discussed with the patient before initiating dental rehabilitation, whether or not it includes minor or major orthodontic treatment (Melsen et al. 1989; Melsen 1991; Melsen and Agerbaek 1994). The patients should be aware that stability cannot be guaranteed, but that much can be done to maintain the treatment result. Maintenance requires the patient's continued compliance. Unfortunately, there seems to be a widespread myth that dental rehabilitation is self-maintaining and remains stable. Orthodontists themselves have contributed to this attitude by the frequent use of the word 'stability' when presenting a special technique or appliance (Reitan 1969; Kahl-Nieke 1996; Russell 2004; Littlewood et al. 2006).

General medical considerations

In relation to all but in particular adult patients, it should be made clear that general health and especially factors controlling the bone turnover and the immune system influence the periodontium and related oral structures. Changes in the occlusion may therefore be the first sign of change in general health. The same applies to unexpected changes in the response of the periodontium to the ongoing treatment. Increased bleeding on probing or loosening of the teeth may be signs of a compromised immune system, and bite opening occurring without any local reason may be the first sign of reduced muscle force and as such the first sign of muscle dystrophy (Kiliaridis et al. 1989) (Figure 19.1). Bite opening may also be caused by local factors such as shortening of the ramus height and is then a sign of an intra-capsular destructive process leading to shortening of the condylar process (Kiliaridis et al. 1989; Kjellberg 1998).

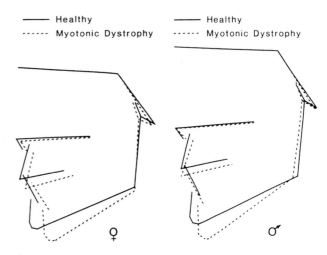

Fig. 19.1 Radiographic tracings of patients demonstrating bite opening due to muscular dystrophy (From Kiliaridis et al. (1989) by permission of Oxford University Press.) (Kiliaridis S, Mejersjo C and Thilander B (1989) Muscle function and craniofacial morphology: a clinical study in patients with myotonic dystrophy. Eur J Orthod 11, 131–138.).

Doubtless, a majority of the post-treatment changes occur as a result of neglect of both biological and mechanical maintenance. Biological maintenance is synonymous with maintenance of the teeth and a healthy periodontium. There is a large variation in the individual resistance to periodontal disease, but the same factors that lead to the destruction of the periodontium and thereby contribute to the development of a malocclusion may also trigger post-treatment changes. In most patients, a three-monthly follow-up appointment with a hygienist would be sufficient to maintain a healthy oral environment, but each patient should also be given an individual oral hygiene cleansing protocol, including the use of, for example, Oral-B Superfloss® (Figure 19.2) where bridges or bonded retainers prevent conventional flossing. Interdental brushes are very useful where the anatomy and restorations can compromise efficiency of normal brushing. Electric brushes may facilitate the brushing, but are not the solution. Each patient should be taught the optimal technique to maintain the healthy periodontium. It is important that the adult patients use a soft toothbrush, as most patients will have exposed cementum, which may further worsen with abrasion of the exposed part due to brushing with a hard toothbrush and incorrect brushing technique (Figure 19.2).

Fibrotomy

When discussing maintenance of a treatment result, most orthodontists only focus on mechanical retention. Mechanical retention is generally used following orthodontic treatment with the purpose of maintaining the positions of the teeth and the occlusion. This may give the patient a false sensation of stability. Following derotation of a rotated tooth, in addition to mechanical retention, circumferential supracrestal fibrotomy (CSF) has been recommended to prevent relapse (Edwards 1993). In a systematic review on retention, Littlewood et al. (2006) concluded that there was a significant increase in stability in the mandibular and maxillary anterior segments when CSF was used in conjunction with a Hawley's retainer, compared with the use of a Hawley's retainer alone. In

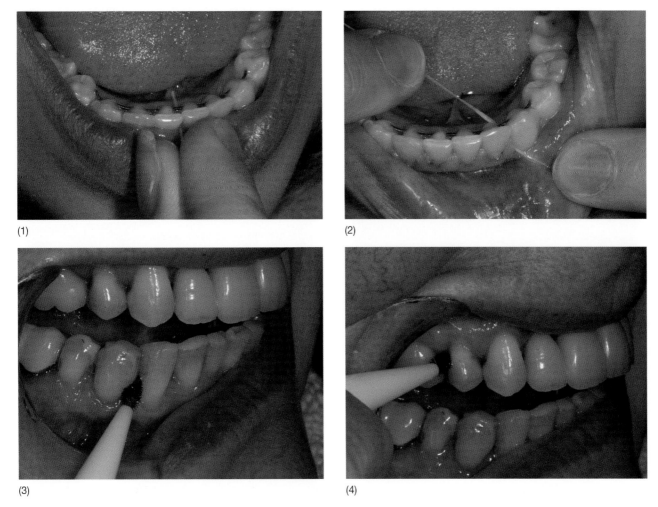

(1)   (2)   (3)   (4)

Fig. 19.2 (1) and (2) Superfloss® can be used for interdental cleansing in spite of the presence of a bonded retainer. (3) Exposure of cementum caused by use of a hard toothbrush and wrong brushing technique. (4) Interdental brushes can be used when the interdental papilla does not fill the interdental space completely and normal brushing cannot remove all debris.

cases of young adults with gingival hyperplasia, both fibrotomy and gingivectomy can be performed for aesthetics and stability, but in adult patients with marginal bone loss, the risk of prolonging the clinical crown goes against this procedure (Figure 19.3).

Mechanical maintenance – retention

Mechanical maintenance comprises fixed and removable retainers. Fixed retainers include bonded flexible wires, bonded rigid wires, stiff cast bonded splints, threaded composite retainers and also fixed prosthetic restorations.

Bonded retainers

Fixed bonded retainers are routinely used in adult patients in the lower arch and frequently in the upper anterior segment. The theoretical basis behind the recommendation of using bonded flexible wires is that these retainers allow micro-movements of the teeth and therefore help maintain the physical properties of the periodontium. Watted et al. (2001) used a periotest and found that the mobility of stabilised teeth decreased but not outside the normal range.

The braided or twisted wire can be bonded to as many teeth as necessary. In the lower arch, the wire most frequently extends from canine to canine or between the premolars on the two sides (Figure 19.4). The latter approach is based on the premise that the contact point between premolar and canine may be a predilection area for relapse of a deep bite.

A comparison between four types of retainers – (1) and (2) a thick plain wire bonded either only to the canines or to all teeth, (3) a twisted wire bonded to all teeth from canine to canine or (4) a removable retainer – did not demonstrate any difference in plaque accumulation or damage to the teeth (Artun et al. 1987). A larger study comparing fixed anterior retainers bonded to only the canines with those bonded to all the teeth favoured the latter (Stormann and Ehmer 2002). Zachrisson (1977) described several generations of the stiffer round wire retainers extending from canine to canine. The retainers were fabricated on plaster models and the teeth to be bonded were sandblasted before bonding. If the wire was adapted to contact the lingual surface of the incisors, the canine-to-canine retainer prevented relapse of irregularities among the incisors (Figure 19.4(1)).

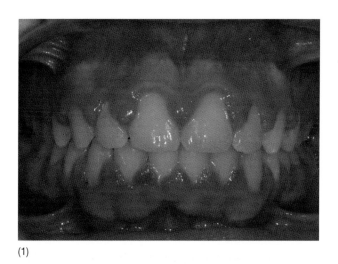

(1)

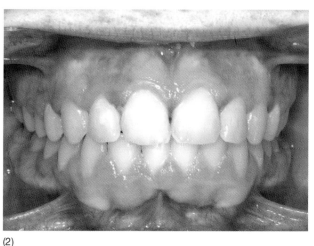

(2)

Fig. 19.3 Young adult patient with severe gingival hypertrophy following orthodontic treatment with fixed appliances. (1) Before gingivectomy and circumferential supracrestal fibrotomy. (2) After the gingival surgery.

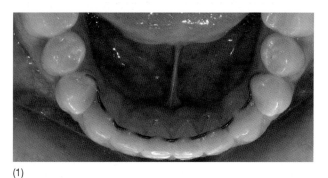

(1)

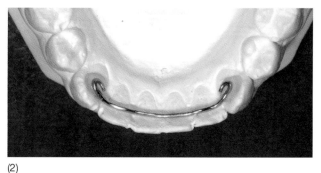

(2)

Fig. 19.4 (1) Premolar to premolar multistrand retainer wire: the position of the bond on the premolar varies according to the occlusion. (2) Model showing a stiff round 0.020-inch wire bonded on the canines only.

An alternative to the metal wires is the use of fibre-reinforced composites, which have also been recommended for temporary bridges (Sidhu and Ali 2001; Arteaga and Meiers 2004). When comparing different materials, Rose et al. (2002) found that longevity of the direct bonded multistranded wire was superior to the resin composite retainers reinforced with plasma-treated woven polyethylene ribbons. This is discussed further in Chapter 10.

When Littlewood et al. (2006) compared the results of fixed versus removable retainers of different fixed retainers and of different removable retainers, they found that there was insufficient evidence to make a valid recommendation for a retention procedure.

The same conclusion was found in a systematic review on the effect of fixed and removable orthodontic retainers by Dalya Al-Moghrabi et al. (2016). They concluded that none of the 24 studies carefully selected from 917 studied papers could answer the essential questions regarding effect on the periodontal health, risk of failure, patient-reported outcomes and cost effectiveness of retention regime.

Bonded retainers are most frequently used in the lower arch, but can also be used in the upper arch, and are recommended in the case of moderate or severe marginal bone loss and to keep spaces from reopening (Figure 19.5). When bonding an upper retainer, interference with occlusal contact should be avoided. In addition, the composite used for bonding can be used to reshape a lingual tuberculum that may have been lost due to abrasion and thus re-establish normal occlusal contacts (Figure 19.5).

It is preferable to bond retainers with the appliances still in place. In this way, the retainer can be ligated to the appliance during bonding (Figure 19.6). Leaving the appliance in the mouth for a few weeks after the retainer has been bonded is advisable, as the majority of failures occur during the first few weeks. Rotational relapse starts immediately when the retainer is lost. Loss of a retainer may be caused by the inability to keep the bonding area dry, thus it may be necessary to apply a rubber dam in these cases. This is especially indicated when the tuberculum on the lingual side of the upper front teeth has to be built up in order to achieve contact in protrusion and laterotrusion.

Fixed retainers and periodontal health

A frequently mentioned drawback of fixed retainers is the potential accumulation of plaque and calculus leading to caries and periodontal disease. This risk, however, seems to be overestimated, as none of the studies focusing on this potential problem have confirmed an increase in caries or pocket formation (Artun et al. 1987; Heier et al. 1997; Butler and Dowling 2005).

Several studies have been carried out and the conclusions are that, according to the currently available literature, orthodontic fixed retainers seem to be a retention strategy compatible with good periodontal health (Storey et al. 2018; Eroglu et al. 2019; Arn et al. 2020; Laursen et al. 2020)

Pros and cons of bonded retainers

A problem related to bonded retainers that has awoken attention the last decennia is that retainers can loosen without being noticed or even be unintentionally activated, resulting in undesirable tooth movements (Oppenheim 1934; Pizarro and Jones 1992; Katsaros et al. 2007; Renkema

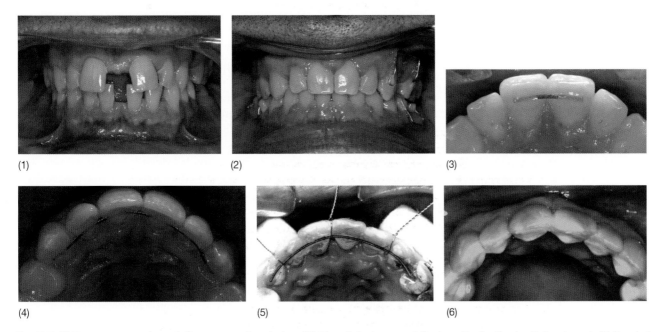

(1) (2) (3)

(4) (5) (6)

Fig. 19.5 (1) Pre-treatment view of diastemas and occlusion. (2) Closed diastema and final result of orthodontic treatment. (3) Bonded retainer between the upper central incisors to prevent reopening of the diastema. (4) Bonded canine to canine retainer. (5) and (6) Bonded retainer in the upper arch built up to simulate the cingula and adjusted for occlusion and protrusion contact, also serving as a bite plane on the four incisors to prevent extrusion of the intruded lower incisors.

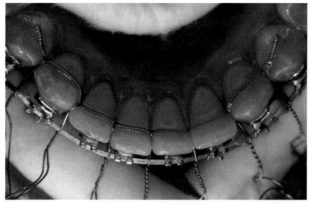

(1)

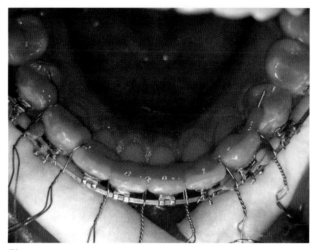

(2)

Fig. 19.6 Ligation of the lower retainer around the fixed appliance still in situ. The retainer is bonded and then after a few weeks the fixed appliance is debonded. Bonding procedure: (1) the multistranded retainer wire is adapted to the lingual surface and maintained by ligatures to the buccal appliance; and (2) etching.

et al. 2011; Pazera et al. 2012; Farret et al. 2015; Laursen et al. 2016, 2020; Jin et al. 2018).

Such displacements can lead to periodontal damage or even root exposure. Even though such displacements can have spontaneous improvement of the gingival recession if the tooth positions are correctly re-established (Machado et al. 2014), some may require the involvement of a periodontist and subsequent mucogingival surgery (Laursen et al. 2016, 2020).

The thin bony coverage of the lower incisor region (Nauert and Berg 1999) – one of the areas most commonly affected by gingival recession (Melsen and Allais 2005; Renkema et al. 2013; Pernet et al. 2019) – constitutes a risk for the development or worsening of fenestrations.

How can unintentional tooth displacements generated by active bonded retainers be avoided? Zachrisson advised the use of a 0.0215-inch five-stranded spiral wire, as opposed to

thinner 0.0195 or 0.0175-inch wire, to avoid side effects caused by distortion (Zachrisson 2007). Renkema and colleagues, on the other hand, found that the type of retainer does not seem to be correlated with the development of labial gingival recession (Renkema et al. 2013). The importance of educating the patient and general dentist in the detection of post-treatment tooth displacement can therefore not be overemphasised (Pazera et al. 2013).

To this end, the family dentist can be provided with digital images or digital models of the final orthodontic results, thus making it possible for them to recognise minor changes. A solution to this problem may also be to provide the patient with a vacuum-formed retainer (VFR). This could be prescribed in addition to bonded retention. Even small tooth movements would be reflected in an improper fit of the VFRs, allowing early detection of undesired tooth movements. The VFR can be worn at nights or once a week, and even minor changes will be detected, and the fixed retainer can be repaired if detached or broken, without any undesirable tooth movements.

One of the authors (Sonil Kalia) had advocated this retention protocol for the last 20 years in private practice with great success.

The choice of retention procedures is mostly based on the orthodontist's personal preference (Lai et al. 2014; Iliadi et al. 2015). Also, survival rate of fixed bonded retainers depends on many factors including personal clinical choice. In a study looking at the survival of maxillary and mandibular bonded retainers 10 to 15 years after orthodontic treatment, attrition was also one of the factors that were seen to create a bias (Kocher et al. 2019).

Cast retainers/retainers forming part of prosthetic rehabilitation

In patients with severely reduced periodontal support (>30%) and consequently increased tooth mobility, it is recommended to use a palatal cast retainer on the upper anterior teeth. This retainer is constructed by a prosthodontist or the general dentist.

The reason for choosing this more complicated approach to retention is the need to create a situation where the remaining periodontium is loaded in an optimal way. This can only be achieved if the retainer is constructed by a build-up of the palatal surface so that a group function of the upper anterior teeth can be established. In the buccal segments, cast onlays or composite fillings may be necessary to maintain the mandibular position. This is especially relevant following the successful treatment in patients with prior temporomandibular disorders (TMDs).

The combined presence of reduced periodontal support and recently finished orthodontic displacement may cause second-degree tooth mobility, and therefore retainers should be placed before debonding or a stiff wire should be bonded to the labial surface after appliance removal. In patients requiring a cast palatal retainer, the orthodontist should complete the treatment with a slight overjet to allow for the restoration of the palatal surface. As in the procedure for a bonded bridge, the palatal surface preparation for such a retainer should be modelled on an individual articulator for group contact in lateral and protrusive movements (Figure 19.7). The buccal wire remains in situ until the palatal retainer has been bonded and, if necessary, equilibrated.

This kind of retainer can also be used when single tooth replacements are also required, whereby the retainer and

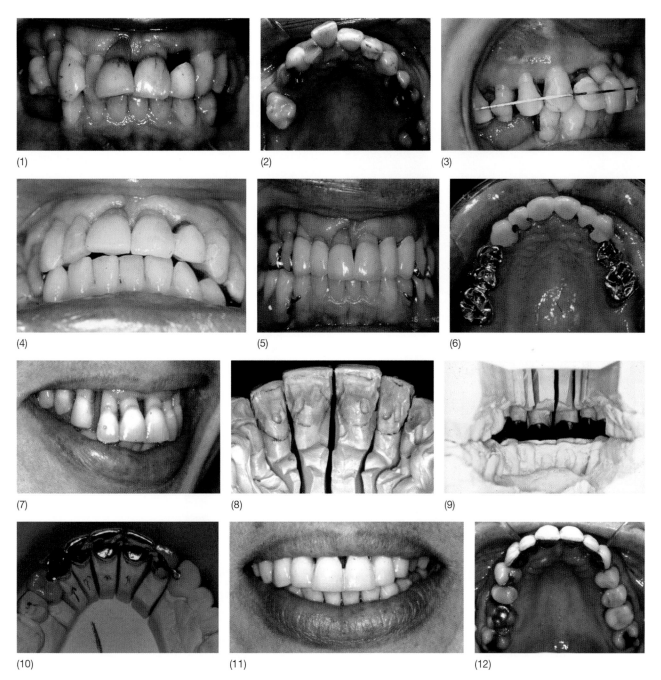

Fig. 19.7 (1) and (2) The situation before commencement of treatment. (3) In order to keep the teeth stable while preparing for a cast retainer, the labial appliance should remain in the mouth or a stiff wire as shown here should be bonded to the labial surface of the anterior teeth. (4) Intraoral image showing that the overjet following treatment allows for the placement of a cast retainer of the lingual surface. (5) and (6) Post-placement view. Single crowns have been adapted to the gold cast retainer bonded to the six anterior teeth and extending to the premolars with an attachment. (7) Pre-treatment image of patient with overerupted upper incisors. (8) Following intrusion and retraction of the anterior teeth, the teeth were prepared for a bonded cast retainer. (9) The cast retainer was modelled on an articulator. (10) Retainer on model. (11) Smile with the bonded retainer in place. (12) Retainer in place.

prosthetic restoration become one. Samama (1995) described a technique whereby the pontic can be replaced when gingival recession occurs in the post-treatment period (see Chapter 14).

In patients in whom teeth have been moved in order to provide space for the insertion of an implant, it is important to stabilise the teeth with a rigid wire bonded to the teeth on either side of the opened space. The wire has to be left in place until the implant has been inserted and fitted with a temporary or permanent crown (Figure 19.8). Even after the implant is inserted, teeth adjacent to the implant can tip into the open space during the healing phase before the crown has been placed.

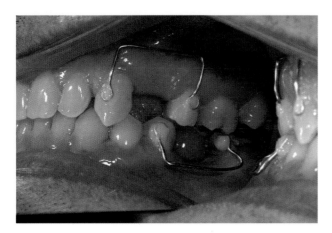

Fig. 19.8 Retainer used to maintain space for an implant.

Removable retention

Removable retainers serve several purposes, but are mainly used to retain the teeth in a fixed mutual position, to maintain arch form and to prevent parafunction. There are many designs and in all cases the original problem that was resolved must be taken into consideration before deciding the design of the retention appliance.

Thermoplastic retainers (Essix)

In adult patients, the first retention appliance may be a thermoplastic clear Essix retainer (Raintree Essix, Metairie) as described by Sheridan et al. (1993). This clear retainer can be fabricated while the patient is waiting and be placed within hours of debonding (Figure 19.9). They are cost-effective and can be remade easily. Therefore, they are ideal as an interim retainer during the rehabilitation treatment for the deteriorated dentition. For example, in cases where missing teeth are replaced or where the dentition and occlusion are reconstructed, a final retainer can be fabricated. This thin splint can be built up for maximal occlusal contact and thus support the mandibular position until final establishment of the occlusal surfaces. A thicker modification of the clear retainers can be used to protect teeth from overloading occurring as a result of parafunction, which often takes place during sleep, especially if the dentition is reduced. Missing teeth can also be replaced in the retainer until a final dental prosthesis can be placed.

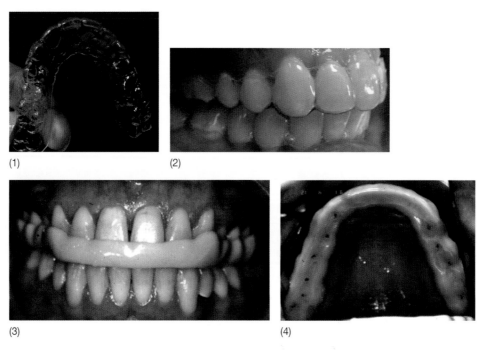

(1)   (2)

(3)   (4)

Fig. 19.9 (1) Upper Essix retainer. (2) Upper and lower Essix retainers in situ. (3) Splint made directly in the mouth from light-cured composite. (4) Distribution of occlusal contacts on the splint.

Fully balanced acrylic splint (tooth pyjamas)

A rather quick and cost-effective solution is the Triad splint light-cured directly in the mouth (Triad VLC Provisional Material, Dentsply) (Figure 19.9). The patient is asked to bite carefully into the splint, to ensure the maximum number of occlusal contacts on the splint. Following light curing, the splint is reduced to an acceptable buccolingual width and can be worn during the period of fabrication of the definitive occlusal restorations.

Splints with occlusal coverage can be produced with occlusal relief or made flat with balanced occlusal contacts (Figure 19.10). The distribution of occlusal contacts seems to be related to symptoms in muscles and joints (Gianniri et al. 1991). A bite-releasing splint would reduce the risk of muscle symptoms caused by asymmetrical distribution of occlusal contacts (Fu et al. 2003; Wassell et al. 2004). An additional advantage of the fully balanced splint is the prevention of overloading of the individual elements of the teeth in cases where we have a reduced dentition or in cases of single implants. From several points of view, it can therefore be recommended to supply elderly patients with what we have chosen to call a 'tooth pyjama' (Figure 19.10). The 'tooth pyjama' is fabricated on a Biostar (Great Lakes Dental Technologies) from 2-mm plastic sheets.

The disadvantage of the occlusal coverage of these splints is that no settling can take place. Settling is an important part of treatments especially in young patients. In adult individuals, the final occlusal adjustment is less dependent on settling, as it is mainly performed by equilibration or restorative adjustments.

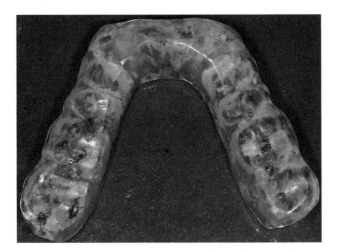

Fig. 19.10 'Tooth pyjamas': 2-mm splint that can be used as the initial full-time retainer and is then rebased while the restorations are being fabricated. Later this splint can be used as night guard for life.

Other types of removable retainers

These include Hawley's and modified Hawley's retainers. With plates, the position of the teeth is maintained by the wires extending from the baseplate. The baseplates are kept in place by various types of clasps crossing the occlusal surfaces. It is important that they do not interfere with occlusal contacts, as this will prevent 'settling', which is the main advantage of plates over splints. The purpose of the labial wire is to maintain the position of the teeth that have been moved and to prevent changes in overbite by eruption. There are various types of retention plates. In cases where the canines have been moved, the anterior wire should encompass these teeth. When only the incisors have been moved, a wire encompassing the four incisors is often sufficient to maintain their respective positions (Figure 19.11). A flat anterior wire or as an alternative a wire covered with composite adjusted to fit tightly to the labial surface is advantageous in maintaining torque corrections of the incisors and to provide better rotational stability.

Maximum settling occurs when patients are wearing a wrap-around retention plate (Figure 19.11). This retainer has no wire passing over the occlusal surfaces, but a precondition for control of the position of the individual teeth is that the long and therefore flexible labial wire is covered with composite for maximum contact with the labial surface of the teeth. Hawley's retainers or splint retainers essentially all aim for the same goal and can be modified based on the needs of the patient (Figure 19.11).

Hawley's retainers can also be modified to replace missing teeth until a final dental prosthesis can be placed (Figure 19.12). Whereas the sagittal and the transverse dimensions of the arch are maintained by all types of retainers, vertical maintenance is still a problem. In patients who have a severe deep bite, the retainer can be manufactured with a palatal bite plane to prevent night-time clenching or composite cingulum can build up lingually on the upper incisors.

Intermaxillary retention

In patients who have had correction of an open bite, the main problem afterwards is the adjustment of the tongue to the closed bite. Maintenance of the treatment results in these patients is known to be rather unpredictable. However, an intermaxillary appliance may prevent the tongue pressure at night. Intermaxillary appliances are of two types: soft and hard.

The soft appliance can be a positioner or two soft splints glued together. The tooth positioner is a one-piece, soft appliance, which may be used for the finishing of orthodontic treatment. The appliance is constructed over a predetermined setup and fills the freeway space and covers the clinical crowns of all the teeth and about 3 mm of the buccal and lingual gingival mucosa. The positioner is fabricated from either rubber or soft plastic and breathing holes can be

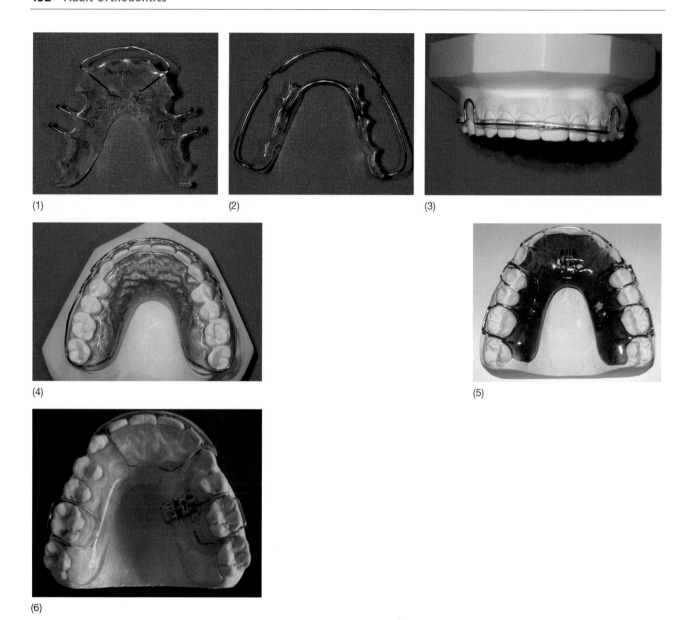

Fig. 19.11 (1) Hawley's retainer. (2) Wrap-around retainer without acrylic covering the labial arch. (3) and (4) Wrap-around retainers with an acrylic-covered labial arch. Modified Hawley's retainer with: (5) a screw in the plate to procline the incisors slightly; and (6) a screw to expand one side only. When the movements are completed, the plate can be rebased to be used as a permanent retainer plate.

included labially to improve tolerance of the appliance during wear. The positioner is used during the first weeks after debonding and can cause minor tipping and changes in the arch form (Bowman and Carano 2002) (Figures 19.13 and 19.14). Though it can be quite bulky, it is well tolerated in most cases; elderly patients however seem not to tolerate it so well. Positioners are constructed on an articulator setup and produced from a soft-rubber-based compound or soft plastic compound. In patients with reduced periodontal support, however, a positioner may also have adverse effects on the dentition, as it may exert abnormal pressures on the

periodontal tissues. This is due to the pure 'tipping' effect on the teeth which may cause unwanted proclination of periodontally compromised teeth (Park et al. 2008; Lochmatter et al. 2012).

Two connected Raintree Essix splints may be used as an alternative intermaxillary appliance, especially in patients with a tendency to open bite. Like the positioner, the two splints are connected on an articulator with an intermaxillary distance corresponding to the freeway space. Intermaxillary appliances have been recommended for use not only after treatment of an open bite but also in

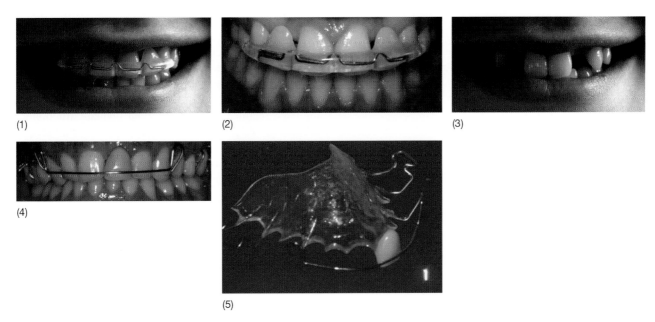

(1) (2) (3)

(4)

(5)

Fig. 19.12 Hawley's retainer with replacement for: (1)–(3) two lateral incisors; and (4) and (5) a central incisor.

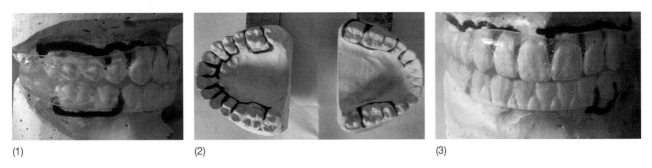

(1) (2) (3)

Fig. 19.13 Positioner: (1) and (2) the articulated setup is completed and then the positioner is fabricated on this setup. (3) Positioner on a model.

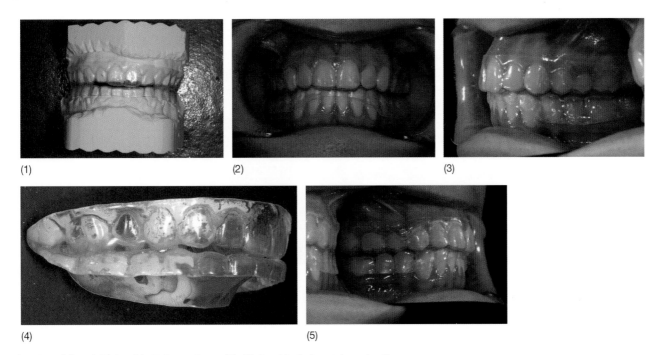

(1) (2) (3)

(4) (5)

Fig. 19.14 (1) and (2) Double Essix retainers. (3)–(5) Double Essix retainers in situ.

Class II and Class III cases that have been corrected with the use of elastics and after treatment of severe crossbite where the mandibular position has been influenced. The double Essix can also help maintain the sagittal and transversal dimensions and can be modified to produce minor tooth movements if needed.

Active retention plates

The commonly used retention plates are excellent at maintaining tooth positions as well as the transverse and sagittal dimensions of the dental arch, and can also be made active for minor correction of either arch form or single teeth. Arch form can be corrected by splitting the retainer into two parts and adding an expansion spring or screw; this can be done in both arches. Correction of single teeth can be performed with a spring retainer (Figure 19.15) (Kuijpers-Jagtman 2002), fabricated on a setup simulating the desired result. A different approach would be the one using the aligners described in Chapter 17.

Latest technology in retainers fabrication (bonded and vacuum-formed)

With the latest, new digital technology and scanning techniques, the dental arches can be scanned after debonding and the scanned digital file of the teeth sent via the Internet to the laboratory instantly. With this scan, a model is printed with 3D printing technology; on this printed model, a vacuum-formed retainer is manufactured and sent to the practice to be fitted.

The advantage of this is that the scanned digital file can be stored digitally for the future, eliminating the need for impressions, that is, if the patient has damaged or lost the retainers.

Bonded retainers can also be fabricated on the printed models as can also a transfer tray; this can be thermoplastically pressed onto the bonded retainer (after spacers and separating material are added to the fixed retainer and model, as not to bond the two components together) forming an indirect bonding tray. This fixed retainer via the bonding transfer tray can then be indirectly bonded in the mouth (Figure 19.16).

As a vacuum-formed retainer is recommended to fit over the fixed retainer, then blocking out lingually the bonded retainer on the printed model is carried out and a vacuum-formed retainer is then manufactured that will then fit over the fixed retainers, and then both retainers can be fitted at the same appointment. So the sequence will be: (a) fit the bonded retainer via the indirect bonding technique, and (b) fit the vacuum formed retainer over this to be worn at nights.

Virtual removal of fixed appliances and or attachments to fabricate retainers

This latest digital technology also gives way to the fact that teeth can be scanned with the fixed appliances in situ as well as attachments in the case of aligner treatments. In the case of fixed appliances, the orthodontic wires need to be removed for the scan, and then replaced to hold the status quo. The scan is sent as a digital file to the lab on the portal via the Internet and the orthodontic laboratory then virtually removes the brackets and appliances with a specific dedicated software. As can be seen (Figure 19.17), Teeth 16 + 15 are where the tubes and brackets have been already digitally removed; brackets on Teeth 13 + 14 are the next to be removed.

After digitally removing the appliances, the models are 3D printed and then the retainers fabricated either vacuum-formed and or bonded retainers as described in the earlier text and sent back to the clinic for the next appointment where then the fixed appliances are removed on the teeth and the retainers fitted directly at the same appointment. This procedure is excellent for avoiding any relapse tendencies straight after debond.

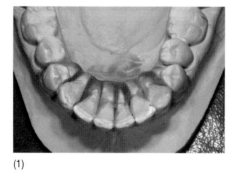
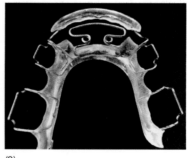

(1) (2)

Fig. 19.15 (1) Setup for treatment of relapse of crowding of the lower incisors. (2) Active 'spring' retainer with a coffin spring to align the lower anterior teeth.

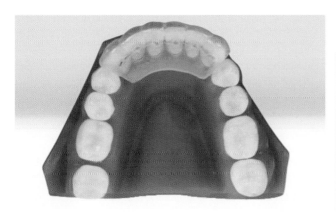

Fig. 19.16 Indirect bonding tray with fixed retainer in situ.

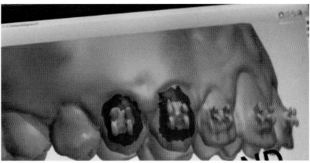

Fig. 19.17 Digital debond: the appliances are 'virtually' removed by a computer software.

In a study comparing direct and indirect bonded retainers, there were fewer unexpected post-treatment changes with indirect bonded retainers as opposed to direct bonded retainers, but there was no difference in the risks of failure between mandibular retainers bonded with direct and indirect methods (Egli et al. 2017).

Retention after aligner orthodontic treatments

The same regime of retention is to be followed after conclusion of a successful aligner orthodontic treatment, as it would be with all successful fixed orthodontic treatments. Bonded retainers with vacuum-formed retainers over the bonded retainers for night-time wear should be advocated. As all aligner company laboratories already have the digital scans of the teeth, they are in the position to print models and fabricate vacuum-formed retainers without the need for new digital scans. Not all aligner companies though offer bonded retainers with indirect bonding trays, but some do (e.g., Orthocaps™).

It is always advocated to have bonded retainers in addition to the vacuum-formed retainers to wear at nights. So, if the aligner company doesn't offer indirect bonding retainer trays and the clinician so wishes, then a fixed retainer should be fitted directly in the mouth and then the scan carried out over the fixed retainer for the laboratory to print models to carry out the vacuum-formed retainer fabrication to ensure a good fit.

Future developments

The use of scanners whereby printed models are fabricated onto which retainers are made will give way to directly printed clear retainers without the need for models. This will be a time-efficient way of fabricating retainers and can therefore be carried out in a practice environment.

Conclusion

Changes of a treatment result over time can only be avoided by combined biological and mechanical maintenance. The changes occurring following orthodontic treatment are a combination of the tendency towards the return to the pre-treatment situation, which occurs predominantly in the early post-treatment period, and lifelong age-related development.

Before commencing any orthodontic treatment, it should be explained to the patient that stability cannot be guaranteed, but that they will be able to retain the treatment result with lifelong maintenance unless local destruction and general diseases contribute to further degeneration of the dentition. If the dentist has reached his treatment goal, for example, an occlusion compatible with normal function, it is advocated to have the patient realise that he or she is responsible for the maintenance. This can be done by asking the patient to sign a form declaring that the retainers have to be used according to the dentist's prescription and that if this is not the case then no guarantee is granted.

The use of scanners and printed models has allowed for a more digital workflow streamlining in retainer fabrication and delivery.

It should be made clear that the responsibility of correct maintenance lies not only with the patients, but also their family dentist should be sufficiently informed and instructed to provide a comprehensive dental service. As in the planning phase, communication between colleagues is desirable. In addition, virtual models, which are now more mainstream, provide an excellent aid in the communication with colleagues and patients. To improve the confidence, a virtual model of the treatment result could be given to the patient and the family dentist.

References

Al-Moghrabi D, Pandis N and Fleming PS (2016) The effects of fixed and removable orthodontic retainers: a systematic review. *Prog Orthod* 2016 Dec;17(1), 24.

Arn ML, Dritsas K, Pandis N and Kloukos D (2020) The effects of fixed orthodontic retainers on periodontal health: a systematic review. *Am J Orthod Dentofacial Orthop* 157(2), 156–164.e17.

Arteaga S and Meiers JC (2004) Single-tooth replacement with a chairside prefabricated fiber-reinforced resin composite bridge: a case study. *Gen Dent* 52, 517–519.

Artun J, Spadafora AT, Shapiro PA, McNeill RW and Chapko MK (1987) Hygiene status associated with different types of bonded, orthodontic canine-to-canine retainers. A clinical trial. *J Clin Periodontol* 14, 89–94.

Bowman SJ and Carano A (2002) Short-term, intensive use of the tooth positioner in case finishing. *J Clin Orthod* 36, 216–219.

Butler J and Dowling P (2005) Orthodontic bonded retainers. *J Ir Dent Assoc* 51, 29–32.

Dahl EH and Zachrisson BU (1991) Long-term experience with direct-bonded lingual retainers. *J Clin Orthod* 25, 619–630.

Dalstra M, Sakima MT, Lemor C and Melsen B (2016) Drifting of teeth in the mandible studied in adult human autopsy material. *Orthod Craniofac Res* 2016 Feb;19(1), 10–17.

Edwards JG (1993) Soft-tissue surgery to alleviate orthodontic relapse. *Dent Clin North Am* 37, 205–225.

Egli F, Bovali E, Kiliaridis S and Cornelis MA (2017) Indirect vs direct bonding of mandibular fixed retainers in orthodontic patients: comparison of retainer failures and posttreatment stability. A 2-year follow-up of a single-center randomized controlled trial. *Am J Orthod Dentofacial Orthop* 151(1), 15-27.

Eroglu AK, Baka ZM and Arslan U (2019) Comparative evaluation of salivary microbial levels and periodontal status of patients wearing fixed and removable orthodontic retainers. *Am J Orthod Dentofacial Orthop* 156(2), 186-192.

Farret MM, Farret MM, da Luz Vieira G, Assaf JH and de Lima EM (2015) Orthodontic treatment of a mandibular incisor fenestration resulting from a broken retainer. *Am J Orthod* 148, 332–337.

Fu AS, Mehta NR, Forgione AG, Al-Badawi EA and Zawawi KH (2003) Maxillomandibular relationship in TMD patients before and after short-term flat plane bite plate therapy. *Cranio* 21, 172–179.

Gianniri AI, Melsen B, Nielsen L and Athanasiou AE (1991) Occlusal contacts in maximum intercuspation and craniomandibular dysfunction in 16- to 17-year-old adolescents. *J Oral Rehabil* 18, 49–59.

Graber TM (1966) Postmortems in posttreatment adjustment. *Am J Orthod* 52, 331–352.

Harris EF and Behrents RG (1988) The intrinsic stability of Class I molar relationship: a longitudinal study of untreated cases. *Am J Orthod Dentofacial Orthop* 94, 63–67.

Heier EE, De Smit AA, Wijgaerts IA and Adriaens PA (1997) Periodontal implications of bonded versus removable retainers. *Am J Orthod Dentofacial Orthop* 112, 607–616.

Hopkins JB and Murphy J (1971) Variations in good occlusions. *Angle Orthod* 41, 55–65.

Humerfelt A and Slagsvold O (1972) Changes in occlusion and craniofacial pattern between 11 and 25 years of age. A follow-up study of individuals with normal occlusion. *Trans Eur Orthod Soc* 1972, 113–122.

Iliadi A, Kloukos D, Gkantidis N, Katsaros C and Pandis N (2015) Failure of fixed orthodontic retainers: a systematic review. *J Dent* 43(8), 876–896.

Jin C, Bennani F, Gray A, Farella M and Mei L (2018) Survival analysis of orthodontic retainers. *Eur J Orthod* 40(5), 531–536.

Kahl-Nieke B (1996) Retention and stability considerations for adult patients. *Dent Clin North Am* 40, 961–994.

Kalia S and Melsen B (2001) Interdisciplinary approaches to adult orthodontic care. *J Orthod* 28, 191–196.

Katsaros C, Livas C and Renkema AM (2007) Unexpected complications of bonded mandibular lingual retainers. *Am J Orthod* 132, 838–841.

Kiliaridis S, Mejersjo C and Thilander B (1989) Muscle function and craniofacial morphology: a clinical study in patients with myotonic dystrophy. *Eur J Orthod* 11, 131–138.

Kjellberg H (1998) Craniofacial growth in juvenile chronic arthritis. *Acta Odontol Scand* 56, 360–365.

Kocher KE, Gebistorf MC, Pandis N, Fudalej PS and Katsaros C (2019) Survival of maxillary and mandibular bonded retainers 10 to 15 years after orthodontic treatment: a retrospective observational study. *Prog Orthod* 20(1), 28. Published 2019 Jul 22.

Kuijpers-Jagtman AM (2002) Repair and revision 8. Relapse of lower incisors: retreatment? *Ned Tijdschr Tandheelkd* 109, 42–46.

Lai CS, Grossen JM, Renkema AM, Bronkhorst E, Fudalej PS and Katsaros C (2014) Orthodontic retention procedures in Switzerland. *Swiss Dent J* 124(6), 655–661.

Laursen MG, Rylev M and Melsen B (2016) Treatment of complications after unintentional tooth displacement by active bonded retainers. *J Clin Orthod* May;50(5), 290–297.

Laursen MG, Rylev M and Melsen B (2020) The role of orthodontics in the repair of gingival recessions. *Am J Orthod Dentofacial Orthop* Jan;157(1), 29–34.

Little RM (1990) Stability and relapse of dental arch alignment. *Br J Orthod* 17, 235–241.

Little RM and Riedel RA (1989) Postretention evaluation of stability and relapse – mandibular arches with generalized spacing. *Am J Orthod Dentofacial Orthop* 95, 37–41.

Little RM, Riedel RA and Artun J (1988) An evaluation of changes in mandibular anterior alignment from 10 to 20 years postretention. *Am J Orthod Dentofacial Orthop* 93, 423–428.

Little RM, Riedel RA and Engst ED (1990) Serial extraction of first premolars – postretention evaluation of stability and relapse. *Angle Orthod* 60, 255–262.

Little RM, Wallen TR and Riedel RA (1981) Stability and relapse of mandibular anterior alignment-first premolar extraction cases treated by traditional edgewise orthodontics. *Am J Orthod* 80, 349–365.

Littlewood SJ, Millett DT, Doubleday B, Bearn DR and Worthington HV (2006) Orthodontic retention: a systematic review. *J Orthod* 33, 205–212.

Lochmatter D, Steineck M and Brauchli L (2012) Influence of material choice on the force delivery of bimaxillary tooth positioners on canine malpositions. *J Orofac Orthop* 73(2), 104–115.

Machado AW, MacGinnis M, Damis L and Moon W (2014) Spontaneous improvement of gingival recession after correction of tooth positioning. *Am J Orthod* 145, 828–835.

Melsen B (1989) Adult orthodontics – specific notice of the choice of biomechanics for adolescents and adults. *Quintessenz* 40, 1639–1655.

Melsen B (1991) Limitations in adult orthodontics. In Melsen B (ed.) *Current Controversies in Orthodontics*, pp. 147–180. Chicago, IL: Quintessence.

Melsen B and Agerbaek N (1994) Orthodontics as an adjunct to rehabilitation. *Periodontol 2000* 4, 148–159.

Melsen B, Agerbaek N and Markenstam G (1989) Intrusion of incisors in adult patients with marginal bone loss. *Am J Orthod Dentofacial Orthop* 96, 232–241.

Melsen B and Allais D (2005) Factors of importance for the development of dehiscences during labial movement of mandibular incisors: a retrospective study of adult orthodontic patients. *Am J Orthod Dentofacial Orthop* May;127(5), 552–561.

Nanda RS and Nanda SK (1992) Considerations of dentofacial growth in long-term retention and stability: is active retention needed? *Am J Orthod Dentofacial Orthop* 101, 297–302.

Nauert K and Berg R (1999) Evaluation of labio-lingual bony support of lower incisors in orthodontically untreated adults with the help of computed tomography. *J Orofac Orthop* 60, 321–334.

Oppenheim A (1934) The crisis in orthodontia, Part I: 2. Tissue changes during retention: Skogsborg's septotomy. *Int J Orthod Dent Child* 20, 639–644.

Park Y, Hartsfield JK, Katona TR and Eugene Roberts W (2008) Tooth positioner effects on occlusal contacts and treatment outcomes. *Angle Orthod* 78(6), 1050–1056.

Pazera P, Fudalej P and Katsaros C (2012) Severe complication of a bonded mandibular lingual retainer. *Am J Orthod* 142, 406–409.

Pazera P, Fudalej PS and Katsaros C (2013) Authors' response. *Am J Orthods* 143, 4.

Pernet F, Vento C, Pandis N and Kiliaridis S (2019) Long-term evaluation of lower incisors gingival recessions after orthodontic treatment. *Eur J Orthod* 2019 Nov 15;41(6), 559–564.

Pizarro K and Jones ML (1992) Crown inclination relapse with multiflex retainers. *J Clin Orthod* 26, 780–782.

Reitan K (1951) The tissue reaction as related to the functional factor. *Dent Rec (London)* 71, 173–183.

Reitan K (1954) Paradental reconstruction in the framework of orthodontics. *Zahnarztl Welt* 9, 2–35.

Reitan K (1967) Clinical and histologic observations on tooth movement during and after orthodontic treatment. *Am J Orthod* 53, 721–745.

Reitan K (1969) Principles of retention and avoidance of posttreatment relapse. *Am J Orthod* 55, 776–790.

Renkema AM, Fudalej PS, Renkema A, Kiekens R and Katsaros C (2013) Development of labial gingival recessions in orthodontically treated patients. *Am J Orthod* 143, 206–212.

Renkema AM, Renkema A, Bronkhorst E and Katsaros C (2011) Long-term effectiveness of canine-to-canine bonded flexible spiral wire lingual retainers. *Am J Orthod* 139, 614–621.

Riedel RA (1960) A review of the retention problem. *Angle Orthod* 30, 179–199.

Riedel RA (1974) A postretention evaluation. *Angle Orthod* 44, 194–212.

Riedel RA and Brandt S (1976) Dr. Richard A. Riedel on retention and relapse. *J Clin Orthod* 10, 454–472.

Riedel RA, Little RM and Bui TD (1992) Mandibular incisor extraction–postretention evaluation of stability and relapse. *Angle Orthod* 62, 103–116.

Rose E, Frucht S and Jonas IE (2002) Clinical comparison of a multistranded wire and a direct-bonded polyethylene ribbon-reinforced resin composite used for lingual retention. *Quintessence Int* 33, 579–583.

Russell K (2004) What type of orthodontic retainer is best? *Evid Based Dent* 5, 106.

Samama Y (1995) Fixed bonded prosthodontics: a 10-year follow-up report. Part I: analytical overview. *Int J Periodontics Restorative Dent* 15, 424–435.

Shah AA, Elcock C and Brook AH (2003) Incisor crown shape and crowding. *Am J Orthod Dentofacial Orthop* 123, 562–567.

Sheridan JJ, LeDoux W and McMinn R (1993) Essix retainers: fabrication and supervision for permanent retention. *J Clin Orthod* 27, 37–45.

Sidhu HK and Ali A (2001) Hypodontia, ankylosis and infraocclusion: report of a case restored with a fibre-reinforced ceromeric bridge. *Br Dent J* 191, 613–616.

Sinclair PM and Little RM (1983) Maturation of untreated normal occlusions. *Am J Orthod* 83, 114–123.

Storey M, Forde K, Littlewood SJ, Scott P, Luther F and Kang J (2018) Bonded versus vacuum-formed retainers: a randomized controlled trial. Part 2: periodontal health outcomes after 12 months. *Eur J Orthod* 40(4), 399–408.

Stormann I and Ehmer U (2002) A prospective randomized study of different retainer types. *J Orofac Orthop* 63, 42–50.

Wassell RW, Adams N and Kelly PJ (2004) Treatment of temporomandibular disorders by stabilising splints in general dental practice: results after initial treatment. *Br Dent J* 197, 35–41.

Watted N, Wieber M, Teuscher T and Schmitz N (2001) Comparison of incisor mobility after insertion of canine-to-canine lingual retainers bonded to two or to six teeth. A clinical study. *J Orofac Orthop* 62, 387–396.

Zachrisson BU (1977) Clinical experience with direct-bonded orthodontic retainers. *Am J Orthod* 71, 440–448.

Zachrisson BU (1997a) Important aspects of long-term stability. *J Clin Orthod* 31, 562–583.

Zachrisson BU (1997b) Orthodontics and periodontics. In Lindhe J, Karring T and Lang NP (eds) *Clinical Periodontology and Implant Dentistry*, 4th edn. Oxford: Blackwell Munksgaard.

Zachrisson BU (2007) Long-term experience with direct-bonded retainers: update and clinical advice. *J Clin Orthod* 41, 728–737.

20

Treatment Duration: Can It be Shortened?

Sabarinath Prasad, Mauro Farella, Birte Melsen

Discipline of Orthodontics, Faculty of Dentistry, University of Otago, Dunedin, New Zealand

Introduction

Treatment time in orthodontics is a key factor that deters many adults from seeking the benefits orthodontic treatment has to offer. Often, the first question that a patient seeking orthodontic treatment asks pertains to the anticipated duration of treatment. Regardless of force magnitude and modality, large inter-individual variations exist in the rate of tooth movement, with an average duration of treatment being over 20 months (range 14–33 months) (Tsichlaki et al. 2016).

Clinical experience indicates that the response to identical force stimuli varies considerably between individuals (Giannopoulou et al. 2016). Pilon and co-workers (Pilon et al. 1996) showed that even dogs of the same litter reacted differently to the same force system, clearly demonstrating the influence of differences in bone metabolism, and turnover in the periodontal ligament.

An effort to predict treatment time has a limited success, as over 50% of the variation is unexplained by pre-treatment characteristics. As treatment time is related to both cost and the likelihood of orthodontic treatment complications such as root resorption, gingival recession and enamel decalcification, many attempts have been made to reduce the duration of treatment.

Adjuncts to accelerate tooth movements

The methods applied to shorten the treatment duration can be classified into surgical interventions, including the timing of orthognathic surgery, various types of corticotomies and micro-osteoperforation (MOP), and non-surgical interventions, such as vibration, laser/photobiomodulation, pharmacological approaches and finally the treatment plan and appliance selection.

It is important to note that studies on the effect of acceleration of tooth movement are always limited to a particular phase of treatment, measuring the rate either of a specific tooth movement or of space closure and not on total treatment time.

Surgical

Surgical intervention may either supplement routine orthodontic treatment as an adjunctive procedure in an attempt to accelerate tooth movement or be a part of the orthodontic treatment plan in the form of extractions or orthognathic surgery.

When surgery is a part of the treatment plan, the timing and/or sequencing of the surgical intervention can be manipulated to shorten treatment time. For instance, the timing of tooth extractions may be optimised to shorten treatment time. Anecdotal evidence shows that space closure tends to be faster when commenced immediately after tooth extraction, possibly owing to the reduced bony resistance offered by the newly healing extraction site to tooth movement.

Orthodontic tooth movement is influenced by bone turnover rate (Verna et al. 2000), with a higher turnover significantly increasing the rate of tooth movement. Frost described the biological mechanisms underlying increased tissue turnover incidental to the repair of an injury, a phenomenon he termed the regional acceleratory phenomenon (RAP) (Frost 1989). Orthodontic forces alone are sufficient to elicit a RAP adjacent to the alveolar wall (Verna et al. 1999). However, the level of RAP expression with orthodontic force alone may be considered as mild to moderate. An intentional surgical insult, at selective sites, enhances the RAP, enabling faster tooth movement. These surgical interventions are undertaken prior to or at the start of orthodontic treatment. Surgical interventions vary considerably in complexity and invasiveness ranging from therapeutic fractures of the anterior alveolus, decortication, corticotomy, transmucosal corticision to MOPs.

Corticotomy

The earliest procedure advocated by Kole in 1959 (Kole 1959) involved reflecting a gingival flap all around the arch, placement of vertical bone cuts on both the facial and lingual aspects between the teeth and immediate activation of orthodontic appliances leading to therapeutic greenstick fractures of the bone followed by alignment of teeth within minutes to hours. Although tooth movement was almost instantaneous, the procedure was extremely invasive and did not allow precise positioning of the teeth.

Selective alveolar decortication (SAD) (Baloul et al. 2011) is less invasive and involves surgical insult on only the buccal cortical bone, limited to sites where acceleration of tooth movement is desired. However, loss of alveolar bone height is a complication which may occur when corticotomy is done without bone grafting. SAD was later broadened to include addition of bioabsorbable bone grafts on the corticotomy-exposed bone and termed 'accelerated osteogenic orthodontics' (AOO) also known as 'Wilckodontics', with the claimed benefits of not just reduction in treatment time but also a facilitation of arch expansion (Wilcko et al. 2009). Since then, corticotomies have been used to facilitate particular stages of comprehensive orthodontic treatment and also assist in correction of isolated tooth problems. Interestingly, majority of the case reports of adjunctive corticotomies in combination with bone grafting show a reduction in treatment time, limited to the aligning stage. What still has not been demonstrated is a reduction in overall orthodontic treatment duration with corticotomy-assisted orthodontics in adult subjects. Unless this happens, exposing adult patients to the costs and risks associated with an additional surgical procedure that has little benefit in shortening overall treatment duration is questionable, and based on the available literature, performing corticotomies on a routine basis is not justified (Buschang et al. 2012). Complications with interdental bone cuts include loss of interdental bone,

subcutaneous haematomas of the face and neck, alterations to pulpal blood flow and decreased width of attached gingiva (Kwon et al. 1985). Additionally, most of the evidence regarding corticotomy as an adjunct to accelerate tooth movement is based on case reports or series of cases and therefore very low in the hierarchy of evidence.

With the premise of less invasive surgery and a more conservative procedure, corticision was advocated and involves using a vibrating piezoelectric knife to injure buccal cortical bone transmucosally, without reflecting a mucoperiosteal flap. However, root damage from contact with the piezoelectric knife has been reported with the use of corticision-assisted orthodontics (Patterson et al. 2017).

Osteoperforations

Using a proprietary device for perforations of the buccal cortical bone in order to generate a RAP phenomenon has also been attempted to shorten treatment time. However, the study citing MOP as a minimally invasive and relatively safe procedure (Alikhani et al. 2013) that could reduce the duration of orthodontic treatment was restricted to only the canine retraction stage and had methodological flaws such as the suitability of the reference points for the canine retraction measurements. A recent systematic review concluded that the clinical effect of MOP was only transient and not clinically significant (Shahabee et al. 2020).

In summary, currently low-level evidence concludes that surgically facilitated orthodontics can accelerate tooth movement, but the acceleration is minimal and transient (Fleming et al. 2015). The clinical significance of this acceleration is thus still dubious, and possible side effects are unclear. The procedures are invasive, and more research is needed (Allareddy et al. 2021) before these can be recommended in the clinical practice.

Orthognathic surgery

Traditional orthognathic surgery has been reported to significantly increase treatment duration (O'Brien et al. 2009). However, altered sequencing of procedures, as in the surgery-first orthognathic approach (SFOA), has been reported to reduce treatment time (Jeong et al. 2016). Unlike the traditional approach, no orthodontic tooth movement is carried out for decompensation in the initial stage of the SFOA. Tooth movement is carried out subsequent to the surgical osteotomies performed for correction of jaw deformities. The temporal pattern of gingival crevicular fluid (GCF) bone marker levels suggests that the accelerated tooth movement after osteotomies in the SFOA is possible due to elevated levels of bone remodelling factors with overlapping functions during fracture healing and tooth movement (Zingler et al. 2017). The biological surge in bone modelling and remodelling activity and associated tooth mobility that happens immediately post osteotomy is utilised to assist faster tooth movement to facilitate a shorter orthodontic treatment duration in the SFOA (Liou et al. 2011).

Although a reduction in treatment duration is claimed by the proponents of the SFOA, this may not always be the case. The initial presenting dentofacial characteristics of the adult patient also need to be borne in mind. Extractions to alleviate crowding, need for transverse expansion and control of vertical dimension are all factors that will influence the duration of the presurgical phase in the traditional approach. Since tooth movements are carried out in the postsurgical phase in the SFOA, the duration of this phase is understandably significantly longer. In instances where there is no need for excessive presurgical preparation, treatment duration in the SFOA and traditional approach may not differ significantly. Therefore, treatment duration in adult patients requiring orthognathic surgery will ultimately be decided by the requirements of the particular set of dentofacial problems needing correction.

Non-surgical
Vibration

Vibration is a mechanical stimulus characterised by oscillatory motion. The key aspects in delineating vibration are frequency (indicates the number of complete up and down movement cycles per second; measured in Hertz), amplitude (the extent of the oscillatory motion; measured in millimetre) and direction of the vibration movement. High-frequency, low-magnitude vibration has been applied to teeth with the aim of increasing the rate of orthodontic tooth movement. Research on vibration and orthodontic tooth movement on animal models, in particular, rats, has shown an increased rate of tooth movement by accelerating periodontal and bony tissue modelling/remodelling (Nishimura et al. 2008). In human experiments, vibratory stimuli have demonstrated only short-term transient accelerated orthodontic tooth movement (Leethanakul et al. 2016).

Devices claiming to increase the rate of orthodontic tooth movement, when used as an adjunct to fixed appliance or aligner treatment, are commercially available (e.g., AcceleDent, Tooth Masseuse, VPro5). One of the first well-designed clinical studies (randomised clinical trial (RCT)) that used a commercially available vibration appliance (Tooth Masseuse), at a frequency of 11 Hz on teeth for 20 minutes daily, failed to find any clinical advantage for the early resolution of crowding (Miles et al. 2012). However, results from another vibration appliance (OrthoAccel Device), which provided vibrational frequency of 30 Hz for 20 minutes, daily showed increased rate of space closure when applied as an adjunct to orthodontic treatment (Pavlin et al. 2015). However, this study had a large dropout rate, included patients of a very wide age range and no reproducibility was reported of the intraoral measurements used in the study. Additionally, the statistically significant differences reported were small in magnitude and of debatable clinical significance. Subsequent systematic reviews have concluded that there is insufficient/absence of any evidence that vibrational stimulus can increase the speed of tooth movement (Aljabaa et al. 2018).

Low-level laser/photobiomodulation

Low-energy laser radiation has been claimed to speed up orthodontic tooth movement (Genc et al. 2013), but the findings are conflicting (Marquezan et al. 2010). Lack of uniformity and the different wavelengths of the lasers, irradiation doses, locations and frequencies used may account for the discrepancies. Although the non-invasiveness and relative ease of operation make low-level laser irradiation seem a popular approach for accelerating orthodontic tooth movement, more research is needed before it can be recommended in daily clinical practice (Gkantidis et al. 2014).

Photobiomodulation (PBM) has been used in the medical field for acceleration of bone healing and used occasionally in clinical orthodontics, as an adjunctive procedure in an attempt to modulate pain response, facilitate maxillary skeletal expansion and encourage the response of the alveolar bone to facilitate tooth movement. However, given the lack of homogeneity of the wavelengths employed and the limited research that has been undertaken, it is premature to offer a PBM therapy protocol to guide clinicians for accelerating tooth movement (Cronshaw et al. 2019).

Pharmacologic agents

Pharmacological agents are used to influence the bone metabolism locally. Several studies have demonstrated the effect of molecules on speeding up the rate of tooth movement in animal models, but limited research has been done on humans. It is difficult to extrapolate the results of animal studies to humans due to differences in periodontal ligament and alveolar bone morphology and physiology.

Prostaglandins are released during the inflammatory process, as they stimulate both osteoclasts and osteoblasts and consequently have repercussions on tooth movement. Increase in the rate tooth movement after multiple local injections of Prostaglandin E_1 (PGE_1) has been reported in human subjects (Spielmann et al. 1989). Even though no negative side effects were observed in this study, the authors did not recommend using PGE_1 injections in routine dental practice, as more data are needed to support their efficacy and safety.

Platelet-rich plasma (PRP) is an autologous concentration of platelets in a minute volume of plasma that contains numerous proteins, including growth factors and chemokines, which are crucial for primary haemostasis and wound healing. PRP has recently been used in an attempt to accelerate the rate of orthodontic tooth movement in human subjects. However, no beneficial and long-term acceleration effects of PRP injections on tooth movement have been demonstrated (El-Timamy et al. 2020).

The problem that remains with the use of pharmacologic agents in attempting to accelerate tooth movement is the potential for concomitant side effects especially in association with systemic administration. However, newer models of drug delivery allowing for sustained, controlled drug release look promising for possible future site-specific applications to control anchorage (Sydorak et al. 2019).

Treatment-related factors

Friction

Most orthodontic treatments are done with sliding mechanics and friction might influence the rate of tooth movements negatively. This idea is reflected in the advertisements where manufacturers promote so-called low-friction 'bracket systems' as an option to reduce treatment time. In particular, self-ligating (SL) brackets have been presented as having lower friction than traditional brackets. Although the initial clinical studies on SL brackets supported the finding of shorter treatment times, these studies were retrospective in design and with a high risk of bias (Eberting et al. 2001). More recent, prospective studies comparing SL brackets and conventional brackets have failed to identify any statistically or clinically significant difference in treatment time or efficacy. Subsequent systematic reviews that combined the evidence from well-designed RCTs also concluded that there was no difference in treatment time between conventional brackets and SL brackets (Chen et al. 2010; Fleming and Johal 2010). Despite claims about the advantages of SL brackets, duration of treatment with SL brackets is similar to that of conventional brackets and shortened chairside time appears to be the only significant time-based advantage of SL systems (Chen et al. 2010). It is important to acknowledge that friction itself plays a relatively minor role in the resistance to sliding of teeth, whereas binding and notching may play a more important role and the latter two do not differ between conventional and SL brackets (Burrow 2009). In conclusion, any orthodontic mechanics that is influenced by surface characteristics and friction will produce resistance to the direction of tooth movement and could prolong treatment time (Burrow 2009).

Appliance selection

With an increasing number of adults seeking orthodontic treatment, the popularity of aesthetic orthodontic appliances including clear aligners and lingual appliances continues to grow. However, differences in treatment details, operator choice and ease with technique make it difficult to compare treatment time between lingual and labial brackets. Nonetheless, low-level evidence suggests that the average treatment duration with lingual brackets is similar to that with labial brackets (Mistakidis et al. 2016).

The duration of treatment with clear aligner therapy was initially found to be shorter than conventional edgewise treatment by a mean duration of 5.5 months, possibly due to the software-assisted positioning of teeth, thus avoiding the need for a separate finishing or detailing phase (Buschang et al. 2013). In terms of treatment duration, a recent systematic review concluded that clear aligner therapy is more efficient than conventional fixed appliances (Zheng et al. 2017). However, the meta-analysis only included non-extraction cases, and when extraction cases were considered, treatment duration with clear aligners was 44% longer (Li et al. 2015). Furthermore, clear aligners appear to be less effective to control root movements and result in a worse treatment outcome than fixed appliance (Papageorgiou et al. 2020).

Custom brackets permit the use of preformed archwires with little or no manual wire bending, whereas wire-bending robots produce custom archwires for a particular patient. Both approaches are targeted at reducing the time spent in the finishing and detailing stage.

In the early days of customised orthodontic appliances, expert opinion and case reports suggested the possibility to achieve shorter active orthodontic treatment duration (Weber et al. 2013). A retrospective study found that a customised CAD/CAM orthodontic appliance that aims to eliminate wire bending significantly reduced treatment time in comparison to directly or indirectly bonded conventional brackets (Brown et al. 2015). Interestingly, the study attributed more of the decrease to indirect bonding than bracket customisation. However, recent studies with more robust designs have concluded that customisation of orthodontic appliances was not significantly associated with reduced treatment duration (Penning et al. 2017).

In order to reduce the clinical time spent in bending wires, the use of computer controlled machines to shape archwires as desired has been attempted. The same orthodontist using robot-formed wires took shorter treatment time (mean duration of 9 months) to finish patients than with manual wire bending (Alford et al. 2011). However, malocclusion severity was lower in the customised wire group and allocation of patients was not randomised in this study.

The 'orthodontist performing treatment' is a key source of variability in treatment time (Penning et al. 2017), particularly the time spent by the orthodontist in the finishing phase of treatment and this could possibly explain why cases treated by specialist orthodontists average a little longer than those of general practitioners.

Delivery of force system

Studies assessing the rate of tooth movement report that a tooth can be displaced 0.3–1 mm per month in experimental studies; nevertheless, superimposing the lateral cephalograms at the end of treatment rarely demonstrates more than 3–4 mm of teeth displacement. It is not before this discrepancy is solved that significant shortening of treatment duration can be obtained.

Burstone in *The Biomechanical Foundation of Clinical Orthodontics* claimed: 'The shortest distance between two points is a straight line' (Burstone and Choy 2015). This

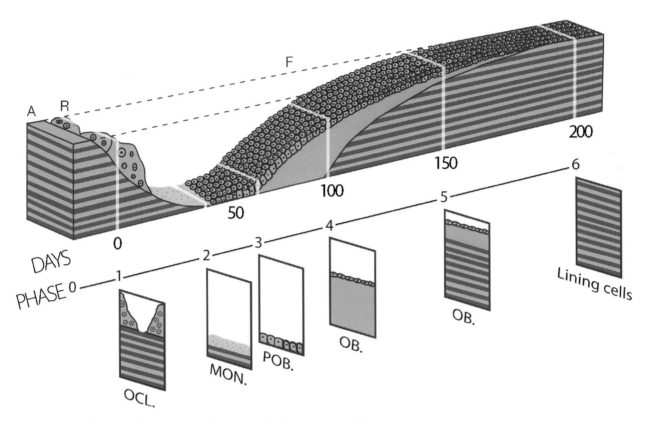

Fig. 20.1 Remodelling cycle (see Figure 3.18 in Chapter 3). The durations of the single phases are added in this version of the image, and as resorption of osteoid-covered unmineralised bone is not possible, changing the force direction will add on an average more than 100 days to the treatment time. It is therefore crucial to minimise the changes in force direction if the treatment time should be reduced.

does however require that we define the treatment goal exactly and define the displacement of each tooth in three dimensions. This can be done by combining the cephalogram and the occlusogram (see Chapter 17). Only when we know where we are going can we find the shortest way. Rarely can the direct road be used and treatment should therefore be separated into phases, and each phase be finished and the result consolidated prior to starting the next phase.

However, this approach is rarely followed when orthodontic treatment is done by sliding tooth/teeth along an archwire. When sliding teeth, displacement occurs as a cycle of initial tipping of the crown followed by root uprighting. During this process, what is an appositional surface of bone becomes a resorptional surface and vice versa. The time factor related to this process has not generally been thought about. A resorptional surface can be turned into an appositional surface within hours, but as osteoclasts can only resorb fully mineralised bone (Chambers and Fuller 1985), resorption will be delayed until the osteoid covering the appositional surface is mineralised. Therefore, it takes longer to turn an appositional surface into a resorptional surface. In addition, the resorption may be indirect involving removal of local necrosis, which may also delay tooth displacement. In summary, every time the distribution of tooth displacement is changing, a delay of at least a month can be expected (Figure 20.1).

Some techniques recommend sliding on a heavy wire in order to avoid or minimise the tipping. Still a force added to

the bracket will always generate a tipping leading to a binding which will generate a moment that ultimately will be big enough for the uprighting. When sliding on a heavy wire, the tipping will be limited, which clinically may appear as translation. On the other hand, when displacement is performed on a more flexible wire, the tipping will be significantly larger before a moment sufficient for uprighting will be generated. It is, as noted in the earlier text, extremely important to set up a detailed treatment goal, define the desired displacement of every tooth and then insert the force system necessary to generate the desired movement. The shortest distance between two points is a straight line and this is not the path taken with an alternation between tipping and uprighting, which is characteristic of sliding mechanics.

The force system delivered by fixed appliances can either be statically indeterminate, when a wire is inserted into more than two brackets, or statically determinate, where the wire is only inserted into one bracket and has a one-point contact to the other unit. Figure 20.2 illustrates how intrusion of a canine to correct a deep curve of Spee can be accomplished with less tooth movement, and thereby faster with a statically determinate force system.

Based on a detailed description of the treatment goal, the displacement of individual teeth can be defined, and a separation between teeth to be moved (the active unit) and teeth to be kept where they are (the passive unit) can be done. Appointments should focus not merely on the reactivation of the forces delivered by the appliance, but also on monitoring the force system to obtain desired tooth movement. Preventing indiscriminate or unnecessary tooth movements, the so-called 'round tripping' (Figure 20.3), helps optimise treatment time, but it has been scarcely investigated in the scientific literature.

Although both orthodontists and orthopaedic surgeons work with bone, the orthodontists' understanding of bone differs from that of the orthopaedic surgeons. Based on orthopaedic research, it is common knowledge that loading leads to increased density of bone, and that unloading, as in the case of space travel, leads to decreased bone density. It therefore seems controversial that the orthodontists associate compression with resorption. Separating bone modelling and bone remodelling is seldom done by orthodontist, but may provide an explanation on the discrepancy between treatment duration and tooth movement. When orthodontists are displacing teeth, it involves both modelling (a change in shape) and remodelling, which is the ongoing process renewing bone and acting to maintain the serum calcium.

(1)   (2)

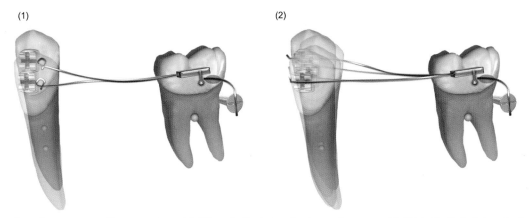

Fig. 20.2 Intrusion of over-erupted lower canine with (1) statically determinate appliance or with (2) statically indeterminate appliance. In the latter case, the geometry will change continuously and therefore the treatment time will be longer. With a one-point contact over the centre of resistance (CR), the canine will be intruded directly and there is no change in the distribution of the cellular activity of the alveolar wall.

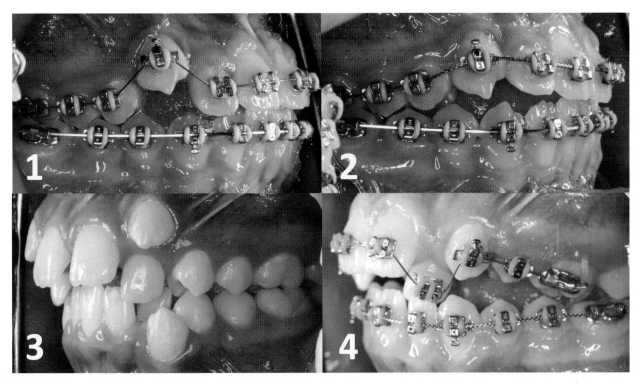

Fig. 20.3 Images depicting the side effects of indiscriminate use of continuous archwires for levelling and aligning. (1) Engaging a flexible 16-mil NiTi archwire in an ectopic canine has resulted in (2) iatrogenic anterior and posterior open bite. Similar use of a flexible round 16-mil archwire with a cinch back has led to loss of sagittal anchorage. (3) and (4) Note the almost complete loss of extraction space without resolving the crowding and the changes in molar relationship. In both instances, orthodontists will first have to spend time to correct unwanted tooth movements and round tripping, thus increasing the overall treatment time.

Conclusions

Undoubtedly, patients and orthodontists will benefit from a shorter treatment duration. A good understanding and application of biomechanical principles help prevent round tripping and unnecessary increase of treatment time. Research continues to be focused at achieving the goal of a shorter treatment duration. Intuitively, biomechanics has a major impact on orthodontic treatment time, but surprisingly this has been only scarcely investigated in the scientific literature. Presently, evidence suggests that most of the interventions that induce faster tooth movements are able to do so only for a short and transient period, with no influence on the overall treatment time. Advances in technology combined with a better understanding of the biology of tooth movement would support to obtain treatment goals with a treatment of a shorter duration.

References

Alford TJ, Roberts WE, Hartsfield JK Jr, Eckert GJ and Snyder RJ (2011) Clinical outcomes for patients finished with the suresmile™ method compared with conventional fixed orthodontic therapy. *Angle Orthod* 81(3), 383–388.

Alikhani M, Raptis M, Zoldan B, Sangsuwon C, Lee YB, Alyami B, Corpodian C, Barrera LM, Alansari S, Khoo E et al (2013) Effect of micro-osteoperforations on the rate of tooth movement. *Am J Orthod Dentofacial Orthop* 144(5), 639–648.

Aljabaa A, Almoammar K, Aldrees A and Huang G (2018) Effects of vibrational devices on orthodontic tooth movement: a systematic review. *Am J Orthod Dentofacial Orthop* 154(6), 768–779.

Allareddy V, Covell DA Jr and Frazier-Bowers SA (2021) American association of orthodontists foundation rapid assessment of evidence: accelerated teeth movement. *Am J Orthod Dentofacial Orthop* 159(3), 396–397.e393.

Baloul SS, Gerstenfeld LC, Morgan EF, Carvalho RS, Van Dyke TE and Kantarci A (2011) Mechanism of action and morphologic changes in the alveolar bone in response to selective alveolar decortication-facilitated tooth movement. *Am J Orthod Dentofacial Orthop* 139(4 Suppl), S83–101.

Brown MW, Koroluk L, Ko CC, Zhang K, Chen M and Nguyen T (2015) Effectiveness and efficiency of a cad/cam orthodontic bracket system. *Am J Orthod Dentofacial Orthop* 148(6), 1067–1074.

Burrow SJ (2009) Friction and resistance to sliding in orthodontics: a critical review. *Am J Orthod Dentofacial Orthop* 135(4), 442–447.

Burstone CJ and Choy K (2015) *The Biomechanical Foundation of Clinical Orthodontics*. Chicago: Quintessence Publ.

Buschang P, Campbell P and Ruso S (2012) Accelerating tooth movement with corticotomies: Is it possible and desirable? *Semin Orthod* 18, 286–294.

Buschang PH, Shaw SG, Ross M, Crosby D and Campbell PM (2013) Comparative time efficiency of aligner therapy and conventional edgewise braces. *Angle Orthod* 84(3), 391–396.

Chambers TJ and Fuller K (1985) Bone cells predispose bone surfaces to resorption by exposure of mineral to osteoclastic contact. *J Cell Sci* 76(1), 155–165.

Chen SS-H, Greenlee GM, Kim J-E, Smith CL and Huang GJ (2010) Systematic review of self-ligating brackets. *Am J Orthod Dentofacial Orthop* 137(6), 726.e721–726.e718.

Cronshaw M, Parker S, Anagnostaki E and Lynch E (2019) Systematic review of orthodontic treatment management with photobiomodulation therapy. *Photobiomodul Photomed Laser Surg* 37(12), 862–868.

Eberting JJ, Straja SR and Tuncay OC (2001) Treatment time, outcome, and patient satisfaction comparisons of damon and conventional brackets. *Clin Orthod Res* 4(4), 228–234.

El-Timamy A, El Sharaby F, Eid F, El Dakroury A, Mostafa Y and Shaker O (2020) Effect of platelet-rich plasma on the rate of orthodontic tooth movement: a split-mouth randomized trial. *Angle Orthod* 90(3), 354–361.

Fleming PS, Fedorowicz Z, Johal A, El-Angbawi A and Pandis N (2015) Surgical adjunctive procedures for accelerating orthodontic treatment. *Cochrane Database Syst Rev* (6), CD010572.

Fleming PS and Johal A (2010) Self-ligating brackets in orthodontics. A systematic review. *Angle Orthod* 80(3), 575–584.

Frost HM (1989) The biology of fracture healing. An overview for clinicians. Part II. *Clin Orthop Relat Res* 248, 294–309.

Genc G, Kocadereli I, Tasar F, Kilinc K, El S and Sarkarati B (2013) Effect of low-level laser therapy (lllt) on orthodontic tooth movement. *Lasers Med Sci* 28(1), 41–47.

Giannopoulou C, Dudic A, Pandis N and Kiliaridis S (2016) Slow and fast orthodontic tooth movement: an experimental study on humans. *Eur J Orthod* 38(4), 404–408.

Gkantidis N, Mistakidis I, Kouskoura T and Pandis N (2014) Effectiveness of non-conventional methods for accelerated orthodontic tooth movement: a systematic review and meta-analysis. *J Dent* 42(10), 1300–1319.

Jeong WS, Choi JW, Kim DY, Lee JY and Kwon SM (2016) Can a surgery-first orthognathic approach reduce the total treatment time? *Int J Oral Maxillofac Surg* 46(4), 473–482.

Kole H (1959) Surgical operations on the alveolar ridge to correct occlusal abnormalities. *Oral Surg Oral Med Oral Pathol* 12(5), 515–529 concl.

Kwon HJ, Pihlstrom B and Waite DE (1985) Effects on the periodontium of vertical bone cutting for segmental osteotomy. *J Oral Maxillofac Surg* 43(12), 952–955.

Leethanakul C, Suamphan S, Jitpukdeebodintra S, Thongudomporn U and Charoemratrote C (2016) Vibratory stimulation increases interleukin-1 beta secretion during orthodontic tooth movement. *Angle Orthod* 86(1), 74–80.

Li W, Wang S and Zhang Y (2015) The effectiveness of the invisalign appliance in extraction cases using the the abo model grading system: a multicenter randomized controlled trial. *Int J Clin Exp Med* 8(5), 8276–8282.

Liou EJ, Chen PH, Wang YC, Yu CC, Huang CS and Chen YR (2011) Surgery-first accelerated orthognathic surgery: postoperative rapid orthodontic tooth movement. *J Oral Maxillofac Surg* 69(3), 781–785.

Marquezan M, Bolognese AM and Araujo MT (2010) Effects of two low-intensity laser therapy protocols on experimental tooth movement. *Photomed Laser Surg* 28(6), 757–762.

Miles P, Smith H, Weyant R and Rinchuse DJ (2012) The effects of a vibrational appliance on tooth movement and patient discomfort: a prospective randomised clinical trial. *Aust Orthod J* 28(2), 213–218.

Mistakidis I, Katib H, Vasilakos G, Kloukos D and Gkantidis N (2016) Clinical outcomes of lingual orthodontic treatment: a systematic review. *Eur J Orthod* 38(5), 447–458.

Nishimura M, Chiba M, Ohashi T, Sato M, Shimizu Y, Igarashi K and Mitani H (2008) Periodontal tissue activation by vibration: intermittent stimulation by resonance vibration accelerates experimental tooth movement in rats. *Am J Orthod Dentofacial Orthop* 133(4), 572–583.

O'Brien K, Wright J, Conboy F, Appelbe P, Bearn D, Caldwell S, Harrison J, Hussain J, Lewis D, Littlewood S et al (2009) Prospective, multi-center study of the effectiveness of orthodontic/orthognathic surgery care in the united kingdom. *Am J Orthod Dentofacial Orthop* 135(6), 709–714.

Papageorgiou SN, Koletsi D, Iliadi A, Peltomaki T and Eliades T (2020) Treatment outcome with orthodontic aligners and fixed appliances: a systematic review with meta-analyses. *Eur J Orthod* 42(3), 331–343.

Patterson BM, Dalci O, Papadopoulou AK, Madukuri S, Mahon J, Petocz P, Spahr A and Darendeliler MA (2017) Effect of piezocision on root resorption associated with orthodontic force: a microcomputed tomography study. *Am J Orthod Dentofacial Orthop* 151(1), 53–62.

Pavlin D, Anthony R, Raj V and Gakunga PT (2015) Cyclic loading (vibration) accelerates tooth movement in orthodontic patients: a double-blind, randomized controlled trial. *Semin Orthod* 21(3), 187–194.

Penning EW, Peerlings RHJ, Govers JDM, Rischen RJ, Zinad K, Bronkhorst EM, Breuning KH and Kuijpers-Jagtman AM (2017) Orthodontics with customized versus noncustomized appliances: a randomized controlled clinical trial. *J Dent Res* 96(13), 1498–1504.

Pilon JJ, Kuijpers-Jagtman AM and Maltha JC (1996) Magnitude of orthodontic forces and rate of bodily tooth movement. An experimental study. *Am J Orthod Dentofacial Orthop* 110(1), 16–23.

Shahabee M, Shafaee H, Abtahi M, Rangrazi A and Bardideh E (2020) Effect of micro-osteoperforation on the rate of orthodontic tooth movement-a systematic review and a meta-analysis. *Eur J Orthod* 42(2), 211–221.

Spielmann T, Wieslander L and Hefti AF (1989) [acceleration of orthodontically induced tooth movement through the local application of prostaglandin (pge1)]. *Schweiz Monatsschr Zahnmed* 99(2), 162–165.

Sydorak I, Dang M, Baxter SJ, Halcomb M, Ma P, Kapila S and Hatch N (2019) Microsphere controlled drug delivery for local control of tooth movement. *Eur J Orthod* 41(1), 1–8.

Tsichlaki A, Chin SY, Pandis N and Fleming PS (2016) How long does treatment with fixed orthodontic appliances last? A systematic review. *Am J Orthod Dentofacial Orthop* 149(3), 308–318.

Verna C, Dalstra M and Melsen B (2000) The rate and the type of orthodontic tooth movement is influenced by bone turnover in a rat model. *Eur J Orthod* 22(4), 343–352.

Verna C, Zaffe D and Siciliani G (1999) Histomorphometric study of bone reactions during orthodontic tooth movement in rats. *Bone* 24(4), 371–379.

Weber DJ 2nd, Koroluk LD, Phillips C, Nguyen T and Proffit WR (2013) Clinical effectiveness and efficiency of customized vs. Conventional preadjusted bracket systems. *J Clin Orthod* 47(4), 261–266;quiz 268.

Wilcko MT, Wilcko WM, Pulver JJ, Bissada NF and Bouquot JE (2009) Accelerated osteogenic orthodontics technique: a 1-stage surgically facilitated rapid orthodontic technique with alveolar augmentation. *J Oral Maxillofac Surg* 67(10), 2149–2159.

Zheng M, Liu R, Ni Z and Yu Z (2017) Efficiency, effectiveness and treatment stability of clear aligners: a systematic review and meta-analysis. *Orthod Craniofac Res* 20(3), 127–133.

Zingler S, Hakim E, Finke D, Brunner M, Saure D, Hoffmann J, Lux CJ, Erber R and Seeberger R (2017) Surgery-first approach in orthognathic surgery: psychological and biological aspects – a prospective cohort study. *J Craniomaxillofac Surg* 45(8), 1293–1301.

21

What are the Limits of Orthodontic Treatment?

Birte Melsen

What determines the limits?

What are the limits of orthodontic treatment? When the dentist is confronted with a situation where the only solution is major implant-based oral rehabilitation or a removable denture? When the degeneration has reached a level where orthodontics no longer plays a viable role as part of oral rehabilitation?

The limitations can be related to:

1. Biology:
   • Dental status.
   • Periodontal status.
   • General health.
2. Configuration:
   • Orthodontic technique.
   • Anchorage.

In relation to the dental status, the quality, the number and the distribution of teeth are of importance. The quality includes the amount of remaining natural tooth substance, and the presence or absence of active caries and periapical pathological processes. The prognosis of each individual tooth has to be taken into consideration before deciding which teeth should be involved in major oral rehabilitation. Therefore, active caries and periapical pathological processes have to be taken care of before the treatment plan is worked out. Teeth with a bad prognosis can, on the other hand still be used to generate bone or to serve as anchorage before extraction.

In relation to periodontal status, the absence of clinically active gingivitis and periodontitis is crucial to move a tooth without further deterioration of its periodontal support. Whereas the quality of the attachment is important, no limit has been proposed for the maximum marginal bone loss beyond which no treatment can be performed. Although the requirements regarding the status of the periodontium differ among authors, optimal periodontal health is a *sine qua non* when intrusion is intended for the purpose of improving the periodontal status. Recently, a clear correlation between the composition of bacteria present on the heart valves and in deep periodontal pockets has been demonstrated. To avoid that the tissue reaction generated by the orthodontic appliance will lead to a negative balance, pocket depths have to be less than 4 mm. The monkey experiments cited in Chapter 11 clearly demonstrate that a gain in attachment can be obtained by intrusion and even further when combined with guided tissue reaction. The pre-condition for such reactions, however, is completely healthy periodontal tissue, which cannot be guaranteed in the presence of pocket depth above 4 mm.

Extrusion can, on the other hand, be carried out in patients with a clinical healthy periodontium even in the presence of increased pocket depths and in the case of minimal attachment. Extrusion of teeth that cannot be saved can be used to generate alveolar bone that can later serve as basis for the insertion of dental implants.

General health is of importance for bone modelling generated by orthodontic forces. The tissue reaction that occurs during orthodontic treatment is an interaction between the general turnover and the reaction to the force systems generated by the appliance. This applies to all patients, but as the maximum age of the patients asking for dental regeneration is increasing, so is the number of

Adult Orthodontics, Second Edition. Edited by Birte Melsen and Cesare Luzi.
© 2022 John Wiley & Sons Ltd. Published 2022 by John Wiley & Sons Ltd.
Companion Website: http://www.wiley.com/go/melsen-adult-orthodontics

patients receiving some kind of medication influencing the bone turnover. Suppression of bone turnover by medication for osteopenia or osteoporosis may be a contraindication to an orthodontic solution being offered as part of oral rehabilitation. Medically induced immune suppression is used in relation to transplantation of kidney, heart or more frequently cornea, as part of treatment of allergies, and, finally, perhaps the most important medication in the orthodontic context is the treatment of osteoporosis with bisphosphonates. Diseases that constitute an increased risk for progressive periodontal pathology will also preclude orthodontics, an alternative may be to use only the minimum tooth movement necessary for a possible prosthetic solution.

Without doubt, the most important limiting factor for tooth movement, even if this is considered essential for the desirable rehabilitation of a deteriorating dentition, is the basic condition of the bone. This is because ultimately it is the response of this bone to the orthodontic force system that determines whether the treatment can be carried out.

The limitation in relation to configuration refers to the difficulty in generating the correct force systems without undesirable side effects. This depends not only on the mutual position of teeth within the individual arches but also on the distribution of teeth with occlusal contact and the marginal bone level.

Treatment of young adult patients with complete dentitions and good occlusal contacts can often be performed with continuous arches. When using superelastic wires, the low force level will be balanced by forces from the soft tissues and the occlusion, thereby obtaining a reasonable vertical control and a desirable occlusion. When treating deteriorated dentitions in adult patients, the treatment goal should be defined in three dimensions and a clear description of the needed displacement of the individual teeth or groups of teeth should be available. This can seldom be achieved with continuous arch treatment, for which reason the technical skills of the individual orthodontist will determine the possibility or limitation of orthodontic treatment in such patients.

Until recently, another limitation related to configuration has been lack of sufficient anchorage. This limitation has been reduced considerably with the introduction of skeletal anchorage (Chapter 8). There are, however, other limitations still present in relation to that type of anchorage. These can be related to the type of skeletal anchorage, as discussed by Melsen (2005), but also how it is manipulated by the dentist and the patient (see Chapter 8). The limitations related to the patient in this context may be local or general limitations. Local limitations include the thickness of the cortical bone and the density of the trabecular bone in addition to the thickness of the mucosa. A thick mucosa increases the distance between the point of application of the force, the head of the mini-implant and the centre of resistance (CR) determined by the bone. The general limitations include the alterations in bone turnover mentioned in the earlier text.

An important development of aligners has occurred since the first edition of this book was published. The most rapid increase of adult treatment has without doubt been treatment performed with aligners with or without interference of trained dentists. The biggest challenge will be to provide patients with sufficient information on the benefits and the damages that can be the result of 'Fast Food' orthodontics. The aligners will most likely replace the use of fixed appliances in a large number of patients and be used separately, but also be part of hybrid appliances. Last year, two and a half million Invisalign* patients were registered, mostly adult patients and there is no reason to belief that it has reached the peak.

A weakness related to aligners used in treatment of degenerated dentitions is that the apically displaced position of the CR due to marginal bone loss is seldom taken into consideration. A second limitation is that the localization of CR will change when the tooth is displaced as it is dependent on the type of bone in which the movement take place, cortical or trabecular bone.

The biggest limitation, however, still lies in the patient's healths, patient's attitude, the general dentist's and frequently also in the orthodontist's capacity and imagination. The expression 'this cannot be done' should be reconsidered, and it is my hope that this book may serve as an encouragement to widen the spectrum of orthodontics.

Reference

Melsen B (2005) Mini-implants: where are we? *J Clin Orthod* 39, 539–547.

Index

Note: Page numbers in **bold** indicate tables and *italics* indicate figures.

Adult Orthodontics, Second Edition. Edited by Birte Melsen and Cesare Luzi.
© 2022 John Wiley & Sons Ltd. Published 2022 by John Wiley & Sons Ltd.
Companion Website: http://www.wiley.com/go/melsen-adult-orthodontics